D U T T O N ' S

ORTHOPEDIC
Survival Guide

Managing
Common Conditions

DUTTON'S
ORTHOPEDIC
Survival Guide
Managing
Common Conditions

Mark Dutton, PT
Allegheny General Hospital
West Penn Allegheny Health System (WPAHS)
Adjunct Clinical Instructor, Duquesne University
School of Health Sciences
Pittsburgh, Pennsylvania

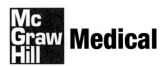

New York Chicago San Francisco Lisbon London Madrid Mexico City Milan
New Delhi San Juan Seoul Singapore Sydney Toronto

The *McGraw·Hill* Companies

1 2 3 4 5 6 7 8 9 10   DOC/DOC   14 13 12 11

ISBN 978-0-0-171510-2
MHID 0-07-171510-X

This book was set in Sabon by Thomson Digital.
The editors were Joe Morita and Christie Naglieri.
The production supervisor was Sherri Souffrance.
The illustration manager was Armen Ovsepyan.
Project management was provided by Pooja Khurana, Thomson Digital.
The interior designer was Eve Siegel; cover image © Guy Cali/Corbis.
RR Donnelley was printer and binder.

This book is printed on acid-free paper.

Library of Congress Cataloging-in-Publication Data

Dutton, Mark.
  Dutton's orthopedic survival guide: managing common conditions / Mark Dutton.
    p. ; cm.
  Other title: Orthopedic survival guide
  Includes bibliographical references and index.
  ISBN-13: 978-0-07-171510-2 (pbk. : alk. paper)
  ISBN-10: 0-07-171510-X (pbk. : alk. paper)
  1. Orthopedics—Handbooks, manuals, etc. I. Title. II. Title:
Orthopedic survival guide.
  [DNLM: 1. Orthopedics—methods—Handbooks. 2. Ambulatory
Care—methods—Handbooks. WE 39]
  RD732.5.D877 2011
  616.7—dc22
                                                    2010029095

McGraw-Hill books are available at special quantity discounts to use as premiums and sales promotions, or for use in corporate training programs. To contact a representative please e-mail us at bulksales@mcgraw-hill.com.

Contents

Preface

This clinic companion was designed to provide physical therapy students and clinicians with a quick reference source for orthopaedics. The book may be used in a number of ways. The beginner should start with the introductory chapters that provide descriptions of anatomy, physiology, and biomechanics in addition to guidelines that steer the clinician through the complex progression of the clinical examination, evaluation, and intervention. The more experienced clinician can brush up on a specific topic by reading the relevant chapter in its entirety or focus on a specific diagnosis. Each of the body area chapters provides quick-reference tables and illustrations to assist the clinician and clinical pearls are provided to highlight the most salient points. At the end of each of the relevant chapters the most common diagnoses are described based on their common subjective and objective findings, confirmatory tests, differential diagnosis, recommended intervention, and prognosis.

The questions provided at the end of each joint chapter are designed to increase the reader's knowledge. Although most of the answers are provided within the text, some are not, so that the reader is encouraged to complete further reading.

Although most clinicians inherently know that the intensity of an intervention is based on the stage of healing, formulating ideas for appropriate intervention beyond the use of heat, cold and the various electrotherapeutic modalities often proves difficult. At the end of each of the body area chapters a hierarchical series of appropriate therapeutic exercises, in the form of a clinical ladder, is presented. The advantage of these exercise steps is that they can be used for any injury regardless of the diagnosis as they are based on patient tolerance. However, for the exercises to be effective, each of the exercise steps must be used in the order they are presented.

It is hoped that this book achieves its aim—to provide the student and clinician with the necessary tools for the comprehensive examination, evaluation, and intervention of the outpatient orthopedic population.

Mark Dutton, PT

Acknowledgments

It is my firm belief that our accomplishments in life are due to a supporting cast of people, who help shape, direct, and inspire. I would therefore like to thank the following:

- My family. Certain sacrifices to family life are always necessary whenever a task of this size is undertaken.
- The production team of McGraw-Hill—Joe Morita for his confidence in this project, and Christie Naglieri for her patience, guidance, and support.
- The team at Thomson Digital, led by Pooja Khurana.
- The staff of Human Motion Rehabilitation, Allegheny General Hospital.

Fundamentals

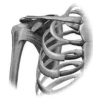

Chapter **1**

Anatomy and Biomechanics of the Musculoskeletal System

OVERVIEW

The musculoskeletal structures involved with human motion include the nerves, muscles, and tendons; the fascia and ligaments that provide support and stability; and the joints around which the motions occur. The neural structures are discussed in Chapter 2. The musculoskeletal system functions intimately with nervous tissue to produce coordinated movement and provide adequate joint stabilization and feedback during sustained positions and movements.

 Clinical Pearl

The basic components of tissue include the following:

1. Collagen. Provides tensile strength of tissue. Over 20 types have been identified, of which type I and type II are the most abundant. Bone, ligaments, tendons, meniscus, and skin are all primarily type I collagen, while articular cartilage is primarily composed of type II collagen.

2. Elastin. Provides elasticity and deformation to tissue.

3. Proteoglycans. Provide the binding properties of tissue.

4. Inorganic components.

5. Extracellular matrix. Formed by a combination of collagen, elastin, proteoglycans, and inorganic components.

6. Water.

7. Cells. Three major types of cells exist in musculoskeletal tissue: blasts (responsible for tissue formation, e.g., osteoblast, fibroblast), cytes (responsible for the maintenance of tissue and the response of tissue to stress, e.g., osteophytes, fibrocytes), and clasts (responsible for resorption of tissue, e.g., osteoclast, fibroclast).

Muscles

There are approximately 430 muscles in the body, each of which can be considered anatomically as a separate organ. Of these 430 muscles, about 75 pairs provide the majority of body movements and postures.[1] Muscle (Figure 1-1) may be classified functionally as either voluntary or involuntary and structurally as either smooth, striated (skeletal), or cardiac (Table 1-1).

 Clinical Pearl

Smooth and cardiac muscles can contract without nervous stimulation, but their contraction is influenced by the nervous system. Skeletal muscles cannot contract unless stimulated by neurons. Therefore, in the presence of weakness, the clinician must include nerve (spinal or peripheral) injury in the differential diagnosis.

 Clinical Pearl

Muscle tissue is responsible for the movement of materials through the body, the movement of one part of the body with respect to another, posture, and locomotion.

Muscle Tissue

Muscle is the only biological tissue capable of actively generating tension. This characteristic enables human skeletal muscle to perform the important functions of maintaining upright body posture, moving body parts, and absorbing

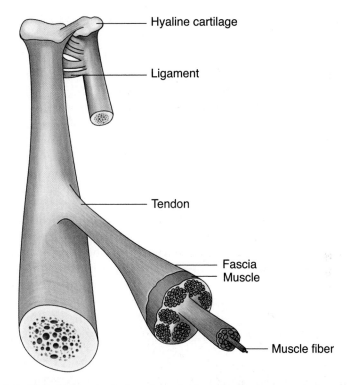

Figure 1-1 Illustration depicting the relationship between muscle, tendon, ligament, fascia, and hyaline cartilage.

shock. Human skeletal muscle possesses four biomechanical properties: extensibility, elasticity, irritability, and the ability to develop tension.

- Extensibility. Extensibility is the ability to be stretched or to increase in length
- Elasticity. Elasticity is the ability to return to normal resting length following a stretch

Table 1-1 Muscle Structure Types

Muscle Type	Example
Striated (skeletal)	Spanning joints and attached to bones via tendons
Smooth	Walls of hollow internal organs
Cardiac	Heart muscle

- Irritability. Irritability is the ability to respond to a stimulus. With reference to skeletal muscle this stimulus is provided electrochemically
- Ability to develop tension. The ability of skeletal muscle is referred to as a contraction. A contraction may or may not result in a muscle's shortening (see later).

The class of tissue labeled *skeletal muscle* consists of individual muscle cells or fibers bound by a plasma membrane (the sarcolemma). The sarcolemma forms a physical barrier against the external environment and also mediates signals between the exterior and the muscle cell. A single muscle cell is called a *muscle fiber* or *myofiber* (Figure 1-1). Individual muscle fibers are wrapped in a connective tissue (CT) envelope called *endomysium*. Bundles of myofibers, which form a whole muscle (fasciculus), are encased in the perimysium. The perimysium is continuous with the deep fascia. Groups of fasciculi are surrounded by a connective sheath called the epimysium. Under an electron microscope, it can be seen that each of the myofibers consists of thousands of *myofibrils*, which extend throughout its length. Each of the myofibrils contains many fibers called *myofilaments*, which run parallel to the myofibril axis. The myofilaments are made up of two different proteins: actin (thin myofilaments) and myosin (thick myofilaments) that give skeletal muscle fibers their striated (striped) appearance (Figure 1-2).[2]

 Clinical Pearl

The sarcomere is the contractile machinery of the muscle. The graded contractions of a whole muscle occur because the number of fibers participating in the contraction varies. Increasing the force of movement is achieved by recruiting more cells into cooperative action.

The striations are produced by alternating dark (A) and light (I) bands that appear to span the width of the muscle fiber. The A bands are composed of myosin filaments, whereas the I bands are composed of actin filaments. The actin filaments of the I band overlap into the A band, giving the edges of the A band a darker appearance than the central region (H band), which contains only myosin. At the center of each I band is a thin, dark Z line. A *sarcomere* represents the distance between each Z line.

Each muscle fiber is limited by a cell membrane called a *sarcolemma*. The protein *dystrophin* plays an essential role in the mechanical strength and stability of the sarcolemma.[3] Dystrophin is lacking in patients with Duchenne muscular dystrophy.

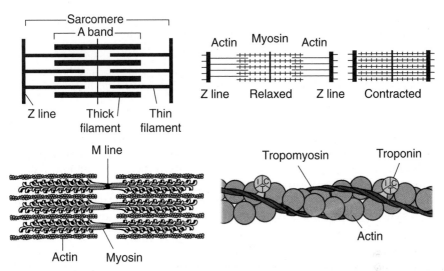

Figure 1-2 (A) Arrangement of thin (actin) and thick (myosin) filaments in skeletal. (B) Sliding of actin on myosin during contraction so that Z lines move closer together. (C) Detail of relation of myosin to actin in an individual sarcomere, the functional unit of the muscle. (D) Diagrammatic representation of the arrangement of actin, tropomyosin, and troponin of the thin filaments in relation to a myosin thick filament. The globular heads of myosin interact with the thin filaments to create the contraction. Note that myosin thick filaments reverse polarity at the M line in the middle of the sarcomere, allowing for contraction. (A and B: Top Left & Right: Reproduced with permission from Ganong WF. *Review of Medical Physiology.* 22nd ed. McGraw-Hill; 2005.) (C and D: Bottom Left & Right: Modified with permission from Kandel ER, Schwartz JH, Jessell TM (eds). *Principles of Neural Science.* 4th ed. McGraw-Hill; 2000.)

When a muscle contracts isotonically, the distance between the Z lines decreases, the I band and H bands disappear, but the width of the A band remains unchanged (Figure 1-2).[4] This shortening of the sarcomeres is not produced by a shortening of the actin and myosin filaments, but by a sliding of actin filaments over the myosin filaments, which pulls the Z lines together.

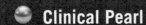

Clinical Pearl

The sarcoplasm is the specialized cytoplasm of a muscle cell that contains the usual subcellular elements along with the Golgi apparatus, abundant myofibrils, a modified endoplasmic reticulum known as the sarcoplasmic reticulum (SR), myoglobin, and mito-chondria. Transverse-tubules (T-tubules) invaginate the sarcolemma, allowing impulses to penetrate the cell and activate the SR.

Structures called *cross-bridges* serve to connect the actin and myosin filaments. The myosin filaments contain two flexible, hinge-like regions, which allow the cross-bridges to attach and detach from the actin filament. During contraction, the cross-bridges attach and undergo power strokes, which provide the contractile force. During relaxation, the cross-bridges detach. This attaching and detaching is asynchronous, so that some are attaching, whereas others are detaching. Thus, at each moment, some of the cross-bridges are pulling, whereas others are releasing.

The regulation of cross-bridge attachment and detachment is a function of two proteins found in the actin filaments: tropomyosin and troponin (Figure 1-2). Tropomyosin attaches directly to the actin filament, whereas troponin is attached to the tropomyosin rather than directly to the actin filament.

 Clinical Pearl

Tropomyosin and troponin function as the switch for muscle contraction and relaxation. In a relaxed state, the tropomyosin physically blocks the cross-bridges from binding to the actin. For contraction to take place, the tropomyosin must be moved.

Each muscle fiber is innervated by a somatic motor neuron. One neuron and the muscle fibers it innervates constitute a motor unit or functional unit of the muscle. Each motor neuron branches as it enters the muscle to innervate a number of muscle fibers.

 Clinical Pearl

The area of contact between a nerve and a muscle fiber is known as the motor end plate or neuromuscular junction.

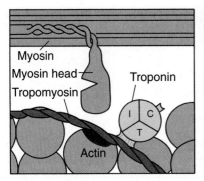 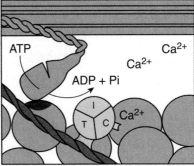

Figure 1-3 Initiation of contraction by Ca^{2+}... When Ca^{2+} binds to troponin C, tropomysonin is displaced laterally, exposing the binding site for myosin on actin (dark area). The myosin head then binds, ATP is hydrolyzed, and the configuration of the head and neck region of myosin changes. For simplicity, only one of the heads of the myosin-II is shown. (Reproduced with permission from Ganong WF. *Review of Medical Physiology*. 22nd ed. McGraw-Hill; 2005.)

The release of a chemical acetylcholine from the axon terminals at the neuromuscular junctions causes electrical activation of the skeletal muscle fibers. When an action potential propagates into the transverse tubule system (narrow membranous tunnels formed from and continuous with the sarcolemma), the voltage sensors on the transverse tubule membrane signal the release of Ca^{2+} from the terminal cisternae portion of the SR (a series of interconnected sacs and tubes that surround each myofibril).[4] The released Ca^{2+} then diffuses into the sarcomeres and binds to troponin, displacing the tropomyosin, and allowing the actin to bind with the myosin cross-bridges (Figure 1-3). At the end of the contraction (the neural activity and action potentials cease), the SR actively accumulates Ca^{2+} and muscle relaxation occurs. The return of Ca^{2+} to the SR involves active transport, requiring the degradation of adenosine triphosphate (ATP) to adenosine diphosphate (ADP)*.[4] Because SR function is closely associated with both contraction and relaxation, changes in its ability to release or sequester Ca^{2+} markedly affect both the time course and magnitude of force output by the muscle fiber.[5]

---

*The most readily available energy for skeletal muscle cells is stored in the form of ATP and phosphocreatine (see Chapter 4). Through the activity of the enzyme ATPase, ATP promptly releases energy when required by the cell to perform any type of work, whether it is electrical, chemical, or mechanical.

Clinical Pearl

The SR forms a network around the myofibrils, storing and providing the Ca^{2+} that is required for muscle contraction.

Activation of varying numbers of motor neurons results in gradations in the strength of muscle contraction. The stronger the electrical impulse, the stronger the muscle twitch. Whenever a somatic motor neuron is activated, all of the muscle fibers that it innervates are stimulated and contract with *all-or-none* twitches. Although the muscle fibers produce all-or-none contractions, muscles are capable of a wide variety of responses.

Terminology

The terminology used to describe the various functions of these paired muscles includes the following:

- Agonist muscle. An agonist muscle contracts to produce the desired movement. Stabilizers provide support in one area so that another area can be moved.
- Synergist muscle. Synergist muscles are muscle groups that work together to produce a desired movement.[6] In essence synergist muscles can be viewed as the agonist's helper muscles as the force generated by the synergists works in the same direction as the agonist.
- The antagonist muscle opposes the desired movement. Antagonists resist the agonist movement by relaxing and lengthening in a gradual manner to ensure that the desired motion occurs, and that it does so in a coordinated and controlled fashion.

Most skeletal muscles span only one joint. However, some skeletal muscles cross two or more joints (Table 1-2).

 Clinical Pearl

A two-joint muscle is more prone to adaptive shortening and thus injury than a one-joint muscle.

Based on contractile properties, two major types of skeletal muscle fibers have been recognized (Table 1-3):

Table 1-2 Examples of Skeletal Muscles That Cross Two or More Joints

Erector spinae
Biceps brachii
Long head of the triceps brachii
The hamstrings
The iliopsoas
Rectus femoris
Gastrocnemius
A number of muscles crossing the wrist/finger and foot/ankle joints

- Type I (slow-twitch): Slow twitch fibers use oxygen to generate fuel (ATP) and are better suited for continuous, extended muscle contractions over a long time.
- Type II (fast-twitch): Fast twitch fibers use anaerobic metabolism to create fuel. They are much better at generating short bursts of strength or speed than slow muscles. However, they fatigue more quickly.
  - Type IIa (fast-twitch white glycolytic): These fast twitch muscle fibers are also known as intermediate fast-twitch fibers. They can use both aerobic and anaerobic metabolism almost equally to create energy.
  - Type IIb (fast-twitch intermediate): These fast twitch fibers use anaerobic metabolism to create energy and excel at producing quick, powerful

Table 1-3 Muscle Fiber Types

Type	Type I	Type IIa	Type IIb
Diameter	Small	Intermediate	Large
Capillaries	Many	Many	Few
Resistance to fatigue	High	Intermediate	Low
Glycogen content	Low	Intermediate	High
Respiration	Aerobic	Aerobic	Anaerobic
Twitch rate	Slow	Fast	Fast
Myosin ATPase content	Low	High	High

bursts of speed. This muscle fiber has the highest rate of contraction (rapid firing) of all the muscle fiber types, but it also has a much faster rate of fatigue.

 Clinical Pearl

Wide functional variations exist in the form of muscles in terms of size and shape. The diameter, length, and arrangement of fascicles vary from muscle to muscle: fine bundles are used in precision muscles, whereas coarse ones are used in power muscles. In a *pennate* muscle, the fascicles form a common angle with the tendon. Three common arrangements are recognized:

• Unipennate: all the muscle fibers insert the same side of the tendon. The resultant force is the result of two vectors. Examples of a unipennate muscle include the flexor pollicis longus and extensor digitorum longus.

• Bipennate: the muscle fibers insert on both sides of the tendon. An example of a bipennate muscle is the rectus femoris.

• Multipennate: the tendon branches within a pennate muscle. One example of a multipennate muscle is the deltoid.

The *angle of pennation* is the angle created between the muscle fiber direction and the line of pull. When the fibers of a muscle lie parallel to the long axis of the muscle, there is no angle of pennation. The number of fibers within a fixed volume of muscle increases with the angle of pennation.[7]

Human muscles contain a genetically determined mixture of both slow and fast fiber type. In humans, most limb muscles contain a relatively equal distribution of each muscle fiber type, whereas the back and trunk demonstrate a predominance of slow twitch fibers.

Clinical Pearl

The use of specific muscle fibers is dependent on the desired activity. Although, the two fiber types generally produce the same amount of force per contraction, the fast twitch fibers produce that force at a higher rate (they fire more rapidly—hence their name).

- Activities that require a limited amount of time to generate maximal force use a predominance of fast twitch fiber recruitment.

- Activities that involve repeated and extended muscle contractions such as those required for endurance events entail more involvement of the slow twitch fibers.

The Type of Muscle Contraction

For motion to take place, the muscles producing movement must have a stable base from which to work from. Muscles perform a variety of roles depending on the required movement. The word *contraction*, used to describe the generation of tension within muscle fibers, conjures up an image of a shortening of muscle fibers. However, a contraction can produce a shortening or a lengthening of the muscle, or no change in the muscle length. In addition, a muscle contraction produces compression at the joint surfaces of neighboring joints.

 Clinical Pearl

By definition, a contractile tissue is a tissue involved with a muscle contraction, and one that can be tested using an isolated muscle contraction. Inert tissues are mainly tested with passive movement and ligament stress tests.

Three types of contraction are commonly recognized: isometric, concentric, and eccentric:

- Isometric contraction. An isometric contraction occurs when there is tension produced in the muscle without any appreciable change in muscle length or joint movement.[8]

- Concentric contraction. A concentric contraction produces a shortening of the muscle. This occurs when the tension generated by the agonist muscle is sufficient to overcome an external resistance, and to move the body segment of one attachment toward the segment of its other attachment.[8]

- Eccentric contraction. An eccentric contraction occurs when a muscle slowly lengthens as it submits to an external force that is greater than the contractile force it is exerting.[8] In reality, the muscle does not actually lengthen, it merely returns from its shortened position to its normal resting length.

 Clinical Pearl

Eccentric muscle contractions, which are capable of generating greater forces than either isometric or concentric contractions,[9–11] are involved in activities that require a deceleration to occur. Because the load exceeds the bond between the actin and myosin filaments during an eccentric contraction, some of the myosin are probably torn from the binding sites on the actin filament, while the remainder are completing the contraction cycle.[7] The resulting force is substantially larger for a torn cross-bridge than for one being created during a normal cycle of muscle contraction. However, eccentric contractions consume less oxygen and fewer energy stores than concentric contractions against similar loads.

A comparison of the three types of muscle actions in terms of force production, according to Elftman proposal, shows that[12]: Eccentric maximum tension > Isometric maximum tension > Concentric maximum tension.

Four other contractions are worth mentioning:

- Isotonic contraction. An isotonic contraction is a contraction in which the tension within the muscle remains constant as the muscle shortens or lengthens.[8] This state is very difficult to produce and measure. Although the term isotonic is used to describe concentric and eccentric contractions alike, its use in this context is erroneous as in most exercise forms the tension produced in muscles will vary with muscle length according to cross bridge formation and with the variation in external torque.[8]

- Isokinetic contraction. An isokinetic contraction occurs when a muscle is maximally contracting at the same speed throughout the whole range of its related lever.[8] Isokinetic contractions require the use of special equipment that produces an accommodating resistance. Both high speed/low resistance, and low speed/high resistance regimens result in excellent strength gains.[13–16] The disadvantage of this type of exercise is its expense. In addition, there is the potential for impact loading and incorrect joint axis alignment.[17] Isokinetic exercises may also have questionable functional carry-over due to their performance in open kinetic chain and training a single motion/muscle group.[18]

- Econcentric contraction. This type of contraction combines both a controlled concentric and a simultaneous eccentric contraction of the same muscle over two separate joints.[19] Examples of an econcentric contraction include the standing hamstring curl and the squat. In the standing hamstring curl, the hamstrings work concentrically to flex the knee, whereas the hip tends to flex eccentrically, lengthening the hamstrings. When rising from a squat the hamstrings work concentrically as the hip extends and work eccentrically as the knee extends. Conversely, the rectus femoris work eccentrically as the hip extends and work concentrically as the knee extends.

- Isolytic contraction. The term isolytic contraction is used in osteopathic circles to describe a type of eccentric isotonic contraction where a greater force than the patient can overcome is used. This type of contraction is used with muscle energy techniques to stretch fibrotic tissue.

 Clinical Pearl

According to Cyriax, pain with a contraction generally indicates an injury to the muscle or a capsular structure (see Chapter 3).[20]

Recruitment of Motor Units[1]

The force and speed of a muscle contraction are based on the requirement of an activity and are dependent on the ability of the central nervous system to control the recruitment of motor units.

 Clinical Pearl

Slow-twitch fiber motor units have low thresholds and are relatively more easily activated than the motor units of the fast-twitch fibers (Table 1-3). Consequently the slow-twitch fibers are the first to be recruited, even when the resulting limb movement is rapid.[21]

 Clinical Pearl

As the force requirement, speed requirement, and/or duration of the activity increases, motor units with higher thresholds are recruited. Type IIa are recruited before Type IIb.[22]

Electromechanical Delay

Following the stimulation of a muscle, a brief period elapses before the muscle begins to develop tension. This period is referred to as the *electromechanical delay* (EMD). The length of the EMD varies considerably between muscles. Fast twitch fibers have shorter periods of EMD when compared with slow twitch fibers.[23]

 Clinical Pearl

It has been suggested that injury increases the EMD and therefore increases the susceptibility to injury.[24] One of the purposes of neuro-muscular reeducation is to return the EMD to a normal level.[25]

Bone

The function of bone is to provide support, enhance leverage, protect vital structures, provide attachments for both tendons and ligaments, and store minerals, particularly calcium. Bones also can serve as useful landmarks during the palpation phase of the examination.

Tendons

Tendons (Figure 1-1) are cordlike structures that function to attach muscle to bone and to transmit the forces generated by muscles to bone to achieve movement or stability of the body in space.[26] The thickness of each tendon varies and is proportional to the size of the muscle from which they originate.

 Clinical Pearl

Some tendons, such as those that wrap around a convex surface or the apex of a concavity, those that cross two joints, those with areas of scant vascular supply, and those that are subjected to repetitive tension, are particularly vulnerable to overuse injuries.

 Clinical Pearl

The term tendonitis implies inflammation, whereas tendinosis results from a degenerative process.

Table 1-4 Major Ligaments of the Upper Quadrant

Joint	Ligament	Function
Shoulder complex	Coracoclavicular	Fixes the clavicle to the coracoid process
	Costoclavicular	Fixes the clavicle to the costal cartilage of the first rib
Glenohumeral	Coracohumeral	Reinforces the upper portion of the joint capsule
	Glenohumeral ("Z")	Reinforces the anterior and inferior aspect of the joint capsule
	Coracoacromial	Protects the superior aspect of the joint
Elbow	Annular	Maintains the relationship between the head of the radius and the humerus and ulna
	Ulnar (medial) collateral	Provides stability against valgus (medial) stress, particularly in the range of 20 degree to 130 degree of flexion and extension
	Radial (lateral) collateral	Provides stability against varus (lateral) stress and functions to maintain the ulnohumeral and radiohumeral joints in a reduced position when the elbow is loaded in supination
Wrist	Extrinsic palmar	Provide the majority of the wrist stability
	Intrinsic	Serve as rotational restraints, binding the proximal carpal row into a unit of rotational stability
	Interosseous	Bind the carpal bones together
Fingers	Anterior (volar) and collateral interphalangeal	Prevent displacement of the interphalangeal joints

Ligaments

Ligaments (Figure 1-1) are densely packed CT structures that consist largely of directionally oriented, high-tensile strength collagen. Ligaments contribute to the stability of joint function by preventing excessive motion, acting as guides to direct motion, and providing proprioceptive information for joint function (Tables 1-4 and 1-5). Because of their function as supporting cables in an environment of high-tensile forces, ligaments must be relatively inextensible to minimize transmission loss of energy.

Fascia

Fascia (Figure 1-1) is viewed as the CT that provides support and protection to the joint, and acts as an interconnection between tendons, aponeuroses, ligaments, capsules, nerves, and the intrinsic components of muscle.

Table 1-5 Major Ligaments of the Lower Quadrant

Joint	Ligament	Function
Spine	Anterior longitudinal ligament	Functions as a minor assistant in limiting anterior translation, and vertical separation of the vertebral body
	Posterior longitudinal ligament	Resists vertebral distraction of the vertebral body
		Resists posterior shearing of the vertebral body
		Acts to limit flexion over a number of segments
		Provides some protection against intervertebral disc protrusions
	Ligamentum flavum	Resists separation of the lamina during flexion
	Interspinous	Resists separation of the spinous processes during flexion
	Iliolumbar (lower lumbar)	Resists flexion, extension, axial rotation, and side bending of L5 on S1
Sacroiliac	Sacrospinous	Creates greater sciatic foramen
		Resists forward tilting of the sacrum on the hip bone during weight bearing of the vertebral column
	Sacrotuberous	Creates lesser sciatic foramen
		Resists forward tilting of the sacrum on the hip bone during weight bearing of the vertebral column
	Interosseous	Resists anterior and inferior movement of the sacrum
	Dorsal sacroiliac (long)	Resists backward tilting of the sacrum on the hip bone during weight bearing of the vertebral column
Hip	Ligamentum teres	Transports nutrient vessels to the femoral head
	Iliofemoral	Limits hip extension, external rotation, and hip adduction
	Ischiofemoral	Limits anterior displacement of the femoral head
	Pubofemoral	Limits hip extension and abduction
Knee	Medial collateral	Stabilizes medial aspect of tibiofemoral joint against valgus stress
	Lateral collateral	Stabilizes lateral aspect of tibiofemoral joint against varus stress
	Anterior cruciate	Resists anterior translation of the tibia and posterior translation of the femur
	Posterior cruciate	Resists posterior translation of the tibia and anterior translation of the femur
Ankle	Medial collaterals (Deltoid)	Provide stability between the medial malleollus, navicular, talus, and calcaneus against eversion
	Lateral collaterals	Static stabilizers of the lateral ankle especially against inversion

(continued on following page)

Joint	Ligament	Function
Foot	Long plantar	Provides indirect plantar support to the calcaneocuboid joint, by limiting the amount of flattening of the lateral longitudinal arch of the foot
	Bifurcate	Supports the medial and lateral aspects of the foot when weight bearing in a plantar flexed position
	Calcaneocuboid	Provides plantar support to the calcaneocuboid joint and possibly helps to limit flattening of the lateral longitudinal arch

Cartilage Tissue

The development of bone is usually preceded by the formation of cartilage tissue. Cartilage tissue exists in three forms: hyaline (Figure 1-1), elastic, and fibrocartilage.

Clinical Pearl

For the purpose of an orthopedic examination, Cyriax subdivided musculoskeletal tissues into those considered to be "contractile" and those considered as "inert" (noncontractile) (refer to Chapter 3).[20]

Joints

Joints (Figure 1-1) are bone regions that are capped and surrounded by CTs that hold the bones together and determine the type and degree of movement between them. Joints may be classified as *diarthrosis*, which permit free bone movement and *synarthrosis*, in which very limited or no motion occurs (Table 1-6).

Diarthrosis (Synovial)

Every synovial joint contained at least one "mating pair" of articular surfaces: one convex and one concave. If only one pair exists, the joint is called simple; more than one pair is called compound; and if the disc is present, the joint is termed complex. Synovial joints have five distinguishing characteristics: joint cavity, articular cartilage, synovial fluid, synovial membrane, and a fibrous capsule. Four types of synovial joint are recognized:

1. Nonaxial—These joints have no planes of motion or primary axes and only permit sliding or gliding motions. Examples include the carpal joints.

2. Uniaxial joint—These joints allow one motion around a single axis and in one plane of the body. Two types are recognized:
   a. Hinge (ginglymus)—the elbow joint.
   b. Pivot joint (trochoid)—atlantoaxial joint.
3. Biaxial joint—These joints allow movement in two planes and around two axes based on their convex/concave surfaces. Two types are recognized:
   a. Condyloid—One bone may articulate with another by one surface or by two, but never more than two. If two distinct surfaces are present, the joint is called condylar or bicondylar. Example, metacarpophalangeal joint of the finger.
   b. Sellar (saddle)—If a section is taken through a sellar surface in one plane, the joint surface can be seen to be convex and the curvature of the joint in the opposite plane is concave. Example: carpometacarpal joint of the thumb.
4. Multiaxial joint—these joints allow movement in three planes and around three axes. Two subtypes are recognized:
   a. Plane (gliding)—carpal joints.
   b. Ball and socket—hip joint.

Synarthrosis (Fibrous)

There are three major types of synarthroses based on the type of tissue uniting the bone surfaces (Table 1-6).[27]

Synovial Fluid

Articular cartilage is subject to a great variation of loading conditions, and joint lubrication through synovial fluid is necessary to minimize frictional

Table 1-6 Joint Types

Type	Characteristics	Examples
Diarthrosis	Fibroelastic joint capsule, which is filled with a lubricating substance called *synovial fluid*	Hip, knee, shoulder, and elbow joints
Synarthrosis		
Synostosis	United by bone tissue	Sutures and gomphoses
Synchondrosis	Joined by either hyaline or fibrocartilage	The epiphyseal plates of growing bones and the articulations between the first rib and the sternum
Syndesmosis	Joined together by an interosseous membrane	The symphysis pubis

resistance between the weight-bearing surfaces. Fortunately, synovial joints are blessed with a very superior lubricating system, which permits a remarkably frictionless interaction at the joint surfaces.

Bursae

Closely associated with some synovial joints are flattened, saclike structures called *bursae* that are lined with a synovial membrane and filled with synovial fluid. The bursa produces small amounts of fluid, allowing for smooth and almost frictionless motion between contiguous muscles, tendons, bones, ligaments, and skin.

Mechanoreceptors

All synovial joints of the body are provided with an array of corpuscular (mechanoreceptors) and noncorpuscular (nociceptors) receptor endings imbedded in articular, muscular, and cutaneous structures with varying characteristic behaviors and distributions depending on articular tissue. Freeman and Wyke categorized the mechanoreceptors into four different types (Table 1-7).[28,29]

The articular mechanoreceptors (types I, II, and III) are stimulated by mechanical forces (soft tissue elongation, relaxation, compression, and fluid tension) and mediate proprioception.[28,30,31] The type IV variety is a nociceptor.[31]

Other receptors found in the joint include proprioceptors. Proprioception is considered a specialized variation of the sensory modality of touch, which plays an important role in coordinating muscle activity, and involves the integration of sensory input concerning static joint position (joint position sensibility), joint movement (kinesthetic sensibility), velocity of movement, and force of muscular contraction, from the skin, muscles, and joints.[32,33] Proprioception can be both conscious, as occurs in the accurate placement of a limb, and unconscious, as occurs in the modulation of muscle function.[33,34]

 Clinical Pearl

The muscle spindle (Box 1-1) functions as a stretch receptor detecting changes in muscle length.

The Golgi Tendon Organ (GTO) (Box 1-2) functions as a monitor for the degree of tension within a muscle and tendon.

Tissue Injury

With the exception of bone tissue, all other tissues of the body can be referred to as *soft tissue*. Injuries to the soft tissues can be classified as primary or secondary:

Table 1-7 Mechanoreceptor Types

Type	Location	Function
I—Small Ruffini endings. Slow-adapting, low threshold stretch receptors	The joint capsule and in ligaments	Important in signaling actual joint position or changes in joint positions
		Contribute to reflex regulation of postural tone, to coordination of muscle activity and to a perceptional awareness of joint position
		An increase in joint capsule tension by active or passive motion, posture or by mobilization or manipulation, causes these receptors to discharge at a higher frequency
II—Pacinian corpuscles. Rapidly adapting, low threshold receptors	In adipose tissue, the cruciate ligaments, the anulus fibrosus, ligaments, and the fibrous capsule	Sense joint motion and regulate motor-unit activity of the prime movers of the joint
		Type II receptors are entirely inactive in immobile joints and become active for brief periods at the onset of movement and during rapid changes in tension
		The Type II receptors fire during active or passive motion of a joint or with the application of traction
III—Large Ruffini. Slowly adapting, high threshold receptors	Ligaments and the fibrous capsule	Detect large amounts of tension
		These receptors only become active in the extremes of motion or when strong manual techniques are applied to the joint
IV—Nociceptors. Slowly adapting, high threshold free nerve endings		Inactive in normal circumstances but become active with marked mechanical deformation or tension
		Also active in response to direct mechanical or chemical irritation

- Primary injuries can be self-inflicted, caused by another individual or entity, or caused by the environment. Primary injuries can be subclassified into acute, chronic, or acute on chronic:
  - Acute. Acute injuries occur as the result of a sudden overloading of the musculoskeletal tissues (macrotrauma), for example, fractures,

Box 1-1 The Muscle Spindle

Muscle Spindle

Within each muscle spindle there are 2 to 12 long, slender, specialized skeletal muscle fibers called *intrafusal fibers*, whose cell bodies lie in the dorsal root ganglia or cranial nerve sensory ganglia (refer to Chapter 2). The central portion of the intrafusal fiber is devoid of actin or myosin and is thus unable to contract; only the intrafusal fibers are capable of putting tension on the spindle.

When the muscle spindle is stimulated by a quick stretch, its receptors are polarized and an impulse volley synapses with α motor neurons that innervate the extrafusal fibers of the stretched muscle and with synergistic muscles. The same afferent supplies inhibitory input to the antagonist muscles by way of interneurons so that as the agonist contracts, the antagonist is relaxed in the process of reciprocal inhibition. This has the effect of producing a smooth contraction and relaxation of muscle and eliminating any jerkiness during movement under normal circumstances. The firing of the α motor neuron fibers is influenced by the rate of stretch; the faster and greater the stimulus, the greater the effect of the associated extrafusal fibers.

Box 1-2 Golgi Tendon Organs

Golgi Tendon Organs

GTOs function to protect muscle attachments from strain or avulsion by using a postsynaptic inhibitory synapse of the muscle in which they are located.

The GTO receptors are arranged in series with the extrafusal muscle fibers and, therefore, become activated by stretch. The signals from the GTO may go both to local areas within the spinal cord and through the spinocerebellar tracts to the cerebellum. The local signals result in excitation of interneurons, which in turn inhibit the anterior α motor neurons of the GTO's own muscle and synergist, while facilitating the antagonists. This is theorized to prevent over-contraction, or stretch, of a muscle.

dislocations, subluxations, sprains (acute injury to a ligament), strains (injury to a muscle), and contusions (excessive compression to the soft tissues with resultant disruption of the muscle fibers and intramuscular bleeding).[35]

- Chronic. Chronic, or overuse injuries occur as the result of a cumulative repetitive overload (overuse), incorrect mechanics, and/or frictional resistance (microtrauma). These microtraumatic injuries include tendonitis, tenosynovitis, bursitis, and synovitis.
- Acute on chronic. This type of injury presents as a sudden rupture of a previously damaged tissue and can occur when the load applied to a tissue is too great for the level of tissue repair or remodeling.
- Secondary injuries are essentially the inflammatory response that occurs with the primary injury.[36]

Muscle Injury

The three most common types of muscle injury include strain (overstretching of muscle tissue), contusion (direct trauma or compressive force to muscle tissue), and laceration (disruption of muscle continuity). Small injuries repair with muscle tissue, whereas large injuries repair with scar tissue (see Tissue Healing).

Tendon Injury

The most common form of tendon injury is overuse, which results from repetitive motion stress or repetitive overload at a rate that exceeds the tissue's ability to repair. Various terms are used to classify tendon injury, including:

- Strain. Defined as an injury to the musculotendinous unit from an abrupt contraction or stretch.
- Tendonitis. Defined as an injury to the tendon accompanied by inflammation.
- Tendinosis. Defined as a tendon injury associated with formation of an extracellular matrix.
- Rupture. Defined as a complete failure of the tendon.

Ligament Injury

The most common mechanism of ligament injury is excessive lengthening of the ligament as a result of the associated joint been moved into an excessive range of motion. Ligament injuries can be classified into three grades:

- Grade I. Involves stretching of the ligament, but no fiber damage.
- Grade II. Involves stretching of the ligament and tearing of some fibers.
- Grade III. Involves almost complete ligament disruption.

Tissue Healing

The musculoskeletal structures commonly injured by patients seen for orthopedic rehabilitation include muscle, tendons, ligaments, bone, cartilage, and nerve.

 Clinical Pearl

The healing process involved three phases and several subphases:

- Phase 1. Inflammatory. Includes two subphases: vascular and cellular.
- Phase 2. Reparative (proliferative, fibroplastic, regenerative).
- Phase 3. Remodeling. Includes two subphases: consolidation and maturation.

A number of factors can have an impact on healing. These include the following:
- Local factors:
  - The degree of tissue damage
  - The type and size of wound
  - The type of tissue involved
  - The presence of swelling
  - The presence of infection
  - The blood supply to the injured site
  - The amount of stress applied to tissue
  - The degree of wound stabilization
- Systemic factors:
  - Age
  - Comorbidities
  - Nutritional state
  - Obesity
- Extrinsic factors:
  - Medications
  - Temperature
  - Humidity

Tissue Healing Phases

- Inflammation (phase 1). The inflammation phase is characterized by the removal of all foreign debris and dead tissue (cellular subphase), increased vascular permeability, and the promotion of fibroblast activity.[37] This process is mediated by chemotactic substances, including anaphylatoxins. Anaphylatoxins serve to attract neutrophils and monocytes:

- Neutrophils. Neutrophils are white blood cells of the polymorphonuclear (PMN) leukocyte subgroup (the others being eosinophils and basophils) that are filled with granules of toxic chemicals (phagocytes) that enable them to bind to microorganisms, internalize them, and kill them.
- Monocytes. Monocytes are white blood cells of the mononuclear leukocyte subgroup (the other being lymphocytes). The monocytes migrate into tissues and develop into macrophages, and provide immunological defences against many infectious organisms. Macrophages serve to orchestrate a "long-term" response to injured cells subsequent to the acute response.

The extent and severity of the inflammatory response depends on the size and the type of the injury, the tissue involved, and the vascularity of that tissue.[38–42] Local vasodilation is promoted by biologically active products of the complement, kinin, and clotting system:[43]

- The complement system involves 20 or more proteins that circulate throughout the blood in an inactive form.[43] After tissue injury, activation of the complement cascade produces a release of histamine from mast cells, which in turn increases vascular permeability.
- The kinin system is responsible for the transformation of the inactive enzyme kallikrein, which is present in both blood and tissue, to its active form, bradykinin. Bradykinin also contributes to the production of tissue exudate through the promotion of vasodilation and increased vessel wall permeability.[44]
- The clotting system is designed to stem the loss of blood from injured tissues.

Clinical Pearl

The inflammation stage of healing is characterized by swelling, redness, heat, and impairment or loss of function. The edema is due to an increase in the permeability of the venules, plasma proteins and leukocytes, which leak into the site of injury.[45,46] Usually there is pain at rest or with active motion, or when specific stress is applied to the injured structure. The pain, if severe enough, can result in muscle guarding and a loss of function. If this phase is interrupted or delayed, chronic inflammation can result, lasting from months to years.

- Reparative phase (phase 2). This phase is responsible for reepithelization, fibroplasia with neovascularization, and the development of a collagenous matrix that facilitates angiogenesis by providing time and protection to new and friable vessels and begins the process of wound contracture. The process of neovascularization during this phase provides a granular appearance to the wound due to the formation of loops of capillaries and migration of macrophages, fibroblasts, and endothelial cells into the wound matrix.

 Clinical Pearl

Upon progressing to the reparative phase, the "active" effusion and local erythema of the inflammatory stage are usually no longer present. However, residual effusion may still be present at this time and resist resorption.[47,48]

- Remodeling (phase 3). The remodeling phase of wound healing involves a conversion of the initial healing tissue to scar tissue—consolidation and maturation. This lengthy phase of contraction, tissue remodeling, and increasing tensile strength in the wound lasts for up to a year.[40,49–53] The application of controlled stresses to the new scar tissue must occur during this stage to help prevent it from shortening.[42,53] If the healing tissues are kept immobile, the fibrous repair is weak, and there are no forces influencing the collagen. Scarring that occurs parallel to the line of force of a structure is less vulnerable to reinjury than a scar, which is perpendicular to those lines of force.[54]

Although simplification of the complex events of healing into these separate categories may facilitate understanding of the phenomenon, in reality these events occur as an amalgamation of different reactions, both spatially and temporally.[43]

 Clinical Pearl

The most important factor regulating the regional time line of healing is sufficient blood flow.[53] The approximate time frames involved with the various phases of tissue healing include:

Phase 1: 0 to 14 days (greatest at 48 hours)

Phase 2: 0 to 21 days

Phase 3: 21 to 360 days

Clinical Pearl

Despite the presence of an intact epithelium at 3 to 4 weeks after the injury, the tensile strength of the wound has been measured at approximately 25% of its normal value. Several months later, only 70% to 80% of the strength may be restored.[55] This would appear to demonstrate that the remodeling process may last many months or even years, making it extremely important to continue applying controlled stresses to the tissue long after healing appears to have occurred.[55]

Tissue-Specific Healing

Muscle Healing

Skeletal muscle has considerable regenerative capabilities, based primarily on the type and extent of injury.[35,56] Broadly speaking, there are three phases in the healing process of an injured muscle: the destruction phase, the repair phase, and the remodeling phase.[57]

- The destruction phase (immediately following injury). The muscle fibers and their CT sheaths are totally disrupted and a gap appears between the ends of the ruptured muscle fibers when the muscle fibers retract.[58] This phase is characterized by the necrosis of muscle tissue, degeneration, and an infiltration by PMN leukocytes as hematoma and edema form at the site of injury.

- The repair phase (occurs after a few days to a few weeks).[58] Usually involves three steps: hematoma formation, matrix formation (gives the initial strength for wound tissue to withstand the forces applied to it),[59] and collagen formation. The production of type I collagen by fibroblasts increases the tensile strength of the injured muscle. An excessive proliferation of fibroblasts can rapidly lead to an excessive formation of dense scar tissue, which creates a mechanical barrier that restricts or considerable delays complete regeneration of the muscle fibers across the gap.[57,58]

 Clinical Pearl

During the first week of muscle tissue healing, the injury site is the weakest point of the muscle-tendon unit.

- The remodeling phase. In this phase, the regenerated muscle matures and contracts with reorganization of the scar tissue. There is often incomplete restoration of the functional capacity of the injured muscle.

 Clinical Pearl

One of the potential consequences of muscle injury is atrophy. The amount of muscle atrophy that occurs depends on the usage before the injury and the function of the muscle.[60] Antigravity muscles (such as the quadriceps) tend to have greater atrophy than antagonist muscles (such as the hamstrings). Research has shown that a single bout of exercise protects against muscle damage, with the effects lasting between 6 weeks[61] and 9 months.[62] Muscle resistance to damage may result from an eccentric exercise-induced morphological change in the number of sarcomeres connected in series.[63] This finding appears to support initiating a reconditioning program with gradual progression from lower intensity activities with minimal eccentric actions to protect against muscle damage.[60,64]

Ligament and Tendon Healing

The process of ligament and tendon healing is complex. Healing of ligaments and tendons generally can be broken down into four overlapping phases:

- Phase I: Hemorrhagic. After disruption of the tissue, the gap is filled quickly with a blood clot. PMN leukocytes and lymphocytes appear within several hours, triggered by cytokines released within the clot. The PMN leukocytes and lymphocytes respond to autocrine and paracrine signals to expand the inflammatory response and recruit other types of cells to the wound.[65]

- Phase II: Inflammatory. Macrophages arrive by 24 to 48 hours and are the predominant cell type within several days. Macrophages perform phagocytosis of necrotic tissues, and also secrete multiple types of growth factors that induce neovascularization and the formation of granulation tissue. Platelets have been shown to release platelet-derived growth factor (PDGF), transforming growth factor (TGF)-β, and epidermal growth factor. Macrophages produce basic fibroblast growth factor, TGF-α, TGF-β, and PDGF. These growth factors are not only chemotactic for fibroblasts and other cells, but also stimulate fibroblast proliferation and the synthesis of types I, III, and V collagen and noncollagenous proteins.[66,67]

- Phase III: Proliferation. Fibroblasts begin producing collagen and other matrix proteins within 1 week of injury. By the second week after disruption, the original blood clot becomes more organized because of cellular and matrix proliferation. Capillary buds begin to form. Total collagen content is greater than in the normal ligament or tendon, but collagen concentration is lower and the matrix remains disorganized.

- Phase IV: Remodeling and maturation. Phase IV is marked by a gradual decrease in the cellularity of the healed tissue. The matrix becomes denser and longitudinally oriented. Collagen turnover, water content, and the ratio of collagen types I to III begin to approach normal levels.[68] The healed tissue continues to mature for many months, but will never attain normal morphological characteristics or mechanical properties. Ligament injuries can take as long as 3 years to heal to the point of regaining near-normal tensile strength,[69] although some tensile strength is regained by about the fifth week following injury, depending on the severity.[51,70-72]

● Clinical Pearl

A ligament may have 50% of its normal tensile strength by 6 months after injury, 80% after 1 year, and 100% only after 1 to 3 years.[73-75] Forces applied to the ligament during its recovery help it to develop strength in the direction that the force is applied.[73-77]

Articular Cartilage Healing

It is well known that the capacity of articular cartilage for repair is limited. Cartilage cells, or chondrocytes, are responsible for the maintenance of the cartilage matrix. The repair response of articular cartilage varies with the depth of the injury.

- Injuries of the articular cartilage that do not penetrate the subchondral bone become necrotic and do not heal. These lesions usually progress to the degeneration of the articular surface.[78] Although a short-lived tissue response may occur, it fails to provide sufficient cells and matrix to repair even small defects.[79,80]

- Injuries that penetrate the subchondral bone undergo repair due to access to the bone's blood supply. These repairs are usually characterized as fibrous, fibrocartilaginous, or hyaline-like cartilaginous, depending on the species, the age of the animal, and the location and size of the injury.[81] However, these reparative tissues differ from normal hyaline cartilage both biochemically and biomechanically. Thus, by 6 months, fibrillation, fissuring, and extensive degenerative changes occur in the reparative tissues of approximately half of the full-thickness defects.[82,83] Similarly, the degenerated cartilage seen in osteoarthrosis does not usually undergo repair but progressively deteriorates.[78]

 Clinical Pearl

Current surgical treatment for damaged cartilage may consist of debridement or removal of loose flaps or pieces of cartilage, abrasion/burr arthroplasty at the site of the lesion, or subchondral drilling.

An experimental technique undergoing active investigation is the transplantation of chondrocytes or chondrogenic cells or periosteal, perichondrial, of mesenchymal origin.[84,85]

Cartilage injuries can be graded as follows[86]:
- Grade 0—normal
- Grade 1—nearly normal: superficial lesions, soft indentations, and/or fissures and cracks
- Grade 2—abnormal: lesions extending less than 50% of the cartilage depth
- Grade 3—severely abnormal: lesions extending greater than 50% of the cartilage depth
- Grade 4—severely abnormal: lesions extending down into the subchondral bone; full thickness injury.

Meniscal Healing

Two pathways for healing in response to a tear in the periphery of the meniscus are described: extrinsic and intrinsic.

- Extrinsic pathway. Once a meniscal tear occurs, a fibrin clot forms within its margins, creating a scaffold into which angiogenesis develops from the perimeniscal capillary plexus. It may take months or even years for the scar tissue to change into fibrocartilage, resembling that of the meniscus. Differences between the newly formed fibrocartilage and mature fibrocartilage are recognizable and include increased cellularity and, at times, increased vascularity in the repair tissue.
- Intrinsic pathway. The chondrocytes within the meniscus have an inherent capability to generate a healing response, even in the avascular region. Chondrocytes are assisted by the fibrin clot, which not only acts as a scaffold but also provides the chemotactic and mitogenic stimuli to promote healing.

Bone Healing

Bone healing is a complex physiological process. The striking feature of bone healing, compared to healing in other tissues, is that repair is by the original tissue, not scar tissue. Regeneration is perhaps a better descriptor than repair. This is linked to the capacity for remodeling that intact bone possesses. Like other forms of healing, the repair of bone fracture includes the processes of inflammation, repair, and remodeling; however, the type of healing varies depending on the method of treatment. According to Wolff law, bone remodels along lines of stress.[87] Bone is constantly being resorbed and replaced as the resorption of circumferential lamellar bone is accomplished by osteoclasts, and replaced with dense osteonal bone by osteoblasts.[88]

In classic histological terms, fracture healing has been divided into two broad phases: primary fracture healing and secondary fracture healing.

- Primary healing, or primary cortical healing, involves a direct attempt by the cortex to reestablish itself once it has become interrupted. In primary cortical healing, bone on one side of the cortex must unite with bone on the other side of the cortex to reestablish mechanical continuity.

- Secondary healing involves responses in the periosteum and external soft tissues with the subsequent formation of a callus. The majority of fractures heal by secondary fracture healing.

Within these broader phases, the process of bone healing involves a combination of intramembranous and endochondral ossification. These two processes participate in the fracture repair sequence by at least four discrete stages of healing: the hematoma formation (inflammation or granulation) phase, the soft callus formation (proliferative) phase, the hard callus formation (maturing or modeling) phase, and the remodeling phase.[89]

- Hematoma formation (inflammation or granulation) phase. This phase is characterized by the release of a variety of products, including fibronectin, PDGF, and TGF, by the activated platelets. These products trigger the influx of inflammatory cells.

- Soft callus formation (proliferative) phase. This phase is characterized by the formation of CTs, including cartilage, and formation of new capillaries from preexisting vessels (angiogenesis). During the first 7 to 10 days of fracture healing, the periosteum undergoes an intramembranous bone formation response, and histological evidence shows formation of woven bone opposed to the cortex within a few millimeters from the site of the fracture. By the middle of the second week, abundant cartilage overlies the fracture site, and this chondroid tissue initiates biochemical preparations to undergo calcification. Thus, the callus becomes a three-layered structure consisting of an outer proliferating part, a middle cartilagenous layer, and an inner portion of new bony trabeculae. The cartilage portion is usually replaced with bone as the healing progresses.

- Hard callus formation (maturing or modeling) phase. This phase is characterized by the production of woven bone. The calcification of fracture callus cartilage occurs by a mechanism almost identical to that which takes place in the growth plate. This can occur either directly from mesenchymal tissue (intramembranous) or via an intermediate stage of cartilage (endochondral or chondroid routes). Osteoblasts can form woven bone rapidly, but it is randomly arranged and mechanically weak. Nonetheless, bridging of a fracture by woven bone constitutes "clinical union." Once cartilage is calcified, it becomes a target for the ingrowth of blood vessels.

- Remodeling phase. By replacing the cartilage with bone, and converting the cancellous bone into compact bone, the callus is gradually remodeled. During this phase, the woven bone is remodeled into stronger lamellar bone by the orchestrated action of osteoclast bone resorption and osteoblast bone formation.

Radiologically, or histologically, fracture gap bridging occurs by three mechanisms[89]:

- Intercortical bridging (primary cortical union). This occurs when the fracture gap is reduced by normal cortical remodeling under conditions of rigid fixation. This mode of healing is the principle behind rigid internal fixation.[90]

- External callus bridging by new bone arising from the periosteum and the soft tissues surrounding the fracture. Small degrees of movement at the fracture stimulate external callus formation.[91] This mode of healing is the aim in functional bracing[92] and intrameduallary (IM) nailing.

- Intramedullary bridging by endosteal callus.

🔵 Clinical Pearl

Normal periods of immobilization following a fracture range from as short as 3 weeks for small bones to around 8 weeks for the long bones of the extremities. During the period of casting, submaximal isometrics are initiated, and once the cast is removed it is important that controlled stresses continue to be applied to the bone, as the period of bone healing continues for up to a year.[93,94] Some fractures heal more slowly than expected or fail to heal at all. Slow healing is known as delayed union and failure to heal is known as nonunion. When a fracture fails to heal, cartilage or fibrocartilage forms over the fracture surfaces (pseudoarthrosis) and a cavity between the fracture surfaces fills with fluid that resembles normal joint or bursal fluid.[95]

The two key determinants of if and how a fracture will heal are the blood supply and the degree of motion experienced by the fracture ends.

- Blood supply: Angiogenesis is the outgrowth of new capillaries from existing vessels. The degree of angiogenesis that occurs depends on well-vascularized tissue on either side of the gap and sufficient mechanical stability to allow new capillaries to survive. Angiogenesis leads to osteogenesis.

- The amount of movement that occurs between fracture ends can be stimulatory or inhibitory depending on their magnitude. Excessive interfragmentary movement prevents the establishment of intramedullary blood vessel bridging. However, small degrees of micromotion have been shown to stimulate blood flow at the fracture site and stimulate periosteal callus.[96]

⬤ Clinical Pearl

A fracture that is rigidly internally fixed produces no periosteal callus, and heals by a combination of endosteal callus and primary cortical union.[89] An IM nail blocks endosteal healing but allows enough movement to trigger periosteal callus.[89] External fixation, particularly with fine wires in a circular fixator, is the least damaging to the medullary blood supply.[89] This type of fixation may provide enough stability to allow rapid endosteal healing without external callus.[97]

⬤ Clinical Pearl

Common risk factors for delayed fracture healing include diabetes mellitus, smoking, long-term steroid use, nonsteroidal anti-inflammatory drugs (NSAIDs) and other medications, and poor nutrition.

Biomechanics

The Anatomical Reference Position

When describing joint movements it is necessary to have a starting position as the reference position. This starting position is referred to as the *anatomical reference position*. The anatomical reference position for the human body is described as the erect standing position with the feet just slightly separated

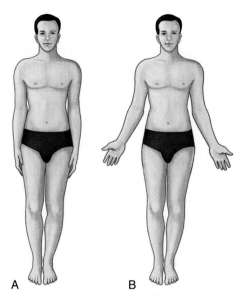

A   B

Figure 1-4 The anatomical reference position of the body. (Reproduced with permission from Luttgens K, Hamilton N. *Kinesiology*. 9th ed. McGraw-Hill; 1997.)

and the arms hanging by the side, the elbows straight and with the palms of the hand facing forward (Figure 1-4).

Directional Terms

Directional terms are used to describe the relationship of body parts or the location of an external object with respect to the body (Table 1-8).[98]

Movements of the Body Segments

Movements of the body segments occur in three dimensions along imaginary planes and around various axes of the body.

Planes of the Body

There are three traditional planes of the body corresponding to the three dimensions of space: sagittal, frontal, and transverse (Figure 1-5).[98]

- Sagittal. The sagittal plane, also known as the anterior–posterior or median plane, divides the body vertically into left and right halves.
- Frontal. The frontal plane, also known as the lateral or coronal plane, divides the body into front and back halves.

Table 1-8 Directional Terms

Term	Explanation
Superior or cranial	Closer to the head
Inferior or caudal	Closer to the feet
Anterior (ventral)	Toward the front of the body
Posterior (dorsal)	Toward the back of the body
Medial	Toward the midline of the body
Lateral	Away from the midline of the body
Proximal	Closer to the trunk
Distal	Away from the trunk
Superficial	Toward the surface of the body
Deep	Away from the surface of the body in the direction of the inside of the body
Volar (anterior)	Pertaining to both the palm and sole
Dorsal (posterior)	Relating to the back or posterior of a structure

- Transverse. The transverse plane, also known as the horizontal plane, divides the body into top and bottom halves.

If movement occurs in a plane that passes through the center of gravity, that movement is deemed to have occurred in a *cardinal* plane. Few movements involved with functional activities occur in pure cardinal planes. Instead, most movements occur in an infinite number of vertical and horizontal planes parallel to the cardinal planes (see below).

Axes of the Body

Three reference axes are used to describe human motion: frontal, sagittal, and longitudinal. The axis around which the movement takes place is always perpendicular to the plane in which it occurs.

- Frontal. The frontal axis, also known as the transverse axis, is perpendicular to the sagittal plane.

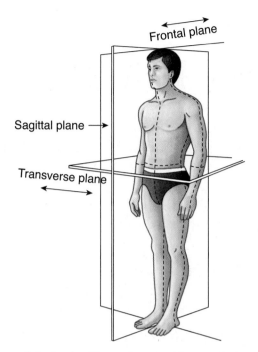

Figure 1-5 Planes of the body. (Reproduced with permission from Luttgens K, Hamilton N. *Kinesiology*. 9th ed. McGraw-Hill; 1997.)

- Sagittal. The sagittal axis is perpendicular to the frontal plane.
- Longitudinal. The longitudinal axis, also known as the vertical axis is perpendicular to the transverse plane.

The planes and axes for the more common planar movements are outlined in Table 1-9.

Both the configuration of a joint and the line of pull of the muscle acting at a joint determine the motion that occurs at a joint:

- A muscle whose line of pull is lateral to the joint is a potential abductor.
- A muscle whose line of pull is medial to the joint is a potential adductor.
- A muscle whose line of pull is anterior to a joint has the potential to extend or flex the joint. At the knee, an anterior line of pull may cause the knee to extend, whereas at the elbow joint, an anterior line of pull may cause flexion of the elbow.
- A muscle whose line of pull is posterior to the joint has the potential to extend or flex a joint (refer to example above).

Table 1-9 Planar Motions and Their Respective Planes and Axes of Motion

Planar Motion	Plane and Axis of Motion
Flexion, extension, hyperextension, dorsiflexion, and plantar flexion	In a sagittal plane around a frontal–horizontal axis
Abduction, adduction; sidebending of the trunk; elevation and depression of the shoulder girdle; radial and ulnar deviation of the wrist; eversion and inversion of the foot	In the frontal plane around a sagittal–horizontal axis
Rotation of the head, neck, and trunk; internal rotation and external rotation of the arm or leg; horizontal adduction and abduction of the arm or thigh; pronation and supination of the forearm	In the transverse plane around the longitudinal axis
Arm circling and trunk circling (circumduction)	Involve an orderly sequence of circular movements that occur in the sagittal, frontal, and intermediate oblique planes, so that segment as a whole incorporates a combination of flexion, extension, abduction, and adduction

Joint Kinematics

Kinematics is the study of motion. In studying joint kinematics, two major types of motion are involved: (1) the osteokinematic and (2) the arthrokinematic.

Osteokinematic Motion

Osteokinematic motion occurs when any object forms the radius of an imaginary circle about a fixed point. All human body segment motions involve osteokinematic motions.

 Clinical Pearl

Examples of osteokinematic motion include abduction or adduction of the arm, flexion of the hip or knee, and sidebending of the trunk.

Arthrokinematic Motion

The motions occurring at the joint surfaces are termed *arthrokinematic* movements. For the sake of simplicity, the shapes of these articulating surfaces in synovial joints are described as being *ovoid* or *sellar* in shape. Under this concept, an articulating surface can be either concave (female) or convex (male) in shape (ovoid), or a combination of both shapes (sellar). An example of an ovoid joint is the glenohumeral joint—the humeral head is the convex surface and the glenoid fossa is the concave surface. An example of a sellar joint is the first carpometacarpal joint.

Normal arthrokinematic motions must occur for full-range physiological motion to take place. A restriction of arthrokinematic motion results in a decrease in osteokinematic motion. The three types of movement that occur at the articulating surfaces include[99]:

- Roll. A roll occurs when the points of contact on each joint surface are constantly changing (Figure 1-6). This type of movement is analogous to a tire on a car as the car rolls forward. The term *rock* is often used to describe small rolling motions.

- Slide. A slide is a pure translation. It occurs if only one point on the moving surface makes contact with varying points on the opposing surface (Figure 1-6). This type of movement is analogous to a car tire skidding when the brakes are applied suddenly on a wet road. This type of motion is also

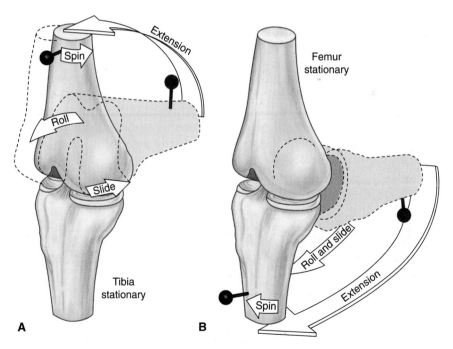

Figure 1-6 Joint movements.

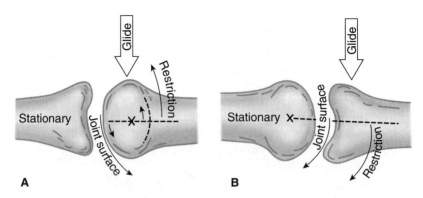

Figure 1-7 Gliding motions according to joint surface shapes.

referred to as *translatory* or *accessory* motion. The roll of a joint always occurs in the same direction as the swing of a bone, whereas the shapes of the articulating surfaces determine the direction of the joint glide (Figure 1-7). This rule is often referred to as the *concave-convex rule*: If the joint surface is convex relative to the other surface, the slide occurs in the opposite direction to the osteokinematic motion (Figure 1-7). If, on the other hand, the joint surface is concave, the slide occurs in the same direction as the osteokinematic motion.

- Spin. A spin is defined as any movement in which the bone moves but the mechanical axis remains stationary. A spin involves a rotation of one surface on an opposing surface around a longitudinal axis (Figure 1-6). This type of motion is analogous to the pirouette performed in ballet. Spin motions in the body include internal and external rotation of the glenohumeral joint when the humerus is abducted to 90 degrees, and at the radial head during forearm pronation and supination.

Osteokinematic and arthrokinematic motions are directly proportional to each other and one cannot occur completely without the other. It therefore follows that if a joint is not functioning correctly, one, or both, of these motions may at fault. When examining a patient with movement impairment, it is critical that the clinician determines whether the osteokinematic motion or the arthrokinematic motion is restricted so that the intervention can be made as specific as possible.

Degrees of Freedom

The number of independent modes of motion at a joint is called the *degrees of freedom* (DOF) (Table 1-10).

Table 1-10 Degrees of Freedom and Joint Examples

Degrees of Freedom	Joint Examples
1	The proximal interphalangeal joint
2	The tibiofemoral joint, temporomandibular joint, proximal and distal radioulnar joints, subtalar joint, and talocalcaneal joint
3	Glenohumeral joint Hip

Clinical Pearl

If a joint can swing in one direction or can only spin, it is said to have 1 DOF.[6,100–102]

If a joint can spin and swing in one way only *or* it can swing in two completely distinct ways, but not spin, it is said to have 2 DOF.[6,100–102]

If the bone can spin and also swing in two distinct directions then it is said to have 3 DOF.[6,100–102]

Most habitual movements, or those movements that occur most frequently at a joint, involve a conjunct rotation. However, the conjunct rotations are not always under volitional control. In fact, the conjunct rotation is only under volitional control in joints with three DOF (glenohumeral, and hip joints). In those joints with fewer than three DOF (hinge joints such as the tibiofemoral and ulnohumeral joints), the conjunct rotation occurs as part of the movement but is not under voluntary control. Joint mobilizing techniques must take into consideration both the relative shapes of the articulating surfaces, in addition to the conjunct rotation that is associated with a particular motion.

Close-Packed and Open-Packed Positions of the Joint

Joint movements are usually accompanied by a relative compression (approximation) or distraction (separation) of the opposing joint surfaces. These relative compression or distractions affect the level of *congruity* of the opposing surfaces. The position of maximum congruity of the opposing joint surfaces is termed the *close-packed* position of the joint. The close-packed positions for the various joints are depicted in Table 1-11. The position of least congruity is termed the *open-packed* position. The open-packed positions for the various

Table 1-11 The Close-Packed Position of the Major Joints

Joint	Position
Zygapophysial (spine)	Extension
Temporomandibular	Teeth clenched
Glenohumeral	Abduction and external rotation
Acromioclavicular	Arm abducted to 90 degrees
Sternoclavicular	Maximum shoulder elevation
Ulnohumeral	Extension
Radiohumeral	Elbow flexed 90 degrees. Forearm supinated 5 degrees
Proximal radioulnar	5 degrees supination
Distal radioulnar	5 degrees supination
Radiocarpal (wrist)	Extension with radial deviation
Metacarpophalangeal	Full flexion
Metacarpophalangeal	Full opposition
Interphalangeal	Full extension
Hip	Full extension, internal rotation, abduction
Tibiofemoral	Full extension, external rotation of tibia
Talocrural (ankle)	Maximum dorsiflexion
Subtalar	Supination
Midtarsal	Supination
Tarsometatarsal	Supination
Metatarsophalangeal	Full extension
Interphalangeal	Full extension

Table 1-12 The Open-Packed (Resting) Position of the Major Joints

Joint	Position
Zygapophysial (spine)	Midway between flexion and extension
Temporomandibular	Mouth slightly open (freeway space)
Glenohumeral	55 degree abduction, 30 degree horizontal adduction
Acromioclavicular	Arm resting by side
Sternoclavicular	Arm resting by side
Ulnohumeral	70 degree flexion, 10 degree supination
Radiohumeral	Full extension, full supination
Proximal radioulnar	70 degree flexion, 35 degree supination
Distal radioulnar	10 degree supination
Radiocarpal (wrist)	Neutral with slight ulnar deviation
Carpometacarpal	Midway between abduction–adduction and flexion–extension
Metacarpophalangeal	Slight flexion
Interphalangeal	Slight flexion
Hip	30 degree flexion, 30 degree abduction, slight external rotation
Knee	25 degree flexion
Talocrural (ankle)	10 degree plantar flexion, midway between maximum inversion and eversion
Subtalar	Midway between extremes of range of movement
Midtarsal	Midway between extremes of range of movement
Tarsometatarsal	Midway between extremes of range of movement
Metatarsophalangeal	Neutral
Interphalangeal	Slight flexion

joints are depicted in Table 1-12. Movements toward the close-packed position of a joint involve an element of compression, whereas movements out of this position involve an element of distraction.

Hypomobility, Hypermobility, and Instability

If a joint moves less than what is considered normal, or when compared to the same joint on the opposite extremity, it may be deemed *hypomobile*. A joint that moves more than considered normal when compared to the same joint on the opposite extremity may be deemed *hypermobile*. Hypermobility may occur as a generalized phenomenon or be localized to just one direction of movement.

The term *stability*, specifically related to the joint, has been the subject of much research.[103–118] In contrast to a hypermobile joint, an unstable joint involves a disruption of the osseous and ligamentous structures of that joint, and results in a loss of function. Joint stability may be viewed as a factor of joint integrity, elastic energy, passive stiffness, and muscle activation:

- Joint integrity. Joint integrity is enhanced in those ball-and-socket joints with deeper sockets, or steeper sides as opposed to those with planar sockets and shallower sides. Joint integrity is also dependent on the attributes of the supporting structures around the joint, and the extent of joint disease.

- Elastic energy. CTs are elastic structures and as such, are capable of storing elastic energy when stretched. This stored elastic energy may then be used to help return the joint to its original position when the stresses are removed.

- Passive stiffness. Individual joints have passive stiffness that increases toward the joint end range. An injury to these passive structures causing inherent loss in the passive stiffness, results in joint laxity.[119]

- Muscle activation. Muscle activation increases stiffness, both within the muscle and within the joint(s) it crosses.[120] However, the synergists and antagonist muscles that cross the joint must be activated with the correct and appropriate activation in terms of magnitude or timing. A faulty motor control system can lead to inappropriate magnitudes of muscle force and stiffness, allowing for a joint to buckle or undergo shear translation.[120]

Pathological breakdown of the above factors may result in *instability*. Two types of instability are recognized: articular and ligamentous. Articular instability can lead to abnormal patterns of coupled and translational movements.[121] Ligamentous instability may lead to multiple planes of aberrant joint motion.[122]

REFERENCES

1. Hall SJ. The biomechanics of human skeletal muscle. In: Hall SJ, ed. *Basic Biomechanics*. New York, NY: McGraw-Hill; 1999:146–185.
2. Jones D, Round D. *Skeletal Muscle in Health and Disease*. Manchester, UK: Manchester University Press; 1990.

3. Armstrong RB, Warren GL, Warren JA. Mechanisms of exercise-induced muscle fibre injury. *Med Sci Sports Exerc.* 1990;24:436–443.
4. Van de Graaff KM, Fox SI. Muscle tissue and muscle physiology. In: Van de Graaff KM, Fox SI, eds. *Concepts of Human Anatomy and Physiology.* New York, NY: WCB/McGraw-Hill; 1999:280–305.
5. Williams JH, Klug GA. Calcium exchange hypothesis of skeletal muscle fatigue. A brief review. *Muscle Nerve* 1995;18:421.
6. MacConnail MA, Basmajian JV. *Muscles and Movements: A Basis for Human kinesiology.* New York, NY: Robert Krieger; 1977.
7. Lakomy HKA. The biomechanics of human movement. In Maughan RJ, ed. *Basic and Applied Sciences for Sports Medicine.* Woburn, MA: Butterworth-Heinemann; 1999:124–125.
8. Luttgens K, Hamilton K. The musculoskeletal system: the musculature. In: Luttgens K, Hamilton K, eds. *Kinesiology: Scientific Basis of Human Motion.* 9th ed. Dubuque, IA: McGraw-Hill; 1997:49–75.
9. Astrand PO, Rodahl K. *The Muscle and Its Contraction: Textbook of Work Physiology.* New York, NY: McGraw-Hill; 1986.
10. Komi PV. *Strength and Power in Sport.* London, UK: Blackwell Scientific; 1992.
11. McArdle WD, Katch FI, Katch VL. *Exercise Physiology: Energy, Nutrition, and Human Performance.* Philadelphia, PA: Lea and Febiger; 1991.
12. Elftman H. Biomechanics of muscle. *J Bone Joint Surg.* 1966; 48A:363.
13. Worrell TW, Perrin DH, Gansneder B, et al. Comparison of isokinetic strength and flexibility measures between hamstring injured and non-injured athletes. *J Orthop Sports Phys Ther.* 1991;13:118–125.
14. Anderson MA, Gieck JH, Perrin D, et al. The relationship among isokinetic, isotonic, and isokinetic concentric and eccentric quadriceps and hamstrings force and three components of athletic performance. *J Orthop Sports Phys Ther.* 1991;14:114–120.
15. Steadman JR, Forster RS, Silfverskold JP. Rehabilitation of the knee. *Clin Sports Med.* 1989;8:605–627.
16. Montgomery JB, Steadman JR. Rehabilitation of the injured knee. *Clin Sports Med.* 1985;4:333–343.
17. Delsman PA, Losee GM. Isokinetic shear forces and their effect on the quadriceps active drawer. *Med Sci Sports Exerc.* 1984;16:151.
18. Albert MS. Principles of exercise progression. In: Greenfield B, ed. *Rehabilitation of the Knee: A Problem Solving Approach.* Philadelphia, PA: FA Davis; 1993.
19. Deudsinger RH. Biomechanics in clinical practice. *Phys Ther.* 1984; 64: 1860–1868.
20. Cyriax J. *Textbook of Orthopaedic Medicine, Diagnosis of Soft Tissue Lesions.* 8th ed. London, UK: Bailliere Tindall; 1982.
21. Desmendt JE, Godaux E. Fast motor units are not preferentially activated in rapid voluntary contractions in man. *Nature.* 1977;267:717.
22. Gans C. Fiber architecture and muscle function. *Exerc Sport Sci Rev.* 1982; 10:160.
23. Nilsson J, Tesch PA, Thorstensson A. Fatigue and EMG of repeated fast and voluntary contractions in man. *Acta Physiol Scand.* 1977;101:194.

24. Sell S, Zacher J, Lack S. Disorders of proprioception of arthrotic knee joint. *Z Rheumatol*. 1993;52:150–155.
25. Mattacola CG, Lloyd JW. Effects of a 6 week strength and proprioception training program on measures of dynamic balance: a single case design. *J Athl Training*. 1997;32:127–135.
26. Teitz CC, Garrett WE Jr, Miniaci A, et al. Tendon problems in athletic individuals. *J Bone Joint Surg*. 1997;79-A:138–152.
27. Junqueira LC, Carneciro J. Bone. In: Junqueira LC, Carneciro J, eds. *Basic Histology*. 10th ed. New York: McGraw-Hill; 2003:141–159.
28. Freeman MAR, Wyke BD. An experimental study of articular neurology. *J Bone Joint Surg*. 1967;49B:185–192.
29. Wyke BD. The neurology of joints. *Ann R Coll Surg Engl*. 1967;41:25–50.
30. Chusid JG. *Correlative Neuroanatomy & Functional Neurology*. 19th ed. Norwalk, CT: Appleton-Century-Crofts; 1985:144–148.
31. Wyke BD. The neurology of joints: a review of general principles. *Clin Rheum Dis*. 1981;7:223–239.
32. McCloskey DI. Kinesthetic sensibility. *Physiol Rev*. 1978;58:763–820.
33. Borsa PA, Lephart SM, Kocher MS, et al. Functional assessment and rehabilitation of shoulder proprioception for glenohumeral instability. *J Sport Rehabil*. 1994;3:84–104
34. Lephart SM, Warner JJP, Borsa PA, et al. Proprioception of the shoulder joint in healthy, unstable and surgically repaired shoulders. *J Shoulder Elbow Surg*. 1994;3:371–380.
35. Zarins B. Soft tissue injury and repair: biomechanical aspects. *Int J Sports Med*. 1982;3:9–11.
36. Prentice WE. Understanding and managing the healing process. In Prentice WE, Voight ML, eds. *Techniques in Musculoskeletal Rehabilitation*. New York: McGraw-Hill; 2001:17–41.
37. Sen CK, Khanna S, Gordillo G, et al. Oxygen, oxidants, and antioxidants in wound healing: an emerging paradigm. *Ann N Y Acad Sci*. 2002;957:239–249.
38. Kellett J. Acute soft tissue injuries: a review of the literature. *Med Sci Sports Exerc*. 1986;18(5):489–500.
39. Amadio PC. Tendon and ligament. In: Cohen IK, Diegelman RF, Lindblad WJ, eds. *Wound Healing: Biomechanical and Clinical Aspects*. Philadelphia, PA: WB Saunders; 1992:384–395.
40. Hunt TK. *Wound Healing and Wound Infection: Theory and Surgical Practice*. New York: Appleton-Century-Crofts; 1980.
41. Peacock EE. *Wound Repair*. 3rd ed. Philadelphia, PA: WB Saunders; 1984.
42. Ross R. The fibroblast and wound repair. *Biol Rev*. 1968;43:51–96.
43. Wong MEK, Hollinger JO, Pinero GJ. Integrated processes responsible for soft tissue healing. *Oral Surg Oral Med Oral Pathol Oral Radiol Endod*. 1996;82:475–492.
44. McAllister BS, Leeb-Lunberg LM, Javors MA, et al. Bradykinin receptors and signal transduction pathways in human fibroblasts: integral role for extracellular calcium. *Arch Biochem Biophys*. 1993;304:294–301.
45. Evans RB. Clinical application of controlled stress to the healing extensor tendon: a review of 112 cases. *Phys Ther*. 1989;69:1041–1049.

46. Emwemeka CS. Inflammation, cellularity, and fibrillogenesis in regenerating tendon: implications for tendon rehabilitation. *Phys Ther.* 1989;69: 816–825.
47. Safran MR, Zachazewski JE, Benedetti RS, et al. Lateral ankle sprains: a comprehensive review part 2: treatment and rehabilitation with an emphasis on the athlete. *Med Sci Sports Exerc.* 1999;31:S438-S447.
48. Safran MR, Benedetti RS, Bartolozzi AR III, et al. Lateral ankle sprains: a comprehensive review: part 1: etiology, pathoanatomy, histopathogenesis, and diagnosis. *Med Sci Sports Exerc.* 1999;31:S429-S437.
49. Oakes BW. Acute soft tissue injuries: nature and management. *Aust Fam Physician.* 1982;10:3–16.
50. Van der Mueulin JHC. Present state of knowledge on processes of healing in collagen structures. *Int J Sports Med.* 1982;3:4–8.
51. Clayton ML, Wier GJ. Experimental investigations of ligamentous healing. *Am J Surg.* 1959;98:373–378.
52. Mason ML, Allen HS. The rate of healing of tendons. An experimental study of tensile strength. *Ann Surg.* 1941;113:424–459.
53. Singer AJ, Clark RAF. Cutaneous wound healing. *N Engl J Med.* 1999;341: 738–746.
54. Farfan HF. The scientific basis of manipulative procedures. *Clin Rheum Dis.* 1980;6:159–177.
55. Orgill D, Demling RH. Current concepts and approaches to wound healing. *Crit Care Med.* 1988;16:899–908.
56. Kasemkijwattana C, Menetrey J, Bosch P, et al. Use of growth factors to improve muscle healing after strain injury. *Clin Orthop Related Res.* 2000;370: 272–285.
57. Kalimo H, Rantanen J, Jarvinen M. Soft tissue injuries in sport. In: Jarvinen M, ed. *Balliere's Clinical Orthopaedics.* WB Saunders; 1997:1–24.
58. Hurme T, Kalimo H, Lehto M, et al. Healing of skeletal muscle injury: an ultrastructural and immunohistochemical study. *Med Sci Sports Exerc.* 1991;23:801–810.
59. Lehto M, Duance VJ, Restall D. Collagen and fibronectin in a healing skeletal muscle injury: an immunohistochemical study of the effects of physical activity on the repair of the injured gastrocnemius muscle in the rat. *J Bone Joint Surg.* 1985;67-B:820–828.
60. Kasper CE, Talbot LA, Gaines JM. Skeletal muscle damage and recovery. *AACN Clinical Issues.* 2002;13:237–247.
61. Byrnes WC, Clarkson PM, White JS, et al. Delayed onset muscle soreness following repeated bouts of downhill running. *J Appl Physiol.* 1985;59:710.
62. Nosaka K, Sakamoto K, Newton M, et al. How long does the protective effect on eccentric exercise-induced muscle damage last. *Med Sci Sports Exerc.* 2001;33:1490–1495.
63. Lynn R, Talbot JA, Morgan DL. Differences in rat skeletal muscles after incline and decline running. *J Appl Physiol.* 1998;85:98–104.
64. Nosaka K, Clarkson P. Influence of previous concentric exercise on eccentric exercise-induced muscle damage. *J Sports Sci.* 1997;15:477.
65. Frank CB, Bray RC, Hart DA, et al. Soft tissue healing. In: Fu F, Harner CD, Vince KG, eds. *Knee Surgery.* Baltimore, MD: Williams and Wilkins; 1994:189–229.

66. Murphy PG, Loitz BJ, Frank CB, et al. Influence of exogenous growth factors on the expression of plasminogen activators by explants of normal and healing rabbit ligaments. *Biochem Cell Biol.* 1993;71:522–529.

67. Pierce GF, Mustoe TA, Lingelbach J, et al. Plateletderived growth factor and transforming growth factor-[beta] enhance tissue repair activities by unique mechanisms. *J Cell Biol.* 1989;109:429–440.

68. Steenfos HH. Growth factors in wound healing. *Scand J Plast Hand Surg.* 1994;28:95–105.

69. Booher JM, Thibodeau GA. The body's response to trauma and environmental stress. In: Booher JM, Thibodeau GA, eds. *Athletic Injury Assessment.* 4th ed. New York: McGraw-Hill; 2000:55–76.

70. Frank G, Woo SL-Y, Amiel D, et al. Medial collateral ligament healing. A multi-disciplinary assessment in rabbits. *Am J Sports Med.* 1983;11:379.

71. Balduini FC, Vegso JJ, Torg JS, et al. Management and rehabilitation of ligamentous injuries to the ankle. *Sports Med.* 1987;4:364–380.

72. Gould N, Selingson D, Gassman J. Early and late repair of lateral ligaments of the ankle. *Foot Ankle.* 1980;1:84–89.

73. Vailas AC, Tipton CM, Mathes RD, et al. Physical activity and its influence on the repair process of medial collateral ligaments. *Connect Tissue Res.* 1981;9:25–31.

74. Tipton CM, Matthes RD, Maynard JA, et al. The influence of physical activity on ligaments and tendons. *Med Sci Sports Exerc.* 1975;7:165–175.

75. Tipton CM, James SL, Mergner W, et al. Influence of exercise in strength of medial collateral knee ligaments of dogs. *Am. J. Physiol.* 1970;218:894–902.

76. Laban MM. Collagen tissue: implications of its response to stress in vitro. *Arch Phys Med Rehab.* 1962;43:461–466.

77. McGaw WT. The effect of tension on collagen remodelling by fibroblasts: a stereological ultrastructural study. *Connect Tissue Res.* 1986;14:229–235.

78. Wakitani S, Goto T, Pineda SJ, et al. Mesenchymal cell-based repair of large, full-thickness defects of articular cartilage. *J Bone Joint Surg.* 1994;76A:579–592.

79. Fuller JA, Ghadially FN. Ultrastructural observations on surgically produced partial-thickness defects in articular cartilage. *Clin Orthop.* 1972;86:193–205.

80. Ghadially FN, Thomas I, Oryschak AF, et al. Long-term results of superficial defects in articular cartilage: a scanning electron-microscope study. *J Pathol.* 1977;121:213–217.

81. Convery FR, Akeson WH, Keown GH. The repair of large osteochondral defects. An experimental study in horses. *Clin Orthop.* 1972;82:253–262.

82. Coletti JM Jr, Akeson WH, Woo SL-Y. A comparison of the physical behavior of normal articular cartilage and the arthroplasty surface. *J Bone Joint Surg.* 1972;54-A:147–160.

83. Furukawa T, Eyre DR, Koide S, et al. Biochemical studies on repair cartilage resurfacing experimental defects in the rabbit knee. *J Bone Joint Surg.* 1980;62-A:79–89.

84. Chu CR, Convery FR, Akeson WH, et al. Articular cartilage transplantation. Clinical results in the knee. *Clin Orthop Relat Res.* 1999;360:159–168.

85. Perka C, Sittinger M, Schultz O, et al. Tissue engineered cartilage repair using cryopreserved and noncryopreserved chondrocytes. *Clin Orthop Relat Res.* 2000;378:245–254.

86. Brittberg M, Winalski CS. Evaluation of cartilage injuries and repair. *J Bone Joint Surg Am*. 2003;85-A(suppl 2):58–69.
87. Monteleone GP. Stress fractures in the athlete. *Orthop Clin North Am*. 1995;26:423–432.
88. Hockenbury RT. Forefoot problems in athletes. *Med Sci Sports Exerc*. 1999;31:S448–S458.
89. Marsh DR, Li G. The biology of fracture healing: optimising outcome. *Br Med Bull*. 1999;55:856–869.
90. Muller ME. Internal fixation for fresh fractures and nonunion. *Proc R Soc Med*. 1963;56:455–460.
91. McKibbin B. The biology of fracture healing in long bones. *J Bone Joint Surg* 1978;60B:150–161.
92. Sarmiento A, Mullis DL, Latta LL, et al. A quantitative comparative analysis of fracture healing under the influence of compression plating vs. closed weight-bearing treatment. *Clin Orthop*. 1980;149:232–239.
93. Bailey DA, Faulkner RA, McKay HA. Growth, physical activity, and bone mineral acquisition. In: Hollosky JO, ed. *Exercise and Sport Sciences Reviews*. Baltimore, MD: Williams and Wilkins; 1996:233–266.
94. Stone MH. Implications for connective tissue and bone alterations resulting from rest and exercise training. *Med Sci Sports Exerc*. 1988;20:S162–S168.
95. Pryde JA, Iwasaki DH. Fractures. In: Cameron MH, Monroe LG, eds. *Physical Rehabilitation. Evidence-Based Examination, Evaluation, and Intervention*. St Louis, MO: Saunders/Elsevier; 2007:194–218.
96. Wallace AL, Draper ER, Strachan RK, et al. The vascular response to fracture micromovement. *Clin Orthop*. 1994;301:281–290.
97. Marsh D. Concepts of fracture union, delayed union, and nonunion. *Clin Orthop*. 1998;355:S22-S230.
98. Hall SJ. Kinematic concepts for analyzing human motion. In: Hall SJ, ed. *Basic Biomechanics*. New York, NY: McGraw-Hill; 1999:28–89.
99. MacConaill MA. Arthrology. In: Warwick R, Williams PL, eds. *Gray's Anatomy*. 35th ed. Philadelphia, PA: WB Saunders: 1975.
100. Lehmkuhl LD, Smith LK. *Brunnstrom's Clinical Kinesiology*. Philadelphia, PA: FA Davis; 1983:361–390.
101. Rasch PJ, Burke RK. *Kinesiology and Applied Anatomy*. Philadelphia, PA: Lea and Febiger; 1971.
102. Steindler A. *Kinesiology of the Human Body under Normal and Pathological Conditions*. Springfield, IL: Charles C Thomas; 1955.
103. Answorth AA, Warner JJP. Shoulder instability in the athlete. *Orthop Clin North Am*. 1995;26:487–504.
104. Bergmark A. Stability of the lumbar spine. *Acta Orthop Scand*. 1989;60:1–54.
105. Boden BP, Pearsall AW, Garrett WE Jr, et al. Patellofemoral instability: evaluation and management. *J Am Acad Orthop Surgeons*. 1997;5:47–57.
106. Callanan M, Tzannes A, Hayes KC, et al. Shoulder instability. Diagnosis and management. *Aust Fam Physician*. 2001;30:655–661.
107. Cass JR, Morrey BF. Ankle instability: current concepts, diagnosis, and treatment. *Mayo Clinic Proc*. 1984;59:165–170.

108. Clanton TO. Instability of the subtalar joint. *Orthop Clin North Am.* 1989;20:583–592.
109. Cox JS, Cooper PS. Patellofemoral instability. In: Fu FH, Harner CD, Vince KG, eds. *Knee Surgery.* Baltimore, MD: Williams & Wilkins; 1994:959–962.
110. Freeman MAR, Dean MRE, Hanham IWF. The etiology and prevention of functional instability of the foot. *J Bone Joint Surg.* 1965;47B:678–685.
111. Friberg O. Lumbar instability: a dynamic approach by traction-compression radiography. *Spine.* 1987;12:119–129.
112. Grieve GP. Lumbar instability. *Physiotherapy.* 1982;68:2–9.
113. Hotchkiss RN, Weiland AJ. Valgus stability of the elbow. *J Orthop Res.* 1987;5:372–377.
114. Kaigle A, Holm S, Hansson T. Experimental instability in the lumbar spine. *Spine.* 1995;20:421–430.
115. Kuhlmann JN, Fahrer M, Kapandji AI, et al. Stability of the normal wrist. In: Tubiana R, ed. *The Hand.* Philadelphia, PA: WB Saunders; 1985:934–944.
116. Landeros O, Frost HM, Higgins CC. Post traumatic anterior ankle instability. *Clin Orthop.* 1968;56:169–178.
117. Luttgens K, Hamilton N. The center of gravity and stability. In: Luttgens K, Hamilton N, eds. *Kinesiology: Scientific Basis of Human Motion.* 9th ed. Dubuque, IA: McGraw-Hill; 1997:415–442.
118. Wilke H, Wolf S, Claes L, et al. Stability of the lumbar spine with different muscle groups: a biomechanical in vitro study. *Spine.* 1995;20:192–198.
119. Panjabi MM. The stabilizing system of the spine. Part 1. Function, dysfunction adaption and enhancement. *J Spinal Disord.* 1992;5:383–389.
120. McGill SM, Cholewicki J. Biomechanical basis for stability: an explanation to enhance clinical utility. *J Orthop Sports Phys Ther.* 2001;31:96–100.
121. Gertzbein SD, Seligman J, Holtby R, et al. Centrode patterns and segmental instability in degenerative disc disease. *Spine.* 1985;10:257–261.
122. Cholewicki J, McGill S. Mechanical stability of the in vivo lumbar spine: implications for injury and chronic low back pain. *Clin Biomech.* 1996;11:1–15.

QUESTIONS

1. What are the three classifications (structural) of muscle?
2. What is a strap or fusiform muscle?
3. Give a definition of a synergist muscle.
4. What is the relationship between an agonist muscle and a synergistic muscle?
5. Give one example of the unipennate muscle.
6. Give one example of a bipennate muscle.
7. Give one example of a multipennate muscle.
8. Which of the skin receptors detect texture/exact location?
9. Which of the skin receptors detect rapid movement and vibration?

10. Which of the joint receptors defined by Wyke are found in fat pads and detect changes in direction or acceleration?

11. What type of muscle fiber uses anaerobic metabolism to create energy and excel at producing quick, powerful bursts of speed?

12. What is the function of the muscle spindle?

13. What are the sensory fibers of the central position of the muscle spindle called?

14. What are the two intrafusal fibers of the muscle spindle called?

15. What are the five major functions of bone?

16. Describe some of the features/factors that make some tendons more prone to overuse injuries than others.

17. Describe the difference between tendonitis and tendinosis.

18. What is the name of the connective tissue that provides support and protection to the joint, and acts as an interconnection between tendons, aponeuroses, ligaments, capsules, nerves, and the intrinsic components of muscle?

19. Describe the anatomical reference position for the human body

20. Which plane of the body divides the body vertically into left and right halves?

21. Which axis of the body is perpendicular to the frontal plane?

22. Give one example of osteokinematic motion.

23. Give one example of an ovoid joint.

24. Give one example of a joint that has 3 degree of freedom.

25. What is the close-packed position of the ulnohumeral joint?

26. What is the open-packed position of the radiohumeral joint?

27. What are the three components of arthrokinematicsmotion at a joint?

28. T__ F__Rolling occurs when the female surface moves?

29. Osteokinematics is the study of what?

30. Arthrokinematics is the study of what?

31. Arthrokinetics is the study of what?

32. Describe the concave–convex rule as it applies to athrokinematic motions.

33. Give one example of motion that occurs through a sagittal plane about a coronal axis?

34. Give one example of a body motion that involves a pure *(cardinal/chordal)* swing.

35. Give two examples of a pure *(unmodified)* sellar joint.

36. Give two examples of a modified sellar joint.

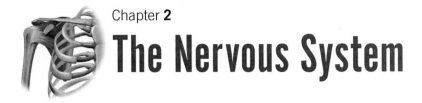

Chapter **2**

The Nervous System

OVERVIEW

Neurons, the basic cells of the nervous system, are highly specialized cells designed for the processing and transmission of electrical and chemical signals. The nervous system can be divided into two anatomical divisions, each with their own subdivisions:

- The central nervous system (CNS)
  - Brain. The brain, contained within the skull (cranium) begins its embryonic development as the cephalic end of the neural tube, before rapidly growing and differentiating into three distinct swellings: the prosencephalon, the mesencephalon, and the rhombencephalon (Table 2-1).
  - Spinal cord. The spinal cord has an external segmental organization (Figure 2-1). Each of the 31 pairs of spinal nerves that arise from the spinal cord has a ventral root and a dorsal root, with each root made up of one to eight rootlets, and each root consisting of bundles of nerve fibers.[1] In the dorsal root of a typical spinal nerve, lies a dorsal root ganglion, a swelling that contains nerve cell bodies.[1]

☉ Clinical Pearl

The spinal cord provides a conduit for the two-way transmission of messages between the brain and the body. These messages may descend, or ascend along pathways, or tracts, which are fiber bundles of similar groups of neurons, each with specific functions (Boxes 2-1 to 2-3). The central gray matter of the spinal cord, which roughly resembles the letter H, contains two anterior (ventral) and two posterior (dorsal) horns united by gray commissure within the central canal.

- Anterior horns: contain cell bodies that give rise to motor (efferent) neurons.

- Gamma motor neurons to muscle spindles (refer to Chapter 1)
- Alpha motor neurons to efferent muscles.
- Posterior horns: contain sensory (afferent) neurons located in the dorsal root ganglia.[1]

⬤ Clinical Pearl

Three membranes, or meninges, envelop the structures of the CNS: the dura, the arachnoid, and the pia. The meninges, and related spaces, are important to both the nutrition and the protection of the spinal cord. The cerebrospinal fluid that flows through the meningeal spaces, and within the ventricles of the brain, provides a cushion for the spinal cord. The meninges also form barriers that resist the entrance of a variety of noxious organisms.

Table 2-1 Derivation and Functions of the Major Brain Structures

	Region	Structure	Function
Prosencephalon (forebrain)	Telencephalon	Cerebrum	Control of most sensory and motor activities; reasoning, memory, intelligence, etc.; instinctual and limbic functions.
	Diencephalon	Thalamus	Relay center; all impulses (except olfactory) going into the cerebrum synapse here; some sensory interpretation; initial autonomic response to pain.
		Hypothalamus	Regulation of food and water intake, body temperature, heartbeat, etc.; control of secretory activity in the anterior pituitary; instinctual and limbic functions.
		Pituitary gland	Regulation of other endocrine glands.
Mesencephalon (midbrain)	Mesencephalon	Superior colliculi	Visual reflexes (hand-eye coordination).
		Inferior colliculi	Auditory reflexes.
		Cerebral peduncles	Reflex coordination; contain many motor fibers.

(continued on following page)

	Region	Structure	Function
Rhombencephalon (hindbrain)	Metencephalon	Cerebellum	Balance and motor coordination.
		Pons	Relay center; contains nuclei (pontine nuclei).
	Myelencephalon	Medulla oblongata	Relay center; contains many nuclei; visceral autonomic center (e.g., respiration, heart rate, vasoconstriction)

- Peripheral nervous system (PNS)
  - Cranial nerves (CN; with the exception of the second CN). The brain stem is literally the stalk of the brain. The brain stem gives rise to 10 of the 12 pairs of CNs.
  - The spinal nerve roots.
  - The dorsal root ganglia (or spinal ganglia).
  - The peripheral nerve trunks and their terminal branches.
  - The peripheral autonomic nervous system.

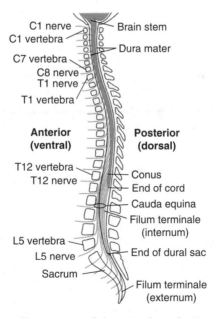

Figure 2-1 Schematic illustration of the spinal cord. (Reproduced with permission from Waxman SG. *Correlative Neuroanatomy.* 24th ed. New York, NY: McGraw-Hill; 2000:70.)

Box 2-1 The Dorsal Medial Lemniscus Tract

The Dorsal Medial Lemniscus Tract:

• Conveys impulses concerned with well-localized touch and with the sense of movement and position (kinesthesis)

• Important in moment-to-moment (temporal) and point-to-point (spatial) discrimination.

• Make it possible for you to put a key in a door lock without light or visualize the position of any part of your body without looking.

• Lesions to the tract from destructive tumors, hemorrhage, scar tissue, swelling, infections, direct trauma, and the like abolish or diminish tactile sensations and movement or position sense.

• The cell bodies of the primary neurons in the dorsal column pathway are in the spinal ganglion. The peripheral processes of these neurons begin at receptors in the joint capsule, muscles, and skin (tactile and pressure receptors).

Box 2-2 The Spinothalamic Tract

Spinothalamic Tract

The spinothalamic tract helps mediate the sensations of pain, cold, warmth, and touch from receptors throughout the body (except the face) to the brain.

• Laterally projecting spinothalamic neurons are more likely to be situated in laminae I and V.

• Medially projecting cells are more likely to be situated in the deep dorsal horn and in the ventral horn.

Most of the cells project to the contralateral thalamus, although a small fraction projects ipsilaterally.

Spinothalamic axons in the anterior-lateral quadrant of the spinal cord are arranged somatotopically—at cervical levels, spinothalamic axons representing the lower extremity and caudal body are placed more laterally, and those representing the upper extremity and anterior body, more anterior-medially.

(continued on following page)

Most of the neurons show their best responses when the skin is stimulated mechanically at a noxious intensity. However, many spinothalamic tract cells also respond, although less effectively, to innocuous mechanical stimuli, and some respond best to innocuous mechanical stimuli.

A large fraction of spinothalamic tract cells also respond to a noxious heating of the skin, whereas others respond to stimulation of the receptors in muscle, joints, or viscera.

Spinothalamic tract cells can be inhibited effectively by repetitive electrical stimulation of peripheral nerves, with the inhibition outlasting the stimulation by 20 to 30 minutes.

Some inhibition can be evoked by stimulation of the large myelinated axons of a peripheral nerve, but the inhibition is much more powerful if small myelinated, or unmyelinated afferents, are included in the volleys. The best inhibition is produced by stimulation of a peripheral nerve in the same limb as the excitatory receptive field, but some inhibition occurs when nerves in other limbs are stimulated. A similar inhibition results when high-intensity stimuli are applied to the skin with a clinical transcutaneous electrical nerve stimulator (TENS unit) in place of direct stimulation of a peripheral nerve. As the spinothalamic tract ascends, it migrates from a lateral position to a posterior-lateral position. In the midbrain, the tract lies adjacent to the medial lemniscus. The axons of the secondary neurons terminate in one of a number of centers in the thalamus.

Box 2-3 The Spinocerebellar Tract

The Spinocerebellar Tract

- Conducts impulses related to the position and movement of muscles to the cerebellum, enabling the cerebellum to add smoothness and precision to patterns of movement initiated in the cerebral hemispheres.

- Spinocerebellar impulses do not reach the cerebrum directly and therefore have no conscious representation.

(continued on following page)

Box 2-3 (*continued*)

- Four tracts constitute the spinocerebellar pathway: posterior spinocerebellar and cuneocerebellar, and anterior and rostral spinocerebellar tracts. The posterior spinocerebellar tract conveys muscle spindle- or tendon organ-related impulses from the lower half of the body (below the level of the T6 spinal cord segment). The cuneocerebellar tract is concerned with such impulses from the body above T6.

- The axons conducting impulses from muscle spindles, tendon organs, and skin in the lower half of the body are large type Ia, Ib, and type II fibers, the cell bodies of which are in the spinal ganglia of spinal nerves T6 and below.

- Primary neurons below L3 send their central processes into the posterior columns. These processes then ascend in the columns to the L3 level. From L3 up to T6, incoming central processes and those in the posterior columns project to the medial part of lamina VII, called Clarke column. Here the central processes of the primary neurons synapse with secondary neurons, the axons of which are directed to the lateral funiculi as the posterior spinocerebellar tracts.

Clinical Pearl

The somatic divisions of the PNS consist of the CNs and the spinal nerves.

Clinical Pearl

Clinical signs and symptoms that may be associated with spinal cord compression include the following:

- Segmental deficits—paraparesis or quadriparesis
- Hyperreflexia
- Extensor plantar response and other pathological reflexes

- Ataxia
- Spasticity
- Loss of sphincter tone (with bowel and bladder dysfunction)
- Sensory deficits

Subacute or chronic spinal cord compression may begin with local back pain, often radiating down the distribution of a nerve root (radicular pain), and sometimes hyperreflexia and loss of sensation. Sensory loss may begin in the sacral segments.

Somatic Division of the Peripheral Nervous System—Cranial Nerves

The CNs are typically described as comprising 12 pairs, which are referred to by the Roman numerals I through XII (Table 2-2). The CN roots enter and exit the brain stem to provide sensory and motor innervation to the head and muscles of the face. CN I (olfactory) and II (optic) are not true nerves but are fiber tracts of the brain. CN testing is described in Chapter 3.

Somatic Division of the Peripheral Nervous System—Spinal Nerves

A total of 31 symmetrically arranged pairs of spinal nerves, exit from all levels of the vertebral column, except for those of C1 and C2,[2] each derived from the spinal cord. The spinal nerves are divided topographically into eight cervical pairs (C1–8), 12 thoracic pairs (T1–12), 5 lumbar pairs (L1–5), 5 sacral pairs (S1–5), and a coccygeal pair (Figure 2-1). Nerve fibers can be categorized according to function: sensory, motor, or mixed (Table 2-3).

 Clinical Pearl

The dorsal and ventral roots of the spinal nerves are located within the vertebral canal. Nerve roots do not have an epineurium and are therefore more susceptible to injury. The portion of the spinal nerve that is not within the vertebral canal, and which usually occupies the intervertebral foramen, is referred to as a peripheral nerve. A dorsal root ganglion is a nodule on a dorsal root that contains cell bodies of neurons in afferent spinal nerves. Dorsal root axons separate into a medial division of large diameter axons and a lateral division of small diameter axons (Table 2-4).

Table 2-2 Cranial Nerves and Their Function

Cranial Nerve	Function
I—Olfactory	The olfactory nerve is responsible for the sense of smell.
II—Optic	The optic nerve is responsible for vision.
III—Oculomotor	The somatic portion of the oculomotor nerve supplies the levator palpabrae superioris muscle, the superior, medial and inferior rectus muscles, and the inferior oblique muscles. These muscles are responsible for some eye movements. The visceral efferent portion of this nerve innervates two smooth intraocular muscles: the ciliary and the constrictor pupillae. These muscles are responsible for papillary constriction.
IV—Trochlear	The trochlear nerve supplies the superior oblique muscle.
V—Trigeminal	All three of these branches contain sensory cells. The ophthalmic and maxillary are exclusively sensory, the latter supplying the soft and hard palate, maxillary sinuses, upper teeth and upper lip, and the mucous membrane of the pharynx. The mandibular branch carries sensory information but also represents the motor component of the nerve, supplying the muscles of mastication, both pterygoids, the anterior belly of digastric, tensor tympani, tensor veli palatine, and mylohyoid.
VI—Abducens	The abducens nerve innervates the lateral rectus muscle.
VII—Facial	The facial nerve is comprised of a sensory (intermediate) root, which conveys taste, and a motor root, the facial nerve proper, which supplies the muscles of facial expression, the platysma muscle, and the stapedius muscle of the inner ear.
VIII—Vestibulocochlear	The cochlear portion is concerned with the sense of hearing. The vestibular portion is part of the system of equilibrium, the vestibular system.
IX—Glossopharyngeal	The glossopharyngeal nerve serves a number of functions, including supplying taste fibers for the posterior third of the tongue.
X—Vagus	The vagus nerve contains somatic motor, visceral efferent, visceral sensory, and somatic sensory fibers. The functions of the vagus nerve are numerous.
XI—Accessory	The cranial root is often viewed as an aberrant portion of the vagus nerve. The spinal portion of the nerve supplies the sternocleidomastoid and the trapezius muscles.
XII – Hypoglossal	The hypoglossal nerve is the motor nerve of the tongue, innervating the ipsilateral side of the tongue, as well as forming the descendens hypoglossi, which anastomosis with other cervical branches to form the ansa hypoglossi, which in turn innervates the infrahyoid muscles

Table 2-3 Nerve Fiber Types and Their Function

Nerve Fiber Type	Function	Example
Sensory	Carry afferents from a portion of the skin. Carry efferents to the skin structures. This area of distribution is called a dermatome, which is a well-defined segmental portion of the skin (Figure 2-2), and generally follows the segmental distribution of the underlying muscle innervation.[1]	Lateral (femoral) cutaneous nerve of the thigh Saphenous nerve Interdigital nerves
Motor	Carry efferents to muscles, and return sensation from muscles, and associated ligamentous structures. Any nerve that innervates a muscle, also mediates the sensation from the joint upon which that muscle acts.	Ulnar nerve Suprascapular nerve Dorsal scapular nerve
Mixed	Combination of skin, sensory, and motor functions	Median nerve Ulnar nerve (at the elbow as it enters the tunnel of Guyon) Common fibular (peroneal) nerve Ilioinguinal nerve

Spinal nerves and peripheral nerves can be injured anywhere along their distribution, although some sites are more commonly injured than others.

Table 2-4 Division of Posterior (Dorsal) Root Axons

	Description	Function
Medial division (posterior/dorsal column system)	Large myelinated axons. These axons enter the lateral and medial aspect of the dorsal columns and terminate in the nucleus proprius	Mediate tactile sense and proprioception
Lateral division (anterolateral system)	Small, unmyelinated axons. These axons enter the cord more laterally than the medial division into the zone of Lissauer, ascend or descend one or two segments and terminate in the dorsal horn. There are two types of dorsal root processes in the lateral division: Delta and C fiber	Mediate pain and temperature Delta fiber: conveys information regarding the sense of cooling, crude touch and fast pain C fibers carry information regarding the sense of warming and slow pain

Clinical Pearl

Neurons are incapable of dividing and migrating; therefore, regeneration occurs only through existing neurons.

Compression and/or irritation of cervical or lumbar nerve roots can cause radiculopathy, a common cause of symptoms. Peripheral nerve injuries can occur at the level of the axon (i.e., axonopathy), the motor neuron or dorsal root ganglion (i.e., neuronopathies).

 Clinical Pearl

Nerve injuries can be classified using the Seddon or Sunderland classification system[3]:

Seddon

Neurapraxia—compression damage of the myelin with temporary disruption of axonal flow (as long as the compression exists).

Axonotmesis—disruption of the axon of the nerve with sparing of the connective tissue sheath, the latter of which allows for quicker nerve regrowth.

Neurotmesis—involves the complete disruption of the nerve, resulting in much slower recovery and regrowth.

Sunderland

Type 1—compression damage of the myelin.

Type 2—disruption of the axon with sparing of the nervous connective tissue (epineurium, perineurium, and endoneurium).

Type 3—disruption of the axon and endoneurium only.

Type 4—disruption of the axon, endoneurium, and perineurium only.

Type 5—complete disruption of the nerve.

Because motor and sensory axons run in the same nerves, disorders of the peripheral nerves (neuropathies) usually affect both motor and sensory functions (Table 2-5). Peripheral symptoms can manifest as abnormal, frequently unpleasant sensations, which are variously described by the patient as numbness, pins and needles and tingling, but more correctly termed *paresthesias* (Table 2-6).[4] Paresthesias can occur anywhere within a dermatomal distribution, or within a peripheral nerve distribution (Figure 2-2). CNS causes of paresthesia include ischemia, obstruction, compression, infection, inflammation, and degenerative conditions. Correct diagnosis of the source of the paresthesias can be elicited by a thorough history and physical examination. Reflex sympathetic dystrophy is an unusual cause of paresthesias, pain, and autonomic dysfunction, occurring after minor soft tissue injuries or fractures and usually affecting the distal extremities.[5]

 Clinical Pearl

Paresthesias that persist are likely to be associated with a serious medical problem and may require appropriate laboratory, radiographic, and special studies to confirm the diagnosis. Electromyography and nerve conduction studies are often the most useful initial laboratory studies.[6] Causalgia is an intense, burning type of paresthesia caused by trauma to a nerve (e.g., the median, ulnar, posterior tibial or fibular nerves). Myelinopathies occur at the level of the myelin sheath and can be inflammatory or hereditary.[6]

 Clinical Pearl

Peripheral neuropathies can be caused by entrapment syndromes, trauma, diabetes, hypothyroidism, vitamin B_{12} deficiency, alcoholism, inflammatory conditions, connective tissue disorders, toxic injury, hereditary conditions, malignancy, infections, and miscellaneous causes.[5]

 Clinical Pearl

The L4–S2 nerve root levels are all assessed with a straight leg raise.

Table 2-5 Signs and Symptoms of a Mixed Peripheral Nerve (LMN) Lesion

Motor	Sensory	Muscle Stretch Reflex
Lower motor neuron paresis or paralysis. Atrophy of specific muscle groups. The muscle or muscle groups involved may become flaccid (hypotonic) with decreased resistance to passive motion.	All modalities of cutaneous sensibility are lost, or become abnormal, only over the area exclusively supplied by the nerve (the autonomous zone). This zone is surrounded by an intermediate zone, which is the area of the nerve's territory overlapped by the sensory supply areas of the adjacent nerves.	As a consequence of sensorimotor loss, the muscle stretch reflex served by each damaged nerve is decreased or absent.

 Clinical Pearl

Calcium, potassium, and sodium are very important in the transmission of nerve impulses.

Table 2-6 Location and Probable Causes of Paresthesia

Paresthesia Location	Probable Cause
Lip (perioral)	Vertebral artery occlusion
Bilateral lower or bilateral upper extremities	Central protrusion of disc impinging on the spine
All extremities simultaneously	Spinal cord compression
One half of the body	Cerebral hemisphere
Segmental (in a dermatomal pattern)	Disc/nerve root
Glove/stocking distribution	Diabetes mellitus neuropathy, lead/mercury poisoning
Half of face and opposite half of body	Brainstem impairment

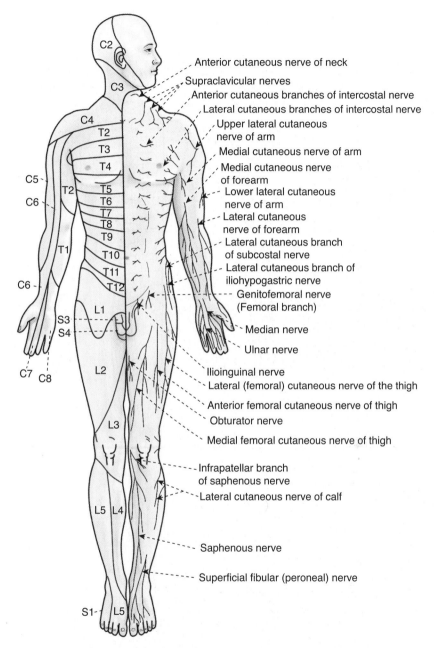

Figure 2-2 Segmental distribution of the body. (Reproduced with permission from Wilkins RH, Rengachary SS, eds. *Neurosurgery.* New York, NY: McGraw-Hill, 1996: 152–153.)

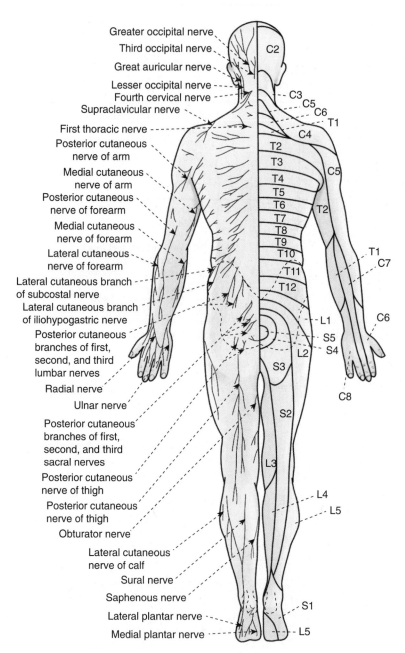

Figure 2-2 (*Continued*)

The Cervical Nerves

The eight pairs of cervical nerves are derived from cord segments between the level of the foramen magnum and the middle of the seventh cervical vertebra.[7]

Posterior Primary Divisions

The C1 (suboccipital) nerve serves the muscles of the suboccipital triangle, with very few sensory fibers.[7]

Anterior Primary Divisions

The anterior primary divisions of the first four cervical nerves (C1–4) form the cervical plexus.

The Cervical Plexus (C1–4)

- Sensory branches (Table 2-7).

- Communicating branches.

- Muscular branches (Figure 2-3). There is a branch to the sterno-cleidomastoid muscle from C2, and branches to the trapezius muscles (C3–4) via the subtrapezial plexus. Smaller branches to the adjacent vertebral musculature supply the rectus capitis lateralis and rectus capitis anterior (C1), the longus capitis (C2, 4) and longus coli (C1–4), the scalenus medius (C3, 4) and scalenus anterior (C4), and the levator scapulae (C3–5).

Table 2-7 Sensory Branches of the Cervical Plexus

Nerve	Supply
The small occipital nerve (C2, 3)	The skin of the lateral occipital portion of the scalp, the upper median part of the auricle, and the area over the mastoid process
The great auricular nerve (C2, 3)	Sensation to the ear and face over the ascending ramus of the mandible
The cervical cutaneous nerve (cutaneous coli) (C2, 3)	Supplies the skin over the anterior portion of the neck
Supraclavicular branches (C3, 4)	Supply the skin over the clavicle and the upper deltoid and pectoral regions, as low as the third rib

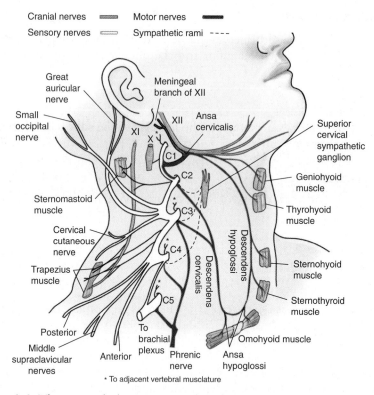

Cranial nerves ━━━━   Motor nerves ━━━
Sensory nerves ⊂⊃   Sympathetic rami - - - -

Figure 2-3 The cervical plexus. (Reproduced with permission from Waxman SG. *Correlative Neuroanatomy*. 24th ed. New York, NY: McGraw-Hill; 2000:357.)

● Clinical Pearl

The phrenic nerve (C3–5) consists of motor and sensory branches.[7] The motor branches supply the diaphragm. Sensory branches supply the pericardium, the diaphragm, and part of the costal and mediastinal pleurae.

The Brachial Plexus

The brachial plexus (Figure 2-4) arises from the anterior primary divisions of the fifth cervical through the first thoracic nerve roots, with occasional contributions from the fourth cervical and second thoracic roots. The roots of the plexus, which consist of C5 and C6, join to form the upper trunk, C7 becomes the middle trunk, and C8 and T1 join to form the lower trunks. Each of the trunks divides into anterior and posterior divisions, which then form cords (Figure 2-4).

 Clinical Pearl

> The anterior divisions of the upper and middle trunk form the lateral cord; the anterior division of the lower trunk forms the medial cord; and all three posterior divisions unite to form the posterior cord.

The three cords, named for their relationship to the axillary artery, split to form the main branches of the plexus. These branches give rise to the peripheral nerves: musculocutaneous (lateral cord) and axillary (Figure 2-5), median (medial and lateral cords) (Figure 2-6), and radial (posterior cord) (Figure 2-7) and ulnar (medial cord) (Figure 2-8).[8] Numerous smaller nerves arise from the roots, trunks, and cords of the plexus:

- From the roots (Table 2-8)
- From the trunks (Table 2-9)
- From the cords (Table 2-10)
- Peripheral nerves of the upper quadrant (Table 2-11).

The Thoracic Nerves

Dorsal Rami
The thoracic dorsal rami travel posteriorly, close to the vertebral zygapophyseal joints, before dividing into medial and lateral branches (Table 2-12).

 Clinical Pearl

> The recurrent meningeal or sinuvertebral nerve, a branch of the spinal nerve, passes back into the vertebral canal through the intervertebral foramen. This nerve supplies the anterior aspect of the dura mater, outer third of the annular fibers of the intervertebral discs, vertebral body, and the epidural blood vessel walls, as well as the posterior longitudinal ligament.[9]

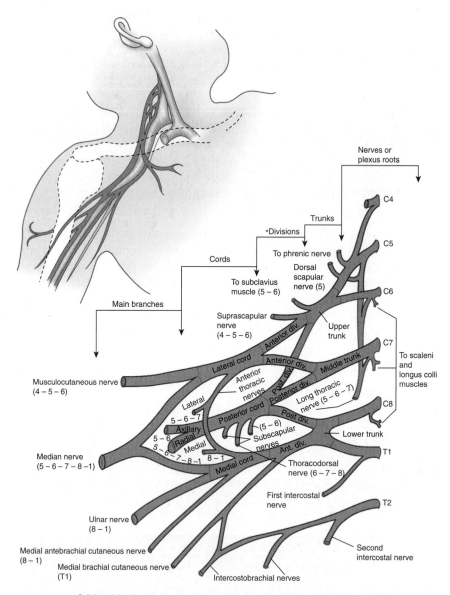

Nerves or
plexus roots

C4

Trunks

*Divisions   C5

To phrenic nerve

Cords   Dorsal
                               scapular   C6
              To subclavius   nerve (5)
              muscle (5 – 6)

Main branches

                  Suprascapular
                  nerve
                  (4 – 5 – 6)   Upper   C7
                                       trunk

                         Anterior div.
                                                              To scaleni
          Lateral cord   Anterior div.   Middle trunk   and
                                                              longus colli
Musculocutaneous nerve   Anterior   muscles
(4 – 5 – 6)   thoracic   Post. div.
                  nerves   Posterior div.
                  Lateral   Long thoracic   C8
                  5 – 6 – 7 Posterior cord nerve (5 – 6 – 7)
                  Axillary
        5 – 6   Radial   (5 – 6)
        5 – 6 – 7 – 8 –1 Medial Subscapular   Lower trunk
Median nerve   nerves   Ant. div.
(5 – 6 – 7 – 8 –1)   8 – 1 Medial cord   T1
                                   Thoracodorsal
                                   nerve (6 – 7 – 8)

                         First intercostal
                         nerve   T2

Ulnar nerve
(8 – 1)

Medial antebrachial cutaneous nerve   Second
(8 – 1)   intercostal nerve
         Medial brachial cutaneous nerve
         (T1)
                         Intercostobrachial nerves

* Splitting of the plexus into anterior and posterior divisions is one of the most significant features
  in the redistribution of nerve fibers, because it is here that fibers supplying the flexor and
  extensor groups of muscles of the upper extremity are separated. Similar splitting is noted
  in the lumbar and sacral plexuses for the supply of muscles of the lower extremity.

Figure 2-4 The brachial plexus. (Reproduced with permission from Waxman SG. *Correlative Neuroanatomy*. 24th ed. New York, NY: McGraw-Hill; 2000:358.)

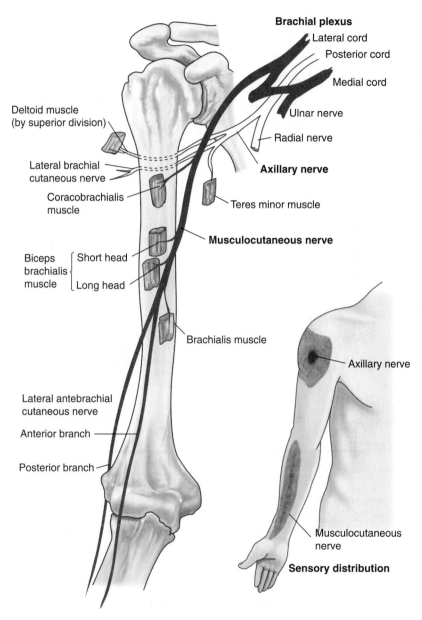

Figure 2-5 The musculocutaneous (C5–6) and axillary (C5–6) nerves. (Reproduced with permission from Waxman SG. *Correlative Neuroanatomy*. 24th ed. New York, NY: McGraw-Hill; 2000:360.)

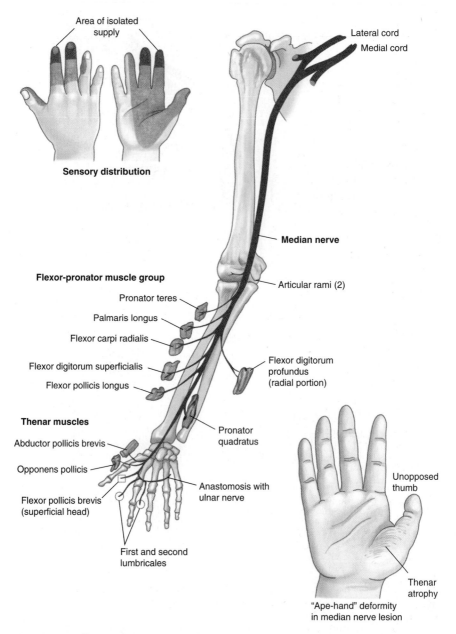

Figure 2-6 The median nerve (C6–8, T1). (Reproduced with permission from Waxman SG. *Correlative Neuroanatomy*. 24th ed. New York, NY: McGraw-Hill; 2000:362.)

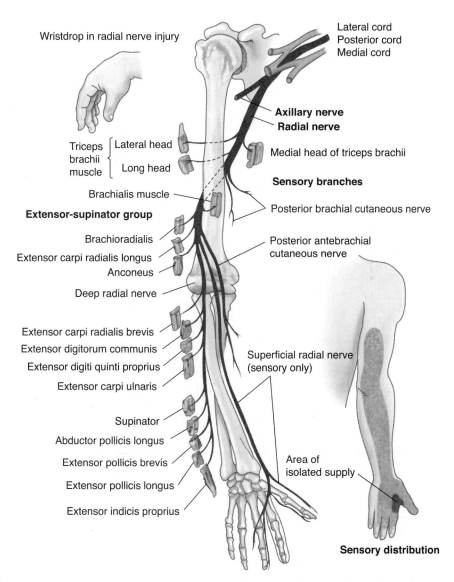

Figure 2-7 The radial nerve (C6–8, T1). (Reproduced with permission from Waxman SG. *Correlative Neuroanatomy.* 24th ed. New York, NY: McGraw-Hill; 2000:361.)

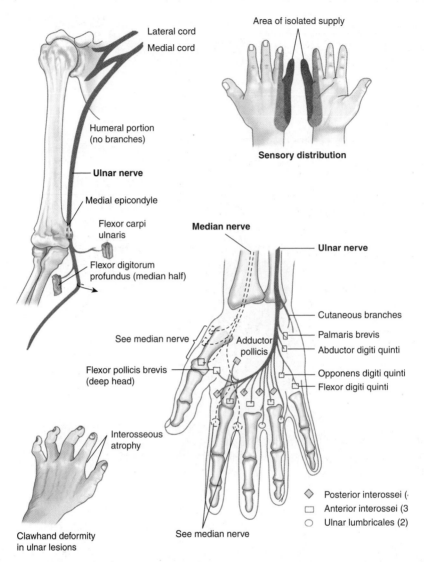

Figure 2-8 The ulnar nerve (C8, T1). (Reproduced with permission from Waxman SG. *Correlative Neuroanatomy*. 24th ed. New York: McGraw-Hill; 2000:363.)

Ventral Rami

There are 12 pairs of thoracic ventral rami, and all but the 12th are located between the ribs serving as intercostal nerves. All of the intercostal nerves

Table 2-8 Nerves That Arise From the Roots of the Brachial Plexus

Nerve	Supply	Action
The dorsal scapular nerve (C5)	Rhomboids	Scapular adduction
	Levator scapulae	Scapular elevation
The long thoracic nerve (C5, C6, and C7)	Serratus anterior (sole innervation)	Scapular abduction
		Scapular upward rotation
		Scapular elevation (weak)
Phrenic nerve (C3, C4, and C5)	Diaphragm	Increases vertical dimension of the chest cavity
		Increases abdominal pressure
Smaller branches from C6, C7, and C8	Scaleni	Rib elevation
		Neck side bending
		Neck rotation
		Neck flexion
	Longus coli	Flexes and rotates the cervical spine
The first intercostal nerve (T1)	Cutaneous	Sensation to anterior chest

mainly supply the thoracic and abdominal walls with the upper two also supplying the upper limb. The thoracic ventral rami of T3–6 supply only the thoracic wall, whereas the lower five rami supply both the thoracic and abdominal walls. The subcostal nerve supplies both the abdominal wall and the gluteal skin.

Table 2-9 Nerves That Arise From the Trunk of the Brachial Plexus

Nerves	Nerve Root	Muscles	Action
Subclavius	C5 and C6	Subclavius	Depresses the clavicle
			Fixates the clavicle during shoulder movements
Suprascapular	C5 and C6	Supraspinatus	Abducts the arm and stabilizes the glenohumeral joint
		Infraspinatus	Externally rotates the arm and stabilizes the glenohumeral joint

Table 2-10 Nerves That Arise From the Cord of the Brachial Plexus

Nerves	Nerve Root	Muscles	Action
Lateral pectoral	C5, C6, and C7	Pectoralis major	Clavicular head: flexes and adducts arm Sternal head: adducts and internally rotates arm Accessory muscle of inspiration
Medial pectoral	C8 and T1	Pectoralis minor	Elevates ribs if the scapula is fixed Protracts scapula (assists the serratus anterior)
Upper subscapular	C7 and C8	Subscapularis	Internally rotates the arm Stabilizes the glenohumeral joint
Middle subscapular (thoracodorsal)	C6, C7, and C8	Latissimus dorsi	Extends, adducts, and internally rotates arm Costal attachment helps with deep inspiration and forced expiration
Lower subscapular	C5 and C6	Teres major	Internally rotates arm Adducts arm Stabilizes the glenohumeral joint
Medial antebrachial cutaneous	C8 and T1	Sensory	
Medial brachial cutaneous	C8 and T1	Sensory	

The Lumbar Plexus

The lumbar plexus (Figure 2-9) is formed from the anterior nerve roots of the second, third, and fourth lumbar nerves (in approximately 50% of cases, the plexus also receives a contribution from the last thoracic nerve) (Table 2-13). Table 2-14 outlines the peripheral nerves of the lumbar plexus.

The Sacral Plexus

The L4 and L5 nerves join medial to the sacral promontory, becoming the lumbosacral trunk. The lumbosacral trunk (L4, 5) descends into the pelvis, where it enters the formation of the sacral plexus (Table 2-15). The S1–4 nerves converge with the lumbosacral trunk in front of the piriformis muscle, forming the broad triangular band of the sacral plexus (Figure 2-10).

Table 2-11 Peripheral Nerves of the Upper Quadrant

Nerves	Nerve Root	Muscles	Action
Musculocutaneous (Figure 2-5)	C5–6	Biceps, brachialis	Flexion of elbow
		Coracobrachialis	Shoulder flexion
Lateral brachial cutaneous nerve of the arm	C5–6	Sensory	Figure 2-5
Median (Figure 2-6)	C5–T1	Flexor carpi radialis	Radial flexion of wrist
		Flexor digitorum sublimis	Flexion of middle phalanges (digiti II–V)
		Flexor digitorum profundus (lateral half)	Flexion of distal phalanges (digiti II, III)
		Pronator teres, pronator quadratus	Pronation of forearm
		Abductor pollicis brevis	Abduction of thumb
		Opponens pollicis brevis	Opposition of thumb
		Flexor pollicis longus	Flexion of distal phalanx of thumb
		Flexor pollicis brevis	Flexion of proximal phalanx of thumb
Axillary (Figure 2-5)	C5–6	Deltoid	Shoulder abduction
		Teres minor	
Radial (Figure 2-7)	C5–T1	Triceps	Extension at elbow
		Brachioradialis	Flexion of forearm
		Extensor carpi radialis/ulnaris	Extension at wrist with radial/ulnar deviation
		Supinator	Supination of forearm
		Extensor pollicis brevis	Extension of thumb (proximal)
		Extensor pollicis longus	Extension of thumb (distal)
		Extensor indicis proprius	Extension of index (proximal)
		Extensor digiti V proprius	Extension of little finger (proximal)
		Extensor digiti communis	Extension of digits (II–V, proximal)
Medial (dorsal) cutaneous (antebrachial) nerve of the forearm	C6–T1	Sensory	Figure 2-7
Lateral cutaneous (antebrachial) nerve of the forearm	C5–6	Sensory	Figure 2-5

Table 2-11 (*Continued*)

Nerves	Nerve Root	Muscles	Action
Ulnar (Figure 2-8)	C8–T1	Flexor carpi ulnaris	Ulnar flexion of wrist
		Flexor digitorum profundus (medial half)	Flexion of distal phalanges (digiti IV, V)
		Abductor digiti minimi	Abduction of digiti V
		All other intrinsics of hand	Finger abduction/adduction

 Clinical Pearl

The upper three nerves of the sacral plexus divide into two sets of branches:

• The medial branches, which are distributed to the multifidi muscles.

• The lateral branches, which become the medial cluneal nerves. The medial cluneal nerves supply the skin over the medial part of the gluteus maximus.

The lower two posterior primary divisions, with the posterior division of the coccygeal nerve, supply the skin over the coccyx.

Table 2-12 The Thoracic Posterior (Dorsal) Rami

Medial Branches	Lateral Branches
Supply the short, medially placed back muscles (the iliocostalis thoracis, spinalis thoracis, semispinalis thoracis, thoracic multifidi, rotatores thoracis, and intertransversarii muscles) and the skin of the back as far as the midscapular line. The medial branches of the upper six thoracic posterior rami pierce the rhomboids and trapezius, and reaching the skin in close proximity to the vertebral spines, which they occasionally supply.	Supply smaller branches to the sacrospinalis muscles. The lateral branches increase in size the more inferior they are. They penetrate, or pass, the longissimus thoracis to the space between it and the iliocostalis cervicis, supplying both of these muscles, as well as the levatores costarum. The 12th thoracic lateral branch sends a filament medially along the iliac crest, which then passes down to the anterior gluteal skin.

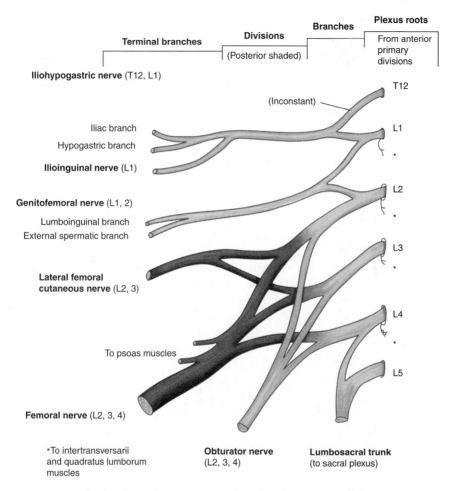

Figure 2-9 The lumbar plexus. (Reproduced with permission from Waxman SG. *Correlative Neuroanatomy*. 24th ed. New York, NY: McGraw-Hill; 2000:364.)

Collateral Branches of the Posterior Division

- Superior gluteal nerve (Table 2-15 and Figure 2-10)
- Inferior gluteal nerve (Table 2-15 and Figure 2-10)
- Superior cluneal nerve
- Posterior cutaneous (femoral) nerve

Table 2-13 Major Nerves of the Lumbosacral Plexus

Nerves	Nerve Root	Muscles	Action
Femoral	L2–4	Iliopsoas	Flexion of hip
		Quadriceps	Extension of knee
Obturator	L2–4	Adductor longus, adductor brevis, adductor magnus	Adduction of hip
Superior gluteal	L4, L5, and S1	Gluteus medius, gluteus minimus, gluteus maximus	Abduction of hip
Sciatic	L4–S3	Biceps femoris, semitendinosus, semimembranosus	Flexion of leg at knee
Sciatic branches: deep fibular	L4–S2	Tibialis anterior	Dorsiflexion of foot
		Extensor digitorum longus	Extension of toes
		Extensor hallucis longus	Extension of great toe
Sciatic branches: superficial fibular	L4–S1	Fibularis group	Eversion of foot
Sciatic branches: tibial	L4–S3	Gastrocnemius, soleus	Plantar flexion of foot
		Flexor digitorum longus	Flexion of distal phalanges (II–IV)
		Flexor hallucis longus	Flexion of distal phalanges (I)
		Flexor digitorum brevis	Flexion of middle phalanges (II–V)
		Flexor hallucis brevis	Flexion of middle phalanges (I)
Lateral cutaneous nerve of the leg	L4–S2	Sensory	
Medial plantar	L4–5		
Sural	S1–2		
Lateral plantar	S1–2		
Pudendal	S2–4	Perineal and sphincters	Closure of sphincters, contraction of pelvic floor

Collateral Branches of the Anterior Division

Collateral branches from the anterior divisions extend to the quadratus femoris and gemellus inferior muscles (from L4, 5, and S1) and to the obturator internus and gemellus superior muscles (from L5 and S1, 2) (Figure 2-10).

Table 2-14 Peripheral Nerves of the Lumbar Plexus

Nerves	Nerve Root	Muscles	Action
The iliohypogastric nerve (Figure 2-9).	T12, L1	Sensory	The lateral (iliac) branch supplies the skin of the upper lateral part of the thigh The anterior (hypogastric) branch supplies the skin over the symphysis.
The ilioinguinal nerve (Figure 2-9)	L1	Sensory	Supplies the skin of the upper medial part of the thigh and the root of the penis and scrotum or mons pubis and labium majores
The genitofemoral nerve (Figure 2-9)	L1, 2	Sensory	The genital branch supplies the cremasteric muscle and the skin of the scrotum or labia. The femoral branch supplies the skin of the middle upper part of the thigh and the femoral artery
Femoral (Figure 2-9)	L2–4	Iliopsoas	Flexion of hip
		Quadriceps	Extension of knee
Saphenous	L3–4		
Obturator (Figure 2-9)	L2–4	Adductor longus, adductor brevis, adductor magnus	Adduction of hip
Lateral cutaneous (femoral) nerve of the thigh	L2–3	Sensory	
Posterior cutaneous nerve of the thigh	L2–3	Sensory	
Anterior cutaneous (femoral) nerve of the thigh	L2–3	Sensory	

Sciatic Nerve

The sciatic nerve (Figure 2-11) is the largest nerve in the body. It arises from the L4, L5, and S1–3 nerve roots as a continuation of the lumbosacral plexus. The nerve is composed of the independent tibial (medial) (Figure 2-12) and common fibular (peroneal) (lateral) (Figure 2-13) divisions, which are usually united as a single nerve down to the lower portion of the thigh.

Table 2-15 Nerves of the Sacral Plexus

Nerves	Nerve Root	Muscles	Action
Superior gluteal (Figure 2-11)	L4, L5, and S1	Gluteus medius Gluteus minimus Tensor of the fascia latae	Abduction of hip
Inferior gluteal	L5–S2	Gluteus maximus	Extension of the hip
Sciatic (Figure 2-11)	L4–S3	Biceps femoris, semitendinosus, semimembranosus	Flexion of leg at knee
Sciatic branches: Deep fibular (peroneal) (Figure 2-11)	L4–S2	Tibialis anterior Extensor digitorum longus Extensor hallucis longus	Dorsiflexion of foot Extension of toes Extension of great toe
Sciatic branches: Superficial fibular (peroneal) (Figure 2-11)	L4–S1	Fibularis (peroneus) muscles	Eversion of foot
Sciatic branches: Tibial (Figure 2-11)	L4–S3	Gastrocnemius, soleus Flexor digitorum longus Flexor hallucis longus Flexor digitorum brevis Flexor hallucis brevis	Plantar flexion of foot Flexion of distal phalanges (II–IV) Flexion of distal phalanges (I) Flexion of middle phalanges (II–V) Flexion of middle phalanges (I)
Lateral cutaneous nerve of the leg	L4–S2	Sensory	Figure 2-13
Medial plantar	L4–5		Figure 2-12
Sural	S1–2		Figure 2-12
Lateral plantar	S1–2		Figure 2-12

● Clinical Pearl

The common fibular nerve, which includes the superficial and deep branches, is formed by the upper four posterior divisions (L4, 5 and S1, 2) of the lumbosacral plexus (Table 2-13).

The tibial nerve is formed from all five anterior divisions (L4, 5 and S1, 2, 3). The tibial division is the larger of the two divisions (Table 2-13).

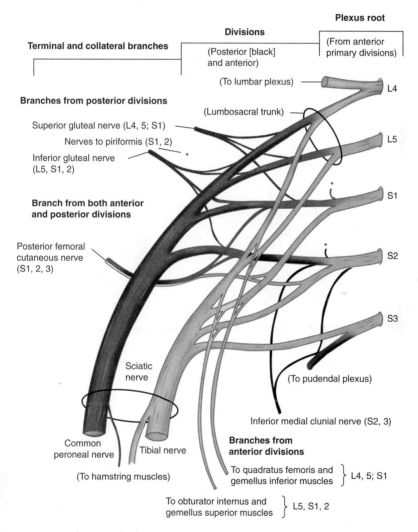

Figure 2-10 The sacral plexus. (Reproduced with permission from Waxman SG. *Correlative Neuroanatomy*. 24th ed. New York, NY: McGraw-Hill; 2000:366.)

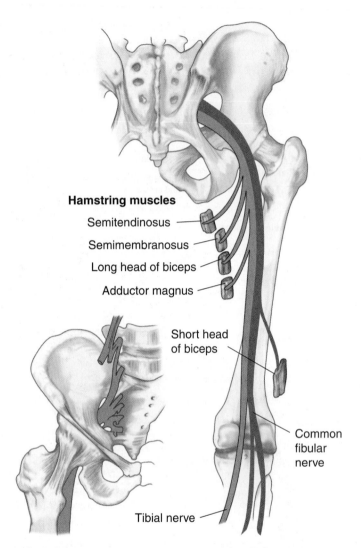

Figure 2-11 The sciatic nerve (L4, 5, S1–3). (Reproduced with permission from Waxman SG. *Correlative Neuroanatomy*. 24th ed. New York, NY: McGraw-Hill; 2000:368.)

Pudendal and Coccygeal Plexuses

The pudendal and coccygeal plexuses are the most caudal portions of the lumbosacral plexus and supply nerves to the perineal structures (Figure 2-14).

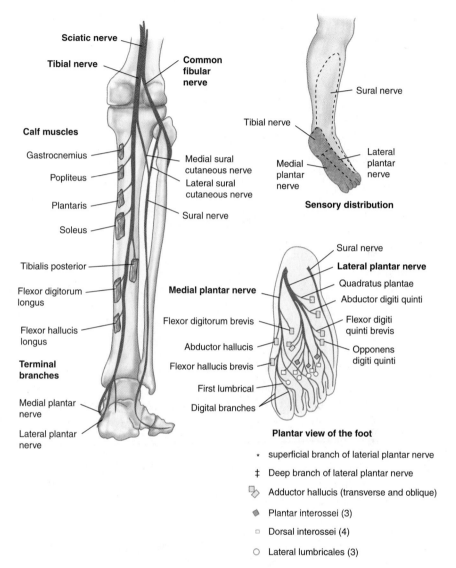

Figure 2-12 The tibial nerve (L4, 5, S1–3). (Reproduced with permission from Waxman SG. *Correlative Neuroanatomy*. 24th ed. New York, NY: McGraw-Hill; 2000:370.)

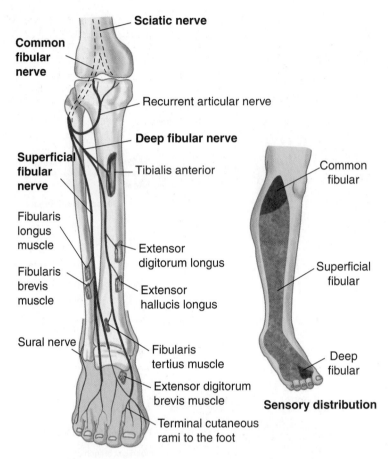

Figure 2-13 The common fibular (peroneal) nerve (L4, 5, S1, 2). (Reproduced with permission from Waxman SG. *Correlative Neuroanatomy*. 24th ed. New York, NY: McGraw-Hill; 2000:369.)

- The pudendal plexus supplies the coccygeus, levator ani, and sphincter ani externus muscles. The pudendal nerve divides into

    a. the inferior hemorrhoidal nerves to the external anal sphincter and adjacent skin

    b. the perineal nerve

    c. the dorsal nerve of the penis.

- The nerves of the coccygeal plexus are the small sensory anococcygeal nerves derived from the last three segments (S4, 5, C). They pierce

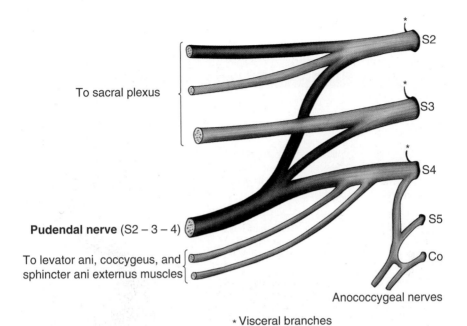

To sacral plexus

S2

S3

S4

S5

Co

Pudendal nerve (S2 – 3 – 4)

To levator ani, coccygeus, and
sphincter ani externus muscles

Anococcygeal nerves

* Visceral branches

Figure 2-14 The pudendal and coccygeal plexuses. (Reproduced with permission from Waxman SG. *Correlative Neuroanatomy*. 24th ed. New York, NY: McGraw-Hill; 2000:371.)

the sacrotuberous ligament and supply the skin in the region of the coccyx.

PERIPHERAL NERVE ENTRAPMENT SYNDROMES

Peripheral nerves are enclosed in three layers of tissue of differing character. From the inside outward, these are the endoneurium, perineurium, and epineurium.[10] The majority of peripheral nerve entrapments result from chronic injury to these nerve layers along their various routes; the compression usually is between ligamentous, muscular, or bony surfaces. Although peripheral nerve entrapments are the most common in the upper extremity (Table 2-16), particularly in the forearm, and wrist, they also occur in the lower extremity (Table 2-17). Neurogenic syndromes are usually incomplete, indicating the absence of severe motor or sensory deficits, but in the typical case they are accompanied by a history of pain or vague sensory disturbances.

Table 2-16 Peripheral Nerve Entrapment Syndromes of the Upper Extremity

Nerve Involved	Entrapment Site	Description of Findings
Axillary	Susceptible to injury at several sites, including the origin of the nerve from the posterior cord, the anterior–inferior aspect of the subscapularis muscle and shoulder capsule, the quadrilateral space, and within the subfascial surface of the deltoid muscle.	A deltoid paralysis—an inability to protract or retract the arm or raise it to the horizontal position, although after some time, supplementary movements may partially take over these functions. Teres minor paralysis causes weakness of shoulder external rotation. Sensation is lost over the deltoid prominence.
Suprascapular nerve	Suprascapular nerve entrapment is by a stout, strong suprascapular ligament that closes over the free upper margins of the suprascapular notch, often in conjunction with a tight, bony notch.	The chief complaint is the insidious onset of a deep, dull aching and noncircumscribed pain in the posterior part of the shoulder and upper periscapular region but does not involve the neck or radiate down the arm. Weakness is confined to the supraspinatus (i.e., in the initiation of shoulder abduction) and to the infraspinatus, the only muscle responsible for external rotation of the humerus.
Musculocutaneous	Reported cases have been associated with positioning during general anesthesia, peripheral nerve tumors, and strenuous upper extremity exercise without apparent underlying disease. Mechanisms proposed for these exercise-related cases include entrapment within the coracobrachialis, as well as traction between a proximal fixation point at the coracobrachialis and a distal fixation point at the deep fascia at the elbow.	Although a musculocutaneous lesion would be expected to demonstrate weakness of elbow flexion, one would not expect to see weakness in all shoulder motions with an injury isolated to the proximal musculocutaneous nerve. Other clinical features of musculocutaneous involvement include a loss of the biceps jerk, muscle atrophy, and loss of sensation to the anterior–lateral surface of the forearm.
Cubital tunnel (ulnar entrapment at the elbow)	Ulnar neuropathy at the elbow may be posttraumatic or nontraumatic. Trauma may be a single event or in mild repetitive form; the pathophysiological basis for the traumatic neuropathy likely is scarring and adhesion. Five potential areas of ulnar nerve injury exist within its course to and out of the elbow. —In 70% of the population, a tense sheet of fascia (the arcade of	Patients with nontraumatic ulnar neuropathy often have jobs that require repetitive elbow flexion and extension or prolonged resting of the elbow on a hard surface, such as a desk. Elbow flexion narrows the cubital tunnel because of traction on the arcuate ligament and bulging of the medial collateral ligament. The nerve also elongates with elbow flexion, increasing intraneural pressure.

(continued on following page)

Nerve Involved	Entrapment Site	Description of Findings
	Struthers) stretches from the medial head of the triceps to insert into the medial intermuscular septum, arching over, and often compressing, the ulnar nerve approximately 6 to 8 cm above the medial epicondyle. —The medial intermuscular septum presents a sharp edge that can indent the nerve, especially following anterior transposition where the nerve may be kinked. —The cubital tunnel, floored by the medial collateral ligament of the elbow, is roofed by the strong arcuate ligament (retinaculum) stretching between the medial humeral epicondyle and the medial aspect of the olecranon. Compression and scarring frequently occur within this tunnel. —The arching band of aponeurosis between the two heads of the flexor carpi ulnaris (Osborne band) often compresses the nerve, especially during repetitive contraction of the muscle. —The aponeurotic covering between the flexors digitorum profundus and superficialis is an occasional site of compression. Other causes include: an increased carrying angle at the elbow, repetitive trauma to the flexed elbow, ruptured ulnar collateral ligament permitting the nerve to sublux.	With scarring and adhesion on the epineurium, elongation accentuates the tethering effect on the axons. Nocturnal paresthesia and pain usually are associated with sleeping with the elbow in flexion. Early symptoms include intermittent paresthesia along the ring and little fingers and discomfort along the medial aspect of the forearm. Pain usually comes later, as a deep ache around the elbow region, and often is exacerbated suddenly when the medial elbow is brushed accidentally. Gentle tapping of the nerve at and around the cubital tunnel elicits distressing electrical shock and/or tingling down the ulnar fingers. There may be diminished sensitivity to pinprick, light touch, and two-point discrimination on the ulnar pad of the fifth finger and along the ulnar split-half of the fourth finger. Provocative test with sustained elbow flexion or combined with gentle digital pressure on the cubital tunnel brings out the symptoms of paresthesia and pain. Weakness of finger abductors and adductors is variable. Late symptoms include dense numbness and profound weakness and atrophy of the intrinsic hand muscles. The last two digits assume the classic ulnar claw hand, with extension at the metacarpal phalangeal joints and flexion at the intraphalangeal joints. The old, "burnt out" neuropathic hand often is atrophic, weak, and thin-skinned but, surprisingly, painless and free of other sensory phenomena
Pronator teres (median nerve)	Compromise of median nerve as it passes through the two heads of the pronator teres. Sites of compression include the lacertus fibrosus (bicipital aponeurosis, superficial forearm fascia), the Struthers ligament (thickened or aberrant origin of pronator teres from distal humerus), the pronator teres	Signs and symptoms: These include pain in the volar forearm that is exacerbated with activity and relieved by rest; decreased sensation in the thumb, index finger, long finger, and radial side of the ring finger; weakness of thenar muscles; and a positive Tinel or Phalen sign in the proximal forearm.

(continued on following page)

Table 2-16 *(continued from previous page)*

Nerve Involved	Entrapment Site	Description of Findings
	(musculofascial band or compression between two muscular heads), and the FDS proximal arch or the flexor digitorum superficialis.	
Anterior interosseous (median nerve)	Causative factors include tendinous bands, a deep head of the pronator teres, accessory muscles (including the Gantzer muscle, which is the accessory head of the FPL), aberrant radial artery branches, and fractures.	Symptoms include vague pain in the proximal forearm and weakness of the FPL and FDP to the index finger. Affected persons cannot form a circle by pinching their thumb and index finger (i.e., hyperextension of index distal interphalangeal joint and thumb interphalangeal joint). Sensory involvement is not described.
Posterior interosseous (radial nerve)	PIN compression most commonly is associated with tendinous hypertrophy of the arcade of Frohse and fibrous thickening of the radiocapitellar joint capsule. Vascular compression by a hypertrophic leash of Henry has been reported. Lesions, such as lipoma, synovial cyst, rheumatoid synovitis, and vascular aneurysms, have been found in some cases. Hobbies or occupations associated with repetitive and forceful supination predispose to PIN neuropathy. Repetitive wrist flexion maneuvers compress the nerve as it enters the dorsal wrist capsule, inciting symptomatic inflammation. Chronic trauma to the flexion surface of the forearm likewise causes problems. For example, the constricting rings of the Canadian crutches, which exert direct pressure over the supinator surface, typically cause PIN neuropathy in paraplegic patients.	Because the posterior interosseous syndrome (PIN) purely affects a motor nerve, sensory symptoms are minor. A dull, aching pain sometimes is present over the front of the elbow, and palpation over the radiohumeral joint often aggravates the pain, probably due to irritation of the nervi nervorum of the PIN. Motor paralysis of the extensor muscles often is heralded by a feeling of fatigue during finger extension and elbow supination. Extension in the metacarpal phalangeal joints is weakened but not in the interphalangeal joints because the latter is affected by the lumbricals. Because the index and fifth fingers receive both their own extensor tendon and tendon branch from the common extensor, they are less affected than extension of the third and fourth digits. Thus, in the early stage of entrapment, the hand exhibits a characteristic pattern on finger extension where the middle two fingers fail to extend, while the index and little fingers hold erect. Progression of paralysis eventually causes weakness in all of the finger extensors and in thumb abduction. Because the radial wrist extensors are spared because of their proximal innervation, wrist extension weakness usually is undetectable in spite of weakness of the ulnar wrist extensor.

Nerve Involved	Entrapment Site	Description of Findings
Radial tunnel	The deep branch of the radial nerve can be compressed by five structures within the radial tunnel. The most common site of compression is at the proximal fibrous edge of the supinator muscle, known as the arcade of Frohse. The most proximal structure that can compress the deep branch of the radial nerve is the fibrous fascia over the radiocapitellar joint. The next structures that can compress the deep branch of the radial nerve are the radial recurrent artery and the venae comitantes, known as the leash of Henry, although this is uncommon. Lastly, the deep branch of the radial nerve can also be compressed by the distal edge of the supinator muscle, which is known to be fibrous in 50% to 70% of patients.	Symptoms: These may include pain in the upper extensor forearm; dysesthesia in a superficial radial nerve distribution; and weakening of the extension of the fingers, thumb, or wrist
Wartenberg syndrome (superficial radial)	A compression of the superficial sensory radial nerve. Inflammation of the tendons of the first dorsal compartment can result in superficial radial neuritis.	Pain, paresthesias, and numbness of the radial aspects of the hand and wrist. In addition, the tendons of the brachioradialis and extensor carpi radialis longus muscles can press on the nerve in a scissor-like fashion when the forearm is pronated, causing a proximal tethering on the distal segment of the nerve at the wrist. Wartenberg sign is described wherein the patient is asked to extend the fingers and abduction or clawing of the little finger occurs.
Guyon canal (deep ulnar nerve)	After entering the Guyon canal, the deep motor branch first supplies the abductor digiti minimi (ADM), then crosses under one head of the flexor digiti minimi (FDM), supplies this muscle, and crosses over to supply the opponens digiti minimi before rounding the hook of the hamate to enter the mid palmar space. Depending on the exact site of compression within the Guyon canal, the ADM or both the ADM and the FDM may be spared. The opponens	The vulnerable candidates include paraplegics using hand crutches that have a horizontal bar across the palm, motorcyclists who firmly grasp the hand bar control, weightlifters, and operators of pneumatic drills. The classic picture is a young man presenting with painless atrophy of the hypothenar muscles and interossei, with sparing of the thenar group. Variable sensory loss over the ulnar fingers or hypothenar eminence, together with aching pain in the palm, may be present in patients whose sensory branch is a recurrent nerve arising from within the proximal canal.

(continued on following page)

Table 2-16 *(continued from previous page)*

Nerve Involved	Entrapment Site	Description of Findings
	always is affected, together with the interossei, ulnar lumbricals, and the adductor pollicis.	
	Proximal compression within the Guyon canal often is attributed to thickening of the tendonous arch stretched between the pisiform and hamate.	
	The hook of the hamate may be sharp-edged and forms an acute angle where the nerve turns radially. Injury to the nerve in this distal part of the canal may be accentuated by fibrous bands. The distal canal also is the common site for ganglions.	
Carpal tunnel (median nerve)	Median nerve compression at the wrist is by the transverse carpal ligament (TCL), which attaches to and arches between the pisiform and hamate ulnarly and the scaphoid and trapezium radially. The palmar fascia is fused to the TCL proximally and then fans out to the soft tissue of the palmar skin as the palmar aponeurosis. The combined layers of the TCL and proximal palmar fascia form the flexor retinaculum. The palmaris longus tendon inserts in the palmar aponeurosis and lies directly over the median nerve just proximal to the TCL. It serves as the most reliable guide to the nerve at operation.	Dull, aching pain at the wrist that extends up the forearm to the elbow. The pain typically is worse at night, disturbing sleep and is often associated with paresthesia in the median fingers and thumb on awakening.
		Sensation is decreased at the palmar pads of the thumb and index finger.
		In long-standing cases, the abductor pollicis brevis (APB) is weak and atrophic, causing thinning of the lateral contour of the thenar bulk.
	The palmaris longus is absent in 25% of healthy individuals, in which case the nerve is beneath a fascial membrane midway between the flexor carpi radialis and the flexor digitorum superficialis tendons. Typically, the median palmar cutaneous nerve originates from the radial side of the median nerve proximal to or just deep to the flexor retinaculum, then tunnels through this structure to innervate the thenar eminence and the palm roughly up to the vertical line overlying the	The flexor pollicis brevis is dually innervated by both the median and ulnar nerves and is unaffected. The opponens pollicis is affected very late.
		Forced wrist flexion causes increasing paresthesia and pain (Phalen sign), as does extreme wrist extension.
		Gentle tapping of the nerve over the flexor retinaculum sets off paresthesia (Tinel sign).

Nerve Involved	Entrapment Site	Description of Findings
	fourth metacarpal. The motor nerve to the thenar muscles also leaves the median nerve radially just beyond the distal edge of the flexor retinaculum, but variant nerves may pierce through the flexor retinaculum or arise from the ulnar aspect of the median nerve and an accessory motor branch may even emerge proximal to the flexor retinaculum. Ten percent of ulnar nerves and 4% of ulnar arteries lie radial to the hook of the hamate outside of the Guyon canal, which places them at risk for injury during carpal tunnel surgery.	

Table 2-17 Peripheral Nerve Entrapment Syndromes of the Lower Extremity

Nerve Involved	Entrapment Site	Description of Findings
Iliohypogastric nerve	The iliohypogastric nerve is rarely injured in isolation. The most common causes of injury are surgical procedures. These include transverse lower abdominal incisions, as in hysterectomies, or injuries from procedures such as inguinal herniorrhaphy and appendectomies. Sports injuries such as trauma or muscle tears of the lower abdominal muscles may also result in injury to the nerve. It may also rarely occur during pregnancy (idiopathic iliohypogastric syndrome) due to the rapidly expanding abdomen in the third trimester.	Symptoms include burning or lancinating pain immediately following the abdominal operation. The pain extends from the surgical incision laterally into the inguinal region and suprapubic region. Occasionally, the pain may extend into the genitalia due to the significant overlap with other cutaneous nerves. Discomfort may occur immediately or up to several years after the procedure and may last for months to years.

Three major criteria are used to diagnose this nerve injury. The first is a history of surgical procedure in the lower abdominal area, although spontaneous entrapment can occur. Pain can usually be elicited by palpating laterally about the scar margin, and the pain usually radiates inferomedially toward the inguinal region and into the suprapubic and proximal genital area. Second, a definite area of hypoesthesia or hyperesthesia should be identified in the region of supply of the |

(continued on following page)

Table 2-17 *(continued from previous page)*

Nerve Involved	Entrapment Site	Description of Findings
		iliohypogastric nerve. Third, infiltration of a local anesthetic into the region where the iliohypogastric and ilioinguinal nerves depart the internal oblique muscle and where symptoms can be reproduced on physical examination by palpation should provide symptomatic relief. If no relief is obtained with injection, a different etiology should be sought for the discomfort. Alternate diagnoses include upper lumbar or lower thoracic nerve root pathology or discogenic etiology of the pain.
Ilioinguinal nerve	Causes of injury include lower abdominal incisions, pregnancy, iliac bone harvesting, appendectomy, inguinal herniorrhaphy, inguinal lymph node dissection, femoral catheter placement, orchiectomy, total abdominal hysterectomy, and abdominoplasty. Nerve injury can also occur idiopathically. The prevalence of injury with surgery has declined due to the use of laparoscopic procedures. Tearing of the lower external oblique aponeurosis may also cause injury to this nerve.	Symptoms could include hyperesthesia or hypoesthesia of the skin along the inguinal ligament. The sensation may radiate to the lower abdomen. Pain may be localized to the medial groin, labia majora or scrotum, and the inner thigh. The characteristics of the pain may vary considerably. Patients may be able to associate their pain clearly with a traumatic event or with the surgical procedure. Pain and tenderness may be present with application of pressure where the nerve exits the inguinal. Sensory impairment is common in the distribution of the nerve supply noted above. Symptoms usually increase with hip extension (patients ambulate with the trunk in a forward-flexed posture). Pain may also be reproduced with palpation medial to the anterosuperior iliac spine (ASIS). The diagnosis can be made on the basis of local infiltration of anesthetic with or without steroid and should result in relief within 10 minutes.
Genitofemoral nerve	Nerve injury may result from hernia repair, appendectomy, biopsies, and cesarean delivery. Injury may also occur due to intrapelvic trauma to the posterior abdominal wall, retroperitoneal hematoma, pregnancy, or trauma to the inguinal ligament. Fortunately, injury to this nerve is rare.	Hypesthesia over the anterior thigh below the inguinal ligament, which is how it is distinguished from the iliohypogastric and ilioinguinal nerve. Groin pain is a common presentation of neuralgia from nerve injury or entrapment. The pain may be worse with internal or external rotation of the hip, prolonged walking, or even with

Nerve Involved	Entrapment Site	Description of Findings
		light touch. Differential diagnoses include injury to the ilioinguinal and genitofemoral nerves as well as L1–2 radiculopathies. Some anatomic overlap may exist with the supply of the ilioinguinal and genitofemoral nerves, making the diagnosis difficult.
Lateral (femoral) cutaneous nerve (LCN) of the thigh (Meralgia paresthetica)	The entrapment may be from intrapelvic causes, extrapelvic causes, or mechanical causes. Intrapelvic causes would include pregnancy, abdominal tumors, uterine fibroids, diverticulitis, or appendicitis. Injury has been described in cases of abdominal aortic aneurism. Examples of extrapelvic causes include trauma to the region of the ASIS (e.g., a seatbelt from a motor vehicle accident), tight garments, belts, girdles, or stretch from obesity and ascites. Mechanical factors include prolonged sitting or standing and pelvic tilt from leg length discrepancy. Diabetes can also cause this neuropathy in isolation or in the clinical setting of a polyneuropathy.	The peak incidence for this condition is in middle age. It is common to encounter meralgia paresthetica in individuals who are obese and in women during their last trimester of pregnancy. A protruding, pendulous abdomen, as seen in obesity and pregnancy, pushes the inguinal ligament forward and downward and drags the nerve with it over the kink. The angulation of the nerve also is exaggerated with extension of the thigh and relaxed with flexion. Extension also tenses the fascia lata and may add to the compression from the front. Differential diagnoses include lumbar radiculopathies and discogenic or nerve root problems at L2 and L3. The main symptoms are an uncomfortable numbness, tingling, and painful hypersensitivity in the distribution of the LCN, usually in the anterolateral thigh down to the upper patella region. The symptoms often are accentuated with walking down gradients and stairs; prolonged standing in the erect posture; and, sometimes, lying flat in bed. The patient learns to relieve symptoms by placing a pillow behind the thighs and assuming a slightly hunched posture while standing. The diagnosis is confirmed with a nerve block. The resulting anesthesia over the sensory territory of the LCN should be concomitant with the complete cessation of pain and tingling.
Piriformis syndrome	Multiple etiologies have been proposed to explain the compression or irritation of the sciatic nerve that occurs with the piriformis syndrome: • *Hypertrophy of the piriformis muscle.*	Six classic findings: 1. A history of trauma to the sacroiliac and gluteal regions. 2. Pain in the region of the sacroiliac joint, greater sciatic notch, and piriformis muscle that usually causes difficulty with walking.

(continued on following page)

Table 2-17 *(continued from previous page)*

Nerve Involved	Entrapment Site	Description of Findings
	• *Trauma.* Trauma, direct or indirect, to the sacroiliac or gluteal region can lead to piriformis syndrome and is a result of hematoma formation and subsequent scarring between the sciatic nerve and the short external rotators. • *Hip flexion contracture.* A flexion contracture at the hip has been associated with piriformis syndrome. This flexion contracture increases the lumbar lordosis, which increases the tension in the pelvic–femoral muscles as these muscles try to stabilize the pelvis and spine in the new position. This increased tension causes the involved muscles to hypertrophy with no corresponding increase in the size of the bony foramina, resulting in neurological signs of sciatic compression. • *Gender.* Females are more commonly affected by piriformis syndrome, with as much as a 6:1 female-to-male incidence. • *Ischial bursitis.* • *Pseudoaneurysm of the inferior gluteal artery.* • *Excessive exercise to the hamstring muscles.* • *Inflammation and spasm of the piriformis muscle.* This is often in association with trauma, infection, and anatomical variations of the muscle. • *Anatomical anomalies.* Local anatomical anomalies may contribute to the likelihood that symptoms will develop.	3. Acute exacerbation of pain caused by stooping or lifting (and moderate relief of pain by traction on the affected extremity with the patient in the supine position). 4. A palpable sausage-shaped mass, tender to palpation, over the piriformis muscle on the affected side. 5. A positive straight leg raise. 6. Gluteal atrophy, depending on the duration of the condition. Other clinical signs include pain and weakness in association with resisted abduction and external rotation of the involved thigh, palpable and local muscle spasm (palpable in the obturator internus or, less commonly, in the piriformis muscle). The neurological examination is usually normal. An examination of the hip and lower leg usually demonstrates restricted external rotation of the hip and lumbosacral muscle tightness.
Femoral nerve	Diabetic amyotrophy is the most common cause of femoral nerve neuropathy. Open injuries can occur from gunshots, knife wounds, glass shards, or	The symptoms of a femoral neuropathy may include pain in the inguinal region that is partially relieved by flexion and external rotation of the hip and dysesthesia over the anterior thigh and

Nerve Involved	Entrapment Site	Description of Findings
	needle puncture in some medical procedures. Pelvic fractures and acute hyperextension of the thigh may also cause an isolated femoral nerve injury. Most entrapment neuropathies occur below the inguinal ligament. Pelvic procedures that require the lower extremity to be positioned in an acutely flexed, abducted, and externally rotated position for long periods can cause compression by angling the femoral nerve beneath the inguinal ligament. The nerve may be compromised by pressure from a fetus in a difficult birth.	anteromedial leg. Patients complain of difficulty with walking and knee buckling depending on the severity of the injury. The nerve gives rise to the saphenous nerve in the thigh; therefore, numbness in this distribution can be present. Anterior knee pain may also be present due to the saphenous nerve supply to the patella. On examination, patients may present with weak hip flexion, knee extension, and impaired quadriceps tendon reflex and sensory deficit in the anteromedial aspect of the thigh. Pain may be increased with hip extension and relieved with external rotation of the hip. If compression occurs at the inguinal region, no hip flexion weakness is present. Sensory loss may occur along the medial aspect of the leg below the knee (saphenous distribution).
Saphenous nerve	The saphenous nerve can become entrapped where it pierces the connective tissue at the roof of Hunter canal, resulting in inflammation from a sharp angulation of the nerve through the structure and the dynamic forces of the muscles in this region. This results in contraction and relaxation of the fibrous tissue that impinges the nerve. The nerve also can be injured from an improperly protected knee or leg support during operation. It may be injured due to neurilemoma, entrapment by femoral vessels, direct trauma, pes anserine bursitis, varicose vein operations, and medial knee arthrotomies and meniscus repairs.	Symptoms of entrapment may include a deep aching sensation in the thigh, knee pain, and possibly paresthesias in the cutaneous distribution of the saphenous distribution in the leg and foot. Saphenous nerve entrapment is a frequently overlooked cause of persistent medial knee pain. As this is a purely sensory nerve, weakness should not be noted with an isolated injury of this nerve. Sensory loss in the saphenous distribution may be present on examination.
Popliteal fossa (tibial nerve)	Compression of tibial nerve as it passes through the popliteal fossa. Usually caused by an enlarged Baker's cyst (which may also compress the common peroneal and sural nerves). Other causes include proliferation of the synovial tissue in patient's with rheumatoid arthritis	Pain behind the knee or in the calf muscles when the foot is dorsiflexed. Hypesthesia or anesthesia of the entire plantar surface of the foot. Incomplete flexion of the knee joint. Weakness of the gastrocnemius, tibialis posterior, flexor hallucis longus, flexor digitorum longus, and the intrinsic muscles of the foot (except for the extensor digitorum brevis)

(continued on following page)

Table 2-17 *(continued from previous page)*

Nerve Involved	Entrapment Site	Description of Findings
Tarsal tunnel	Compression of the posterior tibial nerve behind the medial malleolus, or tarsal tunnel syndrome (TTS), is an uncommon entrapment neuropathy. Numerous fibrous septae between the roof and the floor subdivide the tarsal tunnel into separate compartments at various points. The contents of the tarsal tunnel at its proximal end are, from front to back, (1) the flexor digitorum longus tendon, (2) the posterior tibialis tendon, (3) the posterior tibial artery and vein, (4) the posterior tibial nerve, and (5) the flexor hallucis longus tendon. The nerve has three terminal branches— the medial and lateral plantar nerves and the calcaneal branch. Distally, the medial and lateral plantar nerves travel in separate fascial compartments. The medial branch supplies the intrinsic flexors of the great toe and the sensation over the medial plantar surface of the foot inclusive of at least the first three toes. The lateral branch supplies all of the intrinsics that cause extension of the interphalangeal joints, as well as sensation over the lateral plantar surface of the foot. The calcaneal branch provides sensation to the heel.	Early symptoms include burning, tingling, and dysesthetic pain over the plantar surface of the foot. Characteristically, the pain is set off by pressing or rubbing over the plantar skin, sometimes with after-discharge phenomenon. A Tinel sign often is evident over the course of the main nerve or its branches, and the pain may be aggravated by forced eversion and dorsiflexion of the ankle. In advanced cases, the intrinsic flexors of the great toe are weak and atrophied, producing hollowing of the instep. The lateral toes also may show clawing due to paralysis of the intrinsic toe flexors and the dorsal digital extensions. The calcaneal branch often is spared because of its proximal takeoff.

● Clinical Pearl

Due to presence of mast cells in the epineurium, there is a potential for nerve repair. However, due to the release of inflammatory mediators (histamines) by the mast cells an increase in edema in and around the nerve can occur. On average nerves regenerate at a rate of 1 to 3 mm/day.

PERIPHERAL NERVOUS SYSTEM—AUTONOMIC NERVES

The autonomic system (ANS) is the division of the PNS that is responsible for the innervation of smooth muscle, cardiac muscle, and glands of the body, and functions primarily at a subconscious level.

The ANS has two components: sympathetic (Figure 2-15) and parasympathetic (Figure 2-16), each of which is differentiated by its site of

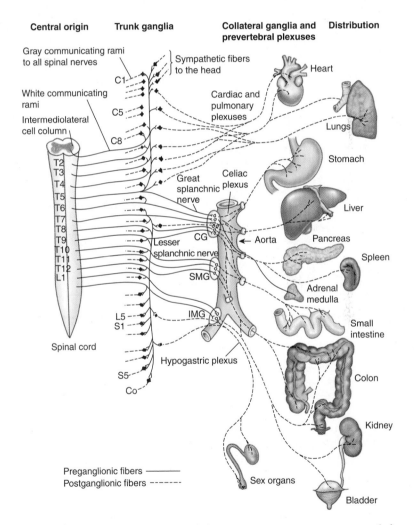

Figure 2-15 Sympathetic division of the autonomic nervous system (left half). (Reproduced with permission from Waxman SG. *Correlative Neuroanatomy*. 24th ed. New York, NY: McGraw-Hill; 2000:250.)

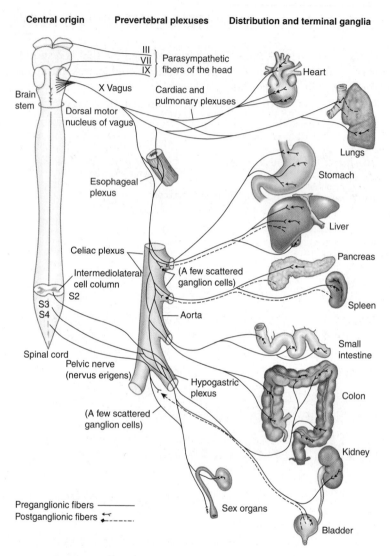

Figure 2-16 Parasympathetic division of the autonomic nervous system (left half). (Reproduced with permission from Waxman SG. *Correlative Neuroanatomy.* 24th ed. New York, NY: McGraw-Hill; 2000:253.)

origin as well as the transmitters it releases (Table 2-18).[11] In general, these two systems have antagonist effects on their end organs.

Table 2-18 Autonomic Nervous System Divisions

	Sympathetic	Parasympathetic
General location	Thoracolumbar	Craniosacral
Specific location	Intermediolateral and medial gray T 1–L 2	CNs III, VII, IX, X, and sacral segments S2–4
Pathway characteristics	Short preganglionic fibers Long postganglionic fibers	Long preganglionic fibers Short postganglionic fibers
Principal neurotransmitter	Norepinephrine (except sweat glands)	Acetycholine

REFERENCES

1. Waxman SG. *Correlative Neuroanatomy*. 24th ed. New York, NY: McGraw-Hill; 1996.

2. Bogduk N. Innervation and pain patterns of the cervical spine. In: Grant R, ed. *Physical Therapy of the Cervical and Thoracic Spine*. New York, NY: Churchill Livingstone; 1988.

3. Seddon H. Nerve injuries. *Med Bull (Ann Arbor)*. 1965;31:4–10.

4. Rowland LP. Diseases of the motor unit. In: Kandel ER, Schwartz JH, Jessell TM, eds. *Principles of Neural Science*. 4th ed. New York, NY: McGraw-Hill; 2000:695–712.

5. McKnight JT, Adcock BB. Paresthesias: a practical diagnostic approach. *Am Fam Physician*. 1997;56:2253–2260.

6. Poncelet AN. An algorithm for the evaluation of peripheral neuropathy. *Am Fam Physician*. 1998;57:755–764.

7. Chusid JG. Correlative *Neuroanatomy & Functional Neurology*. 19th ed. Norwalk, CT: Appleton-Century-Crofts; 1985:144–148.

8. Jenkins DB. *Hollinshead's Functional Anatomy of the Limbs and Back*. 7th ed. Philadelphia, PA: WB Saunders;1998.

9. Mannheimer JS, Lampe GN. *Clinical Transcutaneous Electrical Nerve Stimulation*. Philadelphia, PA: FA Davis; 1984:440–445.

10. Fawcett DW. The nervous tissue. In: Fawcett DW, ed. *Bloom and Fawcett: A Textbook of Histology*. New York, NY: Chapman & Hall; 1984: 336–339.

11. Morgenlander JC. The autonomic nervous system. In: Gilman S, ed. *Clinical Examination of the Nervous System*. New York, NY: McGraw-Hill; 2000:213–225.

QUESTIONS

1. Give four examples of neurological tissue
2. What are the two structural subdivisions of the CNS?
3. What fluid flows through the meningeal spaces, and within the ventricles of the brain, provides a cushion for the spinal cord?
4. Which of the spinal tracts convey motor signals to the cord and pons?
5. Which of the spinal tracts convey motor signals from cortex to the spinal cord?
6. Which of the spinal tracts convey crude touch, pain and temperature, and itching?
7. Which of the spinal tracts convey fine sensation and exact location of stimulus (vibration, posture, etc.)?
8. What are the two types of anterior motor neurons?
9. What is the function of the α motor neurons?
10. What is the function of the γ motor neurons?
11. Which nerve root could be impinged with a disc herniation between C4 and C5?
12. Which nerve root could be impinged with a disc herniation between T4 and T5?
13. Which nerve root could be impinged with a disc herniation between L4 and L5?
14. Give four clinical signs associated with spinal cord compression.
15. How many pairs of cervical nerves are there?
16. Which nerve root levels are assessed with a straight leg raise?
17. Which three minerals are very important in the transmission of nerve impulses?
18. Which of the CN is referred to as the spinal accessory nerve?
19. Which of the CNs is the trochlear nerve?
20. Which two CNs control the gag reflex?
21. With a C6 palsy, which four muscles would you expect to find weak?
22. The motor branches of which nerve supply the diaphragm?
23. Which nerve can be entrapped in the arcade of Frohse?
24. Which nerve can be trapped between the two heads of the pronator teres?
25. Which nerve can be impinged by the ligament of Struthers?
26. Which nerve can be compressed in cubital tunnel syndrome?
27. Atrophy of the hypothenar eminence could indicate a lesion to which nerve?
28. Which nerve lesion results in ape hand deformity?

29. A patient presents with severe weakness of the deltoid muscle and wrist extensors. Where would the lesion probably be located?
   A. C6 nerve root
   B. C7 nerve root
   C. Middle trunk of brachial plexus
   D. Posterior cord of the brachial plexus
   E. Radial nerve

30. A patient was involved in a motorcycle accident and it is suspected that he may have avulsed his C5 nerve root at its origin. To test this impression, what is the best muscle to check electrophysiologically?
   A. biceps
   B. pronator teres
   C. supraspinatus
   D. deltoid
   E. rhomboids

31. Injury to the radial nerve in the spiral groove could result in:
   A. weakness of elbow flexion
   B. inability to initiate glenohumeral abduction
   C. uncontrolled shoulder rotation during glenohumeral abduction
   D. difficulty to hold the humeral head in its socket
   E. all of the above

32. A patient with a musculocutaneous nerve injury is still able to flex the elbow. The major muscle causing this elbow flexion is the
   A. brachioradialis
   B. flexor carpi ulnaris
   C. pronator quadratus
   D. extensor carpi ulnaris
   E. pectoralis major

33. Which of the following muscles is *not* innervated by the median nerve?
   A. abductor pollicis brevis
   B. flexor pollicis longus
   C. medial heads of flexor digitorum profundus
   D. superficial head of flexor pollicis brevis
   E. pronator quadratus

34. The nerve that innervates the first lumbrical muscle in the hand is the
   A. median nerve
   B. ulnar nerve

C. radial nerve

D. anterior interosseus nerve

E. lateral cutaneous nerve of the hand

35. After a nerve injury, regeneration occurs proximally first and then progresses distally at a rate of about 1 mm/day. Following a radial nerve injury in the axilla, which muscle would be the *last* to recover?

    A. long head of the triceps

    B. anconeus

    C. extensor indicis

    D. extensor digiti minimi

    E. supinator

36. A patient complains of a burning sensation in the anterolateral aspect of the thigh. Dysfunction of which nerve could lead to these symptoms?

    A. lateral femoral cutaneous nerve of the thigh

    B. femoral

    C. obturator

    D. genitofemoral

    E. ilioinguinal

37. The sciatic nerve consists of two divisions (medial and lateral) that eventually separate into distinct nerves. The medial and lateral divisions, respectively, form the

    A. femoral and obturator nerves

    B. obturator and femoral nerves

    C. common fibular and tibial nerves

    D. tibial and common fibular nerves

    E. obturator and tibial nerves

38. The saphenous nerve supplies cutaneous sensation to the medial aspect of the leg. From which nerve does the saphenous nerve arise?

    A. obturator

    B. peroneal

    C. sciatic

    D. femoral

    E. the saphenous nerve arises as a direct branch from the sacral plexus

39. The tibial nerve passes into the foot where it divides into its terminal branches. What route does the tibial nerve follow to enter the foot?

    A. it passes along the dorsal aspect of the ankle, then into the foot

    B. it passes anterior to the lateral malleolus

C. it passes under the flexor retinaculum and posterior to the lateral malleolus

D. it passes anterior to the medial malleolus

E. it passes under the flexor retinaculum and posterior to the lateral malleolus

40. Injury to the deep branch of the fibular nerve would result in a sensory deficit to which of the following locations?

A. medial side of the foot

B. lateral side of the foot

C. lateral one and one half toes

D. medial border of the sole of the foot

E. adjacent dorsal surfaces of the first and second toes

41. A brachial plexus injury involving the supper portion of the plexus produces winging of the scapula. Weakness of which of the following muscles would produce the winging observe?

A. long head of the triceps

B. supraspinatus

C. deltoid

D. pectoralis major

E. serratus anterior

42. The anterior interosseus branch of the median nerve innervates which muscles?

A. flexor pollicis longus

B. pronator teres

C. pronator quadratus

D. both A and C

E. all of the above

43. The lumbar plexus is occasionally injured at the point where it passes through a muscle. The muscle causing the compression is the

A. gluteus maximus

B. gluteus medius

C. quadratus lumborum

D. obturator externus

E. psoas major

44. The axillary nerve can occasionally be injured where it passes through a muscle. Which muscle would this be?

A. pronator teres

B. supinator

  C. deltoid

  D. coracobrachialis

  E. biceps

45. Which statement(s) about the brachial plexus is(are) true?

  a. The brachial plexus is formed from the posterior rami of nerves C5–T1.

  b. The cords of the brachial plexus are named with respect to their anatomical position around the axillary artery.

  c. The muscles innervated by the posterior portion of the brachial plexus are primarily flexors.

  d. The nerve to the rhomboid muscles arises from C5 before C5 helps to form the upper trunk.

46. Klumpke palsy involves which trunk of the brachial plexus?

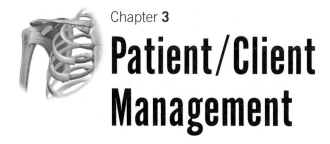

Chapter **3**

Patient/Client Management

The physical therapist integrates the five elements of patient/client management:

1. Examination of the patient
2. Evaluation of the data and identification of problems
3. Determination of the diagnosis
4. Determination of the prognosis and plan of care (POC)
5. Implementation of the POC (intervention).[1]

THE EXAMINATION

The examination (Figure 3-1) consists of three components of equal importance:

- The history
- The systems review
- The tests and measures

The history, systems review, and tests and measures are closely related, in that they often occur concurrently. One further element, observation, occurs throughout.

The History

The history (Table 3-1) usually precedes the systems review and the tests and measures components of the examination, but it may also occur concurrently.

🔵 Clinical Pearl

It is estimated that 80% of the necessary information to explain the presenting patient problem can be provided by a thorough history.

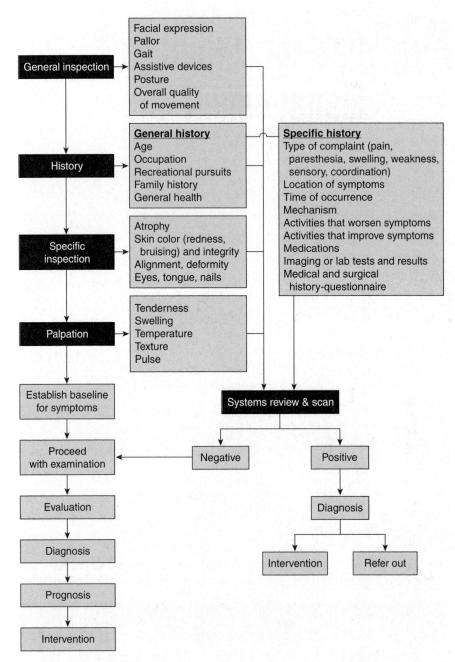

Figure 3-1 Components of the examination and their interrelationships.

Table 3-1 Data Generated From the Patient History

General demographics
Social history
Occupation/employment
Growth and development
Living environment
History of current condition
Functional status and activity level
Medications
Other test and measures
Past history of current condition
Past medical/surgical history
Family history
Social habits (past and present)

Neutral questions should be used whenever possible. These questions are structured in such a way so as not to lead the patient into giving a particular response.

 Clinical Pearl

- Open-ended questions, such as "tell me why you are here" encourage the patient to provide narrative information and decrease the opportunity for biasing on the part of the clinician.[2]
- Close-ended questions are more specific and are asked as the examination proceeds. The specific questions help to focus the examination and deter irrelevant information. Examples include the following:
  - Is the pain becoming worse, better, or is it relatively stable?
  - Does the pain wake you up at night or prevent sleep?
  - Have you experienced any loss of bowel or bladder function?

A sudden onset of pain, associated with trauma, could indicate the presence of an acute injury such as a tear or fracture, whereas immediate pain and "locking" is most likely to result from an intra-articular block (Table 3-2).

Table 3-2 Pain Descriptions and Potentially Related Structures

Type of Pain	Potential Source
Cramping, dull, sore, aching	Muscle
Dull, aching	Ligament, joint capsule
Sharp, shooting, pinching, gnawing	Nerve root
Sharp, burning, shooting	Nerve
Burning, pressure like, sting, smarting	Sympathetic nerve
Deep, nagging, dull	Bone
Sharp, severe, incapacitating	Fracture
Throbbing, pulsing, beating, diffuse	Vasculature

If the onset is gradual or insidious, the clinician must determine whether there are any predisposing factors, such as changes in the patient's daily routines or exercise programs. If there are no such factors, a more serious cause should be suspected until otherwise ruled out.

Clinical Pearl

Acute symptoms (less than 2 weeks' duration) must be differentiated from those of an insidious onset and those of a traumatic onset.

Clinical Pearl

- Musculoskeletal conditions are typically influenced with movements or positions.
- Chemical or inflammatory pain is more constant and is less affected by movements or positions.
- Intermittent pain is usually caused by prolonged postures, by a loose intra-articular body, or by an impingement of a musculoskeletal structure.
- Reports of numbness and tingling suggest a neurological compromise (refer to Chapter 2).

The History of the Current Condition

The clinician must determine whether the condition began insidiously or was trauma involved? If the injury is traumatic, the clinician should determine the specific mechanism, in terms of both the direction and force, and relate the mechanism to the presenting symptoms.

Clinical Pearl

- If the injury is recent, an inflammatory source of pain is likely. An injury of longer duration may indicate an overuse mechanism.

The symptoms need to be carefully evaluated in terms of the site, distribution, quality, onset, frequency, nocturnal occurrence, aggravating factors, and relieving factors.

Clinical Pearl

- Information about how the location of the symptoms has changed since the onset can indicate whether a condition is worsening or improving.

A body chart may be used to record the location of symptoms (Table 3-3).

Clinical Pearl

- Symptoms of pain or limitations of movement, with no apparent reason, can be a result of inflammation, early degeneration, repetitive activity (microtrauma), sustained positioning and postures, or a more insidious cause.

If the extremity appears to be the source of the symptoms, the clinician should attempt to reproduce the symptoms by loading the peripheral tissues. If this proves unsuccessful, a full investigation of the spinal structures must ensue.

Table 3-3 Patient pain evaluation from

Name :_____

Date:_____   **Signature:**_____

Please use the diagram below to indicate where you feel symptoms right now. Use the following key to indicate different types of symptoms.

KEY: Pins and Needles = 000000   Stabbing = ////////   Burning = XXXXX   Deep Ache = ZZZZZZ

Please use the three scales below to rate your pain over the past 24 hours. Use the upper line to describe your pain level right now. Use the other scales to rate your pain at its worst and best over the past 24 hours.

RATE YOUR PAIN: 0 = NO PAIN, 10 = EXTREMELY INTENSE

		0	1	2	3	4	5	6	7	8	9	10
1.	Right now	0	1	2	3	4	5	6	7	8	9	10
2.	At its worst	0	1	2	3	4	5	6	7	8	9	10
3.	At its best	0	1	2	3	4	5	6	7	8	9	10

Clinical Pearl

The term *referred pain* is used to describe those symptoms that have their origin at a site other than where the patient feels them.

 Clinical Pearl

- In general, as a condition worsens, the pain distribution becomes more widespread and distal (peripheralizes). As the condition improves, the symptoms tend to become more localized (centralized).

Questions must be asked to determine whether the symptoms are sufficient to prevent sleep or to wake the patient at night, and the effect that activities of daily living (ADL), work, and recreational activities have on the symptoms.

Past History of Current Condition

If the patient had a similar injury in the past, how was it treated and was the treatment successful or unsuccessful? If it is a recurrent injury, the clinician should note how often, and how easily the injury has recurred, and the success, or failure of previous interventions, and how long did the last episode last?

 Clinical Pearl

A recurrent injury tends to have a detrimental effect on the potential for recovery. The frequency and duration of the patient's symptoms can help the clinician to classify the injury according to its stage of healing (see Chapter 1): acute (inflammatory), subacute (reparative), and chronic (remodeling).

Past Medical/Surgery History

The patient's past medical (PMH) and surgical history, which can provide information with regard to medications, allergies, childhood illnesses, and previous trauma, can be obtained through a questionnaire. In addition, the PMH can provide information on any health conditions that may impact exercise tolerance (cardiac problems, high blood pressure) and speed of healing (diabetes).

 Clinical Pearl

- Certain diseases, such as rheumatoid arthritis, diabetes, cardiovascular disease, and cancer have familial tendencies.

Details about any imaging tests such as x-ray, magnetic resonance imaging (MRI), computed tomography (CT) scan, and bone scan can provide the clinician with useful information.

 Clinical Pearl

A history involving an electromyography (EMG) test, or a nerve conduction velocity (NCV) test, could suggest a compromise to the muscle tissue and/or neurological system.

Review of Systems

The review of systems (ROS) is the part of the history taking that identifies possible health problems that require consultation with, or referral to, another health care provider. The ROS (Table 3-4) can be used to assess either the general health of the patient or a specific system.

 Clinical Pearl

- The clinician must determine whether pain is the only symptom or whether there are other symptoms that accompany the pain, such as dizziness, bowel and bladder changes, radicular pain/numbness, paresthesia, weakness, and increased sweating. Causes of generalized weakness include motor neuron disease, disorders of the neuromuscular junction, and myopathy.

As with other testing procedures, the depth of the review is based on the clinical findings.

Table 3-4 The Components of the ROS (Review of Systems)

Musculoskeletal	Pain, swelling, redness or heat of muscles or joints, gross range of motion, limitation, of motion, symmetry, functional strength/muscular weakness, atrophy, cramps
Neurological	Paralysis, tremor, incoordination, parathesias, difficulties with memory of speech, sensory or motor disturbances, or muscular coordination (ataxia, tremor). General movement patterns
Integumentary	Skin integrity, color, scar, temperature, patient's height and weight
Gastrointestinal	Appetite, dysphagia, indigestion, food idiosyncrasy, abdominal pain, heartburn, nausea, vomiting, hematemesis, jaundice, constipation, or diarrhea, abnormal stools (clay-colored, tarry, bloody, greasy, foul smelling), flatulence, hemorrhoids, recent changes in bowel habits
Cardiovascular	Precordial pain, substernal distress, palpitations, syncope, dyspnea on exertion, orthopnea, nocturnal paroxysmal dyspnea, edema, cyanosis, hypertension, heart murmurs, varicosities, phlebitis, claudication
Pulmonary	Pain (location, quality, relation to respiration), shortness of breath, wheezing, stridor, cough (time of day, productiveness, and color of sputum), hemoptysis, respiratory infections, tuberculosis (or exposure to tuberculosis), fever, or night sweats
Urinary and reproductive	Urgency, frequency, dysuria, nocturia, hematuria, polyuria, oliguria, unusual (or change in) color of urine, stones, infections, nephritis, hesitancy, change in size of stream, dribbling, acute retention or incontinence, libido, potency, genital sores, discharge, venereal disease
	(Female) Age of onset of menses, regularity, last period, dysmenorrhea, menorrhagia, or metrorrhagia, vaginal discharge, postmenopausal bleeding, dyspareunia, number and results of pregnancies (gravida, para)

🔵 Clinical Pearl

The ROS is a form of a decision tree intended to provide a "green light" or "red light" for further physical therapist examination or consultation, or for a referral to another provider. Based on the information gathered, the PT makes one of the following determinations:

1. A more comprehensive physical therapist examination and evaluation is needed;

2. A referral to another health professional is needed;

3. Both 1 and 2 are needed;

4. No problems are identified that require further examination or referral.

Although most serious pathologies can have characteristic findings that alert a clinician, some can occasionally masquerade as a benign condition (Tables 3-5 and 3-6).[2-4]

Table 3-5 Signs and Symptoms of Serious Pathology

Sign or Symptom	Possible Cause
Fevers, chills, or night sweats	Systemic problem (infection, cancer, disease). Increased sweating can have a myriad of causes ranging from increased body temperature due to exertion, fever, apprehension, and compromise to the autonomic system. Night sweats are of particular concern as they can often indicate the presence of a systemic problem*
Recent unexplained weight changes	An unexplained weight gain could be due to congestive heart failure, hypothyroidism, or cancer.† An unexplained weight loss could be due to a gastrointestinal disorder, hyperthyroidism, cancer, or diabetes†
Malaise, or fatigue	Systemic disease Thyroid disease Iron deficiency
Unexplained nausea or vomiting	Never a good sign
Dizziness	Although most causes of dizziness can be relatively benign, dizziness may signal a more serious problem, especially if the dizziness is associated with trauma to the neck or head, or with motions of cervical rotation and extension (vertebral artery compromise). The clinician must ascertain whether the symptoms result from vertigo, nausea, giddiness, unsteadiness, fainting, and the like. Vertigo requires that the patient's physician be informed, for further investigation. However, in of itself, it is not usually a contraindication to the continuation of the examination
Unilateral, bilateral, or quadrilateral paresthesias	The seriousness of the paresthesia depends on its distribution. Quadrilateral paresthesia always indicates the presence of central nervous system involvement.

(continued on following page)

Sign or Symptom	Possible Cause
Shortness of breath	
Bowel or bladder dysfunction	Bowel and bladder dysfunction may indicate involvement of the cauda equina
Night pain	Malignancy
Pain following eating	Gastrointestinal problems
Weakness	Any weakness should be investigated by the clinician to determine whether it is the result of spinal nerve root compression, a peripheral nerve lesion, disuse, inhibition due to pain or swelling, an injury to the contractile or inert tissues (muscle, tendon, bursa, etc.) or a more serious pathology such as a fracture
A gradual increase in the intensity of the pain	Radiating pain refers to an increase in pain intensity and distribution. Radiating pain typically travels distal from the site of the injury
Radicular pain	Nerve root irritation
Numbness	Numbness that is a dermatomal pattern indicates spinal nerve root compression

Data from references [†2] and [*3].

Other tests that may be incorporated as part of the ROS include the Cyriax scanning examination (Tables 3-7 and 3-8).[5]

Clinical Pearl

- The purpose of the scanning examination is to help rule out the possibility of symptom referral from other areas and to ensure that all possible causes of the symptoms are examined (Table 3-9).[6]

The scanning examination is divided into two examinations: one for the lower quarter/quadrant and the other for the upper quarter/quadrant. The tests that comprise the scanning examination are designed to detect neurological weakness (Tables 3-10 and 3-11), the patient's ability to perceive sensations, the inhibition of the deep tendon reflexes (DTRs), and the control of other reflexes by the central nervous system.

Table 3-6 Examination Findings and the Possible Conditions
Causing Them*

Findings	Possible Condition
Dizziness	Upper cervical impairment, vertebrobasilar ischemia, craniovertebral ligament tear. May also be relatively benign
Quadrilateral paresthesia	Cord compression, vertebrobasilar ischemia
Bilateral upper limb paresthesia	Cord compression, vertebrobasilar ischemia
Hyperreflexia	Cord compression, vertebrobasilar ischemia
Babinski or clonus sign	Cord compression, vertebrobasilar ischemia
Consistent swallow on transverse ligament stress tests	Instability, retropharyngeal hematoma, rheumatoid arthritis
Nontraumatic capsular pattern	Rheumatoid arthritis, ankylosing spondylitis, neoplasm
Arm pain lasting >6–9 months	Neoplasm
Persistent root pain <30 years	Neoplasm
Radicular pain with coughing	Neoplasm
Pain worsening after 1 month	Neoplasm
>1 level involved (cervical region)	Neoplasm
Paralysis	Neoplasm or neurological disease
Trunk and limb paresthesia	Neoplasm
Bilateral root signs and symptoms	Neoplasm
Nontraumatic strong spasm	Neoplasm
Nontraumatic strong pain in the elderly patient	Neoplasm
Signs worse than symptoms	Neoplasm
Radial deviator weakness	Neoplasm
Thumb flexor weakness	Neoplasm
Hand intrinsic weakness and/or atrophy	Neoplasm, thoracic outlet syndrome, carpal tunnel syndrome

(continued on following page)

Findings	Possible Condition
Horner syndrome	Superior sulcus tumor, breast cancer, cervical ganglion damage, brainstem damage
Empty end-feel	Neoplasm
Severe posttraumatic capsular pattern	Fracture
Severe posttraumatic spasm	Fracture
Loss of ROM posttrauma	Fracture
Posttraumatic painful weakness	Fracture

*Data from reference 4.

 Clinical Pearl

The entire scanning examination should take no more than a few minutes to complete and is routinely carried out unless there is some good reason for postponing it, such as recent trauma when a modified differential diagnostic examination is used.[4]

Table 3-7 Typical Sequence of the Upper or Lower Quarter Scanning Examinations

Initial observation

This involves everything from the initial entry of the patient including their gait, demeanor, standing and sitting postures, obvious deformities and postural defects, scars, radiation burns, creases, and birth marks

Patient history

Scanning examination

Active range of motion

Passive overpressure

Resistive tests

Deep tendon reflexes

Sensation testing

Special tests

Table 3-8 Components of the Scanning Examination and the Structures Tested

Active ROM	Willingness to move, ROM, integrity of contractile and inert tissues, pattern of restriction (capsular, or noncapsular), quality of motion, and symptom reproduction
Passive ROM	Integrity of inert and contractile tissues, ROM, end-feel, sensitivity
Resisted	Integrity of contractile tissues (strength, sensitivity)
Stress	Integrity of inert tissues (ligamentous/disc stability)
Dural	Dural mobility
Neurological	Nerve conduction
Dermatome	Afferent (sensation)
Myotome	Efferent (strength, fatigability)
Reflexes	Afferent–efferent, and central nervous system

Often the scanning examination does not generate enough signs and symptoms to formulate a working hypothesis or a diagnosis. In which case, further testing with the tests and measures is required to proceed.

Tests and Measures

The tests and measures (Table 3-12) component of the examination (Figure 3-2), which serves as an adjunct to the history and systems review, involves the physical examination of the patient.

Table 3-9 Signs and Symptoms Requiring Neurological Assessment

1. A headache that is sudden, severe, and diffuse; that awakens one from sleep; is worsened with activity or exertion; is associated with projectile vomiting, but no nausea, or begins or worsens with recumbency.*
2. Cognitive impairment
3. Visual disturbances (i.e., blindness, diplopia, distortions, spots, or loss of vision on one side)
4. Sudden loss of strength or coordination; loss or alteration of smell, taste, or hearing*
5. Fever or associated systemic illness
6. Difficulty swallowing
7. Loss or impairment of voice, chronic cough*

*Data from reference 6.

Table 3-10 The Lower Quarter Scanning Motor Examination

Muscle Action	Muscle Tested	Root Level	Peripheral Nerve
Hip flexion	Iliopsoas	L1–L2	Femoral to iliacus and lumbar plexus to psoas
Knee extension	Quadriceps	L2–L4	Femoral
Hamstrings	Biceps femoris, semimembranosus, and semitendinosus	L4–S3	Sciatic
Dorsiflexion with inversion	Tibialis anterior	Primarily L4	Deep fibular
Great toe extension	Extensor hallicus longus	Primarily L5	Deep fibular
Ankle eversion	Fibularis longus and brevis	Primarily S1	Superficial fibular nerve
Ankle plantarflexion	Gastrocnemius and soleus	Primarily S1	Tibial
Hip extension	Gluteus maximus	L5–S2	Inferior gluteal nerve

Table 3-11 The Upper Quarter Scanning Motor Examination

Resisted Action	Muscle Tested	Root Level	Peripheral Nerve
Shoulder abduction	Deltoid	Primarily C5	Axillary
Elbow flexion	Biceps brachii	Primarily C6	Musculocutaneous
Elbow extension	Triceps brachii	Primarily C7	Radial
Wrist extension	Extensor carpi radialis longus, brevis, and extensor carpi ulnaris	Primarily C6	Radial
Wrist flexion	Flexor carpi radialis and flexor carpi ulnaris	Primarily C7	Median n. for radialis and ulnar n. for ulnaris
Finger flexion	Flexor digitorum superficialis, flexor digitorum profundus, and lumbricales	Primarily C8	Median n. superficialis, both median and ulnar n. for profundus and lumbricales
Finger abduction	Dorsal interossei	Primarily T1	Ulnar

Table 3-12 Tests and Measures Related to the Neurological
and Musculoskeletal Preferred Practice Patterns

- Aerobic capacity and endurance
- Anthropometric characteristics
- Circulation
- Cranial and peripheral nerve integrity
- Environmental, home, and work barriers
- Ergonomics and body mechanics
- Gait, locomotion, and balance
- Integumentary integrity
- Joint integrity and mobility
- Motor function
- Muscle performance (including strength, power, and endurance)
- Orthotic, protective, and supportive devices
- Pain
- Posture
- Range of motion
- Reflex integrity
- Sensory integrity
- Work, community, and leisure integration

Clinical Pearl

The decision about which tests to use should be based on the best available research evidence. Before proceeding with the tests and measures, a full explanation must be provided to the patient as to what procedures are to be performed and the reasons for these.

Range of Motion

A normal joint has an available range of active, or physiological, motion, which is limited by a physiological barrier (Figure 3-3) as tension develops within the surrounding tissues. At the physiological barrier, there is an additional amount of passive range of motion (Figure 3-3). Beyond the available passive range of motion, the anatomic barrier (Figure 3-3) is found. This barrier cannot be exceeded without disruption to the integrity of the joint.

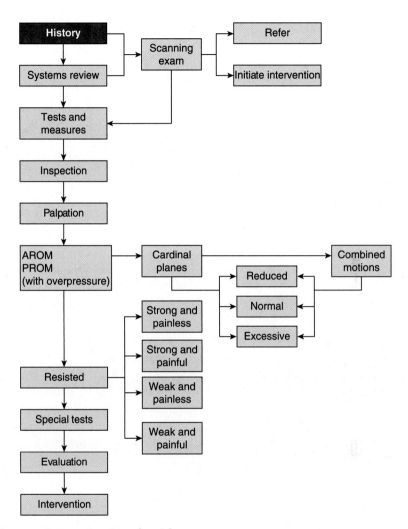

Figure 3-2 Examination algorithm.

Clinical Pearl

Active range of motion testing may be deferred if small and unguarded motions provoke intense pain as this may indicate a high degree of joint irritability.

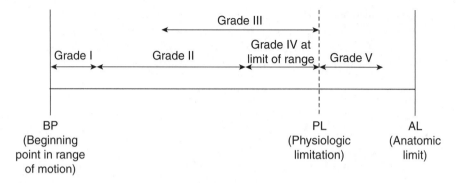

Figure 3-3 Available joint range of motion.

Active Range of Motion

The range of motion examination should determine the exact directions of motion that elicit the symptoms. Any loss of motion compared with the uninvolved joint should be noted. The diagnosis of restricted movement in the extremities can usually be simplified by comparing both sides, provided that at least one side is uninvolved.

Clinical Pearl

The contralateral, nonsymptomatic joint should always be examined first where possible. This allows for a determination of the normal function, allays the patient's anxiety, and allows for a true comparison of function.[7]

Active range of motion testing gives the clinician information about

- the quantity of available physiological motion (Figure 3-3)
- the presence of muscle substitutions
- the willingness of the patient to move
- the integrity of the contractile and inert tissues
- the quality of motion
- symptom reproduction
- the pattern of motion restriction.

For the purpose of an orthopedic examination, Cyriax subdivided musculoskeletal tissues into those considered to be "contractile" and those considered as "inert" (noncontractile).[8]

- Contractile. *Contractile tissue* as defined by Cyriax, is a bit of a misnomer, as the only true contractile tissue in the body is the muscle fiber. However, included under this term are the muscle belly, the tendon, the tenoperiosteal junction, the submuscular/tendinous bursa, and bone (teno-osseous junction), as all are stressed to some degree with a muscle contraction.
- Inert tissue. *Inert tissue* as defined by Cyriax includes the joint capsule, the ligaments, the bursa, the articular surfaces of the joint, the synovium, the dura, bone, and fascia.

The teno-osseous junction and the bursae are placed in each of the subdivisions due to their close proximity to contractile tissue and their capacity to be compressed or stretched during movement.

The normal active range of motion for each of the joints is depicted in Table 3-13.

 Clinical Pearl

- Joint motion can be estimated visually; however, a goniometer enhances accuracy. Knowing the expected zero starting position for each joint is necessary to provide consistent communication between observers.

- Full and pain-free active range of motion suggests normalcy for that movement, although it is important to remember that normal *range* of motion is not synonymous with normal motion.[9] Normal motion implies that the control of motion must also be present.

 Clinical Pearl

If a muscle/tendon crosses two joints, then both joints must be positioned to stretch the injured part. For example if the hamstrings are injured, their involvement will be highlighted by placing these structures on stretch—by flexing the hip to 90 degrees and then extending the knee.

Single motions in the cardinal planes are usually tested first. Dynamic and static testing in the cardinal planes follows if the single motions do not provoke symptoms.

Table 3-13 Active Ranges of Joint Motions

Joint	Action	Degrees of Motion
Shoulder	Flexion	0–180
	Extension	0–40
	Abduction	0–180
	Internal rotation	0–80
	External rotation	0–90
Elbow	Flexion	0–150
Forearm	Pronation	0–75
	Supination	0–85
Wrist	Flexion	0–80
	Extension	0–60
	Radial deviation	0–20
	Ulnar deviation	0–30
Hip	Flexion	0–125
	Extension	0–30
	Abduction	0–40
	Adduction	0–20
	Internal rotation	0–40
	External rotation	0–50
Knee	Flexion	0–140
Ankle	Plantarflexion	0–50
	Dorsiflexion	0–20
Foot	Inversion	0–30
	Eversion	0–20

 Clinical Pearl

Dynamic testing involves repeated movements in specific directions. Repeated movements can give the clinician some valuable insight into the patient's condition[10]:

• Internal derangements tend to worsen with repeated motions.

- The symptoms of a postural dysfunction remain unchanged with repeated motions.

- Pain from a dysfunction syndrome is increased with tissue loading, but ceases at rest.

- Repeated motions can indicate the irritability of the condition.

- Repeated motions can indicate to the clinician the direction of motion to be used as part of the intervention. If pain increases during repeated motion in a particular direction, exercising in that direction is not indicated. If pain only worsens in part of the range, repeated motion exercises can be used for that part of the range that is pain-free, or which does not worsen the symptoms.

- Pain that is increased after the repeated motions may indicate a re-triggering of the inflammatory response, and repeated motions in the opposite direction should be explored.

Static testing involves sustaining a position. Sustained static positions may be used to help detect postural syndromes.[11]

Combined motion testing (e.g., elbow flexion and forearm supination), performed statically and then dynamically, may be used when the symptoms are not reproduced with the cardinal plane motion tests.

The active range of motion will be found to be either abnormal (Figure 3-4) or normal (Figure 3-5). Abnormal motion is typically described as being reduced. It must be remembered though, that abnormal motion may also be excessive.

Clinical Pearl

- Excessive motion is often missed and is erroneously classified as normal motion. To help determine whether the motion is normal or excessive, passive range of motion, in the form of passive overpressure, and the end-feel are assessed (Figure 3-4).

Clinical Pearl

It is important the clinician uses consistent terminology when describing limited range of motion. If a standard form is not available, the clinician should record the date, the patient position (seated, supine, prone, standing), the type of motion (active or passive), the side of the body (right, left), the joint being measured, and any pain or abnormal motion that occurs with the movement.

Using the left knee as an example, and a patient whose available active range of motion is restricted between 20 degrees and 95 degrees of flexion, the documented measurement should be written as: left knee AROM: 20 degrees to 95 degrees.

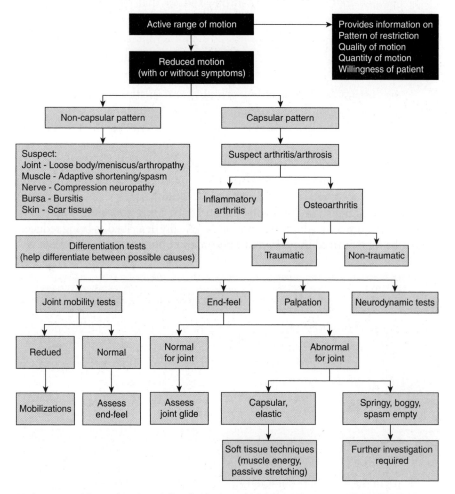

Figure 3-4 Algorithm used for findings of abnormal range of motion.

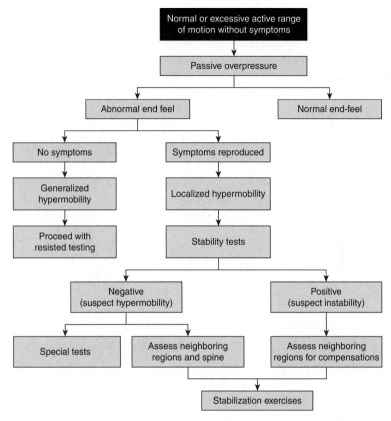

Figure 3-5 Algorithm used for findings of apparent normal range of motion.

If the patient has excessive range of motion, or hypermobility, a minus sign should be used. For example, if a patient has 15 degrees of passive hyperextension of the left knee and full flexion, the documented measurement should be written as: left knee PROM: -15 degrees to 145 degrees

Passive Range of Motion

If the active motions do not reproduce the patient's symptoms, or the active range of motion appears incomplete, it is important to perform gentle passive range of motion, and overpressure, at the end of the active range to fully test the motion (Figure 3-3). The passive overpressure should be applied carefully in the presence of pain. Passive range of motion testing gives the clinician

Table 3-14 Normal End-feels

Type	Cause	Characteristics and Examples
Bony	Produced by bone to bone approximation	Abrupt and unyielding with the impression that further forcing will break something. Examples: Normal: Elbow extension. Abnormal: Cervical rotation (may indicate osteophyte).
Elastic	Produced by the muscle–tendon unit. May occur with adaptive shortening	Stretch with elastic recoil and exhibits constant-length phenomenon. Further forcing feels as if it will snap something. Examples: Normal: Wrist flexion with finger flexion, the straight leg raise, and ankle dorsiflexion with the knee extended. Abnormal: Decreased dorsiflexion of the ankle with the knee flexed.
Soft tissue approximation	Produced by the contact of two muscle bulks on either side of a flexing joint where the joint range exceeds other restraints	A very forgiving end feel that gives the impression that further normal motion is possible if enough force could be applied. Examples: Normal: Knee flexion, elbow flexion in extremely muscular subjects. Abnormal: Elbow flexion with the obese subject.
Capsular	Produced by capsule or ligaments	Various degrees of stretch without elasticity. Stretch ability is dependent on thickness of the tissue. • Strong capsular or extracapsular ligaments produce a hard capsular end feel while a thin capsule produces a softer one. • The impression given to the clinician is, if further force is applied something will tear. Examples: Normal: Wrist flexion (soft), elbow flexion in supination (medium), and knee extension (hard). Abnormal: Inappropriate stretch ability for a specific joint. If too hard, may indicate a hypomobility due to arthrosis; if too soft, a hypermobility.

information about the integrity of the contractile and inert tissues, and the *end-feel*. Cyriax[8] introduced the concept of the end-feel, which is the quality of resistance felt at the end range. The end-feel can indicate to the clinician the cause of the motion restriction (Tables 3-14 and 3-15).

Table 3-15 Abnormal End-feels

Type	Causes	Characteristics and Examples
Springy	Produced by the articular surface rebounding from an intra-articular meniscus or disc. The impression is that if forced further, something will collapse.	A rebound sensation as if pushing off from a Sorbo rubber pad. Examples: Normal: Axial compression of the cervical spine. Abnormal: Knee flexion or extension with a displaced meniscus.
Boggy	Produced by viscous fluid (blood) within a joint.	A "squishy" sensation as the joint is moved toward its end range. Further forcing feels as if it will burst the joint. Examples: Normal: None Abnormal: Hemarthrosis at the knee.
Spasm	Produced by reflex and reactive muscle contraction in response to irritation of the nociceptor predominantly in articular structures and muscle. Forcing it further feels as if nothing will give.	An abrupt and "twangy" end to movement that is unyielding while the structure is being threatened, but disappears when the threat is removed (kicks back). With joint inflammation, it occurs early in the range especially toward the close-pack position to prevent further stress. With an irritable joint hypermobility it occurs at the end of what should be normal range as it prevents excessive motion from further stimulating the nociceptor. Spasm in grade II muscle tears becomes apparent as the muscle is passively lengthened and is accompanied by a painful weakness of that muscle. Note: Muscle guarding is not a true end feel as it involves a co-contraction Examples: Normal: None Abnormal: Significant traumatic arthritis, recent traumatic hypermobility, grade II muscle tears.
Empty	Produced solely by pain. Frequently caused by serious and severe pathological changes that do not affect the joint or muscle and so do not produce spasm. Demonstration of this end feel is, with the exception of acute subdeltoid bursitis, de facto evidence of serious pathology. Further forcing simply increases the pain to unacceptable levels.	The limitation of motion has no tissue resistance component and the resistance is from the patient being unable to tolerate further motion due to severe pain. It is not the same feeling as voluntary guarding but rather it feels as if the patient is both resisting and trying to allow the movement simultaneously. Examples: Normal: None Abnormal: Acute subdeltoid bursitis, sign of the buttock.

(continued on following page)

Table 3-15 *(continued from previous page)*

Type	Causes	Characteristics and Examples
Facilitation	Not truly an end feel as facilitated hypertonicity does not restrict motion. It can, however, be perceived near the end range.	A light resistance as from a constant light muscle contraction throughout the latter half of the range that does not prevent the end of range being reached. The resistance is unaffected by the rate of movement. Examples: Normal: None Abnormal: Spinal facilitation at any level.

Clinical Pearl

The barrier to active motion should occur earlier in the range than the barrier to passive motion.

Clinical Pearl

Pain that occurs at the end range of active and passive movement is suggestive of hypermobility or instability, a capsular contraction, or scar tissue that has not been adequately remodeled.[8]

Clinical Pearl

The type of end-feel can help the clinician determine the presence of dysfunction (Figure 3-4). For example, a hard, capsular end-feel indicates a pericapsular hypomobility, whereas a jammed or pathomechanical end-feel indicates a pathomechanical hypomobility.

A normal end-feel would indicate normal range, whereas an abnormal end-feel would suggest abnormal range, either hypomobile or hypermobile. An association between an increase in pain and abnormal-pathological end-feels compared to normal end-feels has been demonstrated.[12]

 Clinical Pearl

The planned intervention, and its intensity, is based on the type of tissue resistance to movement demonstrated by the end-feel, and the acuteness of the condition (Table 3-16).[8] This information may indicate whether the resistance is caused by pain, muscle, capsule, ligament, disturbed mechanics of the joint, or a combination.

Flexibility

An examination of flexibility is performed to determine whether a particular structure, or group of structures, has sufficient extensibility to perform a desired activity.

Table 3-16 Abnormal Barriers to Motion and Recommended Manual Techniques*

Barrier	End Feel	Technique
Pain	Empty	None
Pain	Spasm	None
Pain	Capsular	Oscillations (I, IV)
Joint adhesions	Early capsular	Passive articular motion stretch (I–V)
Muscle adhesions	Early elastic	Passive physiological motion stretch
Hypertonicity	Facilitation	Hold/relax
Bone	Bony	None

*Data from reference 8.

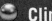 **Clinical Pearl**

A decrease in the length of the soft tissue structures, or adaptive shortening, is very common in postural dysfunctions.

Adaptive shortening can also be produced by the following:
• Restricted mobility
• Tissue damage secondary to trauma
• Prolonged immobilization
• Disease
• Hypertonia. Observation will reveal the muscle to be raised, and the muscle will feel hard and may stand out from those around it.

Capsular and Noncapsular Patterns of Restriction

Cyriax[8] gave us the terms *capsular* and *noncapsular* pattern of restriction, which link impairment to pathology (Table 3-17).

  Clinical Pearl

• A capsular pattern of restriction is a limitation of pain and movement in a joint specific ratio, which is usually present with arthritis, or following prolonged immobilization (Figure 3-4).[8]

  Clinical Pearl

• A noncapsular pattern of restriction is a limitation in a joint in any pattern other than a capsular one, and may indicate the presence of a derangement, a restriction of one part of the joint capsule, or an extra-articular lesion that obstructs joint motion (Figure 3-4).[8]

Joint Integrity and Mobility

The small motion, which is available at the joint surfaces (arthrokinematic motion), is referred to as *accessory* motion. A variety of different measurement

Table 3-17 Capsular Patterns of Restriction*

Joint	Limitation of Motion (Passive Angular Motion)
Glenohumeral	External rotation > abduction > internal rotation (3:2:1)
Acromioclavicular	No true capsular pattern. Possible loss of horizontal adduction, pain (and sometimes slight loss of end range) with each motion
Sternoclavicular	See above: acromioclavicular joint
Humeroulnar	Flexion > extension (±4:1)
Humeroradial	No true capsular pattern. Possible equal limitation of pronation and supination
Superior radioulnar	No true capsular pattern. Possible equal limitation of pronation and supination with pain at end ranges
Inferior radioulnar	No true capsular pattern. Possible equal limitation of pronation and supination with pain at end ranges
Wrist (carpus)	Flexion = extension
Radiocarpal Carpometacarpal Mid carpal	See above (carpus)
First carpometacarpal	Retroposition
Carpometacarpal 2–5	Fan > fold
Metacarpophalangeal 2–5	Flexion > extension (±2:1)
Interphalangeal Proximal (PIP) Distal (DIP)	Flexion > extension (±2:1)
Hip	Internal rotation > flexion > abdduction = extension > other motions
Tibiofemoral	Flexion > extension (±5:1)
Superior tibiofibular	No capsular pattern: pain at end range of translatory movements
Talocrural	Plantar flexion > dorsiflexion
Talocalcaneal (subtalar)	Varus > valgus

(continued on following page)

Table 3-17 *(continued from previous page)*

Joint	Limitation of Motion (Passive Angular Motion)
Midtarsal	
Talonavicular calcaneocuboid	Inversion (plantar flexion, adduction, supination) > dorsiflexion
First metatarsophalangeal	Extension > flexion (±2:1)
Metatarsophalangeal 2–5	Flexion >/= extension
Interphalangeal 2–5	
Proximal	Flexion >/= extension
Distal	Flexion >/= extension

*Data from reference 8.

scales have been proposed for judging the amount of accessory joint motion present between two joint surfaces, most of which are based on a comparison with a comparable contralateral joint using manually applied forces in a logical and precise manner (refer to Passive Accessory Mobility Tests).[13]

 Clinical Pearl

- After assessing the joint glide, joint motion is described as hypo-mobile, normal, or hypermobile (refer to Chapter 1).[14-16]

Passive Accessory Mobility Tests
The passive articular mobility (PAM) tests involve the clinician assessing the accessory motions of a joint.

 Clinical Pearl

The joint glides are tested in the open (loose) pack position of a peripheral joint (refer to Chapter 1) and at the end of available range in the spinal joints, to avoid soft tissue tension affecting the results.

By performing a joint glide, information about the integrity of the inert structures will be given in one of four scenarios (Figure 3-6).

MOBILITY TEST RESULT	SCENARIO	RATIONALE	INTERVENTION
The joint glide is unrestricted	The joint glide is unrestricted	The integrity of both the joint surface and the periarticular tissue is good. If this is the case, the patient's loss of motion must be due to a contractile tissue.	With this scenario, the intervention should emphasize soft tissue mobilization techniques designed to change the length of a contractile tissue.
	The joint glide is both unrestricted and excessive	Stress tests (see Special tests) are then used to assess the integrity of the inert tissues, particularly the ligaments, and to determine whether instability exists at the joint. Instability at a joint may occur if the joint has undergone significant degenerative changes or trauma.	The intervention for excessive motion that is impeding function focuses on stabilizing techniques designed to give secondary support to the joint through muscle action.
The joint glide is restricted	The joint surface and periarticular tissues are implicated as the cause	If the joint surface and periarticular tissues are at fault, a specific joint mobilization to restore the glide should solve the problem.	Distraction and compression can be used to help differentiate the cause of the restriction. If the distraction increases the pain, it may indicate a tear of connective tissue. If the compression increases the pain, a loose body or internal derangement of the joint may be present. The intervention is based on the cause.
	The contractile tissues are adaptively shortened	If after the specific mobilization of the joint, the osteokinematic motion is still reduced, the surrounding tissues have likely adaptively shortened.	The intervention involves addressing the adaptive shortening through stretching and flexibility exercises.

Figure 3-6 Sequence for determining the cause of loss of motion.

Clinical Pearl

By assessing accessory joint motions, the clinician can determine the following[17]:

- The cause of a limitation in a joint's physiological range of motion[18]
- The end-feel response of the tissues[8]
- The stage of healing[19]
- The integrity of the ligaments at a joint (e.g., the Lachman test).

Clinical Pearl

Based on the information gleaned from the joint glide assessment, the clinician makes clinical decisions as to which intervention to use (Figures 3-4 to 3-6).

- If the joint play is felt to be restricted, and there is no indication of a bony end-feel, or severe irritability, joint mobilization techniques are used.
- If the joint play is found to be unrestricted, the clinician may decide to employ a technique that increases the extensibility of the surrounding connective tissues, as abnormal shortness of these connective tissues, including the ligaments, the joint capsule, and the periarticular tissues, can restrict joint mobility.

Clinical Pearl

The same techniques used to assess the joint motion can be used for joint mobilization by adjusting the grade.

Muscle Performance: Strength, Power, and Endurance

Strength testing, generally using manual muscle testing, measures the power with which musculotendinous units act across a bone-joint lever-arm system to actively generate motion, or passively resist movement against gravity and variable resistance.[20]

Clinical Pearl

Voluntary muscle strength testing remains somewhat subjective until a precise way of measuring muscle contraction is generally available.[20] Factors such as pain, motivation, cooperation, fatigue, poor instruction, and fear potentially magnify the subjectivity of muscle testing.[21]

Clinical Pearl

By definition, a contractile tissue is a tissue involved with a muscle contraction, and one that can be tested using an isolated muscle contraction. However, contractile tissues, such as tendons, which have no ability to contract, could be classified as inert, as while they are strongly affected by the contraction of their respective muscle bellies, they are also affected if passively stretched. Conversely, inert tissues, which also have no ability to contract, can be compressed, and therefore affected, during a contraction. Inert tissues are mainly tested with passive movement and ligament stress tests.

According to Cyriax, pain with a contraction generally indicates an injury.

Clinical Pearl

If a muscle contraction causes pain, it is likely that there is an injury to the muscle or a capsular structure.[8] The cause can be determined by assessing passive motion (placing stretch on injured contractile tissue will increase the symptoms) and distraction (to stretch the joint capsule) and compression (to grind the joint surfaces together) of the joint.

In addition to examining the integrity of the contractile and inert structures, strength testing may be used to examine the integrity of the myotomes.

Clinical Pearl

A myotome is defined as a muscle or group of muscles served by a single nerve root. *Key muscle* is a better, more accurate term, as the

Table 3-18 Findings From Muscle Testing

Finding	Possible Explanation
Strong and painless contraction	Normal finding
Strong and painful contraction	Grade I contractile lesion
Weak and painless contraction	• Palsy • Complete rupture of the muscle–tendon unit
Weak and painful contraction	Serious pathology such as a significant muscle tear, fracture, tumor, and so on

muscles tested are the most representative of the supply from a particular segment.

Pain that occurs consistently with resistance, at whatever the length of the muscle, may indicate a tear of the muscle belly. Pain with muscle testing may indicate a muscle injury, a joint injury, or a combination of both (Figure 3-2). Table 3-18 outlines four scenarios of muscle testing based on the work of Cyriax.[8,22]

 Clinical Pearl

Pain that does not occur during the test, but occurs upon the release of the contraction, is thought to have an articular source, produced by the joint glide that occurs following the release of tension.

Manual muscle testing techniques begin by placing the muscle in a shortened position and then proceeding with the examination by resisting the movement. If a position other than the standard position is used, it must be documented.

 Clinical Pearl

The degree of significance with the findings in resisted testing depends on the position of the muscle, and the force applied (Table 3-19). For example, pain reproduced with a minimal contrac-

Table 3-19 Strength Testing Related to Joint Position and Muscle Length

Muscle Length	Rationale/Purpose
Fully lengthened	Muscle in position of passive insufficiency Tightens the inert component of the muscle Tests for muscle tears (tendoperiosteal tears) while using minimal force
Mid-range	Muscle in strongest position Tests overall power of muscle
Fully shortened	Muscle in its weakest position Used for the detection of palsies especially if coupled with an eccentric contraction

tion in the rest position for the muscle is more strongly suggestive of a contractile lesion than pain reproduced with a maximal contraction in the lengthened position for the muscle.

Whenever possible, the same muscle is tested on the opposite side, using the same testing procedure, and a comparison is made.

A number of scales have been devised to assess muscle strength (Tables 3-20, and 3-21).[23,24]

Clinical Pearl

All of the grading systems for manual muscle testing produce ordinal data with unequal rankings between grades and all are innately subjective as they rely on the subject's ability to exert the maximal contraction.

Clinical Pearl

The primary tenet of manual muscle testing is that each muscle should be tested just proximal to the next distal joint of the muscle's insertion and that the clinician must place the subject in positions

Table 3-20 Muscle Grading*

Grade	Value	Movement
5	Normal (100%)	Complete range of motion against gravity with maximal resistance
4	Good (75%)	Complete range of motion against gravity with some (moderate) resistance
3+	Fair +	Complete range of motion against gravity with minimal resistance
3	Fair (50%)	Complete range of motion against gravity
3−	Fair −	Some but not complete range of motion against gravity
2+	Poor +	Initiates motion against gravity
2	Poor (25%)	Complete range of motion with gravity eliminated
2−	Poor −	Initiates motion if gravity eliminated
1	Trace	Evidence of slight contractility but no joint motion
0	Zero	No contraction palpated

*Data from reference 23.

Table 3-21 Muscle Grading According to Janda*

Grade	Interpretation
Grade 5—N (normal)	A normal, very strong muscle with a full range of movement and able to overcome considerable resistance. This does not mean that the muscle is normal in all circumstances (e.g., when at the onset of fatigue or in a state of exhaustion).
Grade 4—G (good)	A muscle with good strength and a full range of movement, and able to overcome moderate resistance.
Grade 3—F (fair)	A muscle with a complete range of movement against gravity only when resistance is not applied.
Grade 2—P (poor)	A very weak muscle with a complete range of motion only when gravity is eliminated by careful positioning of the patient.
Grade 1—T (trace)	A muscle with evidence of slight contractility but no effective movement.
Grade 0	A muscle with no evidence of contractility.

* Data from reference 24.

that will isolate, as much as possible, the specific muscle or muscles being examined and eliminate substitution of agonist muscles.[21]

To be a valid test, strength testing must elicit a maximum contraction of the muscle being tested. Four strategies ensure this:

1. Placing the muscle to be tested in a shortened position. This puts the muscle in an inefficient physiological position and has the effect of increasing motor neuron activity.

2. Having the patient perform an eccentric muscle contraction by using the command "Don't let me move you." As the tension at each cross-bridge and the number of active cross-bridges is greater during an eccentric contraction, the maximum eccentric muscle tension developed is greater with an eccentric contraction than a concentric one (see Chapter 1).

3. Breaking the contraction. It is important to break the patient's muscle contraction to ensure that the patient is making a maximal effort and that the full power of the muscle is being tested.

4. Holding the contraction for at least 5 seconds. Weakness due to nerve palsy has a distinct fatigability and the muscle demonstrates poor endurance as it is usually only able to sustain a maximum muscle contraction for about two to three seconds before complete failure occurs.

   a. This is based on the theories behind muscle recruitment wherein a normal muscle while performing a maximum contraction uses only a portion of its motor units, keeping the remainder in reserve to help maintain the contraction. A palsied muscle with its fewer functioning motor units has very few, if any, in reserve. If a muscle appears to be weaker than normal, further investigation is required.

   b. The test is repeated three times. Muscle weakness resulting from disuse will be consistently weak and should not get weaker with several repeated contractions.

🔵 Clinical Pearl

The key differentiation in manual muscle testing is grade 3/Fair—the ability of the patient to perform complete range of motion of the joint against gravity. Substitutions by other muscle groups during testing, indicates the presence of weakness. It does not, however, tell the clinician the cause of the weakness.

Another muscle that shares the same innervation (spinal nerve or peripheral nerve) is tested. Knowledge of both spinal nerve and peripheral nerve innervation will aid the clinician in determining which muscle to select.

Clinical Pearl

Multiple studies have shown good intertester and intratester reliability with manual muscle testing and a high degree of exact consistency to within one grade using some form of the Medicine Research Council's grading sequence (0–5).[21]

Clinical Pearl

Each peripheral nerve that crosses an acute injury or chronic disorder of the extremity should be evaluated.

The standard manual muscle testing positions as described by Kendall are depicted in Figures 3-7 to Figure 3-41.

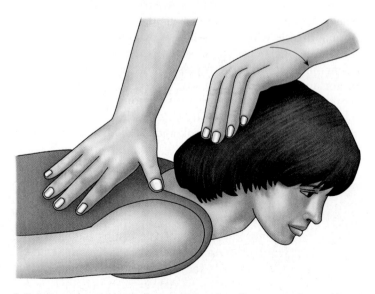

Figure 3-7 Manual muscle testing position for the posterolateral head and neck extensors.

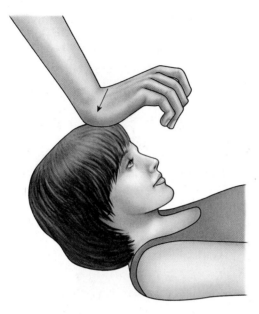

Figure 3-8 Manual muscle testing position for the anterior head and neck flexors.

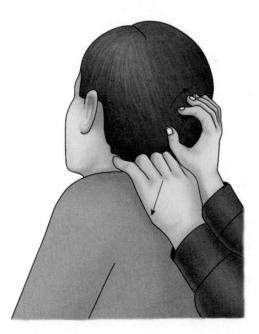

Figure 3-9 Manual muscle testing position for the upper trapezius.

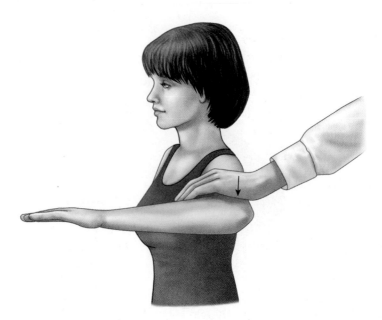

Figure 3-10 Manual muscle testing position for the supraspinatus and middle deltoid.

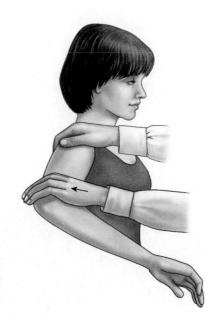

Figure 3-11 Manual muscle testing position for the posterior deltoid.

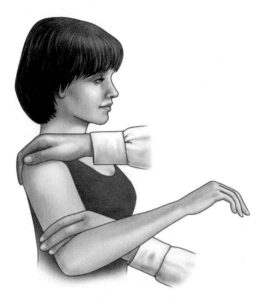

Figure 3-12 Manual muscle testing position for the anterior deltoid.

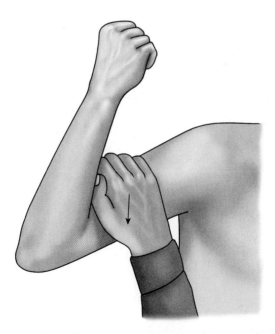

Figure 3-13 Manual muscle testing position for the coracobrachialis.

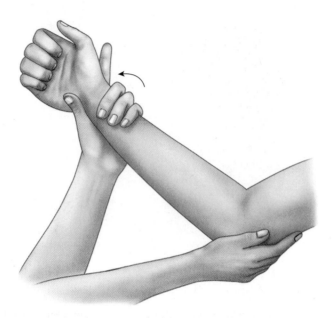

Figure 3-14 Manual muscle testing position for the brachioradialis (forearm in neutral).

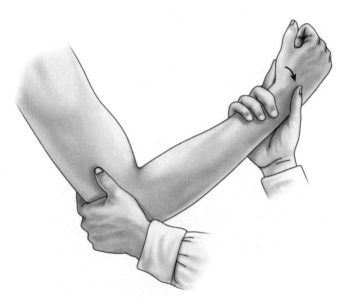

Figure 3-15 Manual muscle testing position for the biceps (forearm supinated).

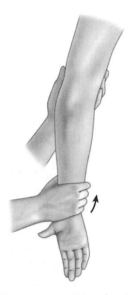

Figure 3-16 Manual muscle testing position for the triceps brachii and anconeus.

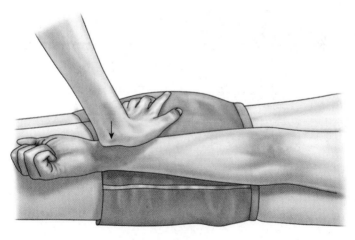

Figure 3-17 Manual muscle testing position for the latissimus dorsi.

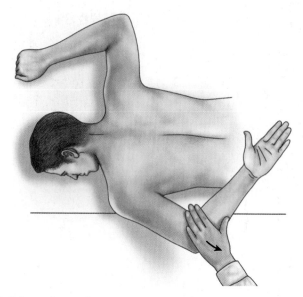

Figure 3-18 Manual muscle testing position for the teres major.

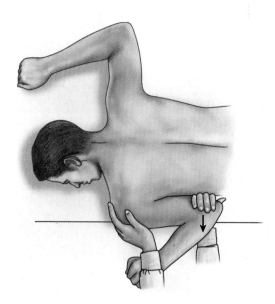

Figure 3-19 Manual muscle testing position for the rhomboids and levator scapulae.

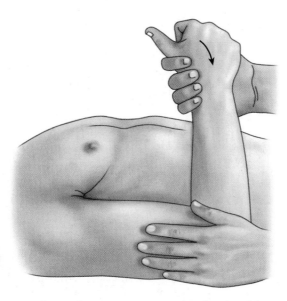

Figure 3-20 Manual muscle testing position for the shoulder internal rotators.

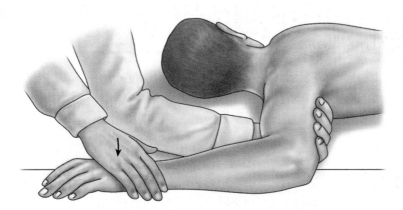

Figure 3-21 Manual muscle testing position for the shoulder external rotators.

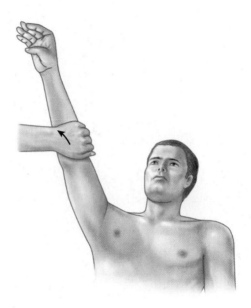

Figure 3-22 Manual muscle testing position for the pectoralis major (lower fibers) with the patient in supine.

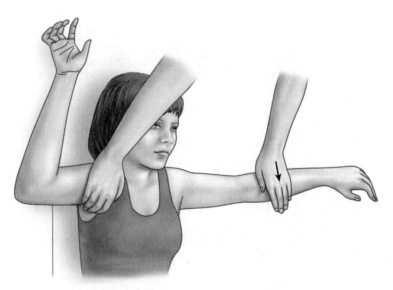

Figure 3-23 Manual muscle testing position for the pectoralis major (upper fibers).

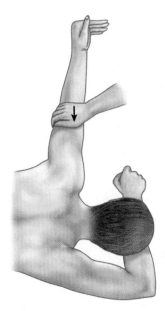

Figure 3-24 Manual muscle testing position for the middle trapezius.

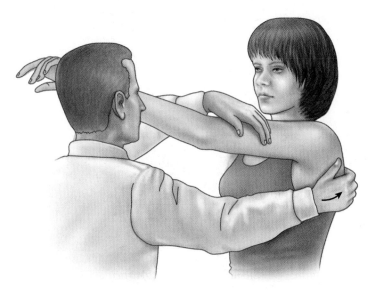

Figure 3-25 Manual muscle testing position for the serratus anterior.

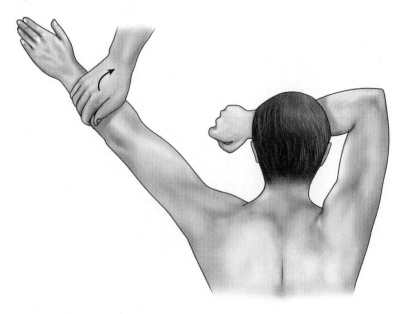

Figure 3-26 Manual muscle testing position for the lower trapezius.

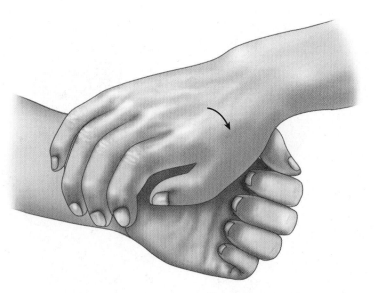

Figure 3-27 Manual muscle testing position for the flexor carpi radialis.

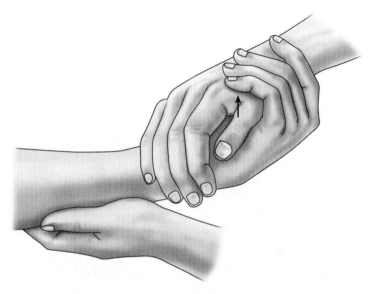

Figure 3-28 Manual muscle testing position for the flexor carpi ulnaris.

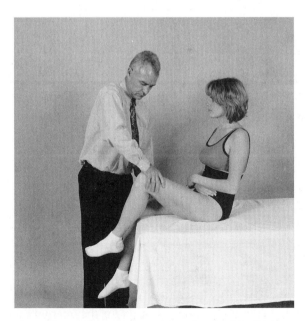

Figure 3-29 Manual muscle testing position for the hip flexors.

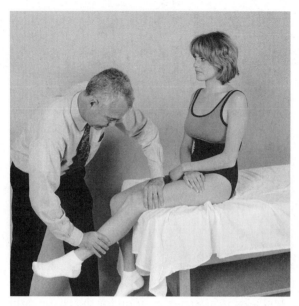

Figure 3-30 Manual muscle testing position for the quadriceps femoris (knee extensors).

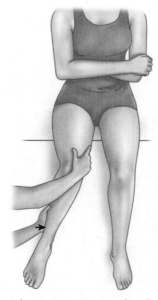

Figure 3-31 Manual muscle testing position for the internal rotators of the hip.

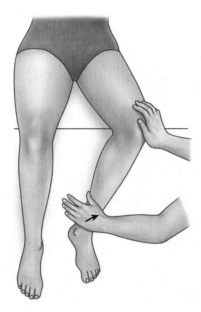

Figure 3-32 Manual muscle testing position for the external rotators of the hip.

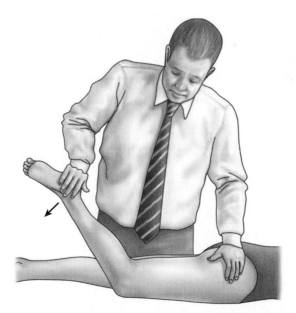

Figure 3-33 Manual muscle testing position for the medial hamstrings.

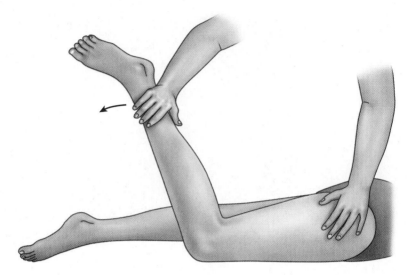

Figure 3-34 Manual muscle testing position for the lateral hamstrings.

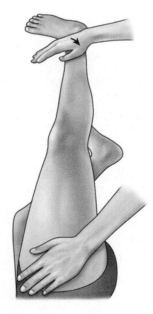

Figure 3-35 Manual muscle testing position for the gluteus medius.

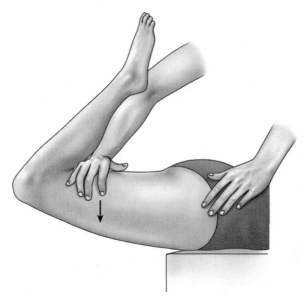

Figure 3-36 Manual muscle testing position for the gluteus maximus.

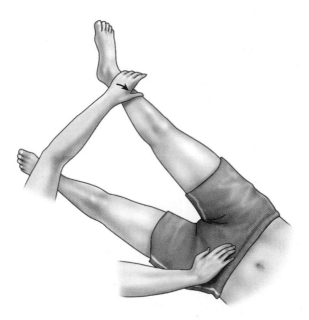

Figure 3-37 Manual muscle testing position for the iliopsoas.

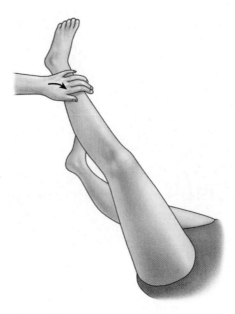

Figure 3-38 Manual muscle testing position for the tensor of the fascia latae

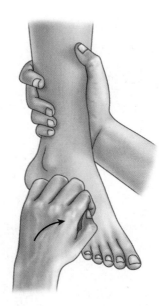

Figure 3-39 Manual muscle testing position for the fibularis (peroneus) tertius.

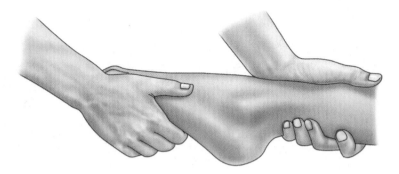

Figure 3-40 Manual muscle testing position for the tibialis posterior.

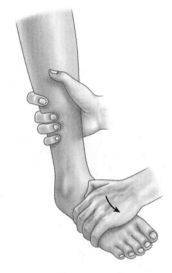

Figure 3-41 Manual muscle testing position for the tibialis anterior.

 Clinical Pearl

There are two major criticisms of manual muscle testing[21]:

1. Grade 4 strength encompasses the ability of the patient to go through full range of motion against gravity with no, little, or

overwhelming clinician resistance. This will obviously differ between clinicians of different strengths and sizes.

2. The overestimation of strength when the muscle is weak as identified by quantitative muscle testing (e.g., isokinetic testing, handheld dynamometer), yet it is graded as normal by manual muscle testing.

Indeed, many studies have shown that reliability in manual muscle testing is dependent on the specific muscle being examined.

As always, these tests cannot be evaluated in isolation, but have to be integrated into a total clinical profile, before drawing any conclusion about the patient's condition.

Neurological Testing

The evaluation of the transmission capability of the nervous system is performed to detect the presence of either an upper motor neuron (UMN) lesion or a lower motor neuron (LMN) lesion.

 Clinical Pearl

- An UMN lesion is also known as a central palsy and is characterized by spastic paralysis or paresis, little or no muscle atrophy, hyperreflexive DTRs in a nonsegmental distribution, and the presence of pathological signs and reflexes.

 Clinical Pearl

- A LMN lesion is also known as a peripheral palsy. These lesions can be due to direct trauma, toxins, infections, ischemia, and compression. The characteristics of a LMN include muscle atrophy and hypotonus, a diminished or absent DTRs of the areas served by a spinal nerve root, or a peripheral nerve and an absence of pathological signs or reflexes.

Muscles Stretch Reflexes

Muscle stretch reflexes (Table 3-22) can be graded as follows:

0 Absent (areflexia)
1+ Decreased (hyporeflexia)
2+ Normal
3+ Hyperactive (brisk)
4+ Hyperactive with clonus (hyperreflexive)

Each of these categories can occur as a generalized, or local, phenomenon. The absence of a reflex signifies an interruption of the reflex arc. A hyperactive reflex with clonus denotes a release from cortical inhibitory influences.

 Clinical Pearl

Even though muscles stretch reflexes have long been assumed to be very objective, the grading of muscle stretch reflexes between

Table 3-22 Common Deep Tendon Reflexes

Reflex	Site of Stimulus	Normal Response	Pertinent Central Nervous System Segment
Jaw	Mandible	Mouth closes	Cranial nerve V
Biceps	Biceps tendon	Biceps contraction	C5–C6
Brachioradialis	Brachioradialis tendon or just distal to the musculotendinous junction	Flexion of elbow and/or pronation of forearm	C5–C6
Triceps	Distal triceps tendon above the olecranon process	Elbow extension	C7–C8
Patella	Patellar tendon	Leg extension	L3–L4
Medial hamstrings	Semimembranosus tendon	Knee flexion	L5, S1
Lateral hamstrings	Biceps femoris tendon	Knee flexion	S1–S2
Tibialis posterior	Tibialis posterior tendon behind medial malleolus	Plantar flexion of foot with inversion	L4–L5
Achilles	Achilles tendon	Plantar flexion of foot	S1–S2

different observers for the same subject is quite variable and subjective due to both patient and clinician factors.[21]

Clinical Pearl

Reflex asymmetry has more pathological significance than the absolute activity of the reflex. For example, a bilateral patella reflex of 3+ is less significant than a 3+ on the left and a 2+ on the right.

Clinical Pearl

The Jendrassik maneuver is the most common method of reinforcing reflexes—the patient is asked to hook together the flexed fingers of his or her right and left hands and pull them apart as strongly as possible while the clinician is attempting to elicit the muscle stretch reflex (Figure 3-42).

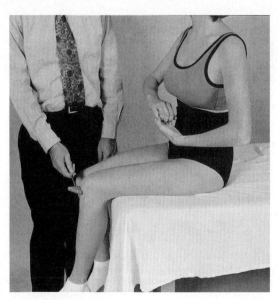

Figure 3-42 The Jendrassik maneuver used during reflex testing.

Hyporeflexia, if not generalized to the whole body, indicates a LMN or sensory paresis, which may be segmental (root), multisegmental (cauda equina), or nonsegmental (peripheral nerve).

True neurological hyperreflexia contains a clonic component and is suggestive of CNS (UMN) impairment such as a brainstem or cerebral impairment, spinal cord compression, or a neurological disease. A brisk reflex is a normal finding, provided that it is not masking a hyperreflexia due to an incorrect testing technique. Unlike hyperreflexia, a brisk reflex does not have a clonic component.

 Clinical Pearl

As with hyporeflexia, the clinician should assess more than one reflex before coming to a conclusion about a hyperreflexia, and can confirm the presence of a UMN with the presence of the pathological reflexes.

Pathological Reflexes

 Clinical Pearl

• The presence of pathological reflexes (Babinski, Oppenheim, Hoffmann) and clonus is suggestive of CNS (UMN) impairment, and requires an appropriate referral.

 Clinical Pearl

The significance of the Hoffmann sign remains disputed in the literature—the validity has not been well studied, although poor to fair sensitivity and fair to good specificity are reported.[25]

Superficial Skin Reflexes
The abdominal and cremaster reflexes are decreased or absent on the side affected by a corticospinal tract lesion and, thus, serve as adjuncts to the muscle stretch and plantar reflexes (Table 3-23).[26]

Table 3-23 Superficial Reflexes

Reflex	Normal Response	Pertinent Central Nervous System Segment
Upper abdominal	Umbilicus moves up and toward area being stroked	T7–T9
Lower abdominal	Umbilicus moves down and toward area being stroked	T11–T12
Cremasteric	Scrotum elevates	T12, L1
Plantar	Flexion of toes	S1–S2
Gluteal	Skin tenses in gluteal area	L4–L5, S1–S3
Anal	Contraction of anal sphincter muscles	S2–S4

Supraspinal Reflexes

A number of processes, which are involved in locomotor function, are oriented around the supraspinal reflexes and referred to as postural reflexes.

 Clinical Pearl

The cervico-ocular reflexes (CORs) and vestibulo-ocular reflexes (VORs) work together to help maintain postural equilibrium and stability during head, trunk, and extremity motions, and *visual fixation* of the eyes during movements of the head and neck.

Sensory Testing

The dorsal roots of the spinal nerves are represented by a series of peripheral sensory regions called dermatomes (Figure 2-2). The peripheral sensory nerves are represented by a number of more distinct and circumscribed areas (Figure 2-2).

 Clinical Pearl

Inouye and Buchthal[27] recorded evoked potentials from C5 to C8 just outside the intervertebral foramen after stimulation of various peripheral nerves and digits. They found dermatomal distributions that were consistent with previous research, although they noted considerable individual variability.

Sensory testing is performed throughout the dermatomal areas. The segmental innervation of the skin has a high degree of overlap, especially in the thoracic spine, necessitating the clinician to test the full area of the dermatome. This is done to seek out the area of sensitivity, or autogenous area, which is a small region of the dermatome with no overlap, and the only area within a dermatome that is supplied exclusively by a single segmental level.[28]

 Clinical Pearl

It is important to start sensory testing using an area of normal sensation before moving toward an area of altered sensation to provide the patient with an appropriate reference point.

Pain sensation is generally tested with a pin or needle, and soft touch is adequately tested with a wisp of cotton.

 Clinical Pearl

Mapping the area of involvement helps to categorize the abnormality into a specifically defined syndrome (i.e., dermatomal, nerve, nerve root, or glove and stocking pattern), a spinal cord lesion, or a peripheral nerve abnormality.[29]

The proximal sensory examination should be compared with the distal examination, paying special attention to areas of numbness. Symmetric distal sensory loss is compatible with a polyneuropathy.

 Clinical Pearl

Overall, the sensitivity, specificity, and reliability of the sensory examination are poorly described in the peer-reviewed literature.

Vibration sense is tested by placing the stem of a 128- or 256-cps (cycles per second) tuning fork against several bony prominences, beginning at the most distal joints.

Clinical Pearl

Loss of vibratory sensation occurs relatively early in a peripheral neuropathy such as those related to diabetes, alcoholism, vitamin B_{12} deficiency, or dorsal column disease.[29]

If the patient does not respond in the distal joints, the more proximal joints should be checked.

Clinical Pearl

The clinician should make sure the patient is responding to the vibration of the tuning fork and not the pressure of the instrument by occasionally dampening the vibration and eliciting a response.[29]

Proprioception is tested by grasping the sides of the finger or toe being tested and asking the patient, whose eyes should be closed, to indicate whether the digit is placed in an up or a down position.

Clinical Pearl

A loss of position sense is associated with a nerve root lesion, a peripheral nerve abnormality, or dorsal column disease.

Thermal sensation is tested with test tubes filled with water of various temperatures. Patients with normal thermal sensation should be able to distinguish between stimuli differing by a few degrees.[29] Unfortunately, this test relies on a subjective patient response, which is dependent on the patient's level of motivation and cognition.

Cranial Nerve Examination

With practice, the entire cranial nerve examination (Table 3-24)[30] can be performed in approximately 5 minutes.[31] The following may

Table 3-24 Cranial Nerves and Methods of Testing*

	Nerve	Afferent (Sensory)	Efferent (Motor)	Test
I	Olfactory	Smell	—	Identify familiar odors (e.g., chocolate, coffee); test visual fields
II	Optic	Sight	—	
III	Oculomotor	—	*Voluntary motor:* levator of eyelid; superior, medial, and inferior recti; inferior oblique muscle of eyeball *Autonomic:* smooth muscle of eyeball	Upward, downward, and medical gaze; reaction to light
IV	Trochlear	—	*Voluntary motor:* superior oblique muscle of eyeball	Downward and lateral gaze
V	Trigeminal	Touch, pain: skin of face, mucous membranes of nose, sinuses, mouth, anterior tongue	*Voluntary motor:* muscles of mastication	Corneal reflex; face sensation; clench teeth, push down on chin to separate jaws
VI	Abducens	—	*Voluntary motor:* lateral rectus muscle of eyeball	Lateral gaze
VII	Facial	Taste: anterior tongue	*Voluntary motor:* facial muscles *Autonomic:* lacrimal, submandibular, and sublingual glands	Close eyes tight; smile and show teeth; whistle and puff cheeks; identify familiar tastes (e.g., sweet, sour)
VIII	Vestibulocochlear (acoustic nerve)	Hearing: ear Balance: ear	— —	Hear watch ticking Hearing tests; balance and coordination test
IX	Glossopharyngeal	Touch, pain: posterior tongue, pharynx Taste: posterior tongue	*Voluntary motor:* unimportant muscle of pharynx *Autonomic:* parotid gland	Gag reflex; ability to swallow
X	Vagus	Touch, pain; pharynx, larynx, bronchi Taste: tongue, epiglottis	*Voluntary motor:* muscles of palate, pharynx, and larynx *Autonomic: thoracic* and abdominal viscera	Gag reflex; ability to swallow; say "Ahhh"

(continued on following page)

Table 3-24 *(continued from previous page)*

	Nerve	Afferent (Sensory)	Efferent (Motor)	Test
XI	Accessory	—	*Voluntary motor:* sternocleidomastoid and trapezius muscles	Resisted shoulder shrug
XII	Hypoglossal	—	*Voluntary motor:* muscles of tongue	Tongue protrusion (if injured, tongue deviates toward injured side)

*Data from reference 30.

be used to help remember the order and tests for the cranial nerve examination[32]:

- Smell and see (CN I and II, respectively)
- And look around (CN III)
- Pupils large and smaller. (CN IV)
- Smile, hear! (CN V–VIII)
- Then say ah… (CN IX–X)
- And see if you can swallow (CN XI)
- If you're left in any doubt
- Shrug and stick your tongue right out (CN XII)

Neurodynamic Mobility Tests

Neurodynamic mobility testing is designed to examine the neurological structures for adaptive shortening and inflammation of the neural structures both centrally and peripherally.

 Clinical Pearl

Neurodynamic mobility tests are only used if a dural adhesion or irritation is suspected.

The tests employ a sequential and progressive stretch to the dura until the patient's symptoms are reproduced.[33] Theoretically, if the dura is scarred, or inflamed, a lack of extensibility with stretching occurs.

Clinical Pearl

Because the sinuvertebral nerve innervates the dural sleeve, the pain due to an inflamed dura, is felt by the patient at multisegmental levels, and is described as having an ache-like quality. If the patient experiences sharp or stabbing pain during the test, a more serious underlying condition should be suspected.

Tests for the lumbosacral plexus stress the sciatic nerve and include the slump test, the straight leg raise (SLR), and the prone knee bend.

Tests for the brachial plexus, the so-called upper limb tension tests (ULTTs), include tests for the median, radial, and ulnar nerve. Tests have also been designed to assess the neurodynamic mobility of the musculocutaneous, axillary, and suprascapular nerve.

Palpation

Palpation can play a central role in the diagnosis.[34]

 Clinical Pearl

Palpation should be performed at three levels of manual pressure: first with light pressure for conformity and temperature (tactile gnosis); second palpation for tissue induration and effusion; and finally palpation for tenderness.[35] By gradually increasing the manual pressure, the clinician will gain the confidence of the patient.

 Clinical Pearl

To help focus the palpation, ask the patient to place one finger on the spot that hurts the most.

The purpose of the palpatory examination is to[36,37]:

- Check for any vasomotor changes such as an increase in skin temperature that might suggest an inflammatory process
- Localize specific sites of swelling
- Identify specific anatomical structures and their relationship to one another

- Identify sites of point tenderness. Hyperalgic skin zones (HAZs) can be detected using skin drag, which consists of moving the pads of the fingertips over the surface of the skin, and attempting to sense resistance or drag
- Identify soft tissue texture changes or myofascial restriction. Normal tissue is soft and mobile and moves equally in all directions. Abnormal tissue may feel hard, or somewhat crunchy or stringy[38]
- Locate changes in muscle tone resulting from, trigger points, muscle spasm, hypertonicity, or hypotonicity
- Determine circulatory status by checking distal pulses
- Detect changes in the moisture of the skin

Aerobic Capacity and Endurance

Clinical indications for the use of the tests and measures for this category are based on the findings of the history and systems review. The aerobic capacity and endurance of a patient can be measured using standardized exercise test protocols (e.g., ergometry, step tests, time/distance walk/run tests, treadmill tests), and the patient's response to such tests.[5]

Anthropometric Characteristics

The use of an anthropometric examination and the subsequent measurements vary. Clearly, if there is a noticeable amount of effusion or swelling present, these measurements serve as an important baseline from which to judge the effectiveness of the intervention.

🌑 Clinical Pearl

- In general, the amount of swelling is related to the severity of the injury.
- A report of rapid swelling (within 2–4 hours) following a traumatic event may indicate bleeding into the joint.
- Swelling that is more gradual, occurring 8 to 24 hours following the trauma is likely caused by an inflammatory process or synovial swelling.
- An edematous limb indicates poor venous return. Pitting edema is characterized by an indentation of the skin after the pressure has been removed.

Clinical Pearl

The more serious reasons for swelling include fracture, tumor, congestive heart failure, and deep vein thombosis (DVT).

Gait, Locomotion, and Balance

Gait analysis is an important component of the examination process and should not just be reserved for those patients with lower extremity dysfunction. Gait, as with posture, varies between individuals, and a gait that differs from normal is not necessarily pathological. The examination of gait is performed to highlight any breakdown, including imbalances of flexibility and/or strength, or compensatory motions (Table 3-25).[39-47]

Table 3-25 Some Gait Deviations and Their Causes*

Gait Deviations	Reasons
Slower cadence than expected for person's age	Generalized weakness
	Pain
	Joint motion restrictions
	Poor voluntary motor control
Shorter stance phase on the involved side and a decreased swing phase on the uninvolved side • Shorter stride length on the uninvolved side • Decrease lateral sway over the involved stance limb • Decrease in cadence • Decrease in velocity • Use of an assistive device	Antalgic gait, resulting from a painful injury to the lower limb and pelvic region
Stance phase longer on one side	Pain
	Lack of trunk and pelvic rotation
	Weakness of lower limb muscles
	Restrictions in lower limb joints
	Poor muscle control
	Increased muscle tone

(continued on following page)

Table 3-25 *(continued from previous page)*

Gait Deviations	Reasons
Lateral trunk lean The purpose is to bring the center of gravity of the trunk nearer to the hip joint.	Ipsilateral lean—hip abductor weakness (gluteus medius/Trendelenburg gait) Contralateral lean—decreased hip flexion in swing limb Painful hip Abnormal hip joint (congenital dysplasia, coxa vara, etc.) Wide walking base Unequal leg length
Anterior trunk leaning Occurs at initial contact to move the line of gravity in front of the axis of the knee	Weak or paralyzed knee extensors, or gluteus maximus Decreased ankle dorsiflexion Hip flexion contracture
Posterior trunk leaning Occurs at initial contact to bring the line of the external force behind the axis of the hip	Weak or paralyzed hip extensors, especially the gluteus maximus (gluteus maximus gait) Hip pain Hip flexion contracture Inadequate hip flexion in swing Decreased knee range of motion
Increased lumbar lordosis Occurs at the end of the stance period	Inability to extend the hip, usually due to a flexion contracture or ankylosis
Pelvic drop during stance	Contralateral gluteus medius weakness Adaptive shortening of quadratus lumborum on the swing side Contralateral hip adductor spasticity
Excessive pelvic rotation	Adaptively shortened/spasticity of hip flexors on same side Limited hip joint flexion

Gait Deviations	Reasons
Circumducted hip Ground contact by the swinging leg can be avoided if it is swung outward (in order for natural walking to occur, the leg which is in its stance phase needs to be longer than the leg which is in its swing phase to allow toe clearance of the swing foot)	Functional leg length discrepancy Arthrogenic stiff hip or knee
Hip hiking The pelvis is lifted on the side of the swinging leg, by contraction of the spinal muscles and the lateral abdominal wall	Functional leg length discrepancy Inadequate hip flexion, knee flexion, or ankle dorsiflexion Hamstring weakness Quadratus lumborum shortening
Vaulting The ground clearance of the swinging leg will be increased if the subject goes up on the toes of the stance period leg	Functional leg length discrepancy Vaulting occurs on the shorter limb side
Abnormal internal hip rotation Produces a 'toe in' gait	Adaptive shortening of the iliotibial band Weakness of the hip external rotators Femoral anteversion Adaptive shortening of the hip internal rotators
Abnormal external hip rotation Produces a 'toe out' gait	Adaptive shortening of the hip external rotators Femoral retroversion Weakness of the hip internal rotators
Increased hip adduction (scissor gait) Results in excessive hip adduction during swing (scissoring), decreased base of support, and decreased progression of opposite foot	Spasticity or contracture of ipsilateral hip adductors Ipsilateral hip adductor weakness Coxa vara
Inadequate hip extension/Excessive hip flexion Results in loss of hip extension in mid stance (forward leaning of trunk, increased lordosis, and increased knee flexion and ankle dorsiflexion) and late stance (anterior pelvic tilt), and increased hip flexion in swing	Hip flexion contracture Iliotibial band contracture Hip flexor spasticity Pain Arthrodesis (surgical or spontaneous ankylosis) Loss of ankle dorsiflexion

(continued on following page)

Table 3-25 *(continued from previous page)*

Gait Deviations	Reasons
Inadequate hip flexion Results in decreased limb advancement in swing, posterior pelvic tilt, circumduction, and excessive knee flexion to clear foot	Hip flexor weakness Hip joint arthrodesis
Decreased hip swing through (psoatic limp) Manifested by exaggerated movements at the pelvis and trunk to assist the hip to move into flexion	Legg-Calve-Perthes disease Weakness or reflex inhibition of the psoas major muscle
Excessive knee extension/ Inadequate knee flexion Results in decreased knee flexion at initial contact and loading response, increased knee extension during stance, and decreased knee flexion during swing	Pain Anterior trunk deviation/bending Weakness of the quadriceps. The hyperextension is a compensation and places the body weight vector anterior to the knee Spasticity of the quadriceps. This is noted more during the loading response and during the initial swing intervals Joint deformity
Excessive knee flexion/Inadequate knee extension At initial contact or around mid stance. Results in increased knee flexion in early stance, decreased knee extension in mid stance and terminal stance, and decreased knee extension during swing	Knee flexion contracture resulting in decreased step length, and decreased knee extension in stance Increased tone/spasticity of hamstrings or hip flexors Decreased range of motion of ankle dorsiflexion in swing period Weakness of plantar flexors resulting in increased dorsiflexion in stance Lengthened limb
Inadequate dorsiflexion control ('foot slap') during initial contact to mid stance	Weak or paralyzed dorsiflexors Lack of lower limb proprioception
Steppage gait during the acceleration through deceleration of the swing phase Exaggerated knee and hip flexion are used to lift the foot higher than usual, for increased ground clearance resulting from a foot drop	Weak, or paralyzed dorsiflexor muscles Functional leg length discrepancy

Gait Deviations	Reasons
Increased walking base (> 20 cm)	
	Deformity such as hip abductor muscle contracture
	Genu valgus
	Fear of losing balance
	Leg length discrepancy
Decreased walking base (<10 cm)	
	Hip adductor muscle contracture
	Genu varum
Excessive eversion of calcaneus during initial contact through mid stance	
	Excessive tibia vara (refers to the frontal plane position of the distal 1/3 of the leg as it relates to the supporting surface)
	Forefoot varus
	Weakness of tibialis posterior
	Excessive lower extremity internal rotation (due to muscle imbalances, femoral anteversion)
Excessive pronation during mid stance through terminal stance	
	Insufficient ankle dorsiflexion (less than 10 degrees)
	Increased tibial varum
	Compensated forefoot or rearfoot varus deformity
	Uncompensated forefoot valgus deformity
	Pes planus
	Long limb
	Uncompensated medial rotation of tibia or femur
	Weak tibialis anterior
Excessive supination during initial contact through mid stance	
	Limited calcaneal eversion
	Rigid forefoot valgus
	Pes cavus
	Uncompensated lateral rotation of the tibia or femur
	Short limb
	Plantar flexed 1st ray
	Upper motor neuron muscle imbalance

(continued on following page)

Table 3-25 *(continued from previous page)*

Gait Deviations	Reasons
Excessive dorsiflexion	
	Compensation for knee flexion contracture
	Inadequate plantar flexor strength
	Adaptive shortening of dorsiflexors
	Increased muscle tone of dorsiflexors
	Pes calcaneus deformity
Excessive plantarflexion	
	Increased plantar flexor activity
	Plantar flexor contracture
Excessive varus	
	Contracture
	Overactivity of the muscles on the medial aspect of the foot
Excessive valgus	
	Weak invertors
	Foot hypermobility
Decreased or absence of propulsion (plantar flexor gait)	Inability of plantar flexors to perform function resulting in a shorter step length on the involved side.

*Data from references 40–47.

 Clinical Pearl

Assistive devices reduce weight-bearing stresses on the lower extremities while augmenting balance and stability. The choice of assistive device is based on patient need and clinical judgment.

- Canes: used on the contralateral side. The optimal length of a cane positions the patient's elbow in 20 degrees to 30 degrees of flexion when the tip of the cane is placed approximately 6 inches in front of and 6 inches lateral to the little toe.

- Crutches: offer more support than a cane, but less than a walker. As a general guideline, the crutch should be 77% of the patient's height. Allow 2 inches of clearance between the anterior axillary fold and the top of the crutch.

- Walkers: provide the greatest support and balance, but lack maneuverability. Rolling walkers require less energy to use, but are less stable than a standard walker.

Special Tests

Special tests for each area are dependent on the special needs and structure of each joint. Numerous tests exist for each joint. These tests are usually only performed if there is some indication that they would be helpful in arriving at a diagnosis. The tests help confirm or implicate a particular structure and may also provide information as to the degree of tissue damage.

Clinical Pearl

- The interpretation of the findings from a special test depends on the skill and experience of the clinician, the specificity of the test, and the degree of familiarity with the test.

Medical Laboratory Tests

Laboratory studies of blood, urine or joint (synovial) fluids are used to identify the presence and amount of chemicals, proteins, and other substances (Table 3-26).

Clinical Pearl

The most important laboratory tests in orthopedics are

- Erythrocyte sedimentation rate (ESR): a nonspecific screening test used to indirectly detect the presence of inflammation, infections, malignancy, and various collagen vascular diseases.
- C-reactive protein (CRP): used to determine a patient's risk for developing heart disease, but also used to detect inflammatory change (rheumatoid arthritis).

Table 3-26 Common Laboratory Values

Laboratory Test	Low Value	High Value
WBC count	<5000/mm3	>10,000/mm3
Neutrophils	<55%	>70%
Lymphocytes	>20%	>40%
Monocytes	<2%	>8%
Eosinophils	<1%	>4%
Basophils	<0.5%	>1%
RBC (male)	<4.7 million/mm3	>6.1 million/mm3
RBC (female)	<4.2 million/mm3	>5.4 million/mm3
Hemoglobin (male)	<14 g/dL	>17 g/dL
Hemoglobin (female)	<12 g/dL	>15 g/dL
Hematocrit (male)	<45%	>52%
Hematocrit (female)	<37%	>47%
Platelets	<150,000 mm3	>400,000 mm3
ESR (male)	Up to 15 mm/hour is normal	
ESR (female)	Up to 20 mm/hour is normal	
CPK (male)	<12 units/mL	>70 units/mL
CPK (female)	<10 units/mL	>55 units/mL
ANA	Normal findings are no ANA detected in a titer with a dilution of >1:32 normal findings are no ANA detected in a titer with a dilution of >1:32	
CRP	------	>1 mg/dL
Rheumatoid factor	Abnormal if present	
Albumin	<35 g/L	>50 g/L

ANA = antinuclear antibody; CPK = Creatine phosphokinase; CRP = C-reactive protein; ESR = erythrocyte sedimentation rate; RBC = red blood cell; WBC = white blood cell.

- Complete blood count (CBC): the white cell count (ordered as part of the CBC) is used to detect infection and conditions such as leukemia.
- Synovial fluid analysis (collected using a procedure called arthrocentesis); can detect the presence of crystals: urate, calcium pyrophosphate.

Imaging Studies

It is important for the clinician to know what relevance to attach to these reports, and the strengths and weaknesses of the various imaging techniques (Table 3-27).

Table 3-27 Strengths and Weaknesses of Various Imaging Studies

Imaging Study	Function	Advantages	Disadvantages
Plain-film or conventional radiograph	Excellent for assessment of bone structures and relationships, bone deformity, arthritic disorders, stages of fracture healing, metabolic disorders, avascular necrosis, and bone tumors. Tissues with the lowest density (air and fat) appear as black or dark grey on the film, whereas higher density structures such as cortical bone, dental fillings, and orthopedic hardware appear white	Helpful in detecting fractures and subluxations in patients with a history of trauma. Highlight the presence of degenerative joint disease. Can provide biomechanical assessment such as leg length	Do not provide an image of soft tissue structures such as muscles, tendons, joint capsule, ligaments and intervertebral disks
Stress radiograph	Used to assess the effect of motion on structures	Helpful in assessing spinal mobility and stability in the spine	Patient may not tolerate stress position
Arthrogram	Conventional arthrography is plain film x-ray technology combined with contrast enhancement for a more detailed assessment of joint injury and pathology	Outlines the soft tissue structures of a joint that would otherwise not be visible with a plain-film radiograph Good for detecting internal derangements	Mildly invasive May require imaging guidance to place the needle
Myelography	Uses radiographic contrast media (dye) that is injected into the subarachnoid space (cerebrospinal fluid, CSF). After the dye is injected, the contrast medium serves to illuminate the spinal canal, cord, and nerve roots during imaging	Provides image of the spinal cord, nerve roots, dura mater and the spinal canal	Potential for a postmyelogram headache Potential for seizure (rare)

(continued on following page)

Table 3-27 *(continued from previous page)*

Imaging Study	Function	Advantages	Disadvantages
CT	An advanced x-ray-based imaging technology that is particular useful for the evaluation of bone pathologies	Provides good visualization of the shape, symmetry and position of structures by delineating specific areas Quicker scan than MRI Better detail of bone than MRI	Generally limited to axial plane Soft tissue contrast not as good as MRI
MRI	MRI utilizes a magnetic field in combination with a radio wave transmitter and receiver to produce images	Excellent tissue contrast No streak artifacts Ability to provide cross-sectional images Noninvasive nature Complete lack of ionizing radiation Can take images of any plane	Expensive Time consuming Poor visualization of cortical bone detail or calcifications Limited spatial resolution compared with CT
Diagnostic ultrasound	As ultrasound waves are transmitted through the body, they are reflected at tissue interfaces, and the time it takes for the waves to be reflected back to the transducing probe allows the computer to produce an image	Readily available Noninvasive Much less expensive than CT or MRI Can be used in any plane (sagittal, coronal, axial, and at any obliquity) Can detect soft tissue injuries, tumors, bone infections, bone mineral density, and arthropathy	Not a sharp, clear image compared to images produced by other radiological modalities Because of the degrees of obliquity, one cannot easily tell what one is looking at without knowledge of cross-sectional anatomy; sonographer identifies anatomic segment Visualization of structures limited by bone and gas (lung, bowel)

Clinical Pearl

- In general, imaging tests have a high sensitivity (few false negatives), but low specificity (high false-positive rate). In other words, misinterpretation of radiographic images is a common source of error.

EVALUATION

Once the history, ROS, and the tests and measures are completed, an evaluation is made based on the information gathered by adding and subtracting the various findings.[48]

 Clinical Pearl

An evaluation is the level of judgment necessary to make sense of the findings to identify a relationship between the symptoms reported and the signs of disturbed function.[19]

 Clinical Pearl

A hypothesis is an impression based on assumption of causality.[49] At the end of the examination the clinician should be able to generate one or more working hypotheses as potential causes for the condition begin to emerge. On those occasions when a hypothesis cannot be generated, treatment cannot be provided in the clinician should refer the patient to another practitioner or consult with a colleague.[49]

When integrating evidence into clinical decision-making, an understanding of how to appraise the quality of the evidence offered by the clinical tests is important. The ideal clinical trial includes a blinded, randomized design and a control group (Table 3-28). The control can be current standard practice, a placebo, or no active intervention.[50]

 Clinical Pearl

Clinicians must constantly remind themselves that without information gathered from controlled clinical trials, they have limited scientific basis for their tests or interventions.[51]

DIAGNOSIS

The best indicator for the correctness of a diagnosis is the quality of the hypothesis considered, for if the appropriate diagnosis is not considered from

Table 3-28 A Hierarchy of Evidence Grading

	Level of Evidence Grading = A	Level of Evidence Grading = B	Level of Evidence Grading = C	Level of Evidence Grading = D	Level of Evidence Grading = E
Type of Study	Randomized clinical trials	Cohort study	Nonrandomized trial with concurrent or historical controls Case study Study of sensitivity and specificity of a diagnostic test Population based descriptive study	Cross-sectional study Case series Case report	Expert consensus Clinical experience

the start, any subsequent inquiries will be misdirected.[52] Once the diagnosis has been determined, one of two scenarios generally exist:

1. The clinical findings warrant a referral to another health care practitioner. A complete and accurate evaluation can only be made when all potential causes for the symptoms have been ruled out. The clinician should resist the urge to categorize a condition based on a small number of findings. In such cases, knowledge of differential diagnosis is essential, so that the clinician can systematically rule out all of the causes for the symptoms. Patients may be referred to physical therapy with a nonspecific diagnosis, an incorrect diagnosis, or no diagnosis at all.[53] Physical therapists are responsible for thoroughly examining each patient and then either treating the patient according to established guidelines or referring the patient elsewhere.[54]

2. The data from the clinical findings are organized into clusters, syndromes, or categories called preferred practice patterns (Table 3-29) and an intervention can be commenced. Most of the time, these patterns do not occur in isolation. Patients often present with a mixture of signs and symptoms that indicate one or more possible problem areas. Once these impairments have been highlighted, a determination can be made as to the reason for those impairments, and the relationship between the impairments, and the patient's functional limitations or disabilities.

Table 3-29 Preferred Practice Patterns*

Musculoskeletal Practice Pattern	Impairments
Pattern 4A	Primary prevention/risk factor reduction for skeletal demineralization
Pattern 4B	*Impaired posture* This pattern is often the result of a combination of other practice patterns including practice patterns C, E, F, and G, and includes impairments of motor function, muscle performance, joint mobility, localized inflammation, and range of motion. The **pathologies** associated with this pattern include vertebral pathology, neural compression syndromes, entrapment syndromes, myofascial syndromes, impingement syndromes, and referred pain. **Clinical findings** can include pain with sustained positions, limited range of motion in a noncapsular pattern of restriction, altered kinematics, positive impingement tests, neurological findings (thoracic outlet, limb tension tests), trigger points, and palpable tenderness of specific muscles.
Pattern 4C	*Impaired muscle performance* This pattern is associated with a combination of other practice patterns including practice patterns D through J, and thus includes impairments of motor function, muscle performance, joint mobility, localized inflammation, and range of motion. The **pathologies** and **clinical findings** associated with this pattern include those that the pattern is associated with (practice patterns D through J).
Pattern 4D	*Impaired joint mobility, motor function, muscle performance, and range of motion associated with connective tissue dysfunction* Pattern D refers to an increased laxity or instability of the joint or hypomobility due to capsular restriction. The primary impairments in pattern D include decreased motor control and muscle performance **Characteristic** of this pattern is the complaint of the joint "slipping" or "popping out" during activities of extreme motion. The **pathologies** associated with this pattern include osteoarthritis, rheumatoid arthropathy, adhesive capsulitis, tendinitis, capsulitis, bursitis, synovitis, and ligament pathology. **Clinical findings** associated with this pattern can include pain, altered kinematics, crepitus, and positive apprehension.

(continued on following page)

Table 3-29 *(continued from previous page)*

Musculoskeletal Practice Pattern	Impairments
Pattern 4E	*Impaired joint mobility, motor function, muscle performance, and range of motion associated with localized inflammation* In addition to those conditions producing impaired range of motion, motor function, and muscle performance attributed to inflammation, practice pattern E includes conditions that cause pain and muscle guarding without the presence of structural changes. The **pathologies** include sprains and strains of the joints, internal derangements of the joint, including muscle tears, and periarticular syndromes—tendonitis, bursitis, capsulitis, and tenosynovitis. The **clinical findings** include pain with active and resisted motions, tenderness to palpation, localized edema, redness, and increased skin temperature.
Pattern 4F	*Impaired joint mobility, motor function, muscle performance, and range of motion, or reflex integrity secondary to spinal disorders* This pattern involves impaired motor function, muscle performance, range of motion, and joint mobility. The pathologies associated with this pattern include adverse neural tension and nerve root irritation. The clinical findings associated with this pattern can include positive limb tension tests, signs and symptoms of nerve, and nerve root compression.
Pattern 4G	*Impaired joint mobility, motor function, muscle performance, and range of motion associated with fracture* The treatment of most fractures is beyond the scope of practice for a physical therapist.
Patterns 4H and 4I	*Impaired joint mobility, motor function, muscle performance, and range of motion associated with joint arthroplasty, or with bony or soft tissue surgical procedures* **Pattern H** is associated with impaired joint mobility, muscle performance, and range of motion due to joint arthroplasty. **Pattern I** involves impaired joint mobility, motor function, muscle performance, and range of motion associated with bony or soft tissue surgical procedures. The clinical findings and treatment following a surgical procedure will vary according to each individual and the procedure performed.
Pattern 4J	*Impaired gait, locomotion, and balance and impaired motor function, secondary to lower extremity amputation*

Musculoskeletal Practice Pattern	Impairments
Pattern 5F	*Impaired peripheral nerve integrity and muscle performance associated with peripheral nerve injury*
	This pattern involves decreased muscle strength, impaired proprioception, impaired sensory integrity, and difficulty with manipulation skills.
	The **pathologies** include carpal tunnel syndrome, cubital tunnel syndrome, radial tunnel syndrome, tarsal tunnel syndrome and paroxysmal positional vertigo.
	The clinical findings can include diminished deep tendon reflexes, positive limb tension tests, signs and symptoms of peripheral nerve compression.

*Data from reference 5.

PROGNOSIS

The prognosis is the predicted level of function that the patient will attain within a certain time frame. This prediction helps guide the intensity, duration, and frequency of the intervention, and aids in justifying the intervention.

Establishing Goals

A goal is what the clinician and patient realistically believes can be achieved with an intervention. Goals should be stated in measurable and behavioral terms, and with a specific time frame.

Clinical Pearl

If the patient's goals have not been met after a determined time frame, the working hypothesis needs to be reexamined and the goals modified, or the patient needs to be referred to another practitioner.

INTERVENTION

The first consideration for rehabilitation is to establish a causal relationship between physical impairments and the pathology. It is then necessary to develop a treatment plan specifically designed to address the impairments.

Clinical Pearl

The types of physical therapy interventions include the following:

• Direct intervention (e.g., therapeutic exercise, manual therapy techniques, electrotherapeutic modalities, etc.)

• Patient-related instruction

• Coordination, communication, and documentation

The most successful intervention programs are those that are custom designed from a blend of clinical experience and scientific data, with the level of improvement achieved related to goal setting and the attainment of those goals (Table 3-30).

 Clinical Pearl

An intervention should be geared toward altering the underlying cause of the condition, and it should be based on sound scientific research that provides an adequate rationale and justification for its use.

The chosen clinical approach is dictated by the stage of healing (Tables 3-31 and 3-32), the tissue involved (Table 3-33), the established goals, and by the patient's tolerance.

Table 3-30 Key Questions for Intervention Planning*

• What is the stage of healing: acute, subacute, or chronic?
• How long do you have to treat the patient?
• What does patient do for activities?
• How compliant is the patient?
• How much *skilled* physical therapy is needed?
• What needs to be taught to prevent recurrence?
• Are there any referrals needed?
• What has worked for other patients with similar problems?
• Are there any precautions?
• What is your skill level?

*Data from reference 5.

Table 3-31 Stages of Healing

Stage	General Characteristics
Acute (inflammatory)	The area is red, warm, swollen, and painful
	The pain is present without any motion of the involved area
	Usually lasts for 48 to 72 hours, but can be as long as 7 to 10 days
Subacute (reparative)	The pain usually occurs with the activity or motion of the involved area
	Usually lasts for 10 days to 6 weeks
Chronic (maturation-remodeling)	The pain usually occurs after the activity
	Usually lasts from 6 weeks to 12 months

 Clinical Pearl

During the acute stage of healing the principles of PRICEMEM (protection, rest, ice, compression, elevation, manual therapy, early motion, and medications) are recommended.

Table 3-32 Goals and Appropriate Approach Based on Stage of Healing

Stage of Healing	Goal of Intervention	Appropriate Modality	Appropriate Manual Technique	Appropriate Exercise
Acute	Control pain, inflammation and swelling (edema)	Cryotherapy, electrical stimulation, pulsed ultrasound, and iontophoresis	Grades I or II joint mobilizations	PROM
	Promote and progress healing			AAROM
Subacute				
Chronic		Thermotherapy, phonophoresis, electrical stimulation, US, iontophoresis, and diathermy		

PROM = passive range of motion; AAROM = active assisted range of motion.

Table 3-33 Intervention of Sprains, Strains, and Overuse Syndromes

Grade	Symptoms	Intervention
I	Pain only after activity Does not interfere with performance Often generalized tenderness Disappears before next exercise session	Modification of activity Assessment of training pattern
II	Minimal pain with activity Does not interfere with intensity or distance Usually localized tenderness	Modification of activity Physical therapy; consider orthotics
III	Pain interferes with activity Usually disappears between sessions Definite local tenderness	Significant modification of activity Assess training schedule Physical therapy; consider orthotics
IV	Pain does not disappear between activity sessions Seriously interferes with intensity of training Significant local sign of pain, tenderness, crepitus, swelling	Usually need to temporarily discontinue aggravating motion Design alternate program May require splinting Physical therapy
V	Pain interferes with sport and activities of daily living Symptoms often chronic or recurrent Signs of tissue changes and altered associated muscle function	Prolonged rest from activity Consider splint or cast Physical therapy May require surgery

Although physical therapy cannot accelerate the healing process, it can ensure that the healing process is not delayed or disrupted, and that it occurs in an optimal environment.[55] In addition to excess stress, detrimental environments include prolonged immobilization, which must also be avoided.

 Clinical Pearl

The electrotherapeutic and thermal modalities, considered as adjunctive interventions, used during the acute phase involve the

application of cryotherapy, electrical stimulation, pulsed ultrasound (US), and iontophoresis (Tables 3-34 and 3-35).

Modalities used during the later stages of healing include thermotherapy, phonophoresis, electrical stimulation, US, iontophoresis, and diathermy.

Therapeutic Exercise

Therapeutic exercise is the foundation of physical therapy, and a fundamental component of the vast majority of interventions.

 Clinical Pearl

The promotion and progression of tissue repair involves a delicate balance between protection, and the application of controlled functional stresses to the damaged structure. The goal of the functional exercise progression is to identify the motion, or motions that the patient is able to exercise into without eliciting symptoms other than postexercise soreness.[56]

 Clinical Pearl

Each exercise should be performed in a slow and controlled fashion and should be repeated for three sets of 8 to 12 reps.

Exercise Ladders

A hierarchy for ROM and resistive exercises exists (see Chapter 4).[57] Based on this hierarchy, a series of appropriate therapeutic exercises, in the form of a clinical ladder, is presented at the end of each of the body area chapters. The purpose of these training ladders is to provide the clinician with a safe and progressive framework of exercises that are designed to allow the patient to improve in an efficient manner. The patient begins at the appropriate step, which is based on the stage of healing and the goal of the intervention.

• Phase 1: Acute—pain management, restoration of full passive range of motion, and restoration of normal accessory motion.

Table 3-34 Electrotherapeutic and Thermal Modalities

Therapeutic Modality	Physiologic Responses
Cryotherapy (cold packs, ice)	Decreased blood flow (vasoconstriction) Analgesia Reduce inflammation Reduce muscle guarding/spasm
Thermotherapy (hot packs, whirlpool, paraffin wax)	Increased blood flow (vasodilation) Analgesia Reduce muscle guarding/spasm Increase metabolic activity
Electrical stimulating currents—high voltage	Pain modulation Muscle reeducation Muscle pumping contractions (retard atrophy) Fracture healing
Electrical stimulating currents—low voltage	Wound healing Fracture healing
Electrical stimulating currents—interferential	Pain modulation Muscle reeducation Muscle pumping contractions Fracture healing
Electrical stimulating currents—Russian	Muscle strengthening
Electrical stimulating currents—MENS	Fracture healing Wound healing
Shortwave diathermy and microwave diathermy	Increase deep circulation Increase metabolic activity Reduce muscle guarding/spasm Reduce inflammation Facilitate wound healing Analgesia Increase tissue temperatures over a large area
Low-power laser	Pain modulation (trigger points) Facilitate wound healing

Therapeutic Modality	Physiologic Responses
Ultrasound	Increase connective tissue extensibility
	Deep heat
	Increased circulation
	Reduce inflammation (pulsed)
	Reduce muscle spasm

Table 3-35 Clinical Decision Making on the Use of Various Therapeutic Modalities During the Various Stages of Healing

Phase	Clinical Presentation	Possible Modalities Used	Examples and Parameters (Where Applicable)	Therapeutic Goals Decrease	Increase
Initial acute	Erythema (rubor), swelling (tumor), elevated tissue temperature (calor) and pain (dolor)	Cryotherapy Electrical stimulation Rest	Ice packs, ice massage, cold whirlpool (15–20° C)	Swelling Pain Inflammation Metabolic rate Muscle tension	Threshold of muscle spindle
Inflammatory response	Swelling subsides, warm to touch, discoloration, pain to touch, pain on motion	Cryotherapy Electrical stimulation Ultrasound	Pulsed	Swelling Pain	
Reparative	Pain to touch, pain on motion, swollen	Thermotherapy Electrical stimulation Ultrasound	Hot packs, paraffin wax, fluidotherapy, and so on (41–45° C)	Pain via muscle pumping	Lymphatic flow Circulation (slightly) Range of motion Strength
Remodeling	Swollen, no more pain to touch, decreasing pain on motion	Thermotherapy Electrical stimulation Ultrasound		Pain	Circulation Range of motion Strength Function

- Phase 2: Subacute—active range of motion exercises and early strengthening.
- Phase 3: Chronic—specific strengthening with a strong emphasis on enhancing dynamic stability.

The degree of movement and the speed of progression are both guided by the signs and symptoms. Once the patient is able to perform an exercise for 8–12 reps without pain, he or she progresses up to the next exercise step. This continues until the patient attempts an exercise that reproduces the pain. At this point, the patient returns to the last exercise that he or she was able to perform without pain and performs that exercise 5 times/day for 1 to 2 days before attempting to progress again. The patient is advanced through the training ladders to the appropriate point, with particular attention paid to patient response to treatment in terms of changes in symptoms, swelling, degree of irritability, or motion. In addition, muscle imbalances are addressed with appropriate flexibility exercises.

Once the patient is able to perform the last exercise of Phase 3 (Step 12 of the ladder), he or she can move on to high-function and sport-specific training (Phase 4) as appropriate, which focus on power and higher-speed exercises similar to sport-specific demands.

Examples of Phase 4 exercises for the upper extremity include

- Hand-walking on a treadmill.
- Rowing machine
- ProFitter
- Plyometric exercises
- Total body training

Examples of Phase 4 exercises for the lower extremity include

- Running, jumping activities
- Speed and agility drills
- Stair stepper/elliptical
- Plyometrics
- Obstacle training
- Total body training

DOCUMENTATION

The three key components when writing in medical records are

- Accuracy: keep the information objective.
- Brevity: use short, succinct sentences while providing enough information.
- Clarity: the meaning of your documentation should be immediately clear to the reader. Avoid using abbreviations that are not standard to the facility.

Clinical Pearl

All notes should be signed with your legal signature (your last name and legal first name or initials) followed by your initials that indicate your status as a physical therapist or student physical therapist based on the facility's requirements.

Empty lines should not be left between one entry and another, nor should empty lines be left within a single entry.

 Clinical Pearl

The SOAP note format includes:

S—Subjective. This includes the patient's current condition/chief complaint, functional status as reported by the patient, growth and development, social history and employment status, living environment, general health status, family health history, surgical/medical history, currently prescribed medications, recent medical and imaging tests, and the patient's goals.

O—Objective. This includes the results of test measurements and objective observations of the various body systems.

A—Assessment. This includes a list of the patient's functional deficits and impairments placed in a diagnostic category or preferred practice pattern.

P—Prognosis/plan. This includes a prediction by the clinician about the level of improvement in function that the patient will obtain (expected outcomes) and the amount of time needed to reach that level.

REFERENCES

1. American Physical Therapy Association. Guide to physical therapist practice: revisions. *Phys Ther*. 2001;9–738.
2. Goodman CC, Snyder TK. Introduction to the interviewing process. In: Goodman CC, Snyder TK, eds. *Differential Diagnosis in Physical Therapy*. Philadelphia, PA: Saunders;WB 1990:7–42.
3. D'Ambrosia R. *Musculoskeletal Disorders: Regional Examination and Differential Diagnosis*. 2nd ed. Philadelphia, PA: J.B. Lippincott; 1986.

4. Meadows J. *Orthopedic Differential Diagnosis in Physical Therapy*. New York, NT: McGraw-Hill; 1999.

5. Guide to physical therapist practice. *Phys Ther*. 2001;81:S13–S95.

6. Isaacs E, Bookout M. Screening for pathological origins of head and facial pain. In: Boissonnault WG, ed. *Examination in Physical Therapy Practice: Screening for Medical Disease*. 2nd ed. Philadelphia, PA: WB Saunders; 1995:175–189.

7. Onieal M-E. Common wrist and elbow injuries in primary care. Lippincott's primary care practice. *Musculoskelet Conditions*. 1999;3:441–450.

8. Cyriax J. *Textbook of Orthopaedic Medicine, Diagnosis of Soft Tissue Lesions*. 8th ed. London, UK: Bailliere Tindall; 1982.

9. Farfan HF. The scientific basis of manipulative procedures. *Clin Rheum Dis*. 1980;6:159–177.

10. McKenzie R, May S. Physical examination. In: McKenzie R, May S, eds. *The Human Extremities: Mechanical Diagnosis and Therapy*. Waikanae, NZ: Spinal Publications New Zealand; 2000:105–121.

11. McKenzie RA. The lumbar spine: mechanical diagnosis and therapy. Waikanae, NZ: Spinal Publication; 1981.

12. Petersen CM, Hayes KW. Construct validity of Cyriax's selective tension examination: association of end-feels with pain ath the knee and shoulder. *J Orthop Sports Phys Ther*. 2000;30:512–527.

13. Riddle DL. Measurement of accessory motion: Critical issues and related concepts. *Phys Ther*. 1992;72:865–874.

14. Maitland G. *Peripheral Manipulation*. 3rd ed. London, UK: Butterworth; 1991.

15. Maitland G. Vertebral Manipulation. Sydney, Australia: Butterworth; 1986.

16. Kaltenborn FM. *Manual Mobilization of the Extremity Joints: Basic Examination and Treatment Techniques*. 4th ed. Oslo, Norway: Olaf Norlis Bokhandel, Universitetsgaten; 1989.

17. Williams PL, Warwick R, Dyson M, et al. *Gray's Anatomy*. 37th ed. London, UK: Churchill Livingstone; 1989.

18. Maitland GD. Passive movement techniques for intra-articular and periarticular disorders. *Aust J Physiother*. 1985;31:3–8.

19. Grieve GP. *Common Vertebral Joint Problems*. New York, NY: Churchill Livingstone Inc; 1981.

20. American Medical Association. *Guides to the Evaluation of Permanent Impairment*. 5th ed. Chicago, IL: American Medical Association; 2001.

21. Nadler SF, Rigolosi L, Kim D, et al. Sensory, motor, and reflex examination. In: Malanga GA, Nadler SF, eds. *Musculoskeletal Physical Examination—An Evidence-based Approach*. Philadelphia, PA: Elsevier-Mosby; 2006:15–32.

22. Cyriax JH, Cyriax PJ. *Illustrated Manual of Orthopaedic Medicine*. London, UK: Butterworth; 1983.

23. Sapega AA. Muscle performance evaluation in orthopedic practice. *J Bone Joint Surg*. 1990;72A:1562–1574.

24. Janda V. *Muscle Function Testing*. London, UK: Butterworths; 1983.

25. Bowen JE, Malanga GA, Pappoe T, et al. Physical examination of the shoulder. In: Malanga GA, Nadler SF, eds. *Musculoskeletal Physical Examination—An Evidence-based Approach*. Philadelphia, PA: Elsevier-Mosby; 2006:59–118.

26. Gilman S. The physical and neurologic examination. In: Gilman S, ed. *Clinical Examination of the Nervous System*. New York, NY: McGraw-Hill; 2000:15–34.

27. Inouye Y, Buchthal F. Segmental sensory innervartion determined by potentials recorded from cervical spinal nerves. *Brain Dev*. 1977;100:731–748.

28. Dutton M. *Manual Therapy of the Spine: An Integrated Approach*. New York, NY: McGraw-Hill; 2002.

29. McKnight JT, Adcock BB. Paresthesias: a practical diagnostic approach. *Am Fam Physician*. 1997;56:2253–2260.

30. Hollinshead WH, Jenkins DB. *Functional Anatomy of the Limbs and Back*. Philadelphia, PA: WB Saunders; 1981.

31. Goldberg S. *The Four Minute Neurological Examination*. Miami, FL: Medmaster; 1992.

32. Judge RD, Zuidema GD, Fitzgerald FT. Head. In: Judge RD, Zuidema GD, Fitzgerald FT, eds. *Clinical Diagnosis*. 4th ed. Boston, MA: Little, Brown and Company; 1982:123–151.

33. Butler DS. *Mobilization of the Nervous Sysytem*. New York, NY: Churchill Livingstone; 1992.

34. Farrell JP. Cervical passive mobilization techniques: The Australian approach. *Phys Med Rehabil: State-of-the-Art Rev*. 1990;4:309–334.

35. Feagin JA Jr. The office diagnosis and documentation of common knee problems. *Clin Sports Med*. 1989;8:453–459.

36. Dyson M, Pond JB, Joseph J, et al. The stimulation of tissue regeneration by means of ultrasound. *Clin Sci*. 1968;35:273–285.

37. Dyson M, Suckling J. Stimulation of tissue repair by ultrasound: a survey of the mechanisms involved. *Physiotherapy*. 1978;64:105–108.

38. Ramsey SM. Holistic manual therapy techniques. *Prim Care*. 1997;24:759–785.

39. Ayub E. Posture and the upper quarter. In: Donatelli RA, ed. *Physical Therapy of the Shoulder*. 2nd ed. New York, NY: Churchill Livingstone; 1991:81–90.

40. Giallonardo LM. Clinical evaluation of foot and ankle dysfunction. *Phys Ther*. 1988;68:1850–1856.

41. Epler M. Gait. In: Richardson JK, Iglarsh ZA, eds. *Clinical Orthopaedic Physical Therapy*. Philadelphia, PA: WB Saunders; 1994:602–625.

42. Hunt GC, Brocato RS. Gait and foot pathomechanics. In: Hunt GC, ed. *Physical Therapy of the Foot and Ankle*. Edinburgh, UK: Churchill Livingstone; 1988.

43. Krebs DE, Robbins CE, Lavine L, et al. Hip biomechanics during gait. *J Orthop Sports Phys Ther*. 1998;28:51–59.

44. Larish DD, Martin PE, Mungiole M. Characteristic patterns of gait in the healthy old. *Ann N Y Acad Sci*. 1987;515:18–32.

45. Levine D, Whittle M. *Gait Analysis: The Lower Extremities*. La Crosse, WI: Orthopaedic Section, APTA, Inc.; 1992.

46. Perry J. *Gait Analysis: Normal and Pathological Function*. Thorofare, NJ: Slack Inc; 1992.

47. Song KM, Halliday SE, Little DG. The effect of limb-length discrepancy on gait. *J Bone Joint Surg*. 1997;79A:1690–1698.

48. Cwynar DA, McNerney T. A primer on physical therapy. *Lippincott's Primary Care Pract*. 1999;3:451–459.

49. Rothstein JM, Echternach JL. Hypothesis-oriented algorithm for clinicians. A method for evaluation and treatment planning. *Phys Ther*. 1986;66:1388–1394.
50. Friedman LM, Furberg CD, DeMets DL. *Fundamentals of Clinical Trials*. 2nd ed. Chicago, IL: Mosby-Year Book; 1985:2, 51, 71.
51. Schiffman EL. The role of the randomized clinical trial in evaluating management strategies for temporomandibular disorders. In: Fricton JR, Dubner R, eds. *Orofacial Pain and Temporomandibular Disorders (Advances in Pain Research and Therapy)*. Vol 21. New York, NY: Raven Press; 1995:415–463.
52. Jones MA. Clinical reasoning in manual therapy. *Phys Ther*. 1992;72:875–884.
53. Clawson AL, Domholdt E. Content of physician referrals to physical therapists at clinical education sites in Indiana. *Phys Ther*. 1994;74:356–360.
54. Leerar PJ. Differential diagnosis of tarsal coalition versus cuboid syndrome in an adolescent athlete. *J Orthop Sports Phys Ther*. 2001;31:702–707.
55. McKenzie R, May S. Introduction. In McKenzie R, May S, eds. *The Human Extremities: Mechanical Diagnosis and Therapy*. Waikanae, NZ: Spinal Publications New Zealand Ltd; 2000:1–5.
56. Hyman J, Liebenson C. Spinal stabilization exercise program. In: Liebenson C, ed. *Rehabilitation of the Spine: A Practitioner's Manual*. Baltimore, MA: Lippincott Williams & Wilkins; 1996:293–317.
57. Ierna GF, Murphy DR. Management of acute soft tissue injuries of the cervical spine. In: Murphy DR, ed. *Conservative Management of Cervical Spine Disorders*. New York, NY: McGraw-Hill; 2000:531–552.

QUESTIONS

1. What are the five elements of care that define patient/client management within physical therapist practice?
2. Which three components comprise the physical therapy examination?
3. List five signs or symptoms that would be considered red flags
4. What term is used to describe those symptoms that have their origin at a site other than where the patient feels them?
5. Give two examples of an inert tissue as defined by Cyriax
6. According to Cyriax, give five examples of contractile tissue.
7. What is a capsular pattern of restriction?
8. List some of the causes of a capsular pattern in a joint.
9. What are some of the causes of a noncapsular pattern?
10. What is the capsular pattern of the hip joint?
11. What is the capsular pattern of the talocrural joint?
12. What is the capsular pattern of the glenohumeral joint?
13. What is the capsular pattern of the humeroulnar joint?
14. What is the optimal amount of time that stretch should be held?
15. Describe the difference between physiological barrier and anatomic barrier.

16. Using the Maitland system, what constitutes a Grade III mobilization?
17. Give three contraindications to manual therapy.
18. Describe the three normal end feels.
19. Which three end feels always indicate pathology?
20. With manual muscle testing, what is implied with a weak and painful finding?
21. With manual muscle testing, what is implied with a weak and painless finding?
22. Which root levels are assessed for dural mobility with the prone knee bend test?
23. What is the key muscle test for L5–S1?
24. What are the two components that contribute to an individual's walking velocity
25. List three positive findings you would find during gait in a patient with a weak tibialis anterior.
26. Describe the findings in a Trendelenburg gait pattern.
27. What are the most common myotomes (key muscles) tested it the upper and lower quarter screening examinations?
28. Which deep tendon reflex is used to assess L3–4?
29. When is the Jendrassik maneuver used?
30. Describe the Oppenheim test
31. What is the function of the CORs and VORs?
32. Which group of tests are designed to examine the neurological structures for adaptive shortening and inflammation of the neural structures both centrally and peripherally.
33. How many imaging views are typically ordered to diagnose injuries?
34. Give three conditions related to orthopedics that result in a decrease in albumin levels.
35. What are antinuclear antibodies (ANA)?
36. What is the ESR and what does its value signify?
37. What is the body's initial response to soft tissue injury and how is it manifested?
38. What are the two key chemical mediators of the inflammatory response?
39. What type of fracture is associated with a sudden increase in physical activity?
40. What is the effect of cryotherapy on metabolic rate?
41. What is the ideal tissue temperature to achieve the optimal physiological effects of cryotherapy?

42. When should ice be used in the treatment of a subacute or chronic injury?

43. What is the ideal tissue temperature to achieve the optimal physiological effects of thermotherapy?

44. What is the effect of cryotherapy on nerve conduction velocity?

45. Give five contraindications for the use of electrotherapy.

46. When using Kaltenborn grades of joint mobilization, which grade accomplishes distraction with slight separation?

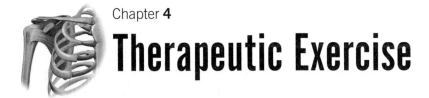

Chapter **4**

Therapeutic Exercise

OVERVIEW

Therapeutic exercise is the foundation of physical therapy, and a fundamental component of the vast majority of interventions. Prescribed accurately, therapeutic exercise can be used to restore, maintain, and improve a patient's functional status by increasing strength, endurance, and flexibility. Therapeutic exercise enables the patient/client to

- remediate or reduce impairments
- enhance function
- optimize overall health
- enhance fitness and well-being.

When prescribing a therapeutic exercise program it is important to consider the functional loss and disability of the patient.

PHYSIOLOGY OF EXERCISE

Energy Systems

Muscles are metabolically active and must generate energy to move. The creation of energy occurs initially from the breakdown of certain nutrients from foodstuffs.

 Clinical Pearl

The energy required for exercise is stored in a compound called adenosine triphosphate (ATP). ATP is produced in the muscle tissue from blood glucose or glycogen. Fats and proteins can also be metabolized to generate ATP. Glucose not needed immediately is stored as glycogen in the resting muscle and liver. Stored glycogen in the liver can later be converted back into glucose and transferred to the blood to meet the body's energy needs.

If the duration or intensity of the exercise increases, the body relies more heavily on fat stored in adipose tissue to meet its energy needs.

 Clinical Pearl

During rest and submaximal exertion, both fat and carbohydrates are used to provide energy in approximately a 60% to 40% ratio.

Two of the most important energy generating systems that function in muscle tissue include the anaerobic and aerobic metabolism, both of which produce ATP:

- Anaerobic metabolism: this process metabolizes glucose to generate small amounts of ATP energy without the need for oxygen.
  - ATP-PCr system: used for ATP production during high-intensity, short duration exercise. Phosphocreatine (PCr) decomposes and releases a large amount of energy that is used to construct ATP.
    - The short-term energy system: provides energy for muscle contraction for up to 15 seconds.
  - Anaerobic glycolysis (glycolytic system): a major supply of ATP during high-intensity, short-duration activities.
    - Muscle glycogen is the initial substrate. Stored glycogen is split into glucose, and through glycolysis, split again into pyruvate acid and lactic acid as the end product, with no oxygen being directly involved. The energy released during this process forms ATP.
    - Although unable to produce as much energy per unit time as the phosphocreatine system (i.e., unable to sustain maximum sprinting speed), it lasts considerably longer before intensity must be further reduced.
    - The intermediate energy system: provides the majority of energy for a sustained performance lasting between 20 seconds and 2 minutes (sprinting 200 to 800 m).
- Aerobic metabolism (oxidative system): if exercise continues beyond a certain point, the body can no longer rely solely on anaerobic metabolism and has to switch to this more complex form of carbohydrate and fat metabolism to generate ATP.
  - The long-term energy system.
  - Ultimately, all exercise has an oxygen cost, and the faster this can be met during recovery, the better the preparation for the next high-intensity exercise bout.

- Delivery of oxygen to the fatigued muscles replenishes stores of creatine phosphate and lowers levels of lactic acid. This means the aerobic system must not be overlooked during rehabilitation.

 Clinical Pearl

In most activities, both aerobic and anaerobic systems function simultaneously with the ratio being determined by the intensity and duration of the activity. In general:

- High-intensity activities of short duration rely more heavily on the anaerobic system.
- Low-intensity activities of longer duration rely more on the aerobic system.

 Clinical Pearl

A metabolic equivalent unit, or MET, is defined as the energy expenditure for sitting quietly, talking on the phone, or reading a book, which, for the average adult, approximates 3.5 mL of oxygen uptake per kilogram of body weight per minute (3.5 mL O_2/kg/min)—1.2 kcal/min for a 70-kg individual). METs are defined as multiples of resting energy metabolism. For example, a 2-MET activity requires two times the metabolic energy expenditure of sitting quietly. The harder the body works during the activity, the higher the MET. Any activity that burns 3 to 6 METs is considered moderate-intensity physical activity. Any activity that burns more than 6 METs is considered vigorous-intensity physical activity.

Normal Exercise Response

The normal response to exercise is an increase in oxygen consumption (VO_2) with an increase in external workload (intensity). There is a direct, almost linear relationship between heart rate (HR) and intensity. Therefore, if a physical therapy intervention requires an increase in systemic oxygen consumption, expressed as either an increase in MET levels, kcal, L/O_2, or mL O_2 per kilogram of body weight per minute, then HR should also increase.[1]

Clinical Pearl

The magnitude at which the HR increases with increasing workloads is influenced by many factors including age, fitness level, type of activity being performed, presence of disease, medications, blood volume, and environmental factors such as temperature, humidity, and altitude. Failure of the HR to increase with increasing workloads (chronotropic incompetence) should be of concern for the clinician, even if the patient is taking β-blockers.[1]

In the normal heart, as workload increases, stroke volume (SV) increases linearly up to 50% of aerobic capacity, after which it increases only slightly.

 Clinical Pearl

Factors that influence the magnitude of change in SV include ventricular function, body position, and exercise intensity.

Cardiac output (CO), the product of HR and SV, increases linearly with workload because of the increases in HR and SV in response to increasing exercise intensity.

Clinical Pearl

Factors that influence the magnitude of change in CO include age, posture, body size, presence of disease, and level of physical conditioning.

Clinical Pearl

- SV: the amount of blood pumped out by the left ventricle of the heart with each beat. The heart does not pump all the blood out of the ventricle—normally, only about two-thirds.

- CO: the amount of blood discharged by each ventricle (not both ventricles combined) per minute, usually expressed as liters per minute.

Blood pressure, a product of CO and peripheral vascular resistance, is defined as the pressure exerted by the blood on the walls of the blood vessels, specifically *arterial blood pressure* (the pressure in the large arteries).

 Clinical Pearl

As with HR, a linear increase in systolic blood pressure is expected with increasing levels of work. Diastolic pressure exhibit limited changes with exercise; it may not change, or either increase or decrease by 10 mm Hg.[1]

Measures of Energy Expenditure

The energy value of the food we eat can be quantified in terms of the calorie. A kilocalorie (kcal) is the amount of heat necessary to raise 1.0 kg of water by 1.0°C.

The Basal Metabolic Rate

The basal metabolic rate (BMR), the sum total of cellular activity in all metabolically active tissues while under basal conditions, is the minimal amount of oxygen utilized to support life.

 Clinical Pearl

A person's BMR varies according to overall body size, gender, age, fat-free mass (FFM), and endocrine function. In general the BMR tends to be 5% to 10% lower in women than in men. There is a decline in BMR of 2% to 3% per decade of life, which is most likely due to the reduction in physical activity associated with aging.

Body Mass Index

Body mass index (BMI) is a measure of body fat based on height and weight.

 Clinical Pearl

BMI can be calculated by dividing the body weight (in kilograms) by the square of the height (in meters) of an individual. Values above 25 are considered abnormal.

> 25 to 30: Overweight
> More than 30: Obese

Body fat can be divided into two types:

- Essential fat: necessary for normal physiological function, serving as a source of energy and a storage site for some vitamins.
- Storage fat: stored in adipose tissue.

 Clinical Pearl

Fat-free mass (FFM) is the total mass of the body minus the fat mass and includes muscle, skin, bone, and viscera.

Separate calculations are used for boys and girls ages 2 to 20 and for adult men and women. Further subdivisions can be made according to gender for adults. The limitations of relying on the BMI include the following:

- It may overestimate body fat in athletes and others who have a muscular build.
- It may underestimate body fat in older persons and others who have lost muscle mass.

 Clinical Pearl

The standard error with estimating percent fat with the BMI is approximately 5%.

Bioelectrical Impedance Analysis

Bioelectrical impedance analysis (BIA) measures body composition by sending a low, safe electrical current through the body fluids contained mainly in the lean and fat tissue. BIA measures the impedance or opposition to the flow of this electric current.

 Clinical Pearl

- Impedance is low in lean tissue, where intracellular fluid and electrolytes are primarily contained.
- Impedance is high in fat tissue.

Impedance is thus proportional to total body water (TBW) volume. Prediction equations, previously generated by correlating impedance measures against an independent estimate of TBW, may be used subsequently to convert the measured impedance into a corresponding estimate of TBW. Lean body mass is then calculated from this estimate using an assumed hydration fraction for lean tissue. Fat mass is calculated as the difference between body weight and lean body mass.

 Clinical Pearl

BIA values are affected by numerous variables including body position, hydration status, consumption of food and beverages, ambient air and skin temperature, recent physical activity, and conductance of the examining table. Reliable BIA requires standardization and control of these variables.

The Kinetic Chain

The expression *kinetic chain* is used to describe the function or activity of an extremity and/or trunk in terms of a series of linked chains. According to kinetic chain theory, each of the joint segments of the body involved in a particular movement constitutes a link along one of these kinetic chains. As each motion of a joint is often a function of other joint motions, the efficiency of an activity can be dependent on how well these chain links work together.[2]

Closed Kinetic Chain

A variety of definitions for a closed kinetic chain (CKC) activity have been proposed:

- Palmitier et al.[3] defined an activity as "closed" if both ends of the kinetic chain are connected to an immovable framework, thus preventing translation of either the proximal or the distal joint center, and creating a situation where movement at one joint produces a predictable movement at all other joints.

- Gray[4] considered a closed-chain activity to involve fixation of the distal segment so that joint motion takes place in multiple planes, and the limb is supporting weight.

- Dillman et al.[5] described the characteristics of closed-chain activities to include relatively small joint movements, low joint accelerations, greater joint compressive forces, greater joint congruity, decreased shear, stimulation of joint proprioception, and enhanced dynamic stabilization through muscle coactivation.[6]

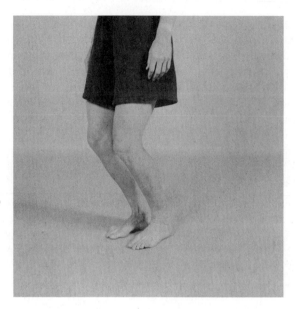

Figure 4-1 Example of a lower extremity CKC activity.

- Kibler[6] defines a closed-chain activity as a sequential combination of joint motions that have the following characteristics:
  - The distal segment of the kinetic chain meets considerable resistance.
  - The movement of the individual joints, and translation of their instant centers of rotation, occurs in a predictable manner that is secondary to the distribution of forces from each end of the chain.

  Examples of a closed kinetic chain exercise (CKCE) involving the lower extremities include the squat (Figure 4-1) and the leg press. The activities of walking, running, jumping, climbing, and rising from the floor, all incorporate CKC components. An example of a CKCE for the upper extremities is the push-up, or when using the arms to rise out of a chair.

Open Kinetic Chain

It is generally accepted that the movement of the end segment determines the difference between open kinetic chain (OKC) and CKC activities. The traditional definition for an "open"-chain activity included all activities that involved the end segment of an extremity moving freely through space, resulting in isolated movement of a joint.

  Examples of an open kinetic chain exercises (OKCEs) involving the lower extremity include the seated knee extension, surgical tubing exercises using

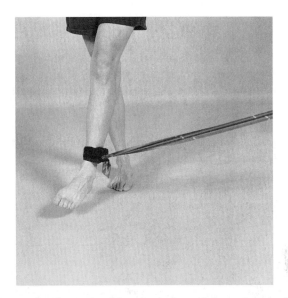

Figure 4-2 Example of an open kinetic chain activity using the left lower extremity.

nonweight-bearing extremity (Figure 4-2), and prone knee flexion. Upper extremity examples of OKCE include the biceps curl and the military press.

Open-chain exercises have traditionally been deemed to be less functional in terms of many athletic movements, primarily serving as a supportive role in strength and conditioning programs. As a result, the use of OKCE in clinical settings declined, and there has been a shift in emphasis toward the use of CKCE, although evidence supports the skillful use of both.

MUSCLE PERFORMANCE

Muscle performance includes strength, endurance, and power.
- Strength. Strength is defined as the maximum force that a muscle can develop during a single contraction. Muscular strength is derived both from the amount of tension a muscle can generate and from the moment arms of contributing muscles with respect to the joint center. Both sources are affected by several factors (see Factors Affecting Muscle Performance). Muscle strength can be measured using a number of methods:
  - Manual muscle testing (MMT): see Chapter 3.
  - Using a dynamometer: a device that measures strength through the use of a load cell or spring-loaded gauge.

- Isokinetic machine: measures the strength of a muscle group during a movement with constant, predetermined speed.
- Endurance. Endurance is defined as the ability of a muscle to sustain or perform repetitive muscular contractions for an extended period. The ability to perform endurance activities is based on the patient's aerobic capacity.
- Power. Power is the rate of performing work. Work is the magnitude of force acting on an object multiplied by the distance through which the force acts. Muscular power is the product of muscular force and velocity of muscle shortening.

 Clinical Pearl

Muscular power is an important contributor to activities requiring both speed and strength. Maximum power occurs at approximately one third of maximum velocity.[7] Individuals with a predominance of fast twitch fibers (see Chapter 1) generate more power at a given load than those with a high composition of slow twitch fibers.[8] The ratio for mean peak power production by Type IIb, Type IIa and Type I fibers in skeletal tissue is 10:5:1.[9]

Factors Affecting Muscle Performance

The maximum tension that is generated within a fully activated muscle is not a constant and depends on a number of factors.[10]

 Clinical Pearl

Factors affecting muscle performance include the following[11]:
- Muscle fiber type
- Muscle fiber size
- Force–length relationships
- Force-velocity relationships
- Muscle design (angle of insertion and angle of pennation)
- Fatigue
- Neural control
- Age
- Level of cognition

Clinical Pearl

For each muscle cell, there is an optimum length, or range of lengths, where the contractile force is strongest. At the natural resting length of the muscle, there is near-optimal overlap of actin and myosin allowing for the generation of maximum tension at this length.

If the muscle is in a shortened position, the overlap of actin and myosin reduces the number of sites available for cross-bridge formation.

 Clinical Pearl

Active insufficiency of a muscle occurs when the muscle is incapable of shortening to the extent required to produce full range of motion at all joints crossed simultaneously.[10,12-14] For example, the finger flexors cannot produce a tight fist when the wrist is fully flexed as when it is in neutral.

If the muscle is in a lengthened position compared to the resting length, the actin filaments are pulled away from the myosin heads, such that they cannot create cross-bridges.[15]

 Clinical Pearl

Passive insufficiency of the muscle occurs when the two-joint muscle cannot stretch to the extent required for full range of motion in the opposite direction at all joints crossed.[10,12-14] For example, a larger range of extension is possible at the wrist when the fingers are not fully extended.

 Clinical Pearl

For maximal effectiveness of muscle force production, slow concentric movements should be emphasized.[16,17]

Just as there are optimal speeds of length change, and optimal muscle lengths, there are optimal insertion angles for each of the muscles. The angle of insertion of a muscle, and therefore its line of pull, can change during dynamic movements.[15]

 Clinical Pearl

Muscles that need to have large changes in length without the need for very high tension, such as the sartorius, do not have pennate (see Chapter 1) muscle fibers.[15] In contrast, pennate muscle fibers are found in those muscles in which the emphasis is on a high capacity for tension generation rather than range of motion (e.g., gluteus maximus).

Skeletal muscle fatigue can compromise exercise tolerance and work productivity while retarding rehabilitation of diseased or damaged muscle. The development of fatigue probably involves several factors that influence force production in a manner dependent on muscle fiber type and activation pattern.[18]

Characteristics of muscle fatigue include reduction in muscle force production capability and shortening velocity, a reduction in the release and uptake of intracellular calcium by the sarcoplasmic reticulum, as well as prolonged relaxation of motor units between recruitment.[18,19]

 Clinical Pearl

Skeletal muscle blood flow increases 20-fold during muscle contractions.[20] The muscle blood flow generally increases in proportion to the metabolic demands of the tissue, a relationship reflected by positive correlations between muscle blood flow and exercise.

Detrimental Effects of Immobilization

Continuous immobilization of skeletal muscle tissues can cause some undesirable consequences. These include the following:

• Weakness or atrophy of muscles (Table 4-1).[21,22] Muscle atrophy is an imbalance between protein synthesis and degradation.

Table 4-1 Structural Changes in the Various Types of Muscle Following Immobilization in a Shortened Position*

	Muscle Fiber Type and Changes		
Structural Characteristics	Slow Oxidative	Fast Oxidative Glycolytic	Fast Glycolytic
Number of fibers	Moderate decrease	Minimal increase	Minimal increase
Diameter of fibers	Significant decrease	Moderate decrease	Moderate decrease
Fiber fragmentation	Minimal increase	Minimal increase	Significant increase
Myofibrils	Minimal decrease and disoriented	—	Wavy
Nuclei	Degenerated and rounded	Degenerated and rounded	Degenerated and rounded
Mitochondria	Moderate decrease, degenerated	Moderate decrease, degenerated	Minimal decrease, degenerated, swollen
Sarcoplasmic reticulum	Minimal decrease, orderly arrangement	Minimal decrease	Minimal decrease
Myofilaments	Minimal decrease, disorganized	Moderate decrease	Minimal decrease, wavy
Z band	Moderate decrease	—	Faint or absent
Vesicles	Abnormal configuration	—	—
Basement membrane	Minimal increase	—	—
Register of sarcomeres	Irregular projections, shifted with time	—	—
Fatty infiltration	Minimal increase	—	—
Collagen	Minimal increase between fibers	—	—
Macrophages	Minimal increased invasion	Minimal increased invasion	Minimal increased invasion
Satellite cells	Minimal increase	—	—
Target cells	Minimal increase	—	—

*From reference 22.

Clinical Pearl

Disuse atrophy of muscle begins within 4 hours of the start of bed rest resulting in decreases in muscle mass, muscle cell diameter, and the number of muscle fibers. However, strenuous exercise of atrophic muscle can lead to muscle damage including sarcolemmal disruption, distortion of the myofibrils' contractile components, and cytoskeletal damage. Thus, a balance must be found.

The cause of muscle damage during exercised recovery from atrophy involves an altered ability of the muscle fibers to bear the mechanical stress of external loads (weight-bearing) and movement associated with exercise. Strenuous exercise can result in primary or secondary sarcolemma disruption, swelling or disruption of the sarcotubular system, distortion of the myofibrils' contractile components, cytoskeletal damage, and extracellular myofiber matrix abnormalities.[23] These pathological changes are similar to those seen in healthy young adults after sprint running or resistance training.[23] It appears that the act of contracting while the muscle is in a stretched or lengthened position, known as an eccentric contraction, is responsible for these injuries.[24]

 Clinical Pearl

The clinician must remember that the restoration of full strength and range of motion may prove difficult if muscles are allowed to heal without early active motion, or in a shortened position, and that the patient may be prone to repeated strains.[25] Thus, range of motion exercises should be started once swelling and tenderness have subsided to the point that the exercises are not unduly painful.[25]

IMPROVING MUSCLE PERFORMANCE

The promotion and progression of tissue repair involves a delicate balance between protection and the application of controlled functional stresses to the damaged structure. The goal of the functional progression is to identify the motion or motions that the patient is able to exercise into without eliciting symptoms other than postexercise soreness.[26] Patients must be advised to let pain be their guide and that pain-free range of motion activities must be continued to prevent loss of function.

Table 4-2 Resistive Exercise Variables

Resistance (load or weight)
Duration and volume (the total number of repetitions performed multiplied by the resistance used)
Frequency (weekly, daily)
Intensity
Point of application
Sequence (exercising large muscle groups before small; perform multijoint before single-joint activities)
Bouts (timed sessions of exercise)
Sets and repetition
Mode (type of contraction)
Rests

 Clinical Pearl

- The dosage of an exercise refers to each particular patient's exercise capability and is determined by a number of variables (Table 4-2) and the goals of the intervention (increasing strength, endurance, or power).[27]

- Intensity and duration are inversely proportional: the higher the intensity, the fewer repetitions that are performed.

A hierarchy for range of motion (ROM) (Table 4-3)[28] and resistive exercise progression (Table 4-4)[29] exists. This hierarchy is based on patient tolerance and response to ensure that any progress made is done in a safe and controlled fashion.

 Clinical Pearl

All of the exercises described at the end of the appropriate chapters are based on exercise progression hierarchies using three phases (see Chapter 3).

Table 4-3 The Hierarchy for the ROM Exercises*

1. Passive ROM
2. Active assisted ROM
3. Active ROM

*Data from reference 28.

Correct Progression

The therapeutic exercise program always begins with an exercise the patient can perform, before progressing in difficulty. Each progression is made more challenging by altering one of the parameters of exercise (type/mode of exercise, intensity, duration, and frequency), which are modified according to patient response.

Intensity

Intensity refers to how much effort is required to perform the exercise. For aerobic activities, the exercise intensity should be at a level that is 40% to 85% maximal aerobic power (VO$_2$ max) or 55% to 90% of maximal HR.[30]

Duration

Duration refers to the length of the exercise session. In most functional exercises, fatigue must be considered when doing exercises so that the patient's

 Clinical Pearl

It is now recognized that an individual's perception of effort (relative perceived exertion) is closely related to the level of physiological effort (Table 4-5).[31,32] It is important therefore, to closely monitor the patient's response to exercise. Any discomfort or reproduction of symptoms that last more than 1 to 2 hours after the intervention is unacceptable. Patient responses that can modify the intensity include increases in pain level, muscle fatigue, time taken to recover from fatigue, cardiovascular response, compensatory movements, insufficient balance, level of motivation, and degree of comprehension.

Table 4-4 The Hierarchy for the Progression of Resistive Exercises*

1. Single angle submaximal isometrics performed in the neutral position
2. Multiple angle submaximal isometrics performed at various angles of the range
3. Multiple angle maximal isometrics
4. Small arc submaximal concentrics
5. Full ROM submaximal concentrics
6. Functional ROM submaximal concentrics

*Data from references 28 and 29.

tolerance is not exceeded. The exercise should be performed in a pain-free range until fatigue occurs. Fatigue may also occur as a lack of coordination observed by the clinician but not perceived by the patient.

Physical conditioning occurs over a period of 15 to 60 minutes depending on the level of intensity. Average conditioning time is 20 to 30 minutes for

Table 4-5 Rating of Perceived Exertion*

Scale	Verbal Rating
6	
7	Very, very light
8	
9	Very light
10	
11	Fairly light
12	
13	Somewhat hard
14	
15	Hard
16	
17	Very hard
18	
19	Very, very hard
20	

*Data from reference 31.

moderate-intensity exercise. However, individuals who are severely compromised are more likely to benefit from a series of short exercise sessions (3–10 minutes) spaced throughout the day.

Frequency

Frequency refers to how often the exercise is performed. Frequency of activity is dependent on intensity and duration; the lower the intensity, the longer the duration, the greater the frequency. The recommended frequency is three to five sessions per week at moderate intensities and duration (>5 METs).

Exercise progression in the following populations is determined by a number of factors including the stage of healing and the degree of irritability of the structure, the patient's response to exercise, and the general health of the patient. Extra care must be taken with the following:

- Patients with an acute illness/fever
- Patients with an acute injury
- Postsurgical patients
- Patients with cardiac disease—edema, weight gain, unstable angina
- Patients who are obese

Overload Principle

The principle of overload states that a greater than normal stress or load on the body is required for training adaptation to take place. To increase strength, the muscle must be challenged at a greater level than it is accustomed to. High levels of tension will produce adaptations in the form of hypertrophy and recruitment of more muscle fibers.

Specificity of Training

Specificity of training is an accepted concept in rehabilitation. This concept involves the principle of the specific adaptation to imposed demand (SAID).

 Clinical Pearl

The focus of the exercise prescription should be to improve the strength and coordination of functional or sport-specific movements with exercises that approximate the desired activity.

For example, resistance training performed concentrically improves concentric muscle strength and the eccentric training improves eccentric muscle strength.

The SAID principle can be applied by exercising the muscles along each extremity and within the trunk in functional patterns.[3]

 Clinical Pearl

The exercise component of the intervention should be as specific as the manual technique used in the clinic.

Delayed Onset Muscle Soreness

Muscular soreness may result from all forms of exercise. Acute muscle soreness develops during or directly after strenuous and aerobic exercise performed to the point of fatigue. The soreness is theoretically related to the decreased blood flow and reduced oxygen that creates a temporary buildup of lactic acid and potassium. A type of soreness that is related to eccentric exercise is delayed onset muscle soreness (DOMS).[27] This type of soreness, which occurs between 48 and 72 hours after exercise, may last for up to 10 days.

 Clinical Pearl

Using a cool-down period of low-intensity exercise that facilitates the return of oxygen to the muscle can minimize the adverse effects of DOMS.

Prevention of this type of muscle soreness involves careful design of the eccentric program including preparatory techniques, accurate training variables, and appropriate aftercare.[27] The intervention for DOMS includes aerobic submaximal exercise with no eccentric component (swimming, biking, or stepper machines), pain-free flexibility exercises, and high-speed (300 degrees/second) concentric only isokinetic training.[27,33]

 Clinical Pearl

Neuromuscular electrical stimulation (NMES) can be an effective component of a rehabilitation program for muscle weakness.

A number of principles are used throughout the exercise phases presented at the end of each of the appropriate chapters[34]:

- The degree of irritability is determined by inquiring about the vigor, duration, and intensity of the symptoms. Greater irritability is associated with very acutely inflamed conditions. The characteristic sign for an acute inflammation is pain at rest, which is diffuse in its distribution and often referred from the site of the primary condition.[35] Chronic conditions usually have low irritability but have an associated loss of active and passive ROM.

 Clinical Pearl

- If pain is reported by the patient before a resistive activity or before the end-feel during passive range of motion, the patient's symptoms are considered irritable. The intervention in the presence of irritability should not be aggressive.[36]

- If pain occurs after resistance, then the patient's symptoms are not considered irritable and exercise, particularly stretching, can be more aggressive.

- The patient is initially taught to exercise in cardinal planes before progressing as quickly as allowed to exercising in the functional planes.
- The exercise protocol is initiated with exercises that utilize a short lever arm. These exercises serve to decrease the amount of torque at the joint. Extremity exercises are adapted to include short levers by flexing the extremity or by exercising with the extremity closer to the body.
- The goal is to achieve the closed pack position at the earliest opportunity. The closed pack position of a joint is its position of maximum stability. However, it is also the position of maximum ligamentous and capsular tautness, so care needs to be taken in achieving this position.
- The prescribed exercises aim to reproduce the forces and loading rates that will approach the patient's functional demands, as the rehabilitation progresses.
- All exercise progressions include the following[37]:
  - Variation. Variation to the exercises is provided by altering
    - the plane of motion
    - the range of motion
    - the body position

- ○ the exercise duration
- ○ the exercise frequency
- A safe progression. A safe progression is ensured as the exercises are progressed from
  - ○ slow to fast
  - ○ simple to complex
  - ○ stable to unstable
  - ○ low to high force.

 Clinical Pearl

At regular intervals, the clinician should ensure that

- the patient is adherent with their exercise program at home

- the patient is aware as to the rationale behind the exercise program

- the patient is performing the exercise program correctly and at the appropriate intensity

- the patient's exercise program is being updated appropriately based on clinical findings and patient response.

Improving Strength

To most effectively increase muscle strength, a muscle must work with increasing effort against progressively increasing resistance.[38,39]

Clinical Pearl

The greatest amount of tension the muscle can achieve is a 20% increase in fiber length measured from the resting length.[40] The clinical implications for this are that the patient can tolerate less resistance in the beginning of range, and at the end of range of contraction, but can overcome more resistance at a point in the range 20% beyond resting contraction.[41]

If a resistance is applied to a muscle as it contracts so that the metabolic capabilities of the muscle are progressively overloaded, adaptive changes occur within the muscle, which make it stronger over time.[16,42] These adaptive changes include the following[17,39,43–47]:

- Remodeling (hypertrophy): The muscle hypertrophies due to an increase in the number and size of the myofilaments (actin and myosin).
- An increase in the efficiency of the neuromuscular system. This increased efficiency results in
  - an increase in the number of motor units recruited
  - an increase in the firing rate of each motor unit
  - an increase in the synchronization of motor unit firing
  - an increase in the endurance of the muscle
- Stimulation of slow twitch (Type I) fibers (when performing workloads of low intensity), and stimulation of fast twitch (Type IIa) fibers (when performing workloads of high intensity and short duration) (see Chapter 1).
- Rhythmic activities increase blood flow to exercising muscles via a contraction and relaxation.
- The power of the muscle improves.
- Improved bone mass (Wolfe law).
- Increase in metabolism/calorie burning/weight control.
- Increased intramuscular pressure results from a muscle contraction of about 60% of its force generating capacity.
- Cardiovascular benefits when using large muscle groups. Strength training of specific muscles has a brief activation period and uses a relatively small muscle mass, producing less cardiovascular metabolic demands than vigorous walking, swimming, and the like.

  Conversely, a muscle can become weak or atrophied through

- disease
- neurological compromise
- immobilization
- disuse.

Types of Exercise

Isometric Exercises

Isometric exercises provide a static contraction with a variable and accommodating resistance without producing a change in muscle length. This type of exercise has an obvious role in which joint movement is restricted, either by pain or by bracing/casting. Their primary role in this regard is to prevent atrophy and prevent a decrease of ligament, bone, and muscle strength. A 6-second hold of 75% of maximal resistance is sufficient to increase strength when performed repetitively. The disadvantages of isometric exercises are as follows:

- The strength gains are developed at a specific point in the range of motion and not throughout the range (unless performed at multiangles).
- Not all of a muscle's fibers are activated—there is predominantly an activation of slow twitch (Type I) fibers.
- There are no flexibility and/or cardiovascular fitness benefits.
- Peak effort can be injurious to the tissues due to vasoconstriction and joint compression forces.
- There is limited functional carry over.[48]
- Considerable internal pressure can be generated, especially if the breath is held during contraction, which can result in
  - further injury to patient's with a weakness in the abdominal wall (hernia).
  - cardiovascular impairment (increase blood pressure through the Valsalva maneuver, even if the exercise is performed correctly).

Concentric/Isotonic Exercises

Concentric contractions are commonly used in the rehabilitation process and occur frequently in activities of daily living (ADLs)—the biceps curl (Figure 4-3) and the lifting of a cup to the mouth are examples, respectively. Isotonic exercise occurs when the tension in the muscle remains constant despite a change in muscle length. This type of contraction is rare.

Concentric exercises are dynamic and allow the clinician to vary the load from constant, using free weights, to variable, using an exercise machine. The speed of contraction can also be manipulated depending on the goal of the intervention.

Eccentric Exercises

Maximum eccentric exercises produce more force than maximal concentric contraction. Eccentric strength is important for many functional activities and can provide a source of shock absorption during closed-chain functional activities. Eccentric exercises involve the development of tension while the muscle length increases. An example of an eccentric exercise includes the reverse arm curl (Figure 4-4). The clinical indications for the use of eccentric exercise are numerous (Table 4-6).[27,49]

Functional Exercises

Functional strength is the ability of the neuromuscular system to perform the various types of contractions involved with multijoint functional activities in an efficient manner and in a multiplanar environment.[50] Functional exercises,

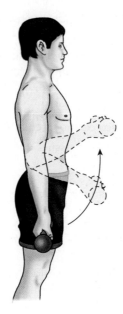

Figure 4-3 A concentric contraction.

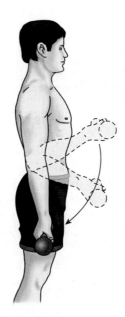

Figure 4-4 An eccentric contraction.

Table 4-6 Clinical Indications for Eccentric-biased Exercise*

Mechanical, reproducible joint pain
Joint pain resistant to modality intervention
Unidirectional joint crepitus or pain arc
De-conditioned or low endurance patients
Plateaus in strength gains
Tendonitis presentations
Late stage rehabilitation and performance training

*Data from references 27 and 49.

such as the step down/step up (Figure 4-5) use combinations of concentric and eccentric contractions in the performance of activities that relate to a patient's needs and requirements (see Specificity of Training). Incremental gains in function should be seen as strength increases.

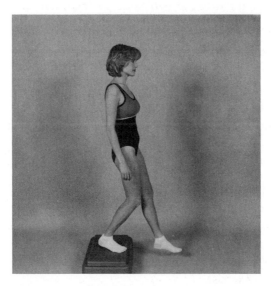

Figure 4-5 Example of a functional exercise.

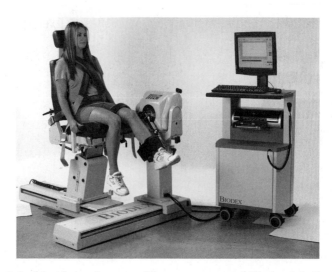

Figure 4-6 Isokinetic equipment. (Photo courtesy of Biodex Medical Systems, Inc.)

Isokinetic Exercise

Isokinetic exercise requires the use of special equipment that produces an accommodating and variable resistance (Figure 4-6). The main principle behind isokinetic exercise is that peak torque (the maximum force generated through the range of motion) is inversely related to angular velocity, the speed that a body segment moves through its range of motion. Thus, an increase in angular velocity decreases peak torque production. Advantages for this type of exercise include the following:

- Both high-speed/low-resistance, and low-speed/high-resistance regimens result in excellent strength gains.[51–54]
- Both concentric and eccentric resistance exercises can be performed on isokinetic machines.
- The machines provide maximum resistance at all point in the range of motion as a muscle contracts.
- The gravity-produced torque created by the machine adds to the force generated by the muscle when it contracts resulting in a higher torque output than it actually created by the muscle. The disadvantages of this type of exercise include
  - Expense
  - The potential for impact loading and incorrect joint axis alignment[55]
  - Questionable functional carry-over[48]
    - Open-chain exercise
    - Single muscle/motion

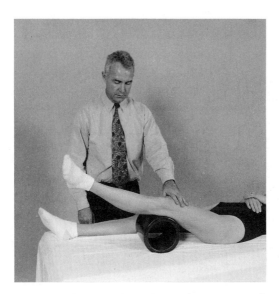

Figure 4-7 Exercising against gravity using a short arc quad.

Types of Resistance

Resistance can be applied to a muscle by any external force or mass, including any of the following.

Gravity

Gravity alone can supply sufficient resistance with a weakened muscle (Figure 4-7). With respect to gravity, muscle actions may occur in

- the same direction of gravity (downward)
- in the opposite direction to gravity (upward)
- in a direction perpendicular to gravity (horizontal)
- in the same or opposite direction to gravity, but at an angle.

Body Weight

A wide variety exercises have been developed using no equipment and relying on the patient's body weight for the resistance. Examples of such exercises include the squat, lunge, and push-up.

Small Weights

Cuff weights and dumbbells are economical ways of applying resistance (Figure 4-8). Small weights are typically used to strengthen the smaller mus-

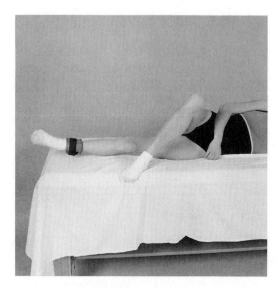

Figure 4-8 Exercise using cuff weight.

cles or to increase the endurance of larger muscles by increasing the number of reps. Free weights also provide more versatility than exercise machines, especially for three-dimensional exercises.

 Clinical Pearl

The disadvantage of free weights is that they offer no variable resistance throughout the range of motion so that the weakest point along the length-tension curve of each muscle limits the amount of weight lifted.

Surgical Tubing/Theraband

Elastic resistance (Figure 4-9) offers a unique type of resistance that cannot be classified within the traditional subcategories of strengthening. The amount of variable resistance offered by elastic bands or tubing is a factor of the internal tension produced by the material. This internal tension is a factor of the elastic material's coefficient of elasticity, the surface area of the elastic material, and how much the elastic material is stretched.[56]

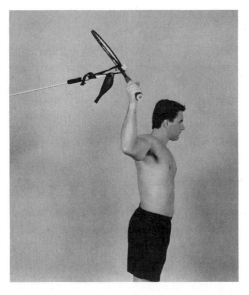

Figure 4-9 Surgical tubing exercise to mimic tennis stroke.

⊚ Clinical Pearl

It is commonly believed that the resistance provided by these bands or tubing increases exponentially at the end range of motion. However, the forces produced by elastic resistance are linear until approximately 500% elongation, at which point the forces increase exponentially.[56] As the elastic resistance is not stretched more than 300% in prescribed exercises, the exponential increase should not be attained.

Exercise Machines

In situations where the larger muscle groups require strengthening, a multitude of specific indoor exercise machines can be used. These machines are often used in the more advanced stages of a rehabilitation program when more resistance can be tolerated, but they can also be used in the earlier stages depending on the size of the muscle undergoing rehabilitation. Examples of these machines include the Multi-hip, the Lat pull-down, the leg extension, and the leg curl machine. Exercise machines are often fitted with an oval-shaped cam or wheel that mimic the length of tension curve of the muscle (Nautilus, Cybex). Although these machines are a more expensive alternative to dumbbell or elastic resistance, they do offer some advantages as they:

- Provide more adequate resistance for large muscle groups that can be achieved with free weights/cuff weights, or manual resistance.
- Are typically safer than free weights as control throughout the range is provided.
- Provide the clinician with the ability to quantify and measure the amount of resistance that the patient can tolerate over time.

The disadvantages of exercise machines include the following:

- The inability to modify the exercise to be more functional or three-dimensional.
- The inability to modify the amount of resistance at particular points of the range.

Manual Resistance

Manual resistance: a type of active exercise in which another person provides resistance manually (Figure 4-10). An example of manual resistance is proprioceptive neuromuscular facilitation (PNF)—refer to section entitled Proprioceptive Neuromuscular Facilitation in the Specialized Exercise Regimes.

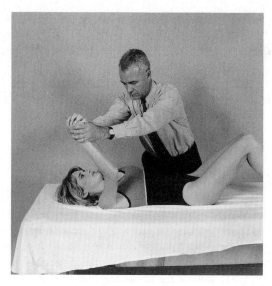

Figure 4-10 Exercising against manual resistance.

The advantages of manual resistance, when applied by a skilled clinician, are as follows[57]:

- Control of the extremity position and force applied. This is especially useful in the early stages of an exercise program when the muscle is weak.
- More effective reeducation of the muscle or extremity, through the use of diagonal or functional patterns of movement.
- Critical sensory input to the patient through tactile stimulation and appropriate facilitation techniques (e.g., quick stretch).
- Accurate accommodation and alterations in the resistance applied throughout the range. For example, an exercise can be modified to avoid a painful arc in the range.
- Ability to limit the range. This is particularly important when the amount of range of motion needs to be carefully controlled (postsurgical restrictions or pain).

The disadvantages of manual resistance include the following:

- The amount of resistance applied cannot be measured quantitatively.
- The amount of resistance is limited by the strength of the clinician/caregiver or family member.
- Difficulty with consistency of the applied force throughout the range, and with each repetition.

Clinical Pearl

Water can be used as a form of resistance (see Specialized Exercise Regimes). Water provides resistance proportional to the relative speed of movement of the patient and the water and the cross-sectional area of the patient in contact with the water.[58]

Prescriptions for Strengthening

Absolute contraindications to strength training include unstable angina, uncontrolled hypertension, uncontrolled dysrhythmias, hypertrophic cardiomyopathy, and certain stages of retinopathy. Patients with congestive heart failure, myocardial ischemia, poor left ventricular function, or autonomic neuropathies must be carefully evaluated before initiating a strength-training program.

A number of precautions must be observed with patients who are performing strength training:

- Substitute motions: Muscles that are weak or fatigued rely on other muscles to produce the movement if the resistance is too high. This results in incorrect stabilization and poor form.
- Overworking of the muscles: This can occur if the exercise parameters (frequency, intensity, duration) are advanced too quickly.
- Adequate rest must be provided (3 to 4 minutes are needed to return the muscle to 90% to 95% of preexercise capacity, with the most rapid recovery occurring in the first minute) after each vigorous exercise.
- The rest period between sets can be determined by the time the breathing rate, or pulse, of the patient returns to the steady state.

Caution must be taken with patients diagnosed with osteoporosis whose bones are unable to withstand normal stresses and are highly susceptible to pathological fracture. Osteoporotic features may also occur as a result of prolonged immobilization, bed rest, inability to bear weight on an extremity and as a result of nutritional, or hormonal factors.

A number of programs have been designed for the progression of concentric exercise programs (Table 4-7). It is important to remember that any exercise progression should always be based on sound rationale (optimal resistance, the number of repetitions, the number of sets, and the frequency of training) and the symptomatic response.

Warm-up and Cool-down Periods

Each exercise session should include a 5- to 15-minute warm-up and a 5- to 15-minute cool-down period.

- Warm-up
  - includes low-intensity cardiorespiratory activities
  - serves to prepare the heart and circulatory system from being suddenly overloaded
- Cool/down
  - includes low-intensity cardiorespiratory activities and flexibility exercises
  - helps prevent abrupt physiological alterations that can occur with sudden cessation of strenuous exercise, such as adaptive shortening, and lactic acid buildup.

The length of the warm-up and cool-down sessions may need to be longer for deconditioned or older individuals.

Progressive Resistive Exercise

Progressive resistive exercises (PREs) use the repetition maximum (RM) or the greatest amount of weight a muscle can move through the range of motion a specific number of times (resistance maximal) (Table 4-7).

Table 4-7 Exercise Progressions

	Set(s) of 10	Amount of Weight	Repetitions
DeLorme program	1	50% of 10 RM	10
	2	75% of 10 RM	10
	3	100% of 10 RM	10
Oxford technique	1	100% of 10 RM	10
	2	75% of 10 RM	10
	3	50% of 10 RM	10
MacQueen technique	3 (beginning/intermediate)	100% of 10 RM	10
	4–5 (advanced)	100% of 2–3 RM	2–3
Sander program	Total of 4 sets (three times per week)	100% of 5 RM	5
	Day 1: 4 sets	100% of 5 RM	5
	Day 2: 4 sets	100% of 3 RM	5
	Day 3: 1 set	100% of 5 RM	5
	2 sets	100% of 3 RM	5
	2 sets	100% of 2 RM	5
Knight DAPRE program	1	50% of RM	10
	2	75% of RM	6
	3	100% of RM	Maximum
	4	Adjusted working weight	Maximum

DAPRE = daily adjustable progressive resistive exercise; RM = repetition maximum.

Repetition maximum
This is based on the premise that whatever exercise progression is used to achieve an increase in the total number of repetitions while maintaining a sufficient effort, the number of sets must also be increased. This increase in

Table 4-8 Adjustment Sequence for DAPRE Isotonic Program

Number of Reps Performed During Set	Adjusted Working Weight for Fourth Set	Next Exercise Session
0–2	−5–10 lb	−5–10 lb
3–4	−0–5 lb	Same weight
5–6	Same weight	+5–10 lb
7–10	+5–10 lb	+5–15 lb
11	+10–20 lb	+10–20 lb

sets must occur in conjunction with a reduction in the number of repetitions per set by 10% to 20%,[41] or a reduction in the resistance.

Resistance maximal
A concept introduced by DeLorme and Watkins[44] that refers to the amount of resistance a group of muscles can overcome exactly 10 times. This amount of resistance is then used for exercise. The various programs are summarized in Tables 4-7 and 4-8.

Circuit Training
Circuit training or cross-training incorporates a wide variety of modes of training and uses high repetitions and low weight to provide a more general conditioning program aimed at improving body composition, muscular strength, and some cardiovascular fitness.

Interval Training
Interval training includes an exercise period followed by a prescribed rest interval. It is perceived to be less demanding than continuous training and tends to improve strength and power more than endurance.

With appropriate spacing of work and rest intervals, a significant amount of high-intensity work can be achieved and is greater than the amount of work accomplished with continuous training.

The longer the work interval, the more the anaerobic system is stressed and the duration of the rest period is not important.

In a short work interval, a work recovery ratio of 1:1 or 1:5 is appropriate to stress the aerobic system.

Tabata Protocol

The Tabata protocol sequence or is a high-intensity training regimen involving an interval training cycle of 20 seconds of maximum intensity exercise, followed by 10 seconds of rest, repeated without pause eight times for a total of 4 minutes (14 minutes when including a 5-minute warm-up and a 5-minute cool-down).[59] A study by Tabata et al.[59] showed that moderate-intensity aerobic training that improves the maximal aerobic power does not change anaerobic capacity and that adequate high-intensity intermittent training may improve both anaerobic and aerobic energy supplying systems significantly, probably through imposing intensive stimuli on both systems.

Maintaining Strength

To maintain the benefits of training, exercise must be maintained. Based on studies of isokinetic and concentric exercise[60,61]:

- Muscle strength recovery follows a steady, nonlinear, and predictable increase over time.[27]
- Reversibility: a lack of training results in decreased muscle recruitment and muscle fiber atrophy.

If an injured patient can maintain some form of strength training, even once per week, their strength can be fairly well maintained over a 3-month period.[62]

Clinical Pearl

When expressed as a weekly percentage, the Albert 5% rule states that a 5% strength increase in a given week can be maintained for many weeks of resistive training providing that the patient trains three times a week at a minimum resistance load of 70% of maximal voluntary muscle contractile force.[27] Although seemingly esoteric, the 5% rule can be used in determining the prognosis. For example, a patient with a 40% deficit in strength of the biceps can be assumed to take approximately 8 weeks to recover, barring any illness, or disease states.[27]

Improving Muscular Endurance

To improve muscle endurance, exercises are performed against light resistance for many repetitions, so that the amount of energy expanded is equal to the amount of energy supplied.

This phenomenon called steady state occurs after some 5 to 6 minutes of exercise at a constant intensity level.

Working at a level to which the muscle is accustomed, improves the endurance of that muscle, but does not increase its strength. However, exercise programs that increase strength also increase muscular endurance.

> ### ⚬ Clinical Pearl
>
> Muscular endurance programs are typically indicated early in a strengthening program as the high-repetition and low-load exercises are more comfortable, enhance the vascular supply to muscle, cause less muscle soreness, less joint irritation, and reduce the risk of muscle injury.

Aerobic Capacity and Cardiorespiratory Endurance

By definition, cardiorespiratory endurance is the ability to perform whole body activities (walking, jogging, biking, swimming, etc.) for extended periods without undue fatigue. A number of training adaptations occur within the circulatory system in response to exercise:

- HR: Monitoring HR is an indirect method of estimating oxygen consumption as, in general, these two factors have a linear relationship.
- SV: The volume of blood being pumped out with each beat increases with exercise, but only to the point when there is enough time between beats for the heart to fill up (approximately 110–120 beats/min).
- CO: CO, calculated by multiplying SV and HR, increases with exercise. A training effect that occurs with regard to CO of the heart is that the SV increases, whereas the exercise HR is reduced at a given standard exercise load.
- Blood pressure: Systolic pressure increases in proportion to oxygen consumption and CO, whereas diastolic pressure shows little or no increase.
- Hemoglobin concentration: The concentration of hemoglobin in circulating blood does not change with training; it may actually decrease slightly.
- Lung changes that occur due to exercise:
  - An increase in the volume of air that can be inspired in a single maximal ventilation.
  - An increase in the diffusing capacity of the lungs.

- Oxygen consumption rises rapidly during the first minutes of exercise and levels off as the aerobic metabolism supplies the energy required by the working muscles.
- Fitter individuals have a respiratory system that is more capable of delivering oxygen to sustain aerobic energy production at increasingly higher levels of intensity.
- In cases of severe pulmonary disease, the cost of breathing can reach 40% of the total exercise oxygen consumption, thereby decreasing the amount of oxygen available for the exercising muscles.
- A decrease in pulmonary resistance to air flow.

A number of precautions need to be taken when exercising patients who have a compromised cardiovascular or pulmonary system:

- An appropriate level of intensity must be chosen.
- Too high a level can overload the cardiorespiratory and muscular systems and potentially cause injuries.
- Exercising at the level it is too high causes the cardiorespiratory system to work anaerobically, not aerobically.
- A sufficient period should be allowed for warm-up and cool-down to permit adequate cardiorespiratory and muscular adaptation.

Techniques for Improving or Maintaining Cardiorespiratory Endurance

The detraining effects of cardiorespiratory endurance occur rapidly, after only 2 weeks, when a person stopped exercising. Several different training factors must be considered when attempting to maintain or improve cardiorespiratory endurance:

- Continuous training: the FITT principle.
  - Frequency: To see at least minimal improvement in cardiorespiratory endurance, it is necessary for the average person to engage in no less than three sessions per week.
    - If the intensity is kept constant, there appears to be no additional benefit from twice a week versus four times or three times a week versus five times per week.
    - If the goal is weight loss, 5 to 7 days/week increases the caloric expenditure more than 2 days/week.
  - Intensity: Recommendations regarding training intensity (overload) vary. Relative intensity for an individual is calculated as a percentage of the maximum function, using VO_2 max or maximum HR (HRmax). To see minimal improvement in cardiorespiratory endurance, the average person

must train with a HR elevated to at least 60% of its maximal rate. Three common methods of monitoring intensity are employed:

- o Monitoring HR: Two formulas are commonly used
    - Karvonen[63] equation: Target training HR = resting HR + (0.6)
    - Maximum HR: 220 – age.
- o Rating of perceived exertion (RPE) (Table 4-5): A cardiorespiratory training effect can be achieved at a rating of "somewhat hard" or "hard" (13 to 16).
- o Calculating the VO_2 max or HR directly or indirectly
    - 3-minute step test.
    - 12-minute run.
    - 1-mile walk test.
- Type of exercise: The type of activity chosen in continuous training must be aerobic—involving large muscle groups activated in a rhythmic manner.
- Time (duration): Duration is increased when intensity is limited, for example, by initial fitness level. For minimal improvement to occur, the patient must participate in continuous activity with a HR elevated to its working level. Three to 5 min/day produces a training effect in poorly conditioned individuals, whereas 20 to 30 minutes, three to five times a week is optimal for conditioned people.

Continuous training at a submaximal energy requirement can be pro-longed for 20 to 60 minutes without exhausting the oxygen transport system. A number of pieces of exercise equipment can be used to improve aerobic capacity and endurance:

- Treadmill walking: Progressing from slow to fast and short distances to longer distances with or without an incline.
- Ergometers: These come in a variety of forms for both the upper extremities and the lower extremities. The pace progression is from slow to fast and the goal is to increase the time spent exercising.
- Free weights and elastic resistance: The use of low resistance and high repetitions can produce an aerobic effect.

Obese individuals should exercise at longer durations and lower intensities—be able to exercise while maintaining a conversation (talk test).

Improving Muscle Power

Plyometric exercises, described next are used to improve the ability of the muscles to perform these actions, by enhancing their power, speed, and agility.

Clinical Pearl

Having a muscle work dynamically against resistance within a specified period increases power.

In the context of rehabilitation, plyometric training is the bridge between strength and power exercises.[64]

Plyometrics

Movement patterns in both athletics and ADL involve repeated stretch shortening cycles, where a downward eccentric movement must be stopped and converted into an upward concentric movement in a desired direction. These patterns occur in activities that require a maximum amount of muscular force in a minimum amount of time.

 Clinical Pearl

The nerve receptors involved in plyometrics are the muscle spindle, the Golgi tendon organ, and the joint capsule/ligamentous receptors. The degree of enhanced muscle performance is dependent on the time frame between the eccentric and concentric contractions.[65]

Acceleration and deceleration are the most important components of all task-specific activities.[41]

 Clinical Pearl

Plyometrics serve to improve the reactivity of neurological receptors by involving muscle stretch-shortening exercises, exposure to increased strength loads, and improvements in the stretch reflex.[66]

Plyometric exercises consist of three distinct phases:
- A setting or eccentric phase in which the muscle is eccentrically stretched and slowly loaded. This phase begins when the athlete mentally prepares for the activity, and lasts until the stretch stimulus is initiated.[66]

- A rapid amortization (reversal) phase. This phase is the amount of time between undergoing the yielding eccentric contraction and the initiation of a concentric force.[66] If the amortization phase is slow, elastic energy is wasted as heat, and the stretch reflex is not activated.[66]
- A concentric response contraction to develop a large amount of momentum and force.

 Clinical Pearl

The goal of plyometric training is to decrease the amount of time required between the yielding eccentric contraction, and the initiation of the overcoming concentric contraction.

Before initiating plyometric exercises, the clinician must ensure that the patient has an adequate strength and physical condition base.[66] Minimal performance criteria for safe plyometrics include the ability to perform one repetition of a parallel squat with a load of body weight on the subjects back (for jumps over 12 inches) for the lower extremity, and a bench press with one-third body weight for the upper extremity.[64] In addition, success in the static stability tests,[64] and dynamic stability tests (vertical jump for the lower extremities and medicine ball throw for the upper extremities) may be used as a measure of preparation.[27]

 Clinical Pearl

Many different activities and devices can be utilized in plyometric exercises. Plyometric exercises may include diagonal and multiplanar motions with tubing or isokinetic machines. These exercises may be used to mimic any of the needed motions and can be performed in the standing, sitting, or supine positions.

Lower Extremity Plyometric Exercises
Lower extremity plyometric exercises involve the manipulation of the role of gravity to vary the intensity of the exercise. Thus, plyometric exercises can be performed horizontally or vertically:

- Horizontal plyometrics are performed perpendicular to the line of gravity. These exercises are preferable for most initial clinical rehabilitation plans as the concentric force is reduced, and the eccentric phase is not facilitated.[27] Examples of these types of exercises include pushing a sled against resistance and a modified leg press that allows the subject to push off and land on the footplate.

- Vertical plyometric exercises (against or with gravitational forces) are more advanced. These exercises require a greater level of control.[27] The drop jump is an example—the subject steps off a box, lands, and immediately executes a vertical jump.

The footwear and landing surfaces used in plyometric drills must have shock-absorbing qualities, and the protocol should allow sufficient recovery time between sets to prevent fatigue of the muscle groups being trained.[49]

Upper Extremity Plyometric Exercises

Plyometric exercises for the upper extremity involve relatively rapid movements in planes that approximate normal joint function. For example, at the shoulder this would include 90-degree abduction in shoulder, trunk rotation and diagonal arm motions, and rapid external/internal rotation exercises.

Plyometrics should be done for all body segments involved in the activity. Hip rotation, knee flexion/extension, and trunk rotation are power activities that require plyometric activation.

 Clinical Pearl

Plyometric exercises for the upper extremity include wall push-offs, corner push-ups, box push-offs, the rebounder, and weighted ball throws (Figure 4-11) using medicine and other weighted balls (the weight of the ball creates a prestretch and an eccentric load when it is caught, creating resistance and demanding a powerful agonist contraction to propel it forward again). The exercises can be performed using one arm or both arms at the same time. The former emphasizes trunk rotation and the latter emphasizes trunk extension and flexion, as well as shoulder motion.

Although force-dependent motor firing patterns should be reestablished, special care must be taken to completely integrate all of the components of the kinetic chain to generate and funnel the proper forces to the appropriate joint.

Clinical Pearl

In general, tonic muscles function as endurance (postural) muscles, whereas phasic muscles function as the power muscles.[67,68]

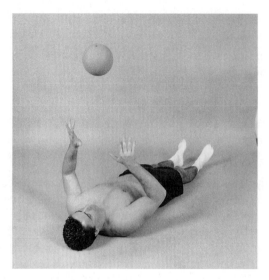

Figure 4-11 Upper extremity plyometric exercise.

IMPROVING JOINT MOBILITY AND RANGE OF MOTION

Normal mobility includes osteokinematic motion, arthrokinematic motion, and neuromuscular coordination. This control is a factor of muscle flexibility, joint stability, and central neurophysiological mechanisms. The amount of available joint motion is based on a number of factors, which include the following:

- Integrity of the joint surfaces and the amount of joint motion.
- Mobility and pliability of the soft tissues that surround a joint.
- Degree of soft tissue approximation that occurs
- Amount of scarring that is present.[69] Interstitial scarring or fibrosis can occur in and around the joint capsules, within the muscles, and within the ligaments as a result of previous trauma.
- Age. Joint motion tends to decrease with increasing age.
- Gender. In general, females have more joint motion than males.

Increasing Joint Mobility

Joint mobility is a function of a number of factors including the arthrokinematic or accessory motions of a joint. The accessory motion at a joint can be assessed by examining the joint glide (see Chapter 3). Joint mobilizations for all of the joints are described in the respective chapters. If the joint glide is not restricted, the surrounding tissues have likely adaptively shortened and the focus shifts to increasing flexibility.

Flexibility Training

Flexibility training has long been recognized as an essential component of any conditioning program as a means to prevent injury and improve performance.

 Clinical Pearl

Whether increased muscle flexibility, or stretching before activity, results in a decrease in muscle injuries has yet to be proven.

The techniques of stretching all involve the stretch reflex. A reflex is a programmed unit of behavior in which a certain type of stimulus from a receptor automatically leads to the response of an effector.

The elasticity of a muscle diminishes with cooling. Optimal flexibility is based on physiological, anatomical, and biomechanical considerations.

 Clinical Pearl

To stretch a muscle appropriately, the stretch must be applied parallel to the muscle fibers. The orientation of the fibers can be determined by palpation. Typically, in the extremities, the muscle fibers run parallel to the bone.

The viscoelastic changes produced by stretching are not permanent, whereas plasticity changes, which are more difficult to achieve, result in a residual or permanent change in length.

 Clinical Pearl

Frequent stretching ensures that the lengthening is maintained before the muscle has the opportunity to recoil to its shortened state.[70]

It is important for the patient to realize that the initial session of stretching may increase symptoms in the stretched muscle.[71] However, this increase in symptoms should only be temporary, lasting for a couple of hours at most.[70,72] The stretch should be performed at the point just shy of the pain, although some discomfort may be necessary to achieve results.[73]

 Clinical Pearl

A muscle usually requires a greater stretching force initially, possibly to break up adhesions or cross-linkages and to allow for viscoelastic and plastic changes to occur in the collagen and elastin fibers.[73]

Static Flexibility

Static flexibility is defined as the passive ROM available to a joint or series of joints.[69,74] Increased static flexibility should not be confused with joint hypermobility, or laxity, which is a function of the joint capsule and ligaments. Decreased static flexibility indicates a loss of motion. The end-feel encountered may help differentiate between adaptive shortening of the muscle (muscle stretch) versus a tight joint capsule (capsular), or arthritic joint (hard).

 Clinical Pearl

Static flexibility can be measured by a goniometer, or by a number of tests, such as the toe-touch and the sit and reach, all of which have been found to be valid and reliable.[75,76]

Dynamic Flexibility

Dynamic flexibility refers to the ease of movement within the obtainable ROM. Dynamic flexibility is measured actively. The important measurement in dynamic flexibility is stiffness, a mechanical term defined as the resistance of a structure to deformation.[77,78] An increase in ROM around a joint does not necessarily equate to a decrease in the passive stiffness of a muscle.[79-81] However, strength training, immobilization, and aging have been shown to increase stiffness.[82-85] The converse of stiffness is pliability. When a soft tissue demonstrates a decrease in pliability, it has usually undergone an adaptive shortening, or an increase in tone, termed *hypertonus*.

Table 4-9 Progressive Velocity Flexibility Program

Static stretching → Slow end-range stretching → Fast end-range stretching → Slow and Fast full-range stretching

Data adapted from reference 86.

Methods of Stretching

A variety of stretching techniques can be used to increase the extensibility of the soft tissues.

Passive Stretching

The clinician or another individual partner can perform passive stretching. Because of the higher risk of injury with this type of stretching with an unskilled operator, it should only be administered with close supervision, and with the assurance that there is excellent communication between the operator and the patient.

Ideally, the passive stretch should involve a gentle, controlled, low-intensity, and prolonged elongation of the tissues.

Static Stretching

Static stretching involves the application of a steady force for a sustained period (Table 4-9).[86]

 Clinical Pearl

Applying small loads to the musculotendinous unit for 20 minutes or more in an exercise session is necessary for adequate soft tissue lengthening to occur.[87,88]

Small loads applied for long periods produce greater residual lengthening than heavy loads applied for short periods.[88] Weighted traction, specific low-load braces, or pulley systems may be modified accordingly to provide this type of stretching.

Ballistic Stretching

This technique of stretching uses bouncing movements to stretch a particular muscle. In comparisons of the ballistic and static methods, two studies[89,90] have found that both produce similar improvements in flexibility. However, this method appears to cause more residual muscle soreness or muscle strain, than those techniques that incorporate relaxation into the technique.[91-93]

Neuromuscular Facilitation

The PNF techniques of "hold-relax," "stretch-relax," and "agonist contract-relax" can be used to actively stretch the soft tissues.

- Hold-relax (HR)—autogenic inhibition: A relaxation technique usually performed at the point of limited range of motion in the agonist pattern:
  - An isometric contraction of the range-limiting antagonist is performed against slowly increasing resistance.
  - This is followed by a voluntary relaxation by the patient and then passive movement of the extremity by the clinician into the newly gained range of the agonist pattern.
- Hold-relax-active (HRA)—reciprocal inhibition.
  - Following application of the hold-relax technique, the patient performs an active contraction into the newly gained range of the agonist pattern.
- Contract-relax (C-R): A relaxation technique usually performed at the point of limited range of motion in the agonist pattern:
  - A concentric movement in rotation is performed followed by an isometric hold of the range-limiting muscles in the antagonist pattern against slowly increasing resistance, voluntary relaxation, and active movement into the new range of the agonist pattern.

The majority of studies have shown the PNF technique to be the most effective stretching technique for increasing ROM through muscle lengthening when compared with the static or slow sustained, and the ballistic or bounce techniques.[94-98]

Clinical Application

Restoration of normal length of the muscles may be accomplished using the following guidelines:

- The muscle activity is inhibited and in the inhibitory period, the muscle should be stretched.
- With true muscle shortness, stronger resistance is used to activate the maximum number of motor units, followed by vigorous stretching of the muscle.
- Stretching should be performed at least three times a week using:
  - Low force, avoiding pain
  - Prolonged duration

Clinical Pearl

Heat should be applied to increase intramuscular temperature before, and during, stretching.[99,100] This heat can be achieved with either through low-intensity warm-up exercise, using relevant muscle groups, or through the use of thermal modalities.[100] The application of a cold pack following the stretch is used to take advantage of the thermal characteristics of connective tissue, by lowering its temperature and thereby theoretically prolonging the length changes.[101]

 Clinical Pearl

Effective stretching, in the early phase, should be performed every hour, but with each session lasting only a few minutes.

Some areas of the body are difficult to stretch adequately using a lengthening technique. In these instances, techniques of localized, manual release, using varying degrees of manual pressure along the length of the muscle and myofascial tissue, may be used.[102]

IMPROVING BALANCE

Balance, or postural equilibrium, is the single most important factor dictating movement strategies, especially in the CKC environment. Postural equilibrium involves synchronization between the neurological system and the musculoskeletal system to maintain a stable weight-bearing and antigravity position for a prolonged period. In order for balance to be effective, an individual must be able to maintain their center of gravity (COG), which is located just above the pelvis, within the body's base of support. A wide base of support provides the best balance.

 Clinical Pearl

Since afferent input is altered after joint injury, the training must focus on the restoration of proprioceptive sensibility to retrain these altered afferent pathways and enhance the sensation of joint movement.[103]

Table 4-10 Progressive Challenges for Balance Training

Position (in order of increasing difficulty)	Target Muscle Groups	Examples of Activities
Supine/Prone	Trunk (all muscles) Neck muscles	Rolling to increase segmentation (a hook lying position is used). Reaching from side lying
Quadruped	Trunk (extensor Upper extremities Proximal lower extremities	Static holding with applied challenges Creeping on all fours
Kneeling	Trunk Lower extremities (except the foot and ankle)	Half-kneeling Tall-kneeling
Sitting	Trunk Lower extremities (hips)	Decreasing upper extremity support Reaching activities Static challenges
Standing	Trunk Lower extremities	Static standing Gait: Bilateral support; parallel bars > walker Single hand support: quad cane > straight cane Narrowing the base of support as with tandem walking

Balance training involving a change in the base of support can be performed with the patient lying, sitting, or standing, depending on the ability of the patient and the goals of the intervention. The usual progression employed involves narrowing of the base of support, raising the COG, and changing the weight-bearing surface from hard to soft, or from flat to uneven, while increasing the perturbation. Challenges to the patient's position can be added in a variety of ways (Table 4-10).

Movement Strategies

The coordination of the body's postural equilibrium is determined by a number of factors:

- Joint position strategies: Three principal joint systems (hip, knee, and ankle) are located between the base of support and the COG.

- Hip—through initiation of large and rapid motions—stepping/stumbling
- Knee—flexes or extends according to need
- Ankle—contracting the anterior tibialis (posterior sway) or gastrocnemius (anterior sway). The primary method of stabilization under normal circumstances.
- The health of the somatosensory, visual, and vestibular systems.

Balance Assessment

A number of methods, ranging from simple to complex and expensive can be used to assess balance:

- Standard Romberg test: standing feet together, arms by the side, and eyes closed. An inability to maintain this position without sway or falling is considered a positive test.
- Balance Error Scoring System (BESS) test[104]
- Computerized force plate/force platform
- Berg balance scale

Restoring Postural Equilibrium

When restoring postural equilibrium, it is important to follow a structured sequence:

1. Static control of trunk without extremity movement: stable base provided by proximal segments and trunk to allow functional movements
   a. Manual perturbation to stable trunk
   b. Weight shifting while maintaining postural equilibrium
2. Dynamic control of trunk without extremity movement
   a. Fixation of distal segments while proximal segments are moved
   b. Gradual increase of range of motion from small range to large
   c. Reverse applies to those patients who have hyperkinetic movement disorders (ataxia) in which the goal is to work from large ranges to small
3. Static control of trunk with extremity movement
4. Maintenance of trunk stability with increasingly ballistic extremity movements
5. Exercises to increase strength, endurance, flexibility, and coordination are prescribed in conjunction with equilibrium exercises
   a. Exercises that challenge the endurance capabilities of the core muscles
   b. Progress from extremity exercises with the spine in neutral to extremity exercises with the spine in a variety of functional positions
   c. Education of the patient about the awareness of how normal alignment of the spine feels in a variety of positions, and how muscles can be used to control those positions

      i. Provision of verbal, visual, tactile, and proprioceptive cues to enhance learning

     ii. Exercises that involve maintaining functional positions to work the correct muscle groups.

The clinician can employ PNF techniques (refer also to Specialized Exercise Regimes) to enhance training:

- Alternating isometrics (AIs) applied in a variety of directions—uniplanar (anterior–posterior, medial–lateral) initially, and the three dimensionally
- Rhythmic stabilization (RS): produces co-contractions of opposing muscle groups
- Dynamic control of trunk with extremity movement

Functional activity progression:

- Simple patterns of movements that encourage safe body mechanics are taught initially, before progressing to more challenging movements.
- Closed-chain activities should be initiated first (wall squats, lunges) then open-chain activities while maintaining trunk control (add extremity motions to the squats and lunges).
- Uniplanar trunk motions are performed first, before progressing to three-dimensional trunk motions, such as PNF rotations, in a variety of positions of lumbar flexion and extension.

Sport-specific progressions as appropriate.

It is important to progress each patient based on the following criteria:

- The required level of strength/endurance is available to perform the activities without fatigue and while maintaining good trunk control.
- The patient has adequate flexibility in those muscles that allow the correct pelvic tilt to occur (adaptively shortened hamstrings can hold the pelvis in a posteriorly rotated position; adaptively shortened hip flexors can hold the pelvis in an anteriorly rotated position) so that a stable base can be created.

Improving Balance Through Exercise and Functional Training

Exercises to improve range of motion, strength, and synergistic responses:

- Stretches of major muscles
- Partial wall squats
- Marching in place
- Single leg kicks
- Shoulder circles
- Head and trunk rotations
- Weight shifts (ankle strategies, hip strategies)

- Stepping activities (forward, backward, sideways)
- Reaching activities
- Practicing of protective fall mechanisms
- Postural awareness training within limits of stability

    Functional training activities:
- Sit-stand-sit activities focusing on moving the body mass forward over the base of support, extending the lower extremities, and raising the body mass over the feet, and then reversing the procedure.
- Stand-to-sit transitions: focusing on balance control while pivoting and changing direction.
- Floor-to-standing raises: using progression of side-sit to quadruped to kneeling to half kneeling to standing.
- Gait activities: ambulating forward, backward, sideward at varying speeds and base of support widths (narrow to wide). Can progress to
    - cross-step walking and braiding, 360-degree turns, obstacle courses.
    - lateral step-ups, stair climbing, walking up and down ramps.
    - performing simultaneous activities with the upper extremities (throwing or bouncing a ball, kicking a ball).

    Community integration:
- Ambulating in open environments, grocery shopping, car transfers, and the like
- Getting on and off escalators, elevators

    Perturbation activities:
- Initiate with manual perturbations with the patient in supine, then sitting, and finally in standing.
- Perturbations should be graded carefully in terms of force and speed.

    Use of stability equipment (Swiss/physio ball, wobble board, etc.):
- The patient performs active weight shifts, upper extremity reaching activities, lower extremity movements such as stepping and marching, and trunk movements with body weight applied through a variety of surfaces.
- Challenges can be added by increasing the range of motion of the movements and by increasing the speed of the movements.

    Sensory training:
- The degree of sensory training will depend on the deficits noted during the examination. Ultimately, the clinician should be able to introduce sensory conflict situations (walking from a cement floor to a carpeted floor while turning the head to the right and left).

Visual deficits:

- The patient should practice standing and walking initially with the eyes open and then progressing to eyes closed.
- Can be made more challenging by reducing the amount of light.

Vestibular deficits:

- The patient should practice standing and walking while moving head side-to-side, up-and-down on both a stationary and moving surface.

Somatosensory deficits:

- The patient should practice standing and walking on a tile floor transitioning to a carpet.
- A variety of under the foot surfaces can be used including differing thicknesses of carpet, dense foam, and uneven terrain outside.

IMPROVING JOINT STABILIZATION

Joint instability implies that a person has increased joint range of motion but does not have the ability to stabilize and control movement of that joint. Stabilization exercises attempt to limit and control any excessive movement. Stabilization activities include patient education, mobility exercises for stiff or hypomobile joints, strengthening exercises in the shortened range for hypermobile segments, and neuromuscular reeducation (NMR). The objective in NMR is to restore proximal stability, muscle control, and flexibility through a balance of proprioceptive retraining and strengthening.

 Clinical Pearl

NMR attempts to improve the nervous system's ability to generate a fast and optimal muscle-firing pattern, to increase joint stability, to decrease joint forces, and to relearn movement patterns and skills.[105]

NMR is initiated with simple activities and progresses to more complex activities requiring proprioceptive and kinesthetic awareness, once the neuromuscular deficits are minimized.[106,107] It is recommended that NMR be initiated as early as possible in the rehabilitative process.[103]

According to Voight and coworkers,[103,108] the standard progression for NMR involves the following:

- Static stabilization exercises with closed-chain loading and unloading (weight shifting). This phase initially employs isometric exercises around the involved joint on solid and even surfaces, before progressing to unstable surfaces. The early training involves balance training and joint repositioning exercises, and is usually initiated (in the lower extremities) by having the patient placing the involved extremity on a 6- to 8-inch stool, so that the amount of weight bearing can be controlled more easily. The proprioceptive awareness of a joint can also be enhanced by using an elastic bandage, orthotic, or through taping.[109-114] As full weight bearing through the extremity is restored, a number of devices such as a mini-trampoline, balance board, Swiss ball, and wobble board can be introduced. Exercises on these devices are progressed from double limb support, to single leg support, to support while performing sport-specific skills.

- Transitional stabilization exercises. The exercises during this phase involve conscious control of motion without impact and replace isometric activity with controlled concentric and eccentric exercises throughout a progressively larger range of functional motion. The physiological rationale behind the exercises in this phase is to stimulate dynamic postural responses and to increase muscle stiffness. Muscle stiffness has a significant role in improving dynamic stabilization around the joint, by resisting and absorbing joint loads.[84]

- Dynamic stabilization exercises. These exercises involve the unconscious control and loading of the joint, and introduce both ballistic and impacts exercises to the patient.

Weight shifting exercises are ideal for enhancing stabilization. For example, the following weight shifting exercises may be used for the upper extremity:

- Standing and leaning against a treatment table or object.

- In the quadruped position, rocking forward and backward with the hands on the floor or on an unstable object.

- Kneeling in the three-point position. A Body Blade can be added to this exercise to increase the difficulty.

- Kneeling in the two-point position.

- Weight shifting on a Fitter while in a kneeling position.

- Weight shifting on a Swiss ball with the feet on a chair, in the push-up position.

- Slide board exercises in the quadruped position moving hands forward and backward, in opposite diagonals and in opposite directions.

Following treatment of any joint, retraining of the muscles must be carried out to reestablish coordination. PNF techniques are especially useful in this regard (see Specialized Exercise Regimes). PNF techniques require motions of the extremities in all three planes.[115] PNF techniques that use combinations of spiral and diagonal patterns are designed to enhance coordination and strength.[116] The diagonal patterns 1 and 2 are appropriate with resistance being added as appropriate.

The Stability Ball

One of the advantages of using the stability ball is that it creates an unstable base, which challenges the postural stabilizer muscles more than using a stable base.

Ball Inflation and Sizing

It is important to choose the correct and appropriate size of ball, which is dependent on patient size:

- 45-cm ball: shorter than 5' (1.52m)
- 55-cm ball: 5' to 5'8" (1.52 to 1.73m)
- 65-cm ball: 5' 9" to 6'3" (1.75 to 1.9m)
- 75-cm ball: taller than 6'3" (1.9m)

    With the patient sitting on the ball with both feet firmly planted on the ground, the patient's thigh should be parallel to the floor (the knee may be slightly above the hips).

- Pumping up the ball increases the level of difficulty in any given exercise.
- The further away the ball is from the support points, the greater the demand for core stability.
- Decreasing the number of support points increases the difficulty of the exercise.

    A wide variety of stability ball exercises are illustrated in the appropriate chapters.

IMPROVING COORDINATION

Coordination involves an intricate and complex sequence of activities, which include

- reacting to sensory input
- choosing and processing the profit motive program from learned skills
- executing the action
- prediction, evaluation, and adjustment.

Table 4-11 Trunk and Lower Extremity Coordination Exercises

Task	Description	Modifications
Simple dynamic movements	The patient reaches in a variety of directions and a variety of distances to a prearranged target. The patient draws an imaginary circle or figure of eight pattern in the air with the upper extremity.	Can be made more challenging by – increasing the height of the center of gravity – increasing the complexity of the dynamic movements
Alternate Heel to knee touching and heel to toe touching	From a supine position, the patient is asked to touch his knee and great toe alternately with the heel of the opposite extremity.	Both the speed of movement and/or the amount of weight can be changed to modify this exercise.

Coordination demands vary from individual to individual—from the world-class athlete to the patient recovering from a stroke. Thus, the type and focus of the coordination training depends on the presenting condition. Tables 4-11 and 4-12 illustrate some examples of commonly employed coordination exercises for the trunk, lower extremities, and the upper extremities (see also Table 4-13).

 Clinical Pearl

Learning requires repetition; however, it is not just a case of "practice makes perfect" but rather "perfect practice makes perfect."

There should be a strong focus on education with patients with coordination and/or balance disorders. The clinician should assist the patient in identifying fall risk factors (medications, postural hypotension, poor lighting, and lack of contrast in surroundings), unsafe activities, and the adverse effects of a sedentary lifestyle. The following progression should be used to improve coordination:

- Postural stability activities:
  - Adopting weight-bearing postures: prone on elbows, sitting, quadruped, kneeling, and standing.
  - The goal is to gradually decrease the base of support while raising the height of the COG.
- Use of PNF manual techniques:
  - AIs and RS to enhance stabilization

Table 4-12 Coordination Exercises for the Upper Extremities

Task	Description	Modifications
Alternate nose to finger	The patient alternately touches the tip of his nose, and the tip of the clinician's finger with the index finger. The position of the clinician's finger may be altered during testing to assess the patient's ability to change distance, direction and the force of movement.	This exercise can be made more challenging by increasing the speed of movement.
Drawing a circle	The patient draws an imaginary circle or figure of eight pattern in the air with the upper extremity.	Having the patient draw smaller circles or tighter figure of 8 patterns make the exercise more challenging
Finger to finger	Both shoulders are abducted to 90°. With the elbows extended, the patient is asked to bring both hands to midline and approximate the index fingers from the opposing hands.	Speed can be used to modify the challenge of this exercise.
Finger to nose	The shoulder is abducted to 90° with the elbows extended. The patient is asked to bring the tip of the index finger to the tip of the nose.	– Alternations are made to the starting position to test the different planes of motion. – Weights can be added to the wrist – The speed of the movement can be increased
Finger opposition	The patient touches the tip of the thumb to the tip of each finger in sequence.	Changing the frequency of movement Changing the target.
Finger to clinician's finger	The patient and clinician sit opposite each other. The clinician's index finger is held in front of the patient and the patient is asked to touch the tip of their index finger to the tip of the clinician's index finger.	– Change the frequency or speed of movement. – Alter the position of the index finger
Mass Grasp	The patient is asked to alternatively open and close the fist	Increase the frequency/speed
Pointing and past pointing	The clinician and the patient are positioned opposite each other (standing or sitting). Both have their shoulders at 90° of flexion, the elbows extended and the index fingers touching. – The patient is asked to flex their shoulder to 180° then return to the starting position. – The patient is asked to move the arm to 0° of shoulder flexion.	Can be modified by: – Using cuff weights – Increasing the frequency/speed – Progressing from sitting to standing.

(continued on following page)

Task	Description	Modifications
Alternating Movements: – Pronation/ Supination	This test is done with the elbows flexed 90°, with the shoulders in neutralshoulder rotation. The patient is asked to supinate and pronate the forearm.	Measuring the level of frequency of movement when ataxia is first observed can modify this.
Alternating Movements: Flexion/extension	Shoulder flexion/extension Elbow flexion/extension Wrist flexion/extension	Can be modified by: – Increasing the speed of movement. – Adding cuff weights
Tapping	The patient is positioned with the elbow flexed to 90°, the forearm pronated, and the hand resting on the knee. The patient is asked to repeatedly tap their hand against their knee	This can be modified by: – Changing the position – Increasing the speed

- Slow reversal (SR) hold to help decrease range of motion with ataxic movements
- Controlled mobility activities: These include weight shifting activities and moving in and out of postures.
  - Specific exercises include the PNF techniques of SRs and SR holds. These techniques are used to
    o enhance synergistic control and reciprocal action of muscles
    o modulate timing and force output
  - Stabilization devices can be used to eliminate unwanted movement and stabilize body segments.
  - Other interventions include aquatic therapy, which increases proprioceptive loading, slows down ataxic movements, and provides light resistance.
- Sensory training: provided for patients with proprioceptive loss.
  - Visual compensation strategies where movements are guided visually.
  - Increased proprioceptive loading through use of light weights/resistance.

SPECIALIZED EXERCISE REGIMES

Aquatic Exercise

In the past decade, widespread interest has developed in aquatic therapy as a tool for rehabilitation. Current research shows aquatic therapy to be

Table 4-13 Frenkel Exercises for Coordination

Techniques for lower extremities	Supine position	Flexion and extension at each leg at hip and knee joint, heel sliding on bed. Abduction and adduction of each leg with knee bent, heel sliding on bed. Repeat same with knee extended. Flexion and extension of one knee at a time with heel raised. Place heel upon some definite part of the opposite leg, for example, on the patella, mid-tibia, ankle, or toes. Slide heel from contralateral knee joint down along shin and back to knee. Flexion and extension of both legs simultaneously, holding knees and ankles together. Draw up one extremity while extending the other: reciprocal flexion and extension. Flexion and extension of one leg and simultaneous abduction and adduction of the other. Reverse procedure.
	Sitting position	Alternately raise each leg, then place foot firmly on a footprint on the floor. Glide each foot alternately over a cross marked on the floor: forward, backward, to left, to right. With a foot in footprint, raise heel, lift foot off floor; in this position extend and flex knee, and bring toes back to original position; bring heel down in corresponding part of footprint. Practice sitting down on chair: avoid falling into chair; allow muscles of hips and knees to ease the body down. Stand in front of chair, with knee slightly flexed and body bent slightly forward. It down by continuing the flexion of knees, hips and trunk. Practice standing up: feet are drawn back until partly under the chair so that the whole foot can be firmly planted. Bend body forward and rise slowly, extending the knees and hips and straightening the body.
	Standing position	Encourage walking on entire foot. Stand on tiptoe, then on the heel of one leg. Walk sideways a few steps in each direction. Walk between two parallel bars 14 inches apart, keeping a distance of 6 inches between the feet. Avoid outward rotation of legs. Walk on straight line; avoid toeing out. Take one half step and bring other foot in apposition. Continue taking several alternate half steps. Repeat with quarter steps. Alternate half and quarter steps, bringing each foot in apposition after each step. Then walk by alternate half steps and quarter steps. Make a complete turn to the left, using left heel as a pivot. Repeat to right. Walk along a circle on the floor, first in one direction, then in the other.

(continued on following page)

Techniques for extremities	Reaching activities	Placing it on marks at different levels on the wall.
		Add marks with chalk to symbols on blackboard, e.g., change minus to plus, cross "t," dot "i," play tic-tac-toe.
		Place small, readily grasped objects on squares of check board which has been numbered.
		Practice writing.
		Practice drawing geometric figures.

beneficial in the treatment of everything from orthopedic injuries to spinal cord damage, chronic pain, cerebral palsy, multiple sclerosis, and many other conditions.[117] Among the psychological aspects, water motivates movement, because painful joints and muscles can be moved more easily and painlessly in water.

 Clinical Pearl

The indications for aquatic therapy include instances when partial weight-bearing ambulation is necessary, to increase range of motion, when standing balance needs to be improved, when endurance/aerobic capacity needs improved, or when the goal is to increase muscle strength via active assisted, gravity assisted, active or resisted exercise.[117]

Contraindications include incontinence, urinary tract infections, unprotected open wounds, heat intolerance, severe epilepsy, uncontrolled diabetes, unstable blood pressure, or severe cardiac and/or pulmonary dysfunction.

Proprioceptive Neuromuscular Facilitation Techniques

The concept of PNF (also termed complex motions) was developed by Dr. Hermann Kabat, then by Sherrington, and finally by Margaret Knott and Dorothy Voss.[118] PNF uses the stimulation of muscle and joint receptors to improve, facilitate, and accelerate the reactions of the neuromuscular mechanism. PNF techniques can be used for a number of purposes including strengthening, increasing range of motion, and improving coordination.

Each of the following definitions includes a description explaining the intent of the techniques:

- Approximation: Joint compression stimulates afferent nerve endings, and encourages extensor muscles and stabilizing patterns (co-contraction), thereby inhibiting tone and enhancing stabilization of the proximal segment.
  - This technique is commonly used with neurologically involved patients.
- Agonist reversals (ARs): A slow isotonic, shortening contraction through the range followed by an eccentric, lengthening contraction using the same muscle groups.
  - Indications include wheat postural muscles, inability to eccentrically control body weight during movement transitions, for example, sitting down.
- AIs: Isometric holding is facilitated first on one side of the joint, followed by alternate holding of the antagonist muscle groups. Can be applied in any direction (anterior–posterior, medial–lateral, and diagonal).
  - Indications include instability in weight bearing and holding, poor anti-gravity control, weakness, and ataxia.
- CR: A relaxation technique usually performed at a point of limited range of motion in the agonist pattern: Isotonic movement in rotation is performed followed by an isometric hold of the range-limiting muscles in the antagonist pattern against slowly increasing resistance, then voluntary relaxation, and active contraction in the newly gained range of the agonist pattern. The patient is then asked to contract the muscle(s) to be stretched (agonists). The clinician resists this contraction except for the rotary component. The patient is then asked to relax and the clinician moves the joint further into the desired range.
  - Indications include limitations in range of motion caused by muscle adaptive shortening, spasticity.
  - Although primarily used as a stretching technique, due to the isometric contractions involved, some strengthening does occur.
- Hold-relax: A similar technique in principle to contract-relax, except that, when the patient contracts, the clinician allows no motion (including rotation) to occur. Following the isometric contraction the patient's own contraction causes the desired movement to occur.
  - Typically used as a relaxation technique in the acute the injured patient as it tends to be less aggressive than the contract/relax technique.
- HRA motion: An isometric contraction performed in the mid-to-shortened range followed by a voluntary relaxation and passive movement into the lengthened range, and resistance to an isotonic contraction through the range.

- May be used with patients who have an inability to initiate movement, hypotonia, weakness, marked imbalances between antagonists.
- Manual contact: A deep but painless pressure is applied through the clinician's contact to stimulate a muscle, tendon, and/or joint afferents.
- Maximal resistance: resistance is applied to stronger muscles to obtain overflow to weaker muscles.
  - Indications include weakness, muscle imbalances.
- Quick stretch: A motion applied suddenly stimulates the tendon receptors resulting in a facilitation of motor recruitment and thus more force.
- Reinforcement: The coordinated use of the major muscle groups, or other body parts, to produce a desired movement pattern.
  - This technique is often used to increase the stability of the proximal segments.
- Repeated contractions (RCs): A unidirectional technique that involves repeated isotonic contractions induced by quick stretch and which is enhanced by resistance performed to the range or part of range at the point of weakness.
  - Indications include weakness, in coordination, muscle imbalances, lack of endurance.
  - Facilitation of the agonist and relaxation the antagonist.
- Resisted progression (RP): A stretch and tracking resistance is applied to facilitate progression in walking, creeping, kneel-walking, or movement transitions.
  - Indications include impaired strength, timing, motor control, and endurance.
- Rhythmic initiation (RI): Unidirectional or bidirectional voluntary relaxation followed by passive movement through increasing range of motion, followed by active-assisted contractions progressing to light tracking resistance to isotonic contractions.
  - Indications include spasticity, rigidity, inability to initiate movement, motor learning deficits, communication deficits.
- Rhythmic rotation: Voluntary relaxation combined with slow, pass it, rhythmic rotation of the body or body part around a longitudinal axis and passive movement into newly gained range. Active holding in the new range is then stressed.
  - Indications include hypertonia with limitations in functional range of motion.
- RS: The application of alternating isometric contractions of the agonist and antagonist muscles to stimulate movement of the agonist, develop joint stability, and relax the antagonist.

- Indications include instability in weight bearing and holding, poor anti-gravity control, weakness, and ataxia.
- May also be used to decrease limitations in range of motion caused by adaptive muscle shortening and painful muscle splinting.
- SR: Uses alternating isotonic contractions of opposing muscle groups to stimulate active motion of the agonist, relaxation of the antagonist, and coordination between agonist and antagonist patterns.
  - Indications include inability to reverse directions, muscle imbalances, weakness, incoordination, and instability.
- SR-hold: Uses alternating activity of opposing muscle groups with a pause between reversals to achieve relaxation of the antagonist and to stimulate the agonist.
- SR-hold-relax: The patient is asked to actively move the involved joint to the point of limitation and then to reverse the direction of the motion, while the clinician resists.
  - This technique is used to increase motion of the agonist.
- Timing for emphasis: The application of maximal resistance in specific parts of the range of motion to the more powerful muscle groups to obtain "overflow" to weaker muscle groups. Can be performed within a limb (ipsilateral from one muscle group to another) or using overflow from one limb to contralateral limb, or trunk to limb.

Table 4-14 PNF Patterns for the Lower Extremity

PNF Patterns for the Lower Extremity				
Joint (proximal to distal)	DIAGONAL ONE (D1) Flexion	DIAGONAL ONE (D1) Extension	DIAGONAL TWO (D2) Flexion	DIAGONAL TWO (D2) Extension
Hip	External rotation, adduction, flexion	Internal rotation, abduction, extension	Internal rotation, abduction, flexion	External rotation, adduction, extension
Knee (may be kept flexed or extended)	Flexion or extension	Extension or flexion	Flexion or extension	Extension or flexion
Ankle	Dorsi flexion	Plantar flexion	Dorsi flexion	Plantar flexion
Subtalar	Inversion	Eversion	Eversion	Inversion
Toes	Extension, abduction to the tibial side	Flexion, adduction to the fibular side	Extension, abduction to the fibular side	Flexion, adduction to the tibial side

Table 4-15 PNF Patterns for the Upper Extremity

PNF Patterns for the Upper Extremity			
Joint (proximal to distal)	DIAGONAL ONE (D1) Flexion	DIAGONAL ONE (D1) Extension	DIAGONAL TWO (D2) Flexion	DIAGONAL TWO (D2) Extension
Scapulothoracic	Rotation, abduction, anterior elevation	Rotation, adduction, posterior depression	Rotation, adduction, posterior elevation	Rotation, abduction, anterior depression
Glenohumeral	External rotation, adduction, flexion	Internal rotation, abduction, extension	External rotation, abduction, flexion	Internal rotation, adduction, extension
Elbow (may be kept flexed or extended)	Flexion	Extension	Flexion	Extension
Radio ulnar	Supination	Pronation	Supination	Pronation
Wrist	Flexion, radial deviation	Extension, ulnar deviation	Extension, radial deviation	Flexion, ulnar deviation
Fingers	Flexion, adduction to the radial side	Extension, abduction to the ulnar side	Extension, abduction to the radial side	Flexion, adduction to the ulnar side
Thumb	Flexion, abduction	Extension, abduction	Extension, adduction	Flexion, abduction

- Typically combined with RCs to the weak components, or superimposed upon normal timing in a distal to proximal sequence.
- Indications include weakness, incoordination.
- Traction: The joint is distracted by use of a traction force, resulting in a decrease of muscular tone and a subsequent increase in range of motion.
  - Indications include stimulation of a fair and nerve endings and facilitation of flexor muscles and mobilizing patterns.
- May also be used to help decrease spasticity.

Proprioceptive Neuromuscular Facilitation Patterns

See Table 4-14.
See Table 4-15.

REFERENCES

1. Grimes K. Heart disease. In: O'Sullivan SB, Schmitz TJ, eds. Physical Rehabilitation. 5th ed. Philadelphia, PA: FA Davis; 2007:589–641.
2. Marino M. Current concepts of rehabilitation in sports medicine. In: Nicholas JA, Herschman EB, eds. The Lower Extremity and Spine in Sports Medicine. St. Louis, MO: Mosby; 1986:117–195.
3. Palmitier RA, An KN, Scott SG, et al. Kinetic chain exercises in knee rehabilitation. Sports Med. 1991;11:402–413.
4. Gray GW. Closed chain sense. Fitness Manage. 1992;8:31–33.
5. Dillman CJ, Murray TA, Hintermeister RA. Biomechanical differences of open and closed chain exercises with respect to the shoulder. J Sport Rehabil. 1994;3:228–238.
6. Kibler BW. Closed kinetic chain rehabilitation for sports injuries. Phys Med Rehabil N Am. 2000;11:369–384.
7. Hill AV. The heat and shortening and the dynamic constants of muscle. Proc R Soc Lond B. 1938;126:136–195.
8. Tihanyi J, Apor P, Fekete GY. Force–velocity–power characteristics and fiber composition in human knee extensor muscles. Eur J Appl Physiol. 1982; 48:331.
9. Fitts RH, Widrick JJ. Muscle mechanics: adaptations with exercise training. Exerc Sport Sci Rev. 1996;24:427.
10. Hall SJ. The biomechanics of human skeletal muscle. In: Hall SJ, ed. Basic Biomechanics. New York, NY: McGraw-Hill; 1999:146–185.
11. Hall C, Thein-Brody L. Impairment in muscle performance. In: Hall C, Thein-Brody L, eds. Therapeutic Exercise: Moving Toward Function. Baltimore, MD: Lippincott Williams & Wilkins; 2005:57–86.
12. Boeckmann RR, Ellenbecker TS. Biomechanics. In: Ellenbecker TS, ed. Knee Ligament Rehabilitation. Philadelphia, PA: Churchill Livingstone; 2000: 16–23.
13. Brownstein B, Noyes FR, Mangine RE, et al. Anatomy and biomechanics. In: Mangine RE, ed. Physical Therapy of the Knee. New York, NY: Churchill Livingstone; 1988:1–30.
14. Deudsinger RH. Biomechanics in clinical practice. Phys Ther. 1984;64:1860–1868.
15. Lakomy HKA. The biomechanics of human movement. In: Maughan RJ, ed. Basic and Applied Sciences for Sports Medicine. Woburn, MA: Butterworth-Heinemann; 1999:124–125.
16. McArdle W, Katch F, Katch V. Exercise Physiology: Energy, Nutrition, and Human Performance. Philadelphia, PA: Lea and Febiger; 1991.
17. Astrand PO, Rodahl K. The Muscle and its Contraction: Textbook of Work Physiology. New York, NY: McGraw-Hill; 1986.
18. Williams JH, Klug GA. Calcium exchange hypothesis of skeletal muscle fatigue. A brief review. Muscle Nerve. 1995;18:421.
19. Allen DG, Lannergren J, Westerblad H. Muscle cell function during prolonged activity: cellular mechanisms of fatigue. Exp Physiol. 1995;80:497.
20. Lash JM. Regulation of skeletal muscle blood flow during contractions. Proc Soc Exp Biol Med. 1996;211:218–235.

21. Gould N, Donnermeyer BS, Pope M, et al. Transcutaneous muscle stimulation as a method to retard disuse atrophy. Clin Orthop. 1982;164:215–220.
22. Gossman MR, Sahrmann SA, Rose SJ. Review of length-associated changes in muscle. Phys Ther. 1982;62:1799–1808.
23. Kasper CE, Talbot LA, Gaines JM. Skeletal muscle damage and recovery. AACN Clinical Issues. 2002;13:237–247.
24. McNeil PL, Khakee R. Disruptions of muscle fiber plasma membranes: role in exercise-induced damage. Am J Pathol. 1992;140:1097–1109.
25. Booher JM, Thibodeau GA. The body's response to trauma and environmental stress. In: Booher JM, Thibodeau GA, eds. Athletic Injury Assessment. 4th ed. New York, NY: McGraw-Hill; 2000:55–76.
26. Hyman J, Liebenson C. Spinal stabilization exercise program. In: Liebenson C, ed. Rehabilitation of the Spine: A Practitioner's Manual. Baltimore, MD: Lippincott Williams & Wilkins; 1996:293–317.
27. Albert M. Concepts of muscle training. In: Wadsworth C, ed. Orthopaedic Physical Therapy: Topic—Strength and Conditioning Applications in Orthopaedics—Home Study Course 98A. La Crosse, WI: Orthopaedic Section, APTA; 1998.
28. Ierna GF, Murphy DR. Management of acute soft tissue injuries of the cervical spine. In: Murphy DR, ed. Conservative Management of Cervical Spine Disorders. New York, NY: McGraw-Hill; 2000:531–552.
29. Davies GJ. Compendium of Isokinetics in Clinical Usage and Rehabilitation Techniques. 4th ed. Onalaska, WI: S & S Publishers; 1992.
30. American College of Sports Medicine. Guidelines for Exercise Testing and Prescription. 4th ed. Philadelphia, PA: Lea & Febiger; 1991.
31. Borg GAV. Psychophysical basis of perceived exertion. Med Sci Sports Exerc. 1992;14:377–381.
32. Borg GAV. Perceived exertion as an indicator of somatic stress. Scand J Rehabil Med. 1970;2:92–98.
33. Hasson S, Barnes W, Hunter M, et al. Therapeutic effect of high speed voluntary muscle contractions on muscle soreness and muscle performance. J Orthop Sports Phys Ther. 1989;10:499.
34. Litchfield R, Hawkins R, Dillman CJ, et al. Rehabilitation of the overhead athlete. J Orthop Sports Phys Ther. 1993;2:433–441.
35. Maitland G. Peripheral Manipulation. 3rd ed. London, UK: Butterworth; 1991.
36. Cyriax J. Textbook of Orthopaedic Medicine, Diagnosis of Soft Tissue Lesions. 8th ed. London, UK: Bailliere Tindall; 1982.
37. Cook G, Voight ML. Essentials of functional exercise: a four-step clinical model for therapeutic exercise prescription. In: Prentice WE, Voight ML, eds. Techniques in Musculoskeletal Rehabilitation. New York, NY: McGraw-Hill; 2001:387–407.
38. Matsen FA III, Lippitt SB, Sidles JA, et al. Strength. In: Matsen FA III, Lippitt SB, Sidles JA, et al. eds. Practical Evaluation and Management of the Shoulder. Philadelphia, PA: WB Saunders; 1994:111–150.
39. Komi PV. Strength and Power in Sport. London, UK: Blackwell Scientific; 1992.
40. Blix M. Length and tension. Scand Arch Physiol. 1892:93–94.

41. Grimsby O, Power B. Manual therapy approach to knee ligament rehabilitation. In: Ellenbecker TS, ed. Knee Ligament Rehabilitation. Philadelphia, PA: Churchill Livingstone; 2000:236–251.
42. Kisner C, Colby LA. Therapeutic Exercise. Foundations and Techniques. Philadelphia, PA: FA Davis; 1997.
43. Astrand PO, Rodahl K. Physical Training: Textbook of Work Physiology. New York, NY: McGraw-Hill; 1986.
44. DeLorme T, Watkins A. Techniques of Progressive Resistance Exercise. New York, NY: Appleton-Century; 1951.
45. Soest A, Bobbert M. The role of muscle properties in control of explosive movements. Biol Cybern. 1993;69:195–204.
46. Komi PV. The stretch-shortening cycle and human power output. In: Jones NL, McCartney N, McComas AJ, eds. Human Muscle Power. Champlain, IL: Human Kinetics; 1986:27.
47. Bandy W, Lovelace-Chandler V, Bandy B, et al. Adaptation of skeltal muscle to resistance training. J Orthop Sports Phys Ther. 1990;12:248–255.
48. Albert MS. Principles of exercise progression. In: Greenfield B, ed. Rehabilitation of the Knee: A Problem Solving Approach. Philadelphia, PA: FA Davis: 1993.
49. Voight ML, Draovitch P, Tippett SR. Plyometrics. In: Albert MS, ed. Eccentric Muscle Training in Sports and Orthopedics. New York, NY: Churchill Livingstone; 1995.
50. Clark MA. Integrated Training for the New Millenium. Thousand Oaks, CA: National Academy of Sports Medicine; 2001.
51. Worrell TW, Perrin DH, Gansneder B, et al. Comparison of isokinetic strength and flexibility measures between hamstring injured and non-injured athletes. J Orthop Sports Phys Ther. 1991;13:118–125.
52. Anderson MA, Gieck JH, Perrin D, et al. The relationship among isokinetic, isotonic, and isokinetic concentric and eccentric quadriceps and hamstrings force and three components of athletic performance. J Orthop Sports Phys Ther. 1991;14:114–120.
53. Steadman JR, Forster RS, Silfverskold JP. Rehabilitation of the knee. Clin Sports Med. 1989;8:605–627.
54. Montgomery JB, Steadman JR. Rehabilitation of the injured knee. Clin Sports Med. 1985;4:333–343.
55. Delsman PA, Losee GM. Isokinetic shear forces and their effect on the quadriceps active drawer. Med Sci Sports Exerc. 1984;16:151.
56. Simoneau GG, Bereda SM, Sobush DC, et al. Biomechanics of elastic resistance in therapeutic exercise programs. J Orthop Sports Phys Ther. 2001;31:16–24.
57. Engle RP, Canner GC. Proprioceptive neuromuscular facilitation (PNF) and modified procedures for anterior cruciate ligament (ACL) instability. J Orthop Sports Phys Ther. 1989;11:230.
58. Manske RC, Reiman MP. Muscle weakness. In: Cameron MH, Monroe LG, eds. Physical Rehabilitation: Evidence-Based Examination, Evaluation, and Intervention. St Louis, MO: Saunders/Elsevier; 2007:64–86.
59. Tabata I, Nishimura K, Kouzaki M, et al. Effects of moderate-intensity endurance and high-intensity intermittent training on anaerobic capacity and VO-2max. Med Sci Sports Exerc. 1996;10:1327–1330.

60. Grimby G, Thomee R. Principles of rehabilitation after injuries. In: Dirix A, Knuttgen HG, Tittel K, eds. The Olympic Book of Sports Medicine. Oxford, UK: Blackwell Scientific; 1984.
61. Thomee R, Renstrom P, Grimby G, et al. Slow or fast isokinetic training after surgery. J Orthop Sports Phys Ther. 1987;8:476.
62. Graves JE, Pollock SH, Leggett SH, et al. Effect of reduced training frequency on muscular strength. Sports Med. 1988;9:316–319.
63. Artalejo AR, Garcia-Sancho J. Mobilization of intracellular calcium by extracellular ATP and by calcium ionophores in the Ehrlich ascites-tumour cell. Biochim Biophys Acta. 1988;941:48–54.
64. Cavagna GA, Disman B, Margarai R. Positive work done by a previously stretched muscle. J Appl Physiol. 1968;24:21–32.
65. Wilk KE, Voight ML, Keirns MA, et al. Stretch-shortening drills for the upper extremities: theory and clinical application. J Orthop Sports Phys Ther. 1993;17:225–239.
66. Wathen D. Literature review: explosive/plyometric exercises. NSCA J. 1993;15:16–19.
67. Janda V. Muscle Function Testing. London, UK: Butterworths; 1983.
68. Jull GA, Janda V. Muscle and motor control in low back pain. In: Twomey LT, Taylor JR, eds. Physical Therapy of the Low Back: Clinics in Physical Therapy. New York, NY: Churchill Livingstone; 1987:258.
69. Gleim GW, McHugh MP. Flexibility and its effects on sports injury and performance. Sports Med. 1997;24:289–299.
70. Kottke FJ. Therapeutic exercise to maintain mobility. In: Kottke FJ, Stillwell GK, Lehman JF, eds. Krusen's Handbook of Physical Medicine and Rehabilitation. Baltimore, MD: WB Saunders; 1982:389–402.
71. Travell JG, Simons DG. Myofascial Pain and Dysfunction—The Trigger Point Manual. Baltimore, MD: Williams & Wilkins; 1983.
72. Swezey RL. Arthrosis. In: Basmajian JV, Kirby RL, eds. Medical Rehabilitation. Baltimore, MD: Williams & Wilkins; 1984:216–218.
73. Joynt RL. Therapeutic exercise. In: DeLisa JA, ed. Rehabilitation Medicine: Principles and Practice. Philadelphia, PA: JB Lippincott; 1988: 346–371.
74. The American Orthopaedic Society for Sports Medicine. Flexibility. Chicago, IL: The American Orthopaedic Society for Sports Medicine; 1988.
75. Kippers V, Parker AW. Toe-touch test: a measure of validity. Phys Ther. 67:1680–1684.
76. Jackson AW, Baker AA. The relationship of the sit and reach test to criterion measures of hamstring and back flexibility in young females. Res Q Exerc Sport. 1986;57:183–186.
77. Litsky AS, Spector M. Biomaterials. In: Simon SR, ed. Orthopaedic Basic Science. Chicago, IL: The American Orthopaedic Society for Sports Medicine; 1994:447–486.
78. Johns R, Wright V. Relative importance of various tissues in joint stiffness. J Appl Physiol. 1962;17:824–830.
79. Toft E, Espersen GT, Kalund S, et al. Passive tension of the ankle before and after stretching. Am J Sports Med. 1989;17:489–494.

80. Halbertsma JPK, Goeken LNH. Stretching exercises: effect of passive extensibility and stiffness in short hamstrings of healthy subjects. Arch Phys Med Rehab. 1994;75:976–981.
81. Magnusson SP, Simonsen EB, Aagaard P, et al. A mechanism for altered flexibility in human skeletal muscle. J Physiol. 1996;497:291–298.
82. Klinge K, Magnusson SP, Simonsen EB, et al. The effect of strength and flexibility on skeletal muscle EMG activity, stiffness and viscoelastic stress relaxation response. Am J Sports Med. 1997;25:710–716.
83. Lapier TK, Burton HW, Almon RF. Alterations in intramuscular connective tissue after limb casting affect contraction-induced muscle injury. J Appl Physiol. 1995;78:1065–1069.
84. McNair PJ, Wood GA, Marshall RN. Stiffness of the hamstring muscles and its relationship to function in ACL deficient individuals. Clin Biomech. 1992;7:131–137.
85. McHugh MP, Magnusson SP, Gleim GW, et al. A cross-sectional study of age-related musculoskeletal and physiological changes in soccer players. Med Exerc Nutr Health. 1993;2:261–268.
86. Zachazewski JE. Flexibility for sports. In: Sanders B, ed. Sports Physical Therapy. Norwalk, CT: Appleton and Lange; 1990:201–238.
87. Bohannon RW. Effect of repeated eight-minute muscle loading on the angle of straight-leg-raising. Phys Ther. 1984;64:491.
88. Yoder E. Physical therapy management of nonsurgical hip problems in adults. In: Echternach JL, ed. Physical Therapy of the Hip. New York, NY: Churchill Livingstone; 1990:103–137.
89. DeVries HA. Evaluation of static stretching procedures for improvement of flexibility. Res Quart. 1962;33:222–229.
90. Logan GA, Egstrom GH. Effects of slow and fast stretching on sacrofemoral angle. J Assoc Phys Ment Rehabil. 1961;15:85–89.
91. Davies CT, White MJ. Muscle weakness following eccentric work in man. Pflugers Arch. 1981;392:168–171.
92. Friden J, Sjostrom M, Ekblom B. A morphological study of delayed muscle soreness. Experientia. 1981;37:506–507.
93. Hardy L. Improving active range of hip flexion. Res Q Exerc Sport. 1985;56:111–114.
94. Markos PD. Ipsilateral and contralateral effects of proprioceptive neuromuscular facilitation techniques on hip motion and electromyographic activity. Phys Ther. 1979;59:1366.
95. Holt LE, Travis TM, Okita T. Comparative study of three stretching techniques. Percep Motor Skills. 1970;31:611–616.
96. Tanigawa MC. Comparison of hold-relax procedure and passive mobilization on increasing muscle length. Phys Ther. 1972;52:725–735.
97. Sady SP, Wortman MA, Blanke D. Flexibility training: ballistic, static or proprioceptive neuromuscular facilitation? Arch Phys Med Rehab. 1982;63:261–263.
98. Prentice WE. A comparison of static stretching and PNF stretching for improving hip joint flexibility. Athl Train. 1983;18:56–59.

99. Murphy P. Warming up before stretching advised. Phys Sports Med. 1986;14:45.

100. Shellock F, Prentice WE. Warm-up and stretching for improved physical performance and prevention of sport-related injury. Sports Med. 1985;2:267–278.

101. Sapega AA, Quedenfeld T, Moyer R, et al. Biophysical factors in range of motion exercise. Phys Sports Med. 1981;9:57–65.

102. Sucher BM. Thoracic outlet syndrome—a myofascial variant: part 2. treatment. JAOA. 1990;90:810–823.

103. Voight M, Blackburn T. Proprioception and balance training and testing following injury. In: Ellenbecker TS, ed. Knee Ligament Rehabilitation. Philadelphia, PA: Churchill Livingstone; 2000:361–385.

104. Guskiewicz KM. Impaired postural stability: regaining balance. In: Prentice WE, Voight ML, eds. Techniques in Musculoskeletal Rehabilitation. New York, NY: McGraw-Hill; 2001:125–150.

105. Risberg MA, Mork M, Krogstad-Jenssen H, et al. Design and implementation of a neuromuscular training program following anterior cruciate ligament reconstruction. J Orthop Sports Phys Ther. 2001;31:620–631.

106. Lephart SM, Borsa PA. Functional rehabilitation of knee injuries. In: Fu FH, Harner C, eds. Knee Surgery. Baltimore, MD: Williams & Wilkins; 1993.

107. Lephart SM, Henry TJ. Functional rehabilitation for the upper and lower extremity. Orthop Clin North Am. 1995;26:579–592.

108. Voight ML, Cook G. Impaired neuromuscular control: reactive neuromuscular training. In: Prentice WE, Voight ML, eds. Techniques in Musculoskeletal Rehabilitation. New York, NY: McGraw-Hill; 2001:93–124.

109. Jerosch J, Prymka M. Propriozeptive Fahigkeiten des gesunden Kniegelenks: Beeinflussung durch eine elastische Bandage. Sportverletz Sportsch. 1995;9:72–76.

110. Jerosch J, Hoffstetter I, Bork H, et al. The influence of orthoses on the proprioception of the ankle joint. Knee Surg Sports Traumatol Arthrosc. 1995;3:39–46.

111. Perlau R, Frank C, Fick G. The effect of elastic bandages on human knee proprioception in the uninjured population. Am J Sports Med. 1995;23:251–255.

112. Robbins S, Waked E, Rappel R. Ankle taping improves proprioception before and after exercise in young men. Br J Sports Med. 1995;29:242–247.

113. Barrett DS. Proprioception and function after anterior cruciate ligament reconstruction. J Bone Joint Surg. 1991;73B:833–837.

114. Lephart SM, Pincivero DM, Giraldo JL, et al. The role of proprioception in the management and rehabilitation of athletic injuries. Am J Sports Med. 1997;25:130–137.

115. Voss DE, Ionta MK, Myers DJ. Proprioceptive Neuromuscular Facilitation: Patterns and Techniques. 3rd ed. Philadelphia, PA: Harper and Row; 1985:1–342.

116. Janda DH, Loubert P. A preventative program focussing on the glenohumeral joint. Clin Sports Med. 1991;10:955–971.

117. Martin G. Aquatic therapy in rehabilitation. In: Prentice WE, Voight ML, eds. Techniques in Musculoskeletal Rehabilitation. New York, NY: McGraw-Hill; 2001:279–287.

118. Kuprian W. Proprioceptive neuromuscular facilitation—PNF complex motions. In: Kuprian W, ed. Physical Therapy for Sports. 2nd ed. Philadelphia, PA: WB Saunders; 1995:99–119.

QUESTIONS

1. What type of contraction occurs when there is tension produced in the muscle without any appreciable change in muscle length or joint movement?

2. What type of contraction occurs when a muscle slowly lengthens as it gives in to an external force that is greater than the contractile force it is exerting?

3. Of the three types of muscle actions, isometric, concentric and eccentric, which one is capable of developing the most force?

4. What are the four biomechanical properties that human skeletal muscle possesses?

5. True or false, rapid lengthening contractions generate less force than do slow ones (slower lengthening contractions).

6. Give two disadvantages of isometric exercise

7. What is the best way to first exercise the postural (or extensor) musculature when it is extremely weak to facilitate muscle control?
   a. Eccentric exercises
   b. Isometric exercises
   c. Isokinetic exercises
   d. Electrical stimulation

8. What are the four parameters of exercise?

9. What is the best gauge of exercise intensity in a healthy individual?
   a. Blood pressure
   b. Heart rate
   c. Rating of perceived exertion
   d. Rate of perspiration

10. You ask a patient to assess his level of exertion using the Rating of Perceived Exertion Scale (RPE). The patient rates the level of exertion as 9 on the 6 to 19 scale. A rating of 9 corresponds to which of the following?
    a. Very, very light
    b. Hard
    c. Very light
    d. Somewhat hard

11. The optimal exercise prescription to improve fast movement speeds and enhance endurance (improving fast-twitch fiber function) is

    a. low-intensity workloads for short durations.

    b. high-intensity workloads for short durations.

    c. low-intensity workloads for long durations.

    d. high-intensity workloads for long durations

12. You have been asked to develop an exercise plan for a pregnant woman. The strengthening of which of the following muscles should be the focus to maintain a strong pelvic floor?

    a. Rectus abdominis, iliococcygeus, and piriformis

    b. Piriformis, obturator internus, and pubococcygeus

    c. Iliococcygeus, pubococcygeus, and coccygeus

    d. obturator internus, piriformis, and external obliques

13. A 35-year-old presents with a prescription to improve aerobic conditioning. Which of the following is not a benefit of aerobic exercise?

    a. Improved cardiovascular fitness

    b. Increased high-density lipoprotein (HDL) cholesterol

    c. Improved flexibility

    d. Improved state of mind

14. You are treating a 15-year-old male soccer player who sustained a Grade II inversion ankle sprain 2 weeks ago. You determine that the patient is now in the early subacute phase of rehabilitation. Which of the following interventions should the patient be performing?

    a. Closed-chain lower extremity strengthening, proprioceptive exercises, and an orthosis

    b. Weaning off crutches to a cane

    c. Protection, rest, ice, compression and elevation (PRICE)

    d. Open-chain lower extremity exercises only

15. You are planning the intervention for a 73-year-old inpatient who received a cemented total hip replacement 2 days ago. Your plan of care should focus on

    a. patient education regarding positions and movements to avoid.

    b. active range of motion exercises and early ambulation using a walker

    c. passive range of motion exercises

    d. tilt table

16. Your first patient of the day has been referred with a prescription stating *Stable humeral neck fracture—Begin functional mobility*. After the examination you decide the best initial intervention for this patient is

    a. pendulum exercises

    b. shoulder isometrics

    c. manual PNF

    d. modalities to control pain

17. You are treating a patient who has been referred to physical therapy to be setup on an exercise program to assist in weight loss. Which type of exercise program promotes weight loss?

18. You have decided to implement PNF exercises with a patient recovering from impingement syndrome of the shoulder. What is the best PNF diagonal pattern to improve function of the shoulder?

    a. D1 flexion

    b. D1 extension

    c. D2 flexion

    d. D2 extension

19. You are planning the intervention for a patient with acute rotator cuff tendonitis and subacromial bursitis. During your examination you found that passive and active glenohumeral motions increased the patient's pain. Your initial intervention should be:

    a. to use modalities to reduce pain and inflammation

    b. to begin rotator cuff strengthening exercises

    c. to begin correcting any muscle imbalances

    d. shoulder isometrics

20. You have been asked to teach a class at a local gym for a group of geriatric athletes. Which of the following is not a general guideline for exercise prescription in this patient population?

    a. Use machines for strength training rather than free weights

    b. Always warm-up before exercise

    c. No pain, no gain

    d. Try to incorporate both aerobic and anaerobic exercises

21. You are assisting a patient in improving anterior stability of the knee joint using exercises to strengthen muscle groups that will assist the anterior cruciate ligament. Which of the following muscle groups provides the most amount of active restraint?

    a. Gastrocnemius

    b. Hamstrings

    c. Quadriceps

    d. Hip adductors

22. You decide to use a contract-relax technique to improve a patient's active straight leg raise. Which of the following muscle groups should you emphasize the contraction of?

a. hip abductors and hip flexors
b. hamstrings and hip extensors
c. quadriceps and hip flexors
d. hip abductors and quadriceps

23. Which of the following exercises is indicated to enhance coordination?
    a. Codman exercises
    b. McKenzie exercises
    c. Frenkel exercises
    d. Williams exercises

24. You have been referred a patient with a prescription that reads *Knee strengthening—open chain exercises only*. Which of the following is not an open chain exercise?
    a. knee extension
    b. hamstring curls
    c. squat
    d. straight leg raise

25. A high school coach asks you which of the best type of exercise to improve an athlete's vertical jump. Which of the following exercise types would be the best to achieve this goal?
    a. Closed chain
    b. Open chain
    c. Plyometrics
    d. DeLorme

26. Give three contraindications to aquatic exercise

27. What should the temperature of the water be for water exercise?

28. You have been asked to set up an exercise program for an obese patient who is 74 pounds overweight and is recovering from a mild myocardial infarction. The most appropriate exercise prescription for this patient is
    a. walking at an intensity of 50% of the patient's maximum heart rate
    b. jogging at an intensity of 60% of the patient's maximum heart rate
    c. swimming at an intensity of 75% of the patient's maximum heart rate
    d. no exercise with a focus on diet

29. You are treating a patient who is beginning recovery stage 4 movements following a right CVA. Which PNF pattern should you use to promote continued recovery of the left upper extremity through the use of out-of-synergy movements?
    a. bilateral symmetrical D1 thrust and reverse thrust
    b. chop, reverse chop with the left upper extremity leading

c. bilateral symmetrical D2 thrust and reverse thrust

d. lift, reverse lift with the left upper extremity leading

30. You have been asked to design an exercise program for a 46-year-old individual who has limited endurance as a result of a sedentary lifestyle. There is no history of cardiorespiratory problems. An appropriate initial exercise intensity for this individual would be:

a. 30% to 60% of the maximum heart rate

b. 60% to 90% of the maximum heart rate

c. 10% to 30% of the maximum heart rate

d. zero to 30% of the maximum heart rate

Peripheral & Spinal Joints

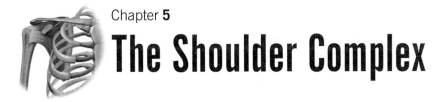

Chapter **5**

The Shoulder Complex

OVERVIEW

The shoulder complex is composed of articulations between the humerus, glenoid, scapula, acromion, clavicle, and the surrounding soft tissue structures that connect them. The shoulder complex allows for a large degree of motion in multiple planes at the expense of stability. As a result, this compound set of articulations can present a diagnostic and treatment challenge.

> **Clinical Pearl**
>
> The rotator interval, according to Neer,[1] is the capsular tissue in the interval between the subscapularis and the supraspinatus tendons. The structures within the rotator interval contribute to the stability of the shoulder by limiting inferior translation and external rotation with the arm adducted, as well as posterior translation when the arm is forward flexed, adducted, and internally rotated.

Anatomy

The specific joints of the shoulder complex include the following:

- Glenohumeral (GH) joint. The most mobile joint in the body.
- Acromioclavicular (AC) joint. The ligaments providing stability to the AC joint include the superior and inferior AC ligaments, and the coracoclavicular ligaments (conoid and trapezoid). The AC ligaments are the principal restraint to anteroposterior translation, whereas the coracoclavicular ligaments restrain vertical motions. The deltoid and trapezius muscles provide dynamic stabilization to the joint.
- Sternoclavicular (SC) joint.
- Scapulothoracic articulation. A pseudojoint critical for normal biomechanics of the shoulder.

277

> ## 🌑 Clinical Pearl
>
> If optimal shoulder function is to occur, motion also has to be available at the cervicothoracic junction and at the connections between the first three ribs and the sternum and spine.

The shoulder complex is endowed with a unique blend of mobility and stability:

- The degree of mobility is contingent on a healthy articular surface, intact muscle–tendon units (Table 5-1), and supple capsuloligamentous restraints (Table 5-2).

Table 5-1 Muscles of the Shoulder Complex According to Their Actions on the Scapula and at the Glenohumeral Joint

Scapula abductors	Trapezius
	Serratus anterior (upper fibers)
Scapula adductors	Levator scapulae
	Rhomboids
Scapula flexors	Serratus anterior (lower fibers)
Scapula extensors	Pectoralis minor
Scapula external rotators	Trapezius
	Rhomboids
The shoulder flexors	Coracobrachialis
	Short-head biceps
	Long-head biceps
	Pectoralis major
	Anterior deltoid
The shoulder extensors	The triceps
	Posterior deltoid
	Teres minor
	Teres major
	Latissimus dorsi

Shoulder abductors	Supraspinatus
	Deltoid
Shoulder adductors	Subscapularis
	Pectoralis major
	Latissimus dorsi
	Teres major
	Teres minor
Shoulder internal rotators	Pectoralis major and minor
	Serratus anterior
	Subscapularis
	Pectoralis major
	Latissimus dorsi
	Teres major
Shoulder external rotators	Infraspinatus
	Supraspinatus
	Deltoid
	Teres minor

Table 5-2 Ligaments of the Shoulder

Ligament	Description	Function
Clavicular Ligaments		
Coracoclavicular ligament	Comprised of the conoid and trapezoid ligaments	Reinforces the connection between the coracoid process Stabilizes the acromioclavicular joint
Acromioclavicular Ligament	Runs between the acromion process and the clavicle	Reinforces the connection between the acromion and the clavicle
Sternoclavicular Ligaments		
Sternoclavicular ligament	Comprised of anterior and posterior ligaments	Reinforces the connection between the sternum and the clavicle
Interclavicular ligament	Connects the superior–medial sternal ends of each clavicle with the capsular ligaments and the upper sternum	Strengthens the articular capsule
Costoclavicular ligament	The strongest of the sternoclavicular ligaments	Reinforces the connection between the first rib and the clavicle and stabilizes the joint

(continued on following page)

Table 5-2 *(continued from previous page)*

Ligament	Description	Function
Glenohumeral Ligaments	Distinct capsular thickenings limiting excessive rotation and translation of the humeral head by reinforcing the connection between the glenoid fossa and the humerus	The primary static stabilizers of the glenohumeral joint
Inferior glenohumeral ligament	A complex—parts include the anterior band, axillary pouch, and the posterior band	Provides anterior stabilization, especially during abduction of the arm
Middle glenohumeral ligament	Strongest of the glenohumeral ligaments	Provides anterior stabilization during external rotation combined with 45 degree of abduction
Superior glenohumeral ligament	Runs from glenoid rim to anatomical neck	Works in conjunction with the coracohumeral ligament to provide inferior stabilization during adduction
Coracohumeral ligament	Runs from the lateral end of the coracoid process and inserts either side of the greater and lesser tuberosities	Provides anterior support by tightening with flexion
Transverse humeral ligament	Traverses the bicipital groove	Maintains the long head of the biceps muscle in the intertubercular groove
Intrinsic Ligaments of the Scapula		
Superior transverse scapular ligament	Attached by one end to the base of the coracoid process, and by the other to the medial end of the scapular notch	Reinforces the connection between the coracoid process and the medial border of the scapular notch
Inferior transverse scapular ligament	An inconstant fibrous band that passes from the lateral border of the spine of the scapula to the posterior margin of the glenoid cavity	Reinforces the connection between the lateral aspect of the root of the spine of the scapula and the margin of the glenoid fossa
Coracoacromial ligament	Runs from the coracoid process to the anterior–inferior aspect of the acromion, with some of its fibers extending to the AC joint	Reinforces the connection between the coracoid process and the acromion, stabilizing the joint

AC joint = acromioclavicular joint

- The degree of stability is dependent upon a combination of ligamentous and capsular restraints, surrounding musculature and the glenoid labrum. Static joint stability is provided by the integrity of the osseous articular structures and the capsulolabral complex, and dynamic stability by the rotator cuff muscles (supraspinatus, infraspinatus, teres minor, and subscapularis) and the scapula pivoters (trapezius, serratus anterior, levator scapulae, and rhomboid major and minor).[2]

Examination of the Shoulder Complex

In the vast majority of cases, an accurate diagnosis can be established with a detailed history and a thorough physical examination supplemented on occasion with appropriate radiographic and laboratory examinations.[3,4]

 Clinical Pearl

An examination of shoulder dysfunction should include the cervical spine, contralateral shoulder, elbow, trunk, and upper limb neurovascular structures.

History

As shoulder pain has a broad spectrum of patterns and characteristics, a good history is the cornerstone of proper diagnosis (Table 5-3). The mechanism of injury can reveal a lot about the structures that may be involved in the injury:

- Direct blow to the shoulder: AC joint separation (see Common Conditions).

Table 5-3 Important Factors in the Patient's History

All Patients	Shoulder Patients
Age	Overhead use—athletics/repetitive work
Hand dominance	Night pain
Occupation	Upper extremity symptoms
Onset	Neck pain
Mechanism?	Previous episodes?
Duration of symptoms	Previous rehabilitation?
	Surgical history

- Insidious onset: adhesive capsulitis (see Common Conditions).
- Direct trauma to the arm (fall onto the outside of the shoulder): humeral fracture. The patient typically complains of a persistent deep ache/pain in the glenohumeral joint and pain or inability to actively move the involved arm.
- Fall on an outstretched hand (FOOSH): clavicular fracture.

 Clinical Pearl

The chief symptom reported by the patient with a shoulder dysfunction is usually related to pain or instability. Associated symptoms include decreased motion, power, and/or function.

Handedness and occupation are key elements to determine during the history.[5] Age can also be an important factor as it is well recognized that certain shoulder pathologies are related to age.

 Clinical Pearl

Impingement, early onset of adhesive capsulitis, and degenerative rotator cuff tears tend to occur more often in the over-45 age group, whereas traumatic tears and instability (glenohumeral dislocations and AC joint separations) are more likely to occur in the younger population.

Determining the location of the pain can provide some clues as to the cause (Figure 5-1). Many shoulder pathologies have key findings that can help guide the examiner (Table 5-4).

 Clinical Pearl

- Questions must be asked about neck pain and previous neck injury, while also attempting to establish a relationship between head and neck movements and symptom reproduction. Symptoms that originate from the neck and which radiate below the elbow are suggestive of a cervical spine disorder.[6]

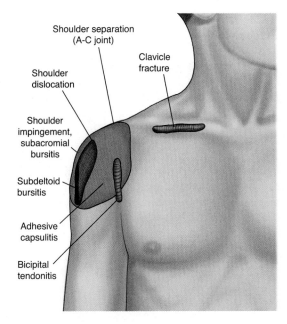

Shoulder separation
(A-C joint)

Clavicle
fracture

Shoulder
dislocation

Shoulder
impingement,
subacromial
bursitis

Subdeltoid
bursitis

Adhesive
capsulitis

Bicipital
tendonitis

Figure 5-1 Determining the location of the pain can provide some clues as to the cause.

Stiffness or loss of motion may be the major symptom in patients with adhesive capsulitis (frozen shoulder), dislocation, or glenohumeral joint arthritis. Pain with throwing (such as pitching a baseball) suggests anterior

Table 5-4 Key Findings in the History and Physical Examination and Their Probable Diagnosis

Finding	Probable Diagnosis
Scapula winging, trauma, recent viral illness	Serratus anterior or trapezius dysfunction
Muscle spasm and inability to passively or actively externally rotate the involved arm	Posterior shoulder dislocation
Supraspinatus/infraspinatus atrophy	Rotator cuff tear; suprascapular nerve entrapment
Loss of active elevation and external rotation	Neurological injury
	Rotator cuff tear
	Neurological injury

glenohumeral instability. The shoulder pathologies that can present with specific subjective complaints are outlined in Table 5-5.

 Clinical Pearl

Two lesions related to glenohumeral instability include the following:

- Bankart lesion: an avulsion of the anteroinferior glenoid labrum at its attachment to the inferior glenohumeral ligament, usually as a result of an anterior shoulder dislocation. It is considered the primary lesion in recurrent anterior instability. Patients typically complain of pain when moving the arm in scaption/flexion with external rotation, particularly with the arm abducted to 90 degrees.

- Hill-Sachs lesion: an osteochondral lesion of the posterolateral humeral head caused by an acute anterior dislocation. Patients typically complain of pain with activities involving resisted external rotation or with overhead activities.

Once the location, quality, distribution, and aggravating and relieving factors of the shoulder symptoms have been established, the possibility of referred pain should be excluded.[6]

Systems Review

Inquiries should be made for a history of rheumatoid arthritis, diabetes, neurofibromatosis, neoplasms, cardiac diseases, and gout as well as other systemic diseases.[5] For example, diaphragmatic irritation from a gallbladder or hepatic disorder will often yield shoulder pain, as can the Pancoast tumor with its coincident Horner syndrome.[5] Pneumonia, cardiac ischemia, and peptic ulcer diseases can also present with shoulder pain.[6] A history of malignancy raises the possibility of metastatic disease.

 Clinical Pearl

- If the clinician is concerned with any signs or symptoms of a systemic disorder that is out of the scope of physical therapy, the patient should be referred back to their physician or another appropriate health care provider.

Table 5-5 Subjective Patient Complaints Related to Specific Diagnoses

Specific Complaint	Pathology
Intermittent mild pain with overhead activities	Impingement (stage I)
Mild to moderate pain with overhead or strenuous activities	Impingement (stage II)
Pain at rest or with activities. Night pain may occur. Weakness is noted	Impingement (stage III)
Night time shoulder pain. Weakness noted predominantly in abductors and external rotators. Loss of motion noted	Rotator cuff tears (Full -thickness)
	Impingement
	Adhesive capsulitis
	Osteoarthritis
Inability to perform activities of daily living due to loss of motion. Loss of motion may be perceived as weakness	Adhesive capsulitis (Frozen shoulder)
Apprehension to mechanical shifting limits activity. Slipping, popping, or sliding may present as subtle instability	Anterior Instability
Apprehension usually associated with horizontal abduction and external rotation. Anterior or posterior pain may be present. Slipping or popping of the humeral head posteriorly. This may be associated with forward flexion and internal rotation while the shoulder is under a compressive load	Posterior Instability
Shoulder pain in throwing athletes; anterior glenohumeral joint pain	Glenohumeral joint instability
Pain or "clunking" sound with overhead motion	Glenoid labrum disorder
Generalized ligamentous laxity and recurrent episodes of subluxations or dislocations with no history of significant trauma. Pain may or may not be present	Multidirectional instability
Localized pain, swelling, deformity, tenderness localized to AC joint or pain localized to the top of the shoulder	AC joint arthritis or chronic separation.
Pain radiating below elbow; decreased cervical range of motion	Cervical disc disease
Pain/numbness and/or tingling in a dermatomal distribution	Cervical nerve root irritation.
Pain along the anterior and posterior G-H joint lines	Degenerative arthritis of the glenohumeral joint
Pain felt in the lateral deltoid region/lateral aspect of the upper arm.	Subacromial bursitis, frozen shoulder, or rotator cuff pathology.

AC joint = acromioclavicular joint.

The patient should be asked about paresthesias and muscle weakness. Brachial plexus lesions and cervical and upper thoracic spine disorders frequently cause shoulder symptoms.

Clinical Pearl

In addition to the cervical and upper thoracic joints, the related joints referring symptoms to the shoulder require clearing. These include the temporomandibular joint (TMJ), costosternal joint, costovertebral and costotransverse joint, and the elbow and forearm.[7,8]

The sympathetic dystrophies can also cause shoulder symptoms.[5,9] The Cyriax scanning examination can help highlight the presence or absence of the more insidious causes of shoulder symptoms and can also help the clinician whether a spinal nerve root or peripheral nerve injury is present (Table 5-6). The patient should be asked about previous corticosteroid injections, particularly in the setting of osteopenia or rotator cuff tendon atrophy.[6]

Tests and Measures

A stepwise approach for evaluating shoulder pain begins with observation and palpation; assessment of range of motion (ROM) and strength; and

Table 5-6 Indications of Peripheral Nerve Damage at the Shoulder

Atrophied Muscle	Peripheral Nerve	Cause	Appearance
Deltoid	Axillary	Anterior dislocation	Squared appearance of the lateral shoulder
Posterior deltoid	Axillary	Multidirectional instability	Atrophy of the deltoid and teres minor
Infraspinatus/ supraspinatus	Suprascapular	Rotator cuff tear Nerve entrapment	Slight indent over fossae. Confirmed by pushing the examining finger into the respective muscle bellies
Trapezius	Spinal accessory	Medical procedures (radical neck dissection and cervical lymph node biopsy)	Appearance of a shoulder girdle that droops in association with a protracted inferior border of the scapula and an elevated acromion
Serratus anterior	Long thoracic	Direct blow or compression	Prominent superior medial border of the scapula and a depressed acromion

Table 5-7 Close-packed, Open-packed, and Capsular Patterns of the Shoulder Complex

	Close-packed	Open-packed	Capsular Pattern
Glenohumeral	90 degrees of glenohumeral abduction and full external rotation; or full abduction and external rotation	55 degrees abduction, 30 degrees horizontal adduction	External rotation, abduction, internal rotation
Acromioclavicular	90° degrees abduction	Arm resting by side	Pain at extremes of range, especially horizontal adduction and full elevation
Sternoclavicular	Full arm elevation and shoulder protraction	Arm resting by side	Pain at extremes of range, especially horizontal adduction and full elevation

provocative testing at the cervical spine, TMJ, SC, AC, and scapulothoracic components of the shoulder joint, then focuses on particular anatomic sites, rotator cuff strength, and impingement signs, followed by glenohumeral tests.

The closed- and open-packed positions and the capsular patterns for the joints of the shoulder complex are outlined in Table 5-7.

Observation

Observation of the shoulder complex can be divided into static and dynamic factors:[3]

- The static factors include physiological age and appearance, posture, generalized diseases such as rheumatoid arthritis, generalized distress, and distress related to the shoulder.

- The dynamic factors include generalized distress with movement, shoulder distress with movements, and the performance of simple functional tasks.

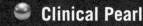 **Clinical Pearl**

Common physical findings include local tenderness, deformity, swelling, and ecchymosis.

Static Observation

Observation of the shoulder requires adequate visualization of the entire upper extremity, shoulder girdle, chest, and back. The examination is performed with the shirt off for male patients and a sleeveless shirt for female patients. Both shoulders should be visible to allow comparative inspection and the observation should be from all views.[5] To ensure this, the observation should be systematically divided into anterior, lateral, posterior, and superior aspects.[3]

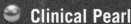

Clinical Pearl

Key focus areas for observation include the following:

- Anterior: abnormal contours and bony prominences (an AC separation produces a "step-off" deformity with prominence of the distal clavicle, whereas an anterior shoulder dislocation reduces a prominent acromion and anterior fullness).

- Posterior: the dominant shoulder often rests slightly lower than the opposite shoulder. Diminished posterior contour from neck to shoulder indicates atrophy of the trapezius, whereas loss of lateral shoulder contour and a prominent suprascapular ridge indicates atrophy of the supraspinatus/infraspinatus muscles.

The clinician initially observes the attitude of the shoulder and notes the overall position of the upper extremity. Symmetry of right and left sides should also be noted.

Clinical Pearl

- A painful shoulder is often held higher than the uninvolved side, or it may be held by the patient in a protective manner across the abdomen, often supported by the opposite extremity.[3]

The clinician should note muscle mass and tone, deformities, scars, masses, ecchymosis, discoloration, swelling, and any venous distention. Examples of deformities are listed in Table 5-8.

Discoloration from bruising may be present from a recent fracture, rotator cuff injury, or biceps rupture.[3] Specific areas of atrophy can imply certain diagnoses. For example, muscle weakness, or atrophy, especially after trauma, might indicate peripheral nerve damage (Table 5-6).[10]

Table 5-8 Shoulder Deformities and Their Possible Reasons

Deformity Present	Possible Reason
Squaring off the shoulder with an anterior prominence of the humeral head	Anterior dislocation of the shoulder
Neck appears fuller, shorter on the affected side An elevated scapula Clavicle tilted superiorly about 25 degrees	Sprengel deformity (most common congenital deformity of the shoulder)
An exaggeration of the AC joint prominence	Third-degree acromioclavicular separation
Excessive prominence of the spine of the scapula	Supraspinatus and infraspinatus wasting
"Popeye" appearance of the biceps muscle belly with elbow flexion	Rupture of the long head of the biceps
Scapular winging	Weakness of the serratus anterior Weakness of the trapezius Glenohumeral joint pathology

AC = acromioclavicular.

The scapula position is initially examined with the arms by the side. The clinician notes any signs of muscle imbalance (Table 5-9) or scapular winging during elevation, depression, adduction, abduction, and rotation of the scapula.

Table 5-9 Common Muscle Imbalances of the Shoulder Complex

Muscles Prone to Tightness	Muscles Prone to Inactivity or Lengthening
Upper trapezius	Middle and lower trapezius
Levator scapulae	Rhomboids
Pectoralis major and minor	Serratus anterior
Upper cervical extensors	Deep neck flexors
Sternocleidomastoid	Subscapularis
Scalenes	Supraspinatus
Teres major and minor	Infraspinatus

● Clinical Pearl

Winging of the scapula is usually evident at the inferior border, but can be found anywhere along the entire border.[3,7,10]

A number of tests can be used to assess the position of the scapula relative to the uninvolved side.

Palpation

Palpation must be systematic and focus on specific anatomical structures (Figure 5-2). The optimal methods of palpating the shoulder tendons occur in regions where there is the least amount of overlying soft tissue.[11] The shoulder girdle should be palpated for warmth, tenderness, deformity, and crepitus. Often, trigger points of pain from myofascial syndromes or isolated muscle spasm will be determined with selective palpation of the shoulder girdle structures.[5]

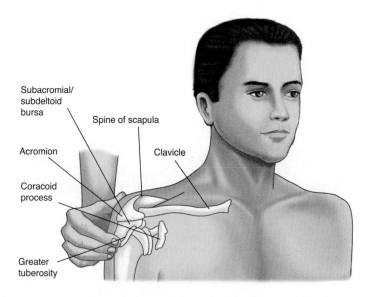

Subacromial/
subdeltoid
bursa
Spine of scapula

Acromion   Clavicle

Coracoid
process

Greater
tuberosity

Figure 5-2 Palpation must be systematic and focus on specific anatomical structures.

Clinical Pearl

Key palpation areas include[6] the following:

- AC joint: identified with palpation of the clavicle and spine of the scapula until they meet laterally.

- The greater and lesser tuberosities.

- The long head of the biceps: anterior between the lesser and greater humeral tuberosities, and more easily palpated with some external rotation of the arm.

- The clavicle.

- The coracoid process: lies medial to the long head of the biceps inferior to the clavicle.

- SC joint.

- The sternal notch.

- Medial scapula.

- Posterior rotator cuff.

- Anterior rotator cuff.

- Deltoid.

- The cervical spinous processes.

- The spine of the scapula.

- The supraclavicular fossa.

- The acromion.

- The subacromial bursa.

- The axilla: should be evaluated for masses, lymph nodes, and palpation of the muscles.

Range of Motion

Due to the complex nature of the arthrokinematics, osteokinematics, and myokinetics of this region, the actual clinical value of active movements are limited if used in isolation. Loss of motion at the shoulder complex is most commonly due to pain. It is important to determine the degree of pain as well as the arc of motion in which the pain occurs.[3,7,10] The potential causes for pain with arm elevation are outlined in Figure 5-3.

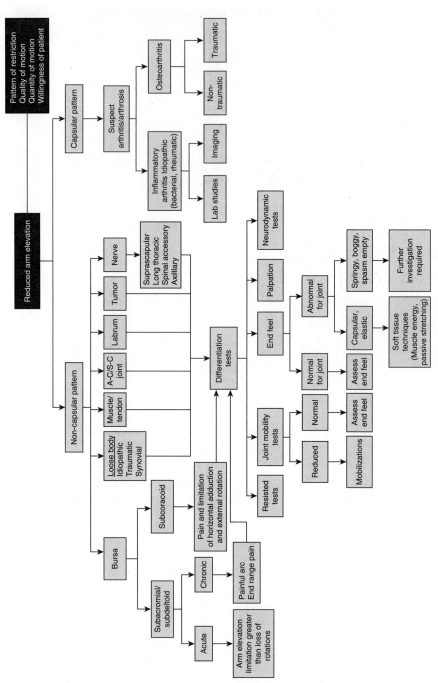

Figure 5-3 The potential causes for pain with arm elevation.

Table 5-10 Normal Ranges for Movements of the Shoulder Complex and Potential Causes of Pain

Motion	Range Norms (Degrees)	End-Feel	Potential Source of Pain
Elevation—Flexion	160–180	Tissue stretch	Suprahumeral impingement
			Stretching of glenohumeral, acromioclavicular, sternoclavicular joint capsule
			Triceps tendon if elbow flexed
Extension	50–60	Tissue stretch	Stretching of glenohumeral joint capsule
			Severe suprahumeral impingement
			Biceps tendon if elbow extended
Elevation—Abduction	170–180	Tissue stretch	Suprahumeral impingement
			Acromioclavicular arthritis at terminal abduction
External rotation	80–90	Tissue stretch	Anterior glenohumeral instability
Internal rotation	60–100	Tissue stretch	Suprahumeral impingement
			Posterior glenohumeral instability

Active Range of Motion

Active motion is assessed first and the patient is asked to move the arm and shoulder actively through the available ROM (Table 5-10). Typically, 170 degrees to 180 degrees of elevation is possible in both flexion and abduction, with the upper portion of the arm able to be placed adjacent to the head. If pain occurs with glenohumeral elevation, the point in the range where the pain occurs can be diagnostic in implicating the cause (Table 5-11)(Figure 5-3 and Figure 5-4).[12]

Clinical Pearl

Normal shoulder motion is a composite movement that couples glenohumeral motion with rotation of the scapula on the thorax with minor contributions from motion at the AC and SC joints.

Ranges of motion that need to be documented are total elevation (forward elevation in the sagittal plane and abduction in the coronal plane), internal

Table 5-11 Diagnosing From the Point in the Range the Pain Is Reproduced

	AROM	AROM	AROM	PROM	PROM	PROM
Findings	Limited range and pain between 70 degrees and 110 degrees of elevation	Full range but pain between 70 degrees and 110 degrees of elevation	Full range but pain at 120 degrees–160 degrees/160 degrees–180 degrees range	Full and pain free	Restriction of all movements	Pain on adduction
Pathology	Rotator cuff impingement Rotator cuff tear Subacromial bursitis	Subacromial bursitis	AC joint pathology	Rotator cuff tear Chronic instability	Adhesive capsulitis	AC joint pathology

AC = acromioclavicular joint; AROM = active range of motion; PROM = passive range of motion.

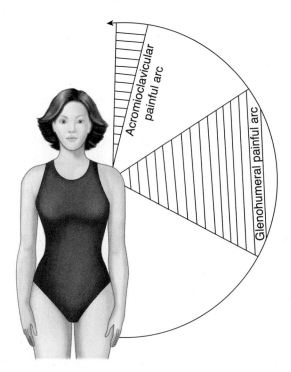

Figure 5-4 The point in the range where the pain occurs can be diagnostic in implicating the cause.

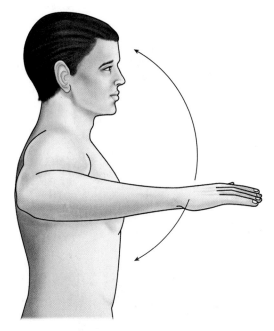

Figure 5-5 Ranges of motion that need to be documented.

and external rotation with the arm by the side and in the 90-degree abducted position (if the patient is able to achieve) (Figure 5-5), horizontal adduction, and shrugging of the shoulders. Internal rotation can be tested further with the patient's arm at the side and the forearm behind their back (Figure 5-6). This measurement for internal rotation is assessed by the position reached with the extended thumb up the posterior aspect of the spine using the spinous processes as landmarks. The patient then completes the motions of shoulder girdle elevation (shrug) and depression, and shoulder protraction and retraction.

Clinical Pearl

An inability to shrug the shoulder may indicate trapezius palsy.[13] Hiking of the shoulder and the scapula during arm elevation is often seen in patients with large rotator cuff tears.[14]

Dynamic Observation

Given the importance of the scapulothoracic joint to overall shoulder function, it is important to examine the scapulothoracic rhythm during humeral abduction.

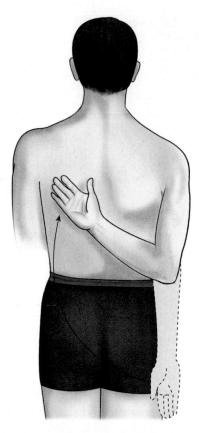

Figure 5-6 Internal rotation can be tested with the patient's arm at the side and the forearm behind their back.

🔵 Clinical Pearl

According to Saha,[15] there are three layers of muscles that stabilize the scapula and assist in force production from the musculature:

- Inner layer: the rotator cuff muscles.

- Middle layer: teres major, pectoralis major, latissimus dorsi, and the short fibers of the anterior and posterior deltoid.

- Superficial layer: triceps, long head of the biceps, coracobrachialis, and the superficial fibers of the anterior and posterior deltoid.

The ability of the patient to perform full abduction will vary according to the presenting pathology and pain.

🔵 Clinical Pearl

During arm elevation, the following force couples are activated:

- The upper trapezius, levator scapula, and superior serratus anterior elevate the scapula.

- The pectoralis minor and major and latissimus dorsi depress the scapula.

- The serratus anterior, pectoralis minor, and levator scapula protract the scapula.

- The trapezius, rhomboids, and latissimus dorsi retract the scapula.

- The superior and inferior portions of the trapezius and inferior portion of the serratus anterior cause lateral scapular rotation.

- The levator scapula, rhomboids, pectoralis minor and major, and latissimus dorsi cause medial scapular rotation.

The first 20 degrees to 30 degrees of abduction do not normally require scapulothoracic motion—the humerus will move upward and the scapula will remain stationary. Frequently in the unstable shoulder, the scapula does not move with its normal rhythm.[3]

🔵 Clinical Pearl

Between 30 degrees and 90 degrees of shoulder flexion, there is a 2:1 ratio of humeral elevation to scapular protraction and upward rotation (60 degrees of the motion has occurred at the glenohumeral joint, with the remaining 30 degrees consisting of scapular motion. Between 90 degrees and 170 degrees, the elevation occurs at a 1:1 glenohumeral to scapula ratio, although this ratio is not consistent throughout the ROM. The final 10 degrees of motion is accomplished through thoracic extension.

On completion of the abduction, the inferior angle of the scapula should be in close proximity to the midline of the thorax, and the vertebral border of the scapula should be rotated 60 degrees. Movement beyond these points may indicate excessive scapula abduction.[16] At the end of range the scapula should slightly depress, posteriorly tilt, and adduct.[16]

Passive Range of Motion

Passive range of motion (PROM) testing follows the active range of motion (AROM) testing even if the AROM appears to be normal. The PROM tests take the form of passive overpressure superimposed on the active motion. PROM is performed to determine the end-feel.[17] Pain often occurs in the extremes of motion in the presence of joint instability.

 Clinical Pearl

A patient with a loss of active motion but normal PROM is more likely to have muscle weakness than joint disease. A discrepancy between active and passive motion may indicate a painful periarticular condition.[14] Loss of active motion with preservation of passive motion is caused by rotator cuff tear[18] or, rarely, suprascapular nerve injury.[19,20] A severely restricted active abduction pattern with no pain is suggestive of a rupture of the supraspinatus or deltoid. Loss of both active and passive motion is usually caused by adhesive capsulitis.[21]

Resisted

In addition to pain, shoulder dysfunction is often caused or exacerbated by loss of motion or weakness (Table 5-12). The resistive tests assess the function and neurological status of the important muscle groups of the upper kinetic chain, including the cervical musculature.

Clinical Pearl

The normal strength ratios of the shoulder are as follows:

• Internal rotation is stronger than external rotation by a 3:2 ratio.

• Adduction is stronger than abduction by a 2:1 ratio.

• Extension is stronger than flexion by a 5:4 ratio.

Women have approximately 45% to 65% of the shoulder strength of men.

Table 5-12 Shoulder Girdle Muscle Function and Innervation

Muscles	Origin	Insertion	Peripheral Nerve	Nerve Root	Motions
Pectoralis major	Anterior surface of the sternal half of the clavicle; anterior surface of the sternum	Intertubercular groove of humerus	Pectoral	Clavicular head: C5 and C6 Sternocostal head: C7, C8, and T1	Adduction, horizontal adduction, and internal rotation; Clavicular fibers—forward flexion; Sternocostal fibers—extension
Pectoralis minor	Ribs three to five	Medial border and superior surface of coracoid process of scapula	Medial pectoral	C8–T1	Stabilizes scapula by drawing it anteriorly and inferiorly against thoracic wall
Latissimus dorsi	Spinous processes of inferior six thoracic vertebrae, thoracolumbar fascia, iliac crest, and inferior three ribs	Floor of intertubercular groove of humerus	Thoracodorsal	C 7 (C 6, C 8)	Adduction, extension, and internal rotation
Teres major	Dorsal surface of inferior angle of scapula	Medial lip of intertubercular groove of humerus	Subscapular	C 5–C 8	Adduction, extension, horizontal abduction, and internal rotation
Teres minor	Superior part of lateral border of scapula	Inferior facet on greater tuberosity of humerus	Axillary	C 5 (6)	Horizontal abduction (also a weak external rotator)
Deltoid	Lateral one third of clavicle, acromion, and spine of scapula	Deltoid tuberosity of humerus	Axillary	C 5 (6)	Anterior—forward flexion, horizontal adduction; Middle—abduction; Posterior—extension, horizontal abduction

(continued on following page)

Table 5-12 (continued from previous page)

Muscles	Origin	Insertion	Peripheral Nerve	Nerve Root	Motions
Supraspinatus	Supraspinatus fossa	Superior facet on greater tuberosity of humerus	Suprascapular	C 5 (6)	Abduction
Subscapularis	Subscapularis fossa	Lesser tuberosity of humerus	Upper and lower subscapular	C 5–C 8	Adduction, and internal rotation
Infraspinatus	Infraspinatus fossa	Middle facet on greater tuberosity of humerus	Suprascapular	C 5 (C 6)	Abduction, horizontal abduction, and external rotation
Serratus anterior	external surfaces of lateral parts of ribs one through eight	Anterior surface of the medial border of scapula	Long thoracic	C5–7	Protracts and rotates scapula and holds it against thoracic wall
Levator scapula	Posterior tubercles of transverse processes of C1-4	Superior part of medial border of scapula	Dorsal scapular	C 4–5	Elevates scapula and tilts glenoid cavity in inferiorly by rotating scapula
Rhomboids	Ligamentum nuchae and spinous processes of C7-T5	Medial border of scapula from level of spine to inferior angle	Dorsal scapular	C 4–5	Retracts scapula and rotates it to depress glenoid cavity
Coracobrachialis	Tip of coracoid process of scapula	Middle medial border of humerus	Musculocutaneous	C5–6	Horizontal flexion and adduction of humerus at shoulder
Biceps brachii	Tip of coracoid and supraglenoid tubercle of scapula	Radial tuberosity and lacertus fibrosis	musculocutaneous	C5–6	Flexes arm and supinates forearm
Trapezius	spinous processes of cervical and thoracic vertebrae	scapula and acromion	spinal accessory, branches of ansa cervicalis	CN XI	Elevates, retracts, and rotates scapula

The comprehensiveness of the strength testing and neurological examination of the shoulder complex is determined by the chief complaint and general status of the patient.

Clinical Pearl

Lesions such as brachial plexus or cervical root injuries may require extensive muscle, sensory and reflex testing.[3] Weakness on isometric testing needs to be analyzed for the type (increasing weakness with repeated contractions of the same resistance indicating a palsy versus consistent weakness with repeated contractions, which could suggest a deconditioned muscle or a significant muscle tear) and the pattern of weakness (spinal nerve root, nerve trunk, or peripheral nerve) (Table 5-12 and Table 5-13).

Localized, individual isometric muscle tests around the shoulder girdle can also give the clinician information about patterns of weakness other than from spinal nerve root or peripheral nerve palsies (eg, instabilities, postural dysfunction, capsular/non-capsular) and also help to isolate the pain generators.

Table 5-13 Peripheral Nerve Tests

Spinal accessory nerve	Inability to abduct the arm beyond 90 degrees
	Pain in shoulder with abduction
Musculocutaneous nerve	Weak elbow flexion with forearm supinated
Long thoracic nerve	Pain on flexing fully extended arm
	Inability to flex fully extended arm
	Winging of scapula at 90 degrees of forward flexion
Suprascapular nerve	Increased pain on forward shoulder flexion
	Pain increased with scapular abduction
	Pain increased with cervical rotation to opposite side
Axillary nerve	Inability to abduct arm with neutral rotation

Clinical Pearl

Increased activity of the upper trapezius muscle, or imbalances between the upper and lower trapezius muscles during shoulder elevation may have adverse effects on the kinematics of the scapula.[22-25]

The supraspinatus can be tested using the "empty can" test; having the patient abduct the shoulders to 90 degrees in forward flexion with the thumbs pointing downward (Figure 5-7). The patient then attempts to elevate the arms against examiner resistance. The function of the infraspinatus and teres minor muscles is tested with the patient's arms at the sides; the patient flexes both elbows to 90 degrees while the examiner provides resistance against external rotation (Figure 5-8).

Clinical Pearl

• The suprascapular nerve (C5–6) innervates the supraspinatus and infraspinatus.

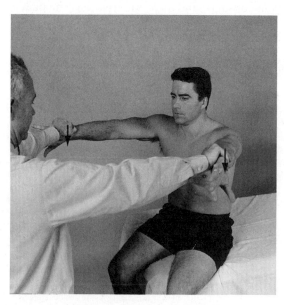

Figure 5-7 The supraspinatus can be tested using the "empty can" test.

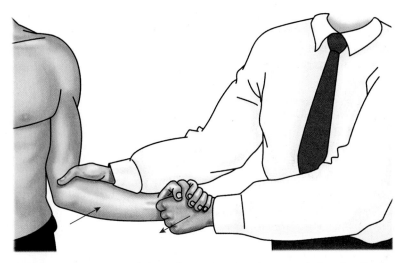

Figure 5-8 The function of the infraspinatus and teres minor muscles is tested with the patient's arms at the sides.

- The axillary nerve (C5–6) innervates the deltoid and teres minor.
- The nerve to the subscapularis (upper and lower) (C5–7) innervates the subscapularis.

The function of the subscapularis is assessed with the Gerber "lift-off test."[26,27] The patient rests the dorsum of the hand on the back in the lumbar area. Inability to move the hand off the back by further internal rotation of the arm suggests injury to the subscapularis muscle or a subscapular nerve injury.[28]

Clinical Pearl

Naredo et al[29] compared findings of the Gerber lift-off test with those of ultrasound and showed the test to have a sensitivity of 50%, specificity of 84.2%, positive predictive value of 66.6, and negative predictive value of 72.7 for detecting subscapularis lesions.

If the patient is unable to place the hand behind the back, a modified version of the lift-off test is used. In this version, the patient places the hand of the affected arm on the abdomen and resists the examiner's attempts to externally rotate the arm. During arm elevation, the greatest activation of the subscapularis occurs with the arm in the scapular plane at 90 degrees of elevation and neutral humeral rotation.[30]

 Clinical Pearl

Dynamic stability of the glenohumeral joint is provided by contraction of the rotator cuff and the long head of the biceps, which increases compression across the glenohumeral joint and dynamically maintains coaptation of the humeral head within the glenoid.[31]

 Clinical Pearl

The deltoid, innervated by the axillary nerve, is tested in forward flexion for the anterior third, straight abduction for the middle third, and in extension for the posterior third.

The serratus anterior, innervated by the long thoracic nerve, is evaluated by having the patient push off a wall while standing. Winging of the scapula during this maneuver is classic when paralysis of the long thoracic nerve is involved.[23,32]

 Clinical Pearl

The rhomboid major and rhomboid minor are innervated by the dorsal scapular nerve (C5).

Rhomboid function is tested by asking the patient to place both hands on the side of the iliac crest as the clinician pushes the patient's arm forward using one hand while palpating the vertebral border of the scapula with the other hand. The test is then repeated on the other side. An intact rhomboid maintains the scapula against the chest wall.

Clinical Pearl

The two components of the pectoralis major, the clavicular and sternocostal divisions, are innervated by the lateral and medial pectoral nerves (clavicular, C5–6 and sternocostal, C7–T1).

- The pectoralis minor is innervated by the lateral and medial pectoral nerves (C6–8).
- The latissimus dorsi is innervated by the thoracodorsal nerve (C6–8).
- The teres major is innervated by the lower subscapular nerve (C6–7).
- The three heads of the triceps are innervated by the radial nerve (C6–8).
- The two heads of the biceps are innervated by the musculocutaneous nerve (C5–6).

Clinical Pearl

A key finding, particularly with rotator cuff problems, is pain accompanied by weakness. True weakness should be distinguished from weakness that is due to pain. A patient with subacromial bursitis with a tear of the rotator cuff often has objective rotator cuff weakness caused by pain when the arm is positioned in the arc of impingement. Conversely, the patient will have normal strength if the arm is not tested in abduction.[33]

Functional Testing

The assessment of shoulder function is an integral part of the examination of the shoulder complex. The term *shoulder function* can include tests for biomechanical dysfunction and tests assessing the patient's ability to perform the basic functions of activities of daily living. In addition to the possibility of nerve pathology, the following pathologies are associated with specific movements:

- Impingement, bursitis, tendinopathy, or rotator cuff tear should be suspected in those patients with difficulty reaching overhead or combing their hair, or with difficulty reaching the arm out to the side.

- Tendinopathy, adhesive capsulitis, or rotator cuff tear should be suspected in those patients who have difficulty reaching backward or with reaching out to the side using external rotation/reaching behind the back using internal rotation.
- AC joint pathology, SC joint pathology, or clavicle fracture should be suspected in those patients who have difficulty reaching across the body using horizontal adduction.

Clinical Pearl

Clavicle fractures typically occur following a high-energy trauma to the shoulder in younger patients and a FOOSH injury in older patients. Common signs and symptoms include pain and obvious deformity at the region of the fracture. Clavicle fractures can be classified as follows:

Class A—middle third fracture.

Class B—lateral third fracture.

Class C—medial third fracture.

Examination of the Passive Restraint System and Neighboring Joints

If following the ROM and the strength and functional movement tests, the clinician is unable to determine a working hypothesis from which to treat the patient, further examination is required. This more detailed examination involves the assessment of the mobility and stability of the passive restraint systems of the shoulder girdle.

Passive Accessory Motion (PAM) Tests

The passive accessory motion tests are performed at the end of the patient's available range to determine whether the joint itself is responsible for the loss of motion. Knowledge of the physiological and accessory motions that accompany each motion is necessary (Table 5-14). For all of these tests, the patient is positioned in supine, with their head supported on a pillow, while the clinician is standing facing the patient.

Distraction/compression of the glenohumeral joint

The clinician palpates and stabilizes the shoulder girdle and the anterior thorax. With the other hand, the clinician gently grasps the proximal 1/3 of the humerus. The clinician distracts (Figure 5-9)/compresses the GH

Table 5-14 Glenohumeral Joint Motions and Their Appropriate Axis and Accessory Motions

Plane/Axis of Motion	Physiological Motion	Accessory Motion
Sagittal/medial–lateral	Flexion/extension	Humeral head moves superiorly, approximately 3 mm at the beginning of elevation and then spins in place with little excursion.
		1. Anterior translation of the humeral head beyond 55 degrees of elevation
		2. Posterior translation of the humeral head beyond 35 degrees of extension
Coronal/anterior–posterior	Abduction	Inferior glide
	Adduction	Superior glide
Transverse/longitudinal	Internal rotation	Posterior glide
	External rotation	Anterior glide

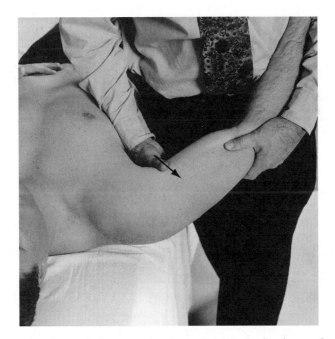

Figure 5-9 The clinician distracts the GH joint perpendicular to the plane of the glenoid fossa.

joint perpendicular to the plane of the glenoid fossa (30 degrees off the sagittal plane). The quantity of motion is noted and compared with the other side.

Inferior glide of the GH joint

The clinician palpates and stabilizes the coracoid process of the scapula and the lateral clavicle. With the other hand, the clinician gently grasps proximal to the patient's elbow. The humerus is glided inferiorly at the GH joint, parallel to the superior–inferior plane of the glenoid fossa (Figure 5-10). The quantity of motion is noted and compared with the other side.

Posterior glide of the GH joint

The clinician palpates and stabilizes the coracoid process and the lateral 1/3 of the clavicle. With the hypothenar eminence of the same hand, the clinician palpates the anterior aspect of the humeral head (Figure 5-11). With the other hand, the clinician gently grasps the distal end of the humerus (Figure 5-11). From this position, the clinician glides the humerus posteriorly at the GH joint, parallel to the anterior–posterior plane of the glenoid fossa. The quantity of motion is noted and compared with the other side.

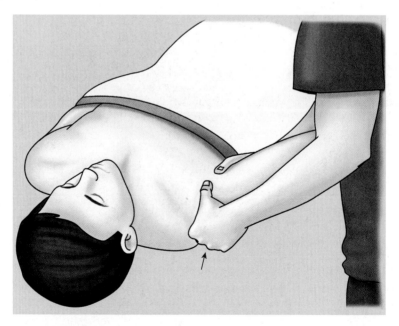

Figure 5-10 The humerus is glided inferiorly at the GH joint, parallel to the superior–inferior plane of the glenoid fossa.

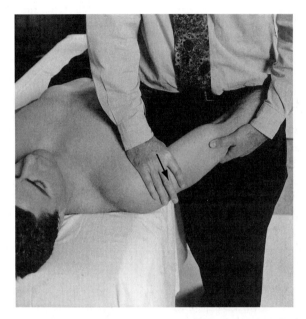

Figure 5-11 With the hypothenar eminence of the same hand, the clinician palpates the anterior aspect of the humeral head and glides the humerus posteriorly at the GH joint.

Passive Accessory Motion Testing of the Acromioclavicular Joint
Anterior and posterior rotations of the clavicle
Anterior and posterior rotations of the clavicle are shown in Figure 5-12.

Passive Accessory Motion Testing of the Sternoclavicular Joint
Anterior and inferior glide
Anterior and inferior glides are depicted in Figure 5-13.

Superior glide
Superior glide is shown in Figure 5-14.

Passive Accessory Motion Testing of the Scapulothoracic Joint
The patient is positioned in side lying. Their head is sufficiently supported to maintain the cervical spine in neutral. The clinician stands in front of the patient. Using one hand the clinician grasps the inferior and medial border of the uppermost scapula. The other hand grasps the anterior aspect of the shoulder. The clinician gently brings both hands together, lifting the scapula (Figure 5-15).[34-44] This position is held until the muscles are felt to relax. Once

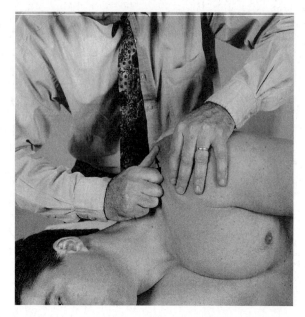

Figure 5-12 Anterior and posterior rotations of the clavicle.

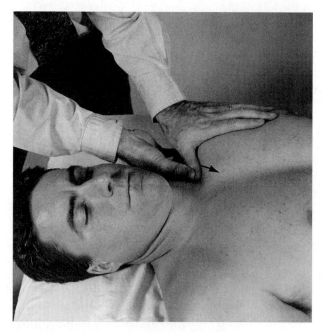

Figure 5-13 Anterior and inferior glides.

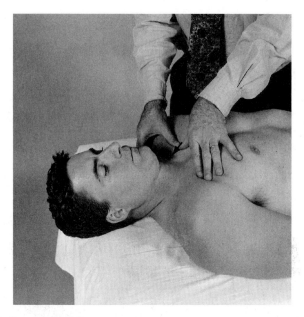

Figure 5-14 Superior glide.

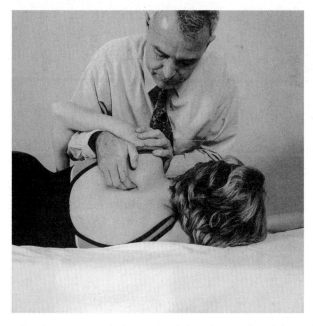

Figure 5-15 The clinician gently brings both hands together, lifting the scapula.

the muscle relaxation has occurred, the clinician moves the scapula into the patterns of restricted scapular motion.

Special Tests of the Shoulder Complex

The special tests for the shoulder are provocative maneuvers designed to assess various structures or confirm a diagnosis. The decision as to which test is used is based on the patient history and clinical findings. The more common special tests used and the significance of their positive findings are outlined in Table 5-15.

Neurological Examination

If the scanning examination is not performed, a thorough sensory examination of all upper extremity dermatomes should be performed, and the deep-tendon reflexes of all extremities should be assessed in those situations where the patient is complaining of neck and or arm pain, and/or when the clinician has been unable to reproduce the symptoms with the shoulder examination.[5]

 Clinical Pearl

Most of the shoulder girdle is supplied by the fifth and sixth cervical roots through the upper trunk of the brachial plexus.

A small number of patients, particularly athletes, have an entirely normal physical examination, but continue to complain of pain. In such cases, the clinician should look for training errors in the athlete's program or a chronic overuse injury. Alternatively, pain may be a normal adaptation to increasing loads placed on the shoulder as it accommodates new demands. It should be stressed that repeated physical examinations over time, particularly with highly competitive athletes, are needed to evaluate changing pain patterns, which may highlight the real diagnostic culprit.

Vascular Examination

A thorough vascular examination is important in patients complaining of vague aching, heaviness, or fatigue radiating down the arm.[3] The vascular status of the upper extremity can be assessed by palpation of the distal

Table 5-15 Special Tests Used and the Estimated Significance of Their Positive Findings

Test	Maneuver	Sensitivity	Specificity	Diagnosis Suggested by Positive Result
Cervical Spine				
Spurling test	Spine extended with head rotated to affected shoulder while axially loaded	Poor	Excellent	Cervical nerve root disorder
Shoulder Complex				
Apley scratch test	Patient reaches behind the back in internal rotation to touch the inferior aspect of the opposite scapula, and behind the neck in abduction and external rotation to touch the superior aspect of the opposite scapula	There are no studies in the literature that discuss the sensitivity, specificity, positive predictive value, or negative predictive value of this maneuver		Loss of ROM within shoulder girdle complex
Scapula				
Lateral slide test	The first position of the test is with the arm relaxed at the side. The second is with the hands on the hips with the fingers anterior and the thumb posterior with about 10 degrees of shoulder extension. The third position is with the palms at or below 90 degrees of arm elevation with maximal internal rotation at the glenohumeral joint.	With 1.5 cm difference as positive:[34] In first position: Sensitivity: 28% Specificity: 53% In second position: Sensitivity: 50% Specificity: 58% In third position: Sensitivity: 34% Specificity: 52%		Weakness of dynamic scapulothoracic stabilizers

(continued on following page)

Table 5-15 *(continued from previous page)*

Test	Maneuver	Sensitivity	Specificity	Diagnosis Suggested by Positive Result
Isometric pinch test	The seated patient is asked to fully retract the shoulders and to hold the position for 20 seconds. Scapular muscle weakness can be noted as a burning pain in less than 15 seconds.	There are no studies in the literature that discuss the sensitivity, specificity, positive predictive value, or negative predictive value of this maneuver		Weakness of scapular muscle strength
Scapular assistance test	The clinician manually stabilizes the upper medial border of the scapula and rotates the inferomedial border as the arm is abducted or adducted. The test is positive when the manual assistance gives relief of symptoms of impingement, clicking, or rotator cuff weakness	There are no studies in the literature that discuss the sensitivity, specificity, positive predictive value, or negative predictive value of this maneuver		Weakness of the lower trapezius
Rotator Cuff				
Empty can[29]	Patient stands with arms elevated to shoulder level in scapula plane, thumbs pointing down. Patient is asked to resist downward force applied by clinician	Good	Fair	Supraspinatus tear
Full can	Patient stands with arms elevated to shoulder level in scapula plane, thumbs pointing up. Patient is asked to resist downward force applied by clinician	Very good	Average	Rotator cuff tear or impingement syndrome

Test	Description	Reliability/Validity	Conditions Assessed
Neer (impingement) sign	Passive flexion of patient's arm to position of full flexion while stabilizing/depressing scapula with other hand	For detecting subacromial impingement:[35] Sensitivity: 88.7% Specificity: 30.5% For assessing subacromial bursitis:[36] Sensitivity: 75% Specificity: 47.5% For detecting rotator cuff pathology:[36] Sensitivity: 83.3% Specificity: 50.8%	Subacromial impingement Subacromial bursitis Rotator cuff pathology
Hornblower signs	Clinician places the seated patient's arm in 90 degrees of scaption (position of isolation for infraspinatus–teres minor) and asks the patient to externally rotate against resistance	Excellent	Excellent	Teres minor injury
Hawkins impingement sign/reinforcement[36]	Passive forward flexion of the shoulder to 90 degrees, support of the patients arm, followed by passive elbow flexion and then internal rotation of the humerus	Excellent	Average	Supraspinatus tendon impingement Rotator cuff tear Subacromial bursitis
Yocum[29]	The patient is asked to place a hand on his or her other shoulder and to raise the elbow without elevating the shoulder. The test is positive when it elicits the pain usually experienced by the patient	For detecting impingement in combination with Hawkins and Neer test: Sensitivity: 65% Specificity: 72.7%	Subacromial impingement

(continued on following page)

Table 5-15 *(continued from previous page)*

Test	Maneuver	Sensitivity	Specificity	Diagnosis Suggested by Positive Result
Drop-arm[37]	Passive abduction of the shoulder to maximum degree possible. Patient then asked to lower arm back to the side. Positive finding when patient unable to control the descent of the arm (usually at around 90–100 degrees)	Poor	Excellent	Large rotator cuff tear, particularly of the supraspinatus Axillary nerve palsy
Acromioclavicular Joint				
Cross-over/cross body	The clinician flexes shoulder to 90 degrees and adducts it towards midline	Good	Good	Acromioclavicular joint arthritis
O'Brien active-compression	Active forward flexion of the shoulder to 90 degrees with the elbow extended. The arm is then brought an additional 15 degrees toward the midline and then maximally internally rotated so that the thumb is pointing down. The patient is then asked to resist a downward force applied by the clinician while noting the presence and location of pain. The patient then externally rotates the shoulder so that the palm is up and the procedure is repeated. Positive finding indicated if patient experiences pain only during the thumbs-down portion of the test	For detecting acromioclavicular joint pathology:[38] Sensitivity: 100% Specificity: 96.6% For detecting both acromioclavicular joint pathology and labral tears:[38] Sensitivity: 100% Specificity: 95.2%		Acromioclavicular joint injury Glenoid labrum tear

Shoulder Stability

Apprehension sign	Shoulder positioned in 90 degrees abduction, and elbow in 90 degrees flexion. Patient's shoulder is progressively externally rotated. Positive if patient reports pain or apprehension	For diagnosing labral pathology:[39] Sensitivity: 69% Specificity: 50% for predicting the labral test in combination with the relocation, load and shift, inferior sulcus sign and crank tests:[40] Sensitivity: 90% Specificity: 85%	Anterior glenohumeral instability. A report of pain without apprehension is less specific Glenoid labral pathology
Fowler sign (relocation)[41]	Shoulder positioned in 90 degrees abduction, and elbow in 90 degrees flexion at the point where the patient feels pain or apprehension. A posterior force is applied to humeral head. Positive if patient reports of pain or apprehension diminish with applied force	Average	Average	Anterior glenohumeral instability
Sulcus sign	Axial load (traction) is applied to the shoulder through the patient's elbow using one hand while palpating the humeral head with the other hand	In predicting labral tears in combination with the relocation, load and shift, apprehension and crank tests: Sensitivity: 90% Specificity: 85%	Inferior glenohumeral instability/laxity if there is widening of the sulcus between the humerus and acromion Glenoid labrum tear

(continued on following page)

Table 5-15 *(continued from previous page)*

Test	Maneuver	Sensitivity	Specificity	Diagnosis Suggested by Positive Result
Jerk test for posterior instability[39]	The patient's arm is passively placed in 90 degrees of flexion and maximum internal rotation with the elbow flexed to 90 degrees. The clinician then adducts the arm across the body in the horizontal plane while pushing the humerus in a posterior direction. Positive if maneuver causes a dislocation, the humeral head can be felt to clunk back into the joint as the arm is then abducted	Poor (19%)	Excellent (95%)	Posterior glenohumeral instability—labral injury
Glenoid Labrum				
Active compression (O'Brien)[38]	Standing patient is asked to flex arm to 90 degrees with elbow in full extension. Patient adducts arm 10 degree and internally rotates humerus. Clinician applies downward force to arm as patient resists. Patient then fully supinates arm and repeats procedure	Excellent (100%)	Excellent (98.5%)	Glenoid labrum tear
Crank[42]	Patient is supine while clinician elevates humerus 160 degress in scapular plane. Axial load is applied to humerus while shoulder is internally and externally rotated	Excellent (91%)	Excellent (93%)	Glenoid labrum tear
Biceps load test	Shoulder positioned in 90 degrees abduction, and elbow in 90 degrees flexion at the point where the patient feels pain or apprehension.	For detecting a SLAP lesion:[43] Sensitivity: 90.9%		Glenoid labral pathology

Test	Procedure	Reliability / Statistics	Indication
	The patient is then asked to flex the elbow while the clinician resists the flexion with one hand and asks how the apprehension has changed, if at all. The test is positive if the shoulder becomes more painful	Specificity: 96.9%	Biceps tendon instability or tendonitis
Biceps Tendon			
Yergason[35]	Elbow flexed to 90 degrees with forearm pronated. Patient is then instructed to actively supinated forearm against resistance. Positive if pain is produced in area of bicipital groove	Very good (86.1%) Poor (37%)	
Ludington	The patient is asked to rest his folded hands, palms down on the top of his/her head and allow the interlocked fingers to support the weight of the arms. The examiner then places to fingers on the tendon of the long head of the biceps in each arm, and asks the patient to simultaneously contract and relax his/her biceps muscles. The contraction of the long head tendon on the sound side is plainly felt while it is absent on the affected side if the tendon is ruptured	There are no studies in the literature that discuss the sensitivity, specificity, positive predictive value, or negative predictive value of this maneuver.	
Speed test	Patient elevates humerus to 60 degrees with elbow flexion and forearm supination. Patient holds this position while clinician applies resistance against elevation	For biceps tendon pathology:[44] Sensitivity: 90% Specificity: 13.8% For subacromial impingement:[35] Sensitivity: 68.5% Specificity: 55.5%	Biceps tendon instability or tendonitis

Data from references. [29, 34-44]

arteries with the arm in various positions.[5] Other tests can include those for thoracic outlet syndrome. In addition, an inspection of the skin color, temperature, hair growth, and alteration in sensation should routinely be assessed.[3]

Diagnostic/Imaging Studies

An A–P view (anterior–posterior view with the humerus in internal rotation and a second A–P view with the humerus in external rotation) of the glenohumeral joint may show calcific tendonitis of the cuff and superior migration of the humeral head, which should prompt requests for further imaging studies if the clinician suspects a rotator cuff tear. However, the conclusions on the radiology reports concerning single plane views should be treated with caution as they have been well documented to result in misdiagnosis.[45]

The "scapular-Y" view, obtained by tilting the x-ray beam approximately 60 degrees relative to the A–P view, provides good visualization of the glenohumeral alignment.[46] A transthoracic lateral is often added.

Arthrography aids in the diagnosis of full-thickness rotator cuff tears (Table 5-16).[47] Bone scans are rarely used in the diagnosis of shoulder pain, but a computed tomography (CT) scan report can be useful in confirming the clinical findings in some cases (Table 5-16).[2] The magnetic resonance imaging is very reliable in detecting lesions of the capsule, and labrum, as well as associated rotator cuff tears (Table 5-16). It can generally indicate the approximate size of a rotator cuff tear, and may also indicate whether the critically important subscapularis tendon is torn.[2,48,49]

Examination Conclusions: Evaluation

Following the examination, and once the clinical findings have been recorded, the clinician must determine a specific diagnosis or a working hypothesis, based on a summary of all of the findings. This diagnosis can be structure-related (medical diagnosis) (Tables 5-17 and 5-18), or a diagnosis based on the preferred practice patterns as described in the *Guide to Physical Therapist Practice*.[50]

INTERVENTION

The rehabilitation procedures chosen to progress the patient will depend on the type of tissue involved, the extent of the damage, and the stage of healing

Table 5-16 Imaging Studies of the Shoulder

Imaging Modality	Advantages	Disadvantages
MRI	Very good at detecting complete rotator cuff tears, cuff degeneration, chronic tendonitis and partial cuff tears No ionizing radiation	Often identifies false positives
Arthrography	Good at identifying complete rotator cuff tear or adhesive capsulitis (frozen shoulder)	Invasive Relatively poor at diagnosing a partial rotator cuff tear
Ultrasonography	Accurately diagnoses complete rotator cuff tears	Less useful in identifying partial cuff tears Operator-dependent interpretation
MRI arthrography	Reliably identifies full-thickness rotator cuff tears and labral tears	Invasive
CT scanning	May be useful in diagnosis of subtle glenohumeral dislocation	Exposes patient to ionizing radiation

MRI = magnetic resonance imaging; CT = computed tomography

Table 5-17 Common Lesions of the Shoulder

Name	Description
Bankart	A lesion of the glenoid labrum involving the detachment of the anchoring point of the anterior band of the inferior glenohumeral ligament and middle glenohumeral ligament from the glenoid rim
Hill-Sachs	Compression fracture of the posterolateral margin of the humeral head caused by impaction on the rim of the glenoid during an anterior shoulder dislocation
HAGL	Avulsion of the humeral attachment of the glenohumeral ligament

HAGL = humeral avulsion of the glenohumeral ligaments.

(see Chapter 3). The intervention must be related to the signs and symptoms present rather than the actual diagnosis.

Table 5-18 Differential Diagnosis for Common Causes of Shoulder Pain

Condition	Approximate Patient Age (y)	Mechanism of Injury	Area of Symptoms	Symptoms Aggravated by	Observation	AROM	PROM	End feel	Pain with Resisted	Tenderness with Palpation
Rotator cuff tendonitis	20–40	Microtrauma/macrotrauma	Anterior and lateral shoulder	Overhead motions	Swelling – anterior shoulder	Limited abduction	Limited abduction		Abduction	Pain below anterior acromial rim
Acute Chronic	30–70	Microtrauma/macrotrauma	Anterior and lateral shoulder	Overhead motions	Atrophy of scapular area Atrophy of shoulder area	Limited abduction and flexion	Pain on IR and ER at 90 degrees abduction		ER Abduction ER IR	Anterior shoulder Pain below anterior acromial rim
Bicipital tendonitis	20–45	Microtrauma	Anterior shoulder	Overhead motions	Possible swelling – anterior shoulder May see signs of concomitant rotator cuff pathology	Limited ER when arm in 90 degrees abduction Pain on full flexion from full extension	Pain on combined extension of shoulder and elbow Biceps stability test may be abnormal (if tendon unstable)		Elbow flexion Speed test painful, Yergason test occasionally painful	Of biceps tendon over bicipital groove

Rotator cuff rupture	40+	Macrotrauma	Posterior/superior shoulder	Arm elevation	Atrophy of scapular area	Limited abduction	Full and pain free	Pain with or without restriction	Abduction ER	Pain below anterolateral acromial rim
Adhesive capsulitis	35–70	Microtrauma/macrotrauma	Shoulder and upper arm – poorly localized	All motions	Atrophy of shoulder area	All motions limited especially ER and abduction	All motions limited especially ER and abd	Capsular	Most/all	Varies
AC joint sprain	Varies	Macrotrauma	Point of shoulder	Horizontal adduction	Step/bump at point of shoulder	Limited abduction; Limited horizontal adduction	Limited abduction; Pain with horizontal adduction		ER; Flexion	Point of shoulder; Soft tissue thickening at point of shoulder
Subacromial bursitis	Varies	Microtrauma	Anterior and lateral shoulder	Overhead motions	Often unremarkable	Limited abduction and IR; May have full range but pain in mid-range of flexion/abd	Pain on IR at 90 degrees abduction; Pain only in mid-range abduction and flexion		Most/all	Pain below anterolateral acromial rim
Glenohumeral arthritis	50+	Gradual onset, but can be traumatic	Poorly localized	Arm activity	Possible posterior positioning of humeral head	Capsular pattern (ER>abduction>IR)	Pain	Capsular	Weakness of rotator cuff, rather than pain	Poorly localized

(continued on following page)

Table 5-18 *(continued from previous page)*

Condition	Approximate Patient Age (y)	Mechanism of Injury	Area of Symptoms	Symptoms Aggravated by	Observation	AROM	PROM	End feel	Pain with Resisted	Tenderness with Palpation
SICK scapula	20-40	Microtrauma	Anterior/superior shoulder Posterosuperior scapular Arm, forearm, hand	Overhead activities	Scapular malposition Inferior medial border prominence Dyskinesia of scapular movement	Decreased forward flexion which diminishes when clinician manually repositions the scapula into retraction and posterior tilt	Normal		Weakness rather than pain	Medial coracoid Superomedial angle of scapula
Cervical radiculopathy	Varies	Typically none but can be traumatic	Upper back, below shoulder	Cervical extension, cervical sidebending, and rotation to ipsilateral side, full arm elevation	May have lateral deviation of head away from painful side	Decreased cervical flexion, cervical sidebending androtation to ipsilateral side. Decreased arm elevation on involved side	Painful into restricted active range of motions Positive Spurling's test	Empty	Weakness rather than pain Other neurological changes	Varies. May have numbness over dermatomal area

COMMON ORTHOPEDIC CONDITIONS

ACROMIOCLAVICULAR JOINT SEPARATION

Diagnosis

Acromioclavicular (AC) joint separation—ICD-9: 831.04 (closed dislocation of AC joint), 831.14 (open dislocation of AC joint), and 840.0 (AC sprain). Also known as shoulder separation, separated shoulder, or closed dislocation of the AC joint.

 Clinical Pearl

AC joint injury commonly occurs in men rather than women and in relatively young, as opposed to older people.

Description

An AC joint separation is typically the result of a traumatic event such as a fall on a outstretched hand (FOOSH), a direct blow to the anterior shoulder, or a fall landing directly on the anterior portion of the shoulder. The trauma can cause the ligaments of the AC joint to be sprained, partially torn, or completely disrupted (first-degree, second-degree, and third-degree AC separations or sprains).

 Clinical Pearl

AC joint injuries are approximately four or five times more prevalent than sternoclavicular injuries.

 Clinical Pearl

AC joint injuries can be classified as one of the six types based on the severity of the injury and the degree of clavicular separation:

• Type I: the AC joint ligaments are partially or completely disrupted but the coracoclavicular ligaments are intact.

- Type II: the AC joint ligaments are torn and in addition the coraco-clavicular ligaments are partially disrupted.
- Type III: the coracoclavicular ligaments are completely disrupted, and there is complete separation of the clavicle from the acromion.
- Type IV-VI: these types are uncommon. In these injuries, the periosteum of the clavicle and/or the deltoid and trapezius muscle are also torn, causing wide displacement.

Subjective Findings

An accurate history includes the description of the onset of symptoms, duration and progression of pain, history of a traumatic event, activities that worsen the pain, and previous treatments and outcomes. Typical findings for this condition include the following:

- Relief is reported with cradling of the involved arm —this position reduces the gravitational pull of the weight of the arm inferiorly.
- Very localized pain over the AC joint and pain on lifting the arm.

Objective Findings

The patient is examined for joint inflammation, arthritic change, and disruption of the ligaments that support joint.

- With type III injuries, there is an obvious deformity.
- Patients supports the arm in an adducted position.
- Swelling at the AC joint.
- Pain is consistently aggravated by passively adducting the arm across the chest.

 Clinical Pearl

Severe osteophytic enlargement of the AC joint can contribute to subacromial impingement.

Confirmatory/Special Tests

- Cross-over test (Table 5-14).
- O'Brien test (Table 5-14).

Medical Studies

X-rays of the shoulder (including posteroanterior, external rotation, Y-outlet, and weighted views of the AC joint) are recommended. Special radiographic angles may be ordered (a 10 degrees to 15 degrees superior angulation view, a supine notch view, or a scapulolateral view). Plain films of the shoulder may show degenerative change, such as narrowing, sclerosis, or osteophytic spurring.

Differential Diagnosis

- Fracture of the acromion (positive radiograph).
- Fracture of the end of the clavicle (positive radiograph).
- Rotator cuff tear (most tenderness over the subacromial space, not the AC joint; no visible deformity or radiographic findings).

Intervention

The ultimate treatment decision is based on a variety of factors, including the patient's overall medical condition, severity, and duration of symptoms, expectations, associated shoulder pathology, and surgeon preference. The treatment goal for this condition is to reduce direct pressure and traction at the AC joint to allow the ligaments to reattach to their respective bony insertions.

- Type I and II: protection and rest—wearing a sling for a few days until the pain subsides (type II), ice, and analgesics. Gentle range of motion can be initiated as tolerated within pain-free limits. Progress to nonpainful strengthening exercises, especially to deltoid and trapezius muscles. Unrestricted activity is usually achieved 2 to 4 weeks after the injury.
- Type III: treatment is controversial—can be treated nonsurgically; surgical repair may be considered in a young manual laborer.
- Types IV-VI: require evaluation for surgical repair.

 Clinical Pearl

Immobilization using an immobilizer that holds the humerus superiorly and the clavicle inferiorly so as to approximate the torn ends, thereby approximating the soft tissue so as to provide maximum stability.

Prognosis

Second-degree and third-degree separations are most likely to remain symptomatic. A variety of surgical stabilization procedures are available to eliminate the movement of the clavicle against the acromion.

Clinical Pearl

If left untreated, an AC joint injury may result in permanent residual deformity, weakened shoulder abduction, and eventual traumatic arthritis.

ADHESIVE CAPSULITIS: FROZEN SHOULDER

Diagnosis

Adhesive capsulitis of the shoulder—ICD-9: 726.0. Also known as frozen shoulder, frozen shoulder syndrome, and Duplay disease.

Description

Adhesive capsulitis or frozen shoulder is a distinct clinical syndrome that can be described as primary or secondary:

- Primary. Characterized by an idiopathic, progressive, and painful loss of active and passive shoulder motion, particularly external rotation, which causes the individual to gradually limit the use of the arm.
- Secondary. Either traumatic in origin or related to a disease process, neurological, or cardiac condition.

Subjective Findings

The subjective findings vary according to the stage of the condition, but typically include the following:

- Diffuse aching at the shoulder.
- Difficulty sleeping on the involved shoulder.
- Difficulty with dressing and grooming.

 Clinical Pearl

Adhesive capsulitis classically presents as a cycle of three distinct stages:

- Freezing: characterized by acute constant shoulder pain and muscle spasm that restricts movement in all directions, particularly in a capsular pattern. Pain is usually worse at night and is exacerbated when the patient lies on the involved side.

- Frozen: characterized by subsiding pain and progressive loss of shoulder movement in a capsular pattern.
- Thawing: characterized by gradual regaining of shoulder movement and shoulder function.

Objective Findings

Findings vary according to the stage of the condition.

- Inability to elevate the involve shoulder correctly.
- Point tenderness may be present over the bicipital groove (the glenohumeral joint capsule bridges the gap between the lesser and greater tuberosities).
- External rotation is more limited than abduction which, in turn, is more limited than internal rotation.
- Restriction of anterior and inferior glide of the glenohumeral joint.
- Neurologic tests are negative.
- Pain at the end range of shoulder motions with resisted testing, but no pain at midrange.

Confirmatory/Special Tests

No specific confirmatory/special tests —diagnosis based on findings from history and physical examination.

Imaging Studies

- Radiographs usually are negative in patients with frozen shoulder, although there may be evidence of disuse osteopenia.
- Magnetic resonance imaging (MRI) has been used for investigation purposes in patients with adhesive capsulitis.
- Arthrography is the standard diagnostic test—an arthrogram reveals at least a 50% reduced volume of the involved glenohumeral joint capsule.

Differential Diagnosis

- Glenohumeral arthritis.
- Acute bursitis.
- Calcific tendonitis.
- Long-standing rotator cuff disease.

- Painful acromioclavicular joint.
- Primary or secondary malignancy.

Intervention

Conventional management for adhesive capsulitis, which is based on the degree of inflammation and irritability, includes patient education, analgesics, nonsteroidal anti-inflammatory drugs (NSAIDs), steroid injection, and a wide variety of physical therapy methods. The primary goal of conservative intervention is the restoration of the range of motion and focuses on the application of controlled tensile stresses to produce elongation of the restricting tissues.

 Clinical Pearl

As a general guideline, the patient with capsular restriction and low irritability may require aggressive soft tissue and joint mobilization, whereas patients with high irritability may require pain-easing manual therapy techniques. In contrast, the emphasis on intervention of limited ROM due to nonstructural changes is aimed at addressing the cause of the pain.

Prognosis

The outcome of the patient depends on their level of compliance to the recommended intervention plan, as well as other recommended lifestyle changes. Studies have indicated that a gradual return of full mobility occurs within 18 months to 3 years in most patients, even without specific intervention.

 Clinical Pearl

Manipulation under anesthesia is a source of much controversy because of complications, such as fracture, dislocation, brachial plexus injury, and gross tearing of soft tissue causing severe scarring.

BICEPS TENDONITIS

Diagnosis

Biceps (long head) tendonitis—ICD-9: 726.12. Also referred to as bicipital tendonitis, bicipital tendinosis, bicipital tenosynovitis, biceps tear, and biceps tendon rupture. Tendonitis is a misnomer because histological inflammatory changes in the tendon are rarely seen—tenosynovitis would be more accurate.

> ### 🔘 Clinical Pearl
>
> The function of the long head of the biceps tendon (LHBT) at the shoulder is controversial and incompletely understood. The biceps musculotendinous junction is particularly susceptible to overuse injuries, especially in individuals performing lifting activities. LHBT pathology can be a significant cause of anterior shoulder pain, but is rarely seen in isolation—it is typically found with rotator cuff pathology, subdeltoid bursitis, or glenohumeral instability.

Description

Pathological disorders of the LHBT can be divided into three categories:

1. Inflammatory/degenerative conditions. Associated with subacromial impingement, and repetitive motion in overhead athletes.
2. Instability of the biceps tendon. Can vary from subluxation to dislocation, and from intermittent to fixed. Rarely occurs in isolation—usually associated with injury to the rotator cuff.
3. SLAP (superior labrum anterior posterior) lesions/bicep tendon anchor abnormalities. These have several proposed causes:
   a. FOOSH (fall on an outstretched hand) with the outstretched arm abducted and flexed and slightly forward.
   b. Traction mechanism where the eccentric firing of the long head of the biceps muscle causes injury to the superior labrum complex and its attachment during the deceleration phase of overhead throwing.
   c. Peel-back: the arm is abducted and maximally externally rotated, and the twisting of the biceps tendon may result in the peel-back of the anchor and its subsequent gradual or acute detachment from the superior glenoid.

Subjective Findings

An accurate history includes the description of the onset of symptoms, duration and progression of pain, history of a traumatic event, activities that worsen the pain, and previous treatments and outcomes.

- Pain, which is diffuse and vague, localized to the anterior shoulder over the bicipital groove. Pain is aggravated with:
  - Resisted elbow flexion.
  - Passive shoulder abduction (painful arc).
- Similar mechanism of injury that would cause rotator cuff impingement syndrome.

Objective Findings

- Point tenderness over the bicipital groove.
- Possible loss of shoulder ROM, similar to what is seen with rotator cuff tendinopathy.

 Clinical Pearl

> Pinpoint tenderness in the biceps groove is best localized with the humerus in about a 10 degrees of internal rotation, which places the long tendon directly anteriorly and located 6 cm below the acromion.

Confirmatory/Special tests

- Speed test: resisted elevation of the supinated arm with the elbow extended. Positive for pain localized to the proximal biceps area.
- Yergason test: resisted supination with elbow flexed is positive for pain at the bicipital groove. May be specific but lacks sensitivity.
- O'Brien active-compression test: the patient elevates the arm to 90 degrees and adducts the arm 10 to 15 degrees, with the elbow in full extension and the arm internally rotated so that the thumb is pointing to the floor. The patient then resists downward pressure applied by the clinician. The palm is then fully supinated and the patient resists downward pressure again. A positive test for labral pathology is *deep* shoulder pain in the thumb down position, relieved in the supinated position.
- Crank test. The patient's arm is elevated to 160 degrees in the scapular plane of the body and is in maximal internal or external rotation. The clinician then applies an axial load along the humerus. A positive test is indicated by the re-

production of a painful click in the shoulder during the maneuver. This test has been found to have a high sensitivity and specificity in detecting labral tears.

- Load and shift test. The clinician's index finger is placed across the anterior glenohumeral joint (GH) joint line and humeral head, and the long finger over the coracoid process. The clinician then applies a "load and shift" of the humeral head across the stabilized scapula in an anteromedial direction to assess anterior stability, and in a posterolateral direction to assess posterior instability. The normal motion anteriorly is half of the distance of the humeral head. Although attempts have been made to grade or quantify the degree of instability more specifically, the literature supports no consistency in the grading to date. This test has been reported to be 100% sensitive for the detection of instability in patients with recurrent dislocation, but not in cases of recurrent subluxation.

Based on the fact that no one test offers acceptable sensitivity and specificity, the clinician must utilize multiple examination findings in combination with the patient history, differential injections, and imaging to determine the appropriate treatment course.

Medical Studies

Imaging begins with standard plain radiographs consisting of a true anterior posterior, axillary, and outlet view. The bicipital groove view determines medial wall angle; the width of the groove, coexisting degenerative changes in the greater or lesser tuberosity; presence, or absence of bicipital groove spurs; and the presence or absence of a supratubercular ridge. A caudal tilt view may reveal the degree of anterior acromial prominence or spurring. Ultrasound imaging has the advantage of being inexpensive and noninvasive.

 Clinical Pearl

The radiological study of choice for biceps tendon pathology is MRI due to its high sensitivity and specificity.

Differential Diagnosis

- Rotator cuff tendonitis. Pain is often diffuse, located more proximally, and is accompanied by tenderness in the arm, anterior acromion, coracoacromial ligament, coracoid process, and supraspinatus insertion.
- Anterior shoulder instability. In addition to there often being an obvious swelling within the patient's armpit, the maximum point of apprehension

and clicking should be at 90-degree abduction and maximum external rotation (positive apprehension sign).

- Rotator cuff tear.
- Biceps tendon rupture. History of an audible pop in the shoulder, change of contour of the biceps muscle, weakness of the forearm supinators and elbow flexors.
- Biceps tendon subluxation.
- Brachial neuritis. Extremely painful condition that frequently presents as anterior shoulder pain.
- Thoracic outlet syndrome. Positive thoracic outlet syndrome tests.
- Coracoid impingement syndrome. Symptoms, which are consistently provoked by forward flexion and internal rotation or abduction and internal rotation, include dull pain in the front of the shoulder with referral to the front of the arm and occasionally extending into the forearm.
- Glenoid labrum tears without instability. Should demonstrate an audible or palpable clunk occurring as the tear flips in and out of the joint, impinging on normal humeral head excursion during rotation above the horizontal plane.
- Cervical radiculopathy. Can be ruled out by careful neurological examination.

Intervention

The ultimate treatment decision is based upon a variety of factors, including the patient's overall medical condition, severity and duration of symptoms, expectations, associated shoulder pathology, and surgeon preference. Treatment is initiated with a period of rest, withdrawal from aggravating activities, ice, and a course of anti-inflammatory medication.

- Phase 1: pain and inflammation management, restoration of full passive ROM, and restoration of normal accessory joint motion.
- Phase 2: consists of active ROM exercises and early strengthening. The early exercises focus on stabilizing the GH joints and preventing anterior translation of the humeral head.
- Phase 3: specific strengthening with a strong emphasis on enhancing dynamic stability. Close-kinetic chain exercises are generally started first, with open-kinetic chain exercises initiated later.
- Phase 4: return to sport or high workloads, focusing on power higher-speed exercises similar to specific demands.

Prognosis

This condition usually responds well to conservative measures. Surgical release with or without tenodesis may be beneficial in refractory cases.

GLENOHUMERAL JOINT INSTABILITY

Diagnosis

Glenohumeral joint instability—ICD-9: 755.59.

 Clinical Pearl

The majority of glenohumeral dislocations and subluxations are in the anteroinferior direction.

Description

Chronic unidirectional or multidirectional instability of the glenohumeral joint is more common in young women with poor muscular support of the shoulder, in patients with large rotator cuff tendon tears, and in athletic patients younger than age 40.

 Clinical Pearl

TUBS: instability caused by a Traumatic event, is Unidirectional, associated with a Bankart lesion, and often requires Surgery.

AMBRI: Atraumatic, Multidirectional, may be Bilateral, best treated by Rehabilitation, Inferior capsular shift is the surgery performed if rehabilitation fails.

ALPSA: Anterior Labroligamentous Periosteal Sleeve Avulsion.

Subjective Findings

An accurate history includes the description of the onset of symptoms, duration and progression of pain, history of a traumatic event, activities that worsen the pain, and previous treatments and outcomes. The typical findings for this condition include:

- Complaints of looseness of the shoulder, a "noisy" shoulder.
- May or may not have history of trauma.

- Patients with anterior instability typically describe the sensation of the shoulder slipping out of joint when the arm is abducted and externally rotated. They also tend to support the arm in a neutral position.
- Patients with multidirectional instability may have vague symptoms but these symptoms tend to be activity related.

Objective Findings

- Sulcus sign (appears when downward traction is applied to the upper arm) is suggestive for multidirectional instability (also inferior laxity).
- Variable degrees of crepitation or popping.
- Apprehension when performing the extremes of ROM, especially internal or external rotation.
- May have evidence of generalized ligamentous laxity.

Confirmatory/Special Tests

- Anterior instability: apprehension test is positive when arm is externally rotated. Other tests include crank, sulcus, and fulcrum.
- Posterior instability: apprehension test is positive when arm is internally rotated. The jerk test may also be used.

Clinical Pearl

In a **provocation test**, the humeral head is placed in a position of imminent subluxation or dislocation, which makes the patient recognize the pain-provoking movement and react with anticipated fear and/or pain.

In a **relief test**, the humeral head is placed in such a position that the pain of subluxation or dislocation is relieved.

Medical Studies

Plain radiographs of the shoulder (including posteroanterior, external rotation, Y-outlet, and axillary views) are highly recommended for patients with persistent pain, loss of ROM, or persistent signs of rotator cuff tendonitis.

CT arthrography is the test of choice to assess the integrity of the glenoid labral cartilage and to determine the degree of early osteoarthritis of the glenohumeral joint.

Differential Diagnosis

- SLAP lesion.
- Glenohumeral arthritis (confirmed with radiographs).
- Impingement syndrome (pain with negative apprehension tests).
- Rotator cuff tear (pain and weakness with negative apprehension tests).

Intervention

The ultimate treatment decision is based upon a variety of factors, including the patient's overall medical condition, severity and duration of symptoms, expectations, associated shoulder pathology, and surgeon preference. The mainstay of the physical therapy program emphasizes strengthening of the rotator cuff muscles, especially the subscapularis muscle, and a shoulder stabilization exercise progression.

Prognosis

The risk of recurrent instability is greater in younger patients and in those with multiple episodes.

GLENOHUMERAL JOINT OSTEOARTHRITIS

Diagnosis

Glenohumeral osteoarthritis —ICD-9: 715.11 (primary osteoarthrosis, shoulder), 715.21 (osteoarthrosis localized secondary involving shoulder region). Also known as shoulder degenerative joint disease.

Description

Glenohumeral osteoarthritis, characterized by destruction of joint cartilage with loss of joint space, is typically a long-term consequence of trauma to the shoulder (previous dislocation, humeral head or neck fracture, large rotator cuff tendon tears, and rheumatoid arthritis). As the cartilage degrades and the joint space narrows, the ligaments become more lax decreasing the stability of the joint and encouraging the growth of osteophytes.

Clinical Pearl

Less common causes of glenohumeral osteoarthritis include osteone-crosis, infection, seronegative spondyloarthropathies, and rotator cuff tear arthropathy.

Subjective Findings

The subjective findings typically include the following:

- Gradual onset of deep-seated shoulder pain and stiffness. The worst pain is typically localized to the posterior aspect of the shoulder, but can also be reported in the lateral upper arm, upper trapezius region, and interscapular region.
- Progressive loss of shoulder motion and therefore function.
- History of trauma to the shoulder.

 Clinical Pearl

There appears to be no apparent relationship between the development of osteoarthritis in the shoulder and a patient's previous level of physical activity.

Objective Findings

The physical examination typically reveals the following findings:

- Forward humeral head, protracted scapula.
- Glenohumeral (GH) joint line tenderness, located anteriorly, just under the coracoid process.
- Swelling around the joint, usually in the infraclavicular fossa, may or may not be present.
- Decreased active and passive range of motion into abduction and external rotation.
- Crepitation with circumduction may or may not be present.

Confirmatory/Special Tests

Confirmatory/special testing is unnecessary in moderate to advanced cases.

Medical Studies

Plain radiographs of the shoulder including posteroanterior, external rotation, Y-outlet, and axillary views are strongly recommended. The axillary view most reliably demonstrates the joint space narrowing.

 Clinical Pearl

As the disease progresses, the distance between the inferior glenoid and humeral head gradually decreases, and spurring of the inferior portion of the humeral head gradually increases.

 Clinical Pearl

Rheumatoid arthritis is suggested by the presence of periarticular erosions, osteopenia, and central wear of the glenoid.

Differential Diagnosis

- Adhesive capsulitis.
- Rotator cuff tear.
- Fracture of the humerus.
- Infection.
- Cervical disk herniation.
- Tumor of the shoulder girdle.

Intervention

The physical therapy intervention for GH joint osteoarthritis is aimed at improving glenohumeral flexibility, emphasizing those directions in which the patient has suffered the greatest loss, and general rotator cuff tendon strengthening exercises.

Prognosis

GH joint osteoarthritis is a slowly progressive process. Chronic shoulder pain and loss of strength in motion can develop. Total shoulder replacement is indicated when overall function is impaired, activities of daily living are significantly affected, and pain is intractable.

IMPINGEMENT SYNDROME

Diagnosis

Impingement syndrome—ICD-9: 840.6 (supraspinatus strain). Also referred to as subacromial impingement syndrome, and subacromial compression.

Description

Subacromial impingement syndrome (SIS) is a recurrent and troublesome condition closely related to rotator cuff disease. Impingement syndrome is a mechanical impingement of the rotator cuff between the coracoacromial arch and the humeral head. Anything that decreases the volume of this space such as calcifications in the acromioclavicular ligament and anterior acromial spur formation can cause impingement. Hypertrophy of the acromioclavicular (AC) joint secondary to arthritis has also been implicated in the cause of impingement.

 Clinical Pearl

The coracoacromial (subacromial) arch is a tunnel whose walls are formed by two scapular processes—the acromion located posteriorly and laterally, and the coracoid process located anteriorly and medially. The contents of this tunnel include the supraspinatus tendon, the tendon of the long head of the biceps, the subacromial (subdeltoid) bursa, and the coracohumeral ligament.

Subjective Findings

A detailed history is important to diagnose a rotator cuff injury and can help to rule out other diagnoses in the differential (eg, referred pain from the cervical spine, more serious referred symptoms of cardiac origin), and to determine if the patient's symptoms are related to a specific injury or event, or to a repetitive motion, or are of a more insidious onset. Typical subjective findings include:

- Pain felt down the lateral aspect of the upper arm near the deltoid insertion, over the anterior proximal humerus, or in the periacromial area.
- Functional loss of the shoulder attributable to pain, stiffness, weakness, and catching especially when the arm is used in the flexed and internally rotated position.
- Difficulty sleeping on the involved side.
- Pain provoked by everyday activities such as putting on a coat, pouring coffee, and so on.

Objective Findings

The objective findings depend on the stages:

- Stage 1: tenderness at the supraspinatus insertion and anterior acromion, a painful arc, and weakness of the rotator cuff secondary to pain, particularly when tested at 90-degree abduction or flexion.
- Stage 2: The physical examination reveals crepitus or catching at approximately 100 degrees and restriction of passive range of motion (due to fibrosis).
- Stage 3: Atrophy of the infraspinatus and supraspinatus, and more limitation in active and passive range of motion than the other stages. If a rotator cuff tear is present, weakness may be present—the amount of weakness is directly related to the size of the tear.

Confirmatory/Special Tests

A combination of the Hawkins–Kennedy impingement sign, the painful arc sign, and the infraspinatus muscle test yield the best posttest probability (95%) for any degree of impingement syndrome.*

Imaging Studies

Routine x-rays at the shoulder (including posteroanterior, external rotation, Y-outlet, and axillary views) are optional in patients presenting with a first episode of impingement. Patients with recurrent or persistent cases should undergo radiographic testing. Diagnostic ultrasound, arthrography, and MRI often are ordered in persistent or chronic cases to exclude the possibility of rotator cuff tendon tear.

Differential Diagnosis

- Rotator cuff tendon tears.
- Adhesive capsulitis.
- Acromioclavicular osteoarthritis/separation.
- Glenohumeral osteoarthritis.
- Multidirectional instability of the shoulder.
- Referred pain from cervical spine, lung, diaphragm, and upper abdomen.

Intervention

The exercises prescribed should be as specific as possible, and tailored to the patient's functional and recreational goals. The goals of the exercise progression are to strengthen:

- The rotator cuff (in order to increase the depressor effect on the humeral head).

---

*Park HB, Yokota A, Gill HS, et al. Diagnostic accuracy of clinical tests for the different degrees of subacromial impingement syndrome. *J Bone Joint Surg Am*. 2005;87:1446–1455.

- Internal and external rotation exercises initially performed as isometric exercises at various parts of the range.
- The scapular pivoters, while avoiding any increase in the elevating effect of the deltoid beginning with manual resistance and progressing to free weights.
- The lower extremity and trunk muscles that provide core stability.
  - Deficits in strength, strength imbalances, and flexibility in the legs, hips, and trunk should be addressed. This is particularly so in throwing athletes, where restrictions of the hip and back motion are common.

 Clinical Pearl

Care should be taken with exercises that involve the use of weights with the arm flexed or abducted away, or overhead, as these may exacerbate supraspinatus impingement and tendonitis symptoms if performed in the early stages of rehabilitation.

- Manual techniques can be used to address any tightness in the capsule (usually the posterior and inferior aspects) or motion restrictions of the sternoclavicular (SC) or AC joints.

Prognosis

This condition usually responds well to conservative measures.

Clinical Pearl

Surgery is considered only in those patients who, after having undergone a conservative regimen for a minimum of 6 months, and having explored vocational rehabilitation, continue to experience substantial impingement symptoms.

ROTATOR CUFF TEAR

Diagnosis

Rotator cuff tear—ICD-9: 727.61 (rotator cuff tear, nontraumatic). Also known as rotator cuff rupture.

Description

Rotator cuff tears, which can be acute and traumatic or chronic and degenerative, are described by size, location, direction, and depth. The proposed causes of a rotator cuff tendon failure include trauma (including overuse), attrition, ischemia, and impingement. Tears of the rotator cuff are usually longitudinal but may be transverse. They occur in a critical zone situated at the anterior portion of the cuff located within the subacromial space between the supraspinatus tendon and the coracohumeral ligament. Wear of the anterior aspect of the acromion on the greater tuberosity and the supraspinatus tendon eventually results in a full-thickness tear of the rotator cuff.

 Clinical Pearl

A rotator cuff tear is uncommon before 40 years unless associated with high-energy trauma. Most tears occur in the supraspinatus tendon as it passes directly under the acromion..

Subjective Findings

The typical subjective findings include the following:

- Patient complains of significant weakness and pain with activities that involve abduction and external rotation.
- Localized pain over the upper back, deltoid, shoulder, and arm.
- A popping sensation may be present.

 Clinical Pearl

In throwers, repetitive hyperextension together with internal impingement causes fraying of the deep layers of infraspinatus, ultimately establishing a partial-thickness tear. A similar situation is seen on the articular surface of the supraspinatus.

Objective Findings

The physical examination typically reveals the following:

- Observation may reveal muscle asymmetry, atrophy, or obvious deformity.

- Palpation should be used to locate tenderness. Point tenderness is typically located at the greater tuberosity.
- Loss of passive/active ROM to varying degrees depending on extent of injury.
- Positive special tests (Table 5-15) specific to injury.
- Weakness to some extent always accompanies rotator cuff tears—the amount of weakness is directly related to the size of the tear.
  - With small tears, the weakness may not be detected and the patient may have full ROM, although there may be a painful arc. Massive tears of the rotator cuff present with sudden profound weakness with an inability to raise the arm overhead, and exhibit a positive "drop arm" sign (see Special Tests).

Confirmatory/Special Tests

- Drop arm (Codman) test
- Empty can test

Medical/Imaging Studies

- Plain radiographs are usually normal in small cuff tears, but usually highlight full-thickness tears.
- A rotator cuff tear is typically diagnosed radiographically by MRI.
- Diagnostic ultrasonography reliably demonstrates the location and extent of cuff tears greater than 1 cm.
- Arthrography shows intravasation of dye into the subacromial space after injection and vigorous exercise that extends beyond the normal cuff attachment at the greater tuberosity.
- A subacromial injection (9 mL lidocaine/1 mL dexamethasone) can be used as a diagnostic tool—alleviation of the patient's pain supports a diagnosis of subacromial bursitis.

Differential Diagnosis

- Rotator cuff impingement.
- Acromioclavicular joint arthritis/abnormalities.
- Glenohumeral arthritis.
- SLAP lesion.
- Shoulder instability (anterior).
- Cervical strain or cervical radiculopathy.
- A snapping scapula.
- External impingement.
- Internal impingement (pain with the cocking motion of throwing).

Intervention

The conservative intervention for patients with a small or partial tear is directed toward strengthening the rotator cuff and scapula stabilizer muscles. Full-thickness tears likely require surgery depending on the patient's age and activity level.

Prognosis

The prognosis depends on the extent of the injury (small- to medium-sized tears have a good prognosis, whereas medium-size to large tears have a poor prognosis without surgery), the age of the patient, and if the dominant side is affected.

 Clinical Pearl

Criteria for operative intervention includes the following:

- A patient who is younger than 60 years of age.
- Failure to improve after a conservative regimen of not less than 6 weeks.
- Presence of a full-thickness tear, either clinically or by imaging techniques.
- The patient's need to use the involved shoulder in a vocation or an avocation.
- The ability and willingness of the patient.

SLAP LESION

Diagnosis

Superior labrum anterior to posterior (SLAP) lesion —ICD-9: 840.7. Also known as biceps labral complex injuries, shoulder sprain, or superior glenoid labrum tear.

Description

The labrum is a fibrocartilaginous ring that fits around the glenoid fossa. It functions to increase the fit of the humeral head and to provide stability to the humeral head. SLAP lesions involve an injury to the superior glenoid labrum and the biceps. There are several injury mechanisms that are speculated to be responsible for creating SLAP lesions ranging from single traumatic events to repetitive microtraumatic injuries.

Clinical Pearl

A SLAP lesion typically results from a fall on an outstretched hand (FOOSH injury), sudden deceleration or traction forces such as catching a falling heavy object, or chronic anterior and posterior instability.

 Clinical Pearl

SLAP lesions can be classified by signs and symptoms:

- Type I. This type involves a fraying and degeneration of the edge of the superior labrum. The patient loses the ability to horizontally abduct or externally rotate with the forearm pronated without pain.

- Type II. This type involves a pathological detachment of the labrum and biceps tendon anchor, resulting in a loss of the stabilizing effect of the labrum and the biceps.

- Type III. This type involves a vertical tear of the labrum, similar to the bucket-handle tear of the meniscus, although the remaining portions of the labrum and biceps are intact.

- Type IV. This type involves an extension of the bucket-handle tear into the biceps tendon, with portions of the labral flap and biceps tendon displaceable into the GH joint.

- Type V. This type is characterized by the presence of a Bankart lesion of the anterior capsule that extends into the anterior superior labrum.

- Type VI. This type involves a disruption of the biceps tendon anchor with an anterior or posterior superior labral flap tear.

- Type VII. This is described as the extension of a SLAP lesion anteriorly to involve the area inferior to the middle glenohumeral ligament.

Subjective Findings

The subjective findings typically include the following:

- History of trauma or overuse.
- Complaints of pain and/or instability with overhead activities and symptoms of painful clicking, catching, or locking.

Clinical Pearl

Athletes performing overhead movements, particularly baseball pitchers, may report a "dead arm" syndrome in which they have a painful shoulder with throwing and can no longer throw a baseball with their preinjury velocity.

Objective Findings

Diagnosis of a SLAP lesion can often be difficult as the symptoms are very similar to those of instability and rotator cuff disease. The physical examination typically reveals positive findings of pain or clicking with maneuvers that place tensile or torsional load on the biceps, thereby stressing the loose anchor of the biceps-superior labrum complex.

Confirmatory/Special Tests

Several special tests can be used to help identify the presence of a SLAP lesion, including the O'Brien (active-compression) test, the crank test, the clunk test, the Speed test, the Jobe relocation test, the biceps load test and the anterior slide test (Table 5-15).

Medical/Imaging Studies

Plain radiographs should be obtained because they are part of a thorough workup of any shoulder disorder, but they cannot confirm a diagnosis of a SLAP lesion.
MR arthrography is the gold standard to evaluate for a SLAP lesion.

Differential Diagnosis

- Shoulder instability.
- Rotator cuff disease.
- Subacromial impingement.
- Acromioclavicular joint arthritis.
- Biceps tendonitis.
- Suprascapular nerve entrapment.

Intervention

Conservative intervention should address the underlying hypermobility or instability of the shoulder using dynamic stabilization exercises of the GH joint to effectively return function and symptomatic relief to the patient.

Prognosis

If conservative management fails and symptoms persist, diagnostic shoulder arthroscopy is recommended.

 Clinical Pearl

Studies of surgical labral repairs are generally good to excellent in terms of returning patients to their prior level of activity, whether sports or work.

SUBSCAPULAR BURSITIS

Diagnosis

Subscapular bursitis—ICD-9: 727.3. Also referred to as scapulothoracic syndrome

Description

Subscapular bursitis is a focal inflammation caused by mechanical pressure and friction between the superomedial angle of the scapula and the second and third ribs.

 Clinical Pearl

Conditions associated with subscapular bursitis include frozen shoulder, glenohumeral osteoarthritis, and chronic rotator cuff tendonitis.

Subjective Findings

The typical subjective findings include the following:
- Complaints of localized pain over the upper back.
- Reports of a popping sound whenever the shoulder is shrugged.
- Difficulty sitting against a hard-backed chair or sleeping supine.

Objective Findings

The findings from the physical examination typically include the following:
- Localized tenderness under the superomedial angle of the scapula along the second or third rib.

Confirmatory/Special Tests

No special testing is indicated. The diagnosis is usually confirmed using a local anesthetic block at the level of the adjacent rib.

Medical Studies

No medical studies are indicated in an uncomplicated case.

Differential Diagnosis

- Rhomboid or levator scapular muscle irritation.
- Cervical radiculopathy.
- Glenohumeral instability.

Intervention

The intervention is aimed at reducing the acute inflammation, treating any underlying cause, and to prevent further episodes by improvement in posture and in shoulder muscle tone.

 Clinical Pearl

Theoretically, by increasing the tone and bulk of the subscapularis, a natural padding is provided between the ribs and the under surface of the scapula.

Prognosis

Conservative intervention is highly effective in both treating and avoiding recurrences.

THORACIC OUTLET SYNDROME

Diagnosis

Thoracic outlet syndrome (TOS)—ICD-9: 724.4. The other names used for TOS are based on descriptions of the potential sources for its compression. These names include cervical rib syndrome, scalenus anticus syndrome, hyperabduction syndrome, costoclavicular syndrome, pectoralis minor syndrome, and first thoracic rib syndrome.

Description

- TOS is a clinical syndrome characterized by symptoms attributable to compression of the neural or vascular anatomic structures (brachial plexus, subclavian artery or vein) that pass through the thoracic outlet.
- The bony boundaries of the outlet include the clavicle, first rib, and scapula, and the outlet passage is further defined by the interscalene interval, a triangle with its apex directed superiorly. This triangle is bordered anteriorly by the anterior scalene muscle, posteriorly by the middle scalene muscle, and inferiorly by the first rib.
- TOS is more common in women, with onset of symptoms usually between 20 and 50 years.

 Clinical Pearl

An insidious onset of symptoms could suggest postural (e.g., thoracic outlet syndrome), degenerative, or myofascial origins; or a disease process, such as ankylosing spondylitis, cervical spondylosis, or facet syndrome. An insidious onset may also indicate the presence of a serious pathology such as a tumor.

Subjective Findings

- Symptoms are often vague and variable—the chief complaint is one of diffuse arm and shoulder pain, especially when the arm is elevated beyond 90 degrees.
  - Potential symptoms include pain localized in the neck, face, head, upper extremity, chest, shoulder, or axilla; and upper extremity paresthesias, numbness, weakness, heaviness, fatigability, swelling, discoloration, ulceration, or Raynaud phenomenon, especially when the arm is elevated beyond 90 degrees.
  - Neural compression symptoms occur more commonly than vascular symptoms.[57]

Objective Findings

- Swelling or discoloration of the arm.
- Auscultation may reveal the presence of bruits, especially while doing the provocative maneuvers listed under special tests.
- Difference in distal pulses with those on the opposite side.
- Differences in sensory and motor function in any of the peripheral nerves, especially the ulnar nerve.
- Positive special tests.

Clinical Pearl

The lowest trunk of the brachial plexus, which is made up of rami from the C8 and T1 nerve roots, is the most commonly compressed neural structure in TOS. These nerve roots provide sensation to the fourth and fifth fingers of the hand and motor innervation to the hand intrinsic muscles.

Confirmatory/Special Tests

TOS is a clinical diagnosis, made almost entirely on the basis of the history and physical examination. Despite their widespread use, no studies documenting the reliability of the common thoracic outlet maneuvers have been performed. Tests include the following:

- Adson vascular test.
- Allen pectoralis minor test.
- Costoclavicular test.
- Hallstead maneuver.
- Roos test (EAST).
- Overhead test.
- Hyperabduction maneuver (Wright test).
- Passive shoulder shrug.

 Clinical Pearl

Because the false-positive rates for the thoracic outlet tests are relatively high, the clinician should perform at least three different tests.

 Clinical Pearl

When performing thoracic outlet syndrome tests, either the diminution or disappearance of pulse or reproduction of neurologic symptoms indicates a positive test. However, the aim of the tests should be to reproduce the patient's symptoms rather than to obliterate the radial pulse, because more than 50% of normal, asymptomatic people exhibit obliteration of the radial pulse during classic provocative testing.

Medical Studies

No laboratory studies currently exist to confirm the diagnosis. Chest radiographs (apical lung tumor or infection), shoulder films, EMG/NCS, Doppler studies.

 Clinical Pearl

Characteristic electrodiagnostic changes include but are not limited to prolonged latency of the ulnar F wave and reduced amplitude of the ulnar sensory evoked amplitude.

Differential Diagnosis

- C8-T1 cervical radiculopathy (neck pain and stiffness with unilateral or bilateral pain and neurologic findings in a radicular pattern).
- Carpal tunnel syndrome (numbness on the radial side of the hand, positive Phalen maneuver)
- Ulnar nerve neuropathy (numbness on the ulnar side of the hand, positive Tinel's sign)
- Peripheral neuropathy
- Connective tissue diseases or infection
- Brachial plexus neuritis (sudden onset, severe pain, proximal muscle weakness)
- Pancoast tumors (venous congestion, lesion on apical lordotic chest radiograph).

To help rule out other conditions that can mimic TOS, the physical examination should include the following:

- Careful inspection of the spine, thorax, shoulder girdles, and upper extremities for postural abnormalities, shoulder asymmetry, muscle atrophy, excessively large breasts, obesity, and drooping of the shoulder girdle.
- Palpation of the supraclavicular fossa for fibromuscular bands, percussion for brachial plexus irritability, and auscultation for vascular bruits that appear by placing the upper extremity in the position of vascular compression.
- Assessment of the neck and shoulder girdle for active and passive ROMs, areas of tenderness, or other signs of intrinsic disease.
- A thorough neurological examination of the upper extremity, including a search for sensory and motor deficits and abnormalities of deep tendon reflexes.
- Assessment of respiration to ensure the patient is using correct abdominodiaphragmatic breathing.

- Assessment of the suspensory muscles: the middle and upper trapezius, levator scapulae, and SCM (thoracic outlet "openers"). These muscles typically are found to be weak.
- Assessment of the scapulothoracic muscles: the anterior and middle scalenes, subclavius, pectoralis minor and major (thoracic outlet "closers"). These muscles typically are found to be adaptively shortened.
- First rib position or presence of cervical rib.
- Clavicle position and history of prior fracture, producing abnormal callous formation or malalignment.
- Scapula position, acromioclavicular joint mobility, and sternoclavicular joint mobility.

Intervention

The focus of the intervention is the correction of postural abnormalities of the neck and shoulder girdle (corner stretches, shoulder rolls, neck retractions, and neck stretches) strengthening of the scapula suspensory muscles, stretching of the scapulothoracic muscles (levator scapular, pectoralis minor) and neck muscles (scalenes, sternocleidomastoid), and mobilization of the whole shoulder complex and the first and second ribs.

Prognosis

Fifty percent to 90% of patients with thoracic outlet syndrome respond rapidly and favorably to a conservative intervention and regain normal pain-free function of the upper extremity.

 Clinical Pearl

The criteria for surgical intervention include the following:
- Failure to respond to conservative intervention within 4 months.
- Signs of muscle atrophy.
- Intermittent paresthesias being replaced by sensory loss.
- Pain becoming incapacitating.

Surgical intervention can include depression of the scalene muscles and resetting of the first rib, removal of the cervical rib (if present), removal of the clavicle, severing the pectoralis minor muscle, and trisection of the subclavius muscle above the coracoid ligament.

REHABILITATION LADDER

SHOULDER

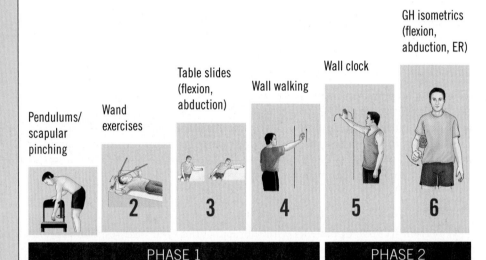

The purpose of these training ladders is to provide the clinician with a safe and progressive framework of exercises that are designed to allow the patient to improve in an efficient manner. The patient begins at the appropriate step, which is based on the stage of healing and the goal of the intervention.

- Phase 1: Acute—pain management, restoration of full passive range of motion, and restoration of normal accessory motion.
- Phase 2: Subacute—active range of motion exercises and early strengthening.
- Phase 3: Chronic—specific strengthening with a strong emphasis on enhancing dynamic stability.

The degree of movement and the speed of progression are both guided by the signs and symptoms. Once the patient is able to perform an exercise

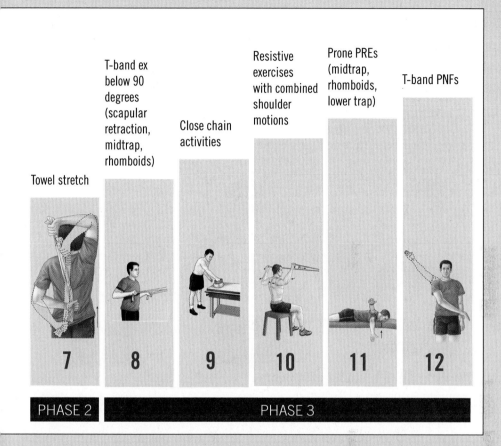

for 8–12 reps without pain, he or she progresses up to the next exercise step. This continues until the patient attempts an exercise that reproduces the pain. At this point, the patient returns to the last exercise that he or she was able to perform without pain and performs that exercise five times per day for 1 to 2 days before attempting to progress again. The patient is advanced through the training ladders to the appropriate point, with particular attention paid to patient response to treatment in terms of changes in symptoms, swelling, degree of irritability, or motion. In addition, muscle imbalances are addressed with appropriate flexibility exercises.

Once the patient is able to perform the last exercise of Phase 3 (Step 12 of the ladder), he or she can move on to functional and sport-specific training (Phase 4) as appropriate, which focus on power and higher-speed exercises similar to sport-specific demands.

1a. Pendulums

The patient is positioned in standing, with the uninvolved arm resting on a table and the trunk flexed at the hips about 90 degrees. The patient's arm hangs loosely downward in a position between 60 degrees and 90 degrees of flexion or scaption. The patient is asked to produce a pendulum swinging motion of the arm by moving the trunk slightly back and forth. The motions of flexion, extension, and horizontal abduction, adduction and circumduction can all be performed in this manner. This exercise can also be performed with the patient in prone and the arm hanging over the edge of the table.

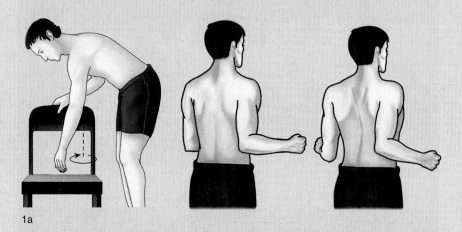

1a

🔵 Clinical Pearl

Codman pendulum exercises are commonly prescribed after shoulder surgery and injury to provide grade I and grade II distraction and oscillation resulting in decreased pain, increased flow of nutrients into the joint space, and early joint mobilization. Many shoulder protocols suggest that weight may be added to the pendulum exercises late in the subacute and chronic stages as the added weight produces a grade III distraction.

This exercise is not appropriate for patients with peripheral edema or for those who get dizzy when bending forward.

1b. Scapular pinches

The patient is positioned standing with the arms resting by the side and the elbows flexed to 90 degrees. The patient is asked to squeeze the "shoulder blades" together and to hold the contraction for 20 seconds. Alternatively, patient can be asked to clasp the hands together behind the low back and to hold this position for 20 seconds. This exercise can also be performed with the patient in prone and asking the patient to raise his or her extended arms toward the ceiling.

2. Wand exercises

The patient is positioned in the supine position. By grasping one end of a cane or wand with the hand of the involved arm, the patient then uses the uninvolved arm to move the involved arm into flexion, abduction, scaption, and rotation.

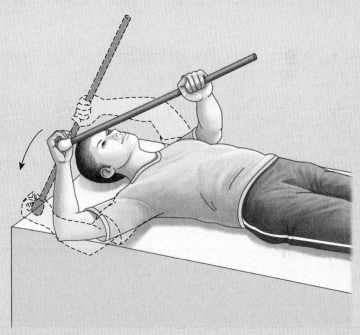

2

 Clinical Pearl

When the patient is performing internal or external rotation exercises, a towel can be placed under the humerus of the involved arm to position the humerus anterior to the midline of the body thereby relieving stress on the anterior capsule.

3. Table slides

The patient is positioned sitting with the involved side next to a table or flat surface. Using the back of the hand, or placing the hand of the involved extremity on top of a duster or towel, the patient uses the duster to slide the hands away from his or her body as they slowly stretch forward or sideways, thereby increasing GH flexion or abduction respectively. The patient then returns to the starting position. The exercise is repeated 8 to 10 times.

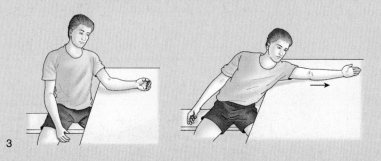

3

● Clinical Pearl

This exercise can be modified to increase glenohumeral motion in the direction of abduction, extension, external rotation, and internal rotation:

Abduction: the patient is positioned in sitting with the involved side next to a table, and with forearm resting in supination and pointing toward the opposite side of the table. The patient is asked to slide his or her arm across the table as the head is moved down toward the arm and the trunk moves away from the table.

Extension: the patient stands with his or her back to the table, and both hands grasping the edge so that the palms are facing away. The patient is then asked to perform a squat while letting the elbows flex. Caution must be used with this exercise with any patient who is prone to anterior subluxation/dislocation of the shoulder.

External rotation: the patient stands facing a doorframe with the palm of the hand against the edge of the frame and elbow flexed to 90 degrees. A rolled towel is placed in the axilla between the humerus and trunk to maintain slight abduction. The patient is then asked to turn away from the fixed hand. This exercise can also be done with the patient sitting at the side of a table with the anterior aspect of the forearm resting on the table, and elbow flexed to 90 degrees. The patient is then asked to bend from the waist, which brings the head and shoulder level with the table.

Internal rotation: the patient is positioned standing facing a doorframe with the elbow flexed to 90 degrees and the back of the hand against the doorframe. The patient is then asked to turn his trunk toward the fixed hand. This exercise can also be done with the patient in sidelying on the involved side, and the shoulder and elbow each flexed to 90 degrees, and the involved arm internally rotated to its end position. Using the uninvolved hand, the patient is then asked to push the forearm toward the table.

4. Wall walking
The patient is positioned standing with the hand placed against the wall at about chest height supporting a towel or a ball. The patient is asked to move the hand up the wall as far as tolerated without causing symptoms. Wall markings can be used to provide visual feedback.

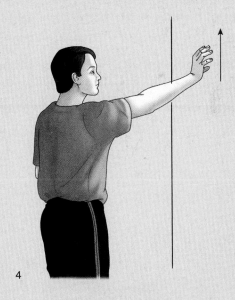

4

5. Wall clocks
The patient is positioned standing with the hand placed against the wall at about chest height supporting a towel or a ball. The patient is asked to move

the hand in both clockwise and counterclockwise direction in ever-increasing circles as far as tolerated without causing symptoms.

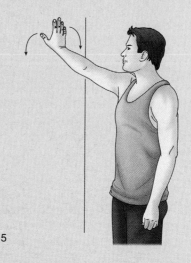

5

6. Glenohumeral isometrics

The patient is positioned in sitting or standing. Using the uninvolved arm and hand, the patient applies an isometric resistance at the distal end of the humerus of the involved arm. Using sufficient intensity consistent with the therapeutic goals, the patient attempts to move the involved arm against the isometric block into shoulder flexion, abduction, and internal and external rotation.

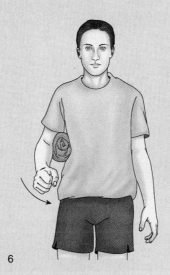

6

7. Towel stretch

The patient is positioned in standing with a towel grasped by the hand of the uninvolved arm and draped over the upper trapezius of the uninvolved side. Using the involved hand, the patient is asked to grasp the other end of the towel at the position of the maximum pain-free motion behind the back. The patient is then asked to pull on the towel with the uninvolved hand thereby drawing the involved hand up the back.

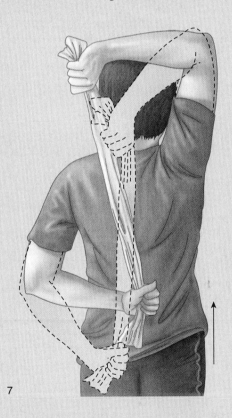

7

8. T-band exercises

The patient is positioned in standing with the involved arm at the patient's side (with a rolled towel placed in the axilla), or in various positions of abduction, scaption, or flexion. Using the hand of the involved arm, the patient grasps the end of the T-band and, using proper technique, pulls against the resistance of the T-band into forward flexion, abduction, internal and external rotation, horizontal abduction, and abduction. This exercise can also be modified so that the patient performs seated rowing using a narrow grip, middle grip, and wide grip.

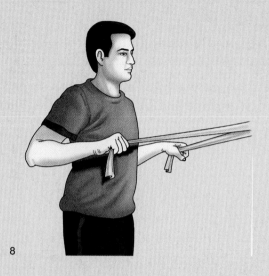

8

9. Closed-chain activities

A number of close chain activities can be used in shoulder rehabilitation. These include the prayer and quadruped positions initially using two hands and progressing to one hand. These exercises can also be performed in standing with the shoulder placed in various positions and with one or both hands leaning against a wall or an object, such as a ball.

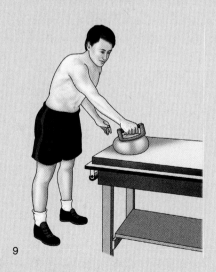

9

Clinical Pearl

More advanced techniques include having the patient on all fours with the hands on a rocker or wobble board or on a Swissball. The patient varies the amount of resistance by adjusting the trunk position—leaning forward produces more resistance, while leaning backward reduces the resistance. In addition, the exercises can be made more difficult by asking the patient to just use the involved arm.

10. Resistive exercises with combined motions

The patient is positioned sitting or standing with shoulders in the 90-90 position. The middle of a piece of elastic resistance is secured in front of the patient slightly above the shoulders. The patient is asked to grasp each end of the elastic resistance and is then asked to pull the hands and elbows back performing a combination of scapular abduction with shoulder horizontal abduction and external rotation.

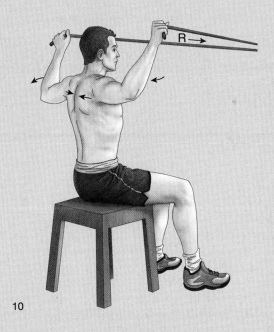

10

11. Prone Progressive Resistive Exercises (PREs)

The patient is positioned in prone with the involved arm hanging over the edge of the table in a dependent position and an appropriate weight in the hand.

The patient is asked to keep the elbow extended and to raise the arm toward the ceiling.

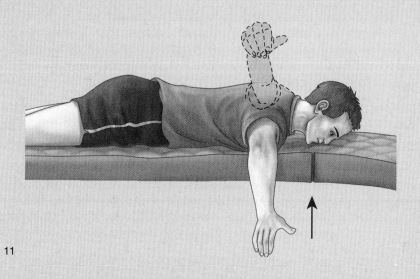

11

🌀 Clinical Pearl

By adjusting humeral rotation, different muscle groups can be targeted. External rotation of the shoulders (thumbs pointing upward) emphasizes the middle and lower trapezius, whereas internal rotation of the shoulders (thumbs pointing downward) emphasizes the rhomboids.

12. T-band PNF

Proprioceptive neuromuscular facilitation (PNF) patterns utilize the entire upper extremity. Elastic resistance is secured to the floor, or placed under the patient's foot (a dumbbell held in the hand can also be used). The following patterns can be performed:

D_1 flexion pattern—the arm begins in extension, internal rotation, and slight abduction. The patient is asked to bring the arm into flexion, adduction, and external rotation.

D_2 flexion pattern—the arm begins in extension, internal rotation, and slight adduction. The patient is asked to bring the arm into flexion, external rotation, and abduction.

Elastic resistance is secured above the head (a weighted pulley system can also be used).

D_1 extension pattern—the arm begins in flexion, adduction, and external rotation. The patient is asked to pull against the resistance into a combination of extension, abduction and internal rotation

D_2 extension pattern—the arm begins in flexion, abduction, and external rotation. The patient is asked to pull against the resistance into a combined motion involving extension, adduction, and internal rotation

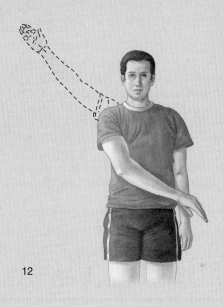

12

REFERENCES

1. Neer C. Impingement lesions. *Clin Orthop.* 1983;173:71–77.
2. Burkhart SS. A 26-year-old woman with shoulder pain. *JAMA.* 2000;284:1559–1567.
3. Boublik M, Hawkins RJ. Clinical examination of the shoulder complex. *J Orthop Sports Phys Ther.* 1993;18:379–385.
4. Hawkins RJ, Bokor DJ. Clinical evaluation of shoulder problems. In: Rockwood CA, Matsen FA, eds. *The Shoulder.* Philadelphia, PA: WB Saunders; 1990.
5. Yocum LA. Assessing the shoulder. History, physical examination, differential diagnosis, and special tests used. *Clin Sports Med.* 1983;2:281–289.
6. Woodward TW, Best TM. The painful shoulder: part I. Clinical evaluation. *Am Fam Physician.* 2000;61:3079–3088.

7. Cappel K, Clark MA, Davies GJ, et al. Clinical examination of the shoulder. In: Tovin BJ, Greenfield B, eds. *Evaluation and Treatment of the Shoulder—An Integration of The Guide to Physical Therapist Practice*. Philadelphia: FA Davis; 2001:75–131.

8. Davies GJ, DeCarlo MS. Examination of the shoulder complex. In: Bandy WD, ed. *Current Concepts in the Rehabilitation of the Shoulder, Sports Physical Therapy Section—Home Study Course*. La Crosse, WI, Orthopaedic Section, APTA, 1995.

9. Minter WW. A shoulder hand syndrome in coronary disease. *J Med Assoc GA*. 1967;56:45–49.

10. Silliman FJ, Hawkins RJ. Clinical examination of the shoulder complex. In: Andrews JR, Wilk KE, eds. *The Athlete's Shoulder*. New York, NY: Churchill Livingstone; 1994.

11. Mattingly GE, Mackarey PJ. Optimal methods for shoulder tendon palpation: a cadaver study. *Phys Ther*. 1996;76:166–174.

12. Kessel L, Watson M. The painful arc syndrome: clinical classification as a guide to management. *J Bone Joint Surg Br*. 1977;59:166–172.

13. Warner JJ, Navarro RA. Serratus anterior dysfunction. Recognition and treatment. *Clin Orthop Relat Res*. 1998;349:139–148.

14. Daigneault J, Cooney LM, Jr. Shoulder pain in older people. *J Am Geriatr Soc*. 1998;46:1144–1151.

15. Saha AK. Mechanisms of shoulder movements and a plea for the recognition of "Zero Position" of the glenohumeral joint. *Clin Orthop*. 1983;173:3–10.

16. Sahrmann SA. Movement impairment syndromes of the shoulder girdle. In: Sahrmann SA, ed. *Movement Impairment Syndromes*. St Louis, MO: Mosby; 2001:193–261.

17. Cyriax J. *Textbook of Orthopaedic Medicine, Diagnosis of Soft Tissue Lesions*. 8th ed. London, UK: Bailliere Tindall; 1982.

18. Codman EA. *The Shoulder, Rupture of the Supraspinatus Tendon and Other Lesions in or About the Subacromial Bursa*. Boston, MA: Thomas Todd; 1934.

19. Post M, Mayer J. Suprascapular nerve entrapment: diagnosis and treatment. *Clin Orthop*. 1987;223:126–130.

20. Cohen RB, Williams GR Jr. Impingement syndrome and rotator cuff disease as repetitive motion disorders. *Clin Orthop Relat Res*. 1998;351:95–101.

21. Cuomo F. Diagnosis, classification, and management of the stiff shoulder. In: Iannotti JP, Williams GR, eds. *Disorders of the Shoulder: Diagnosis and Management*. Philadelphia, PA; Lippincott Williams & Wilkins; 1999:397–417.

22. Kamkar A, Irrgang JJ, Whitney S. Non-operative management of secondary shoulder impingement syndrome. *J Orthop Sports Phys Ther*. 1993;17:212–224.

23. Kuhn JE, Plancher KD, Hawkins RJ. Scapular winging. *J Am Acad Orthop Surg*. 1995;3:319–325.

24. Paine RM, Voight M. The role of the scapula. *J Orthop Sports Phys Ther*. 1993; 18:386–391.

25. Dunleavy K. *Relationship Between the Shoulder and the Cervicothoracic Spine*. La Crosse, WI: Orthopedic Section, APTA; 2001.

26. Kelly BT, Roskin LA, Kirkendall DT, et al. Shoulder muscle activation during aquatic and dry land exercises in nonimpaired subjects. *J Orthop Sports Phys Ther*. 2000;30:204–210.

27. Kelly BT, Kadrmas WR, Kirkendall DT, et al. Optimal normalization tests for shoulder muscle activation: an electromyographic study. *J Orthop Res.* 1996;14:647–653.

28. Gerber C, Krushell RJ. Isolated rupture of the tendon of the subscapularis muscle: clinical features in 16 cases. *J Bone Joint Surg.* 1991;73B:389–394.

29. Naredo E, Aguado P, De Miguel E, et al. Painful shoulder: comparison of physical examination and ultrasonographic findings. *Ann Rheum Dis.* 2002;61:132–136.

30. Jenp Y, Malanga GA, Growney ES, et al. Activation of the rotator cuff in generating isometric shoulder rotation torque. *Am J Sports Med.* 1996;24:477–485.

31. Bowen JE, Malanga GA, Pappoe T, et al. Physical examination of the shoulder. In: Malanga GA, Nadler SF, eds. *Musculoskeletal Physical Examination—An Evidence-based Approach.* Philadelphia, PA: Elsevier-Mosby; 2006:59–118.

32. Babyar SR. Excessive scapular motion in individuals recovering from painful and stiff shoulders: causes and treatment strategies. *Phys Ther.* 1996;76:226–247.

33. Miniaci A, Salonen D. Rotator cuff evaluation: imaging and diagnosis. *Orthop Clin North America.* 1997;28:43–58.

34. Odom CJ, Taylor AB, Hurd CE, Denegar CR. Measurement of scapular asymetry and assessment of shoulder dysfunction using the Lateral Scapular Slide Test: a reliability and validity study. *Phys Ther.* 2001;81:799–809.

35. Calis M, Akgun K, Birtane M, Karacan I, Calis H, Tuzun F. Diagnostic values of clinical diagnostic tests in subacromial impingement syndrome. *Ann Rheum Dis.* 2000;59:44–47.

36. MacDonald PB, Clark P, Sutherland K. An analysis of the diagnostic accuracy of the Hawkins and Neer subacromial impingement signs. *J Shoulder Elbow Surg.* 2000;9:299–301.

37. Bryant L, Shnier R, Bryant C, Murrell GA. A comparison of clinical estimation, ultrasonography, magnetic resonance imaging, and arthroscopy in determining the size of rotator cuff tears. *J Shoulder Elbow Surg.* 2002;11:219–224.

38. O'Brien SJ, Pagnani MJ, Fealy S, et al. The active compression test; a new and effective test for diagnosing labral tears and acromioclavicular abnormality. *Am J Sports Med.* 1998;26:610–613.

39. Holovacs T, Osbahr DC. The sensitivity and specificity of the physical examination to detecting glenoid labrum tears. *Scientific Program AAOS, 67th annual meeting.* Orlando, FL; 2000.

40. Liu SH, Henry MH, Nuccion SL. A prospective evaluation of a new physical examination in predicting glenoid labral tears. *Am J Sports Med.* 1996;24:721–725.

41. Speer KP, Hannafin JA, Altchek DW, et al. An evaluation of the shoulder relocation test. *Am J Sports Med.* 1994;22:177–83.

42 Liu SH, Henry MH, Nuccion S, Shapiro MS, Dorey F. Diagnosis of glenoid labral tears: a comparison between magnetic resonance imaging and clinical examinations. *Am J Sports Med.* 1996;24:149–154.

43 Kim SH, Ha KI, Han KY. Biceps load test: a clinical test for superior labrum anterior and posterior lesions (SLAP) in shoulders with recurrent anterior dislocations. *Am J Sports Med.* 1999;27:300–303.

44 Bennett WF. Specificity of the Speed's test: arthroscopic technique for evaluating the biceps tendon at the level of the bicipital groove. *Arthroscopy.* 1998;14:789–796.

45. Rockwood CA Jr, Szalay EA, Curtis RJ, et al. X-ray evaluation of shoulder problems. In: Rockwood CA Jr, Matsen FA III, eds. *The Shoulder*. Philadelphia, Pa: WB Saunders Co; 1990:178–207.
46. Rubin SA, Gray RL, Green WR. The scapular "Y" view: a diagnostic aid in shoulder trauma. A technical note. *Radiology*. 1974;110:725–726.
47. Swen WA, Jacobs WG, Neve WC, et al. Is sonography performed by the rheumatologist as useful as arthrography executed by the radiologist for the assessment of full thickness rotator cuff tears? *J Rheum*. 1998;25:1800–1806.
48. Kneeland JB. Magnetic resonance imaging: general principles and techniques., In: Iannotti JP, Williams GR, eds. *Disorders of the Shoulder: Diagnosis and Management*. Philadelphia, PA: Lippincott Williams & Wilkins; 1999:911–925.
49. Tirman PF, Feller JF, Janzen DL, et al. Association of glenoid labral cysts with labral tears and glenohumeral instability: radiologic findings and clinical significance. *Radiology*. 1994;190:653–658.
50. Guide to physical therapist practice. *Phys Ther*. 2001;81:S13–S95.

QUESTIONS

1. Define the "rotator interval" as described by Neer.
2. What is considered to be the average ratio of the scapulohumeral rhythm?
3. What effect does the rotator cuff has on the humeral head?
4. What structure(s) pass through the triangular space?
5. What is the normal version or tilt angle of the glenoid?
6. What four articulations make up the shoulder complex?
7. Give three medical conditions that can refer pain to the shoulder.
8. What are the two close-packed positions of the glenohumeral joint?
9. Name the five scapular pivoter muscles.
10. An injury to which peripheral nerve of the shoulder causes medial scapular winging?
11. A severely restricted active abduction pattern with no pain is suggestive of a lesion to what structures?
12. Which osteokinematics glenohumeral motion is associated with an inferior glide of the humeral head?
13. What is os acromiale?
14. Which neurovascular structure is a greatest risk during anterior shoulder surgery?
15. What does a positive empty can test indicate?
16. Describe a posterior (internal) impingement.
17. What is the Mumford procedure?
18. What is the usual cause of a painful arc in the shoulder?

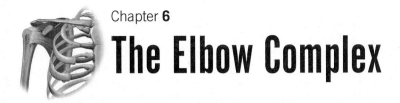

Chapter **6**

The Elbow Complex

OVERVIEW

The elbow serves as the central link in the kinetic chain of the upper extremity. The management of elbow symptoms requires a thorough appreciation of the intricate anatomy and biomechanics of the joint complex to diagnose the cause of these symptoms correctly.

Anatomy

The elbow joint comprises three distinct articulations: the ulnohumeral, radiohumeral (radiocapitellar), and proximal radioulnar joints.

- The ulnohumeral and radiohumeral joints provide flexion/extension of the elbow and pronation/supination of the forearm.
- The proximal radioulnar joint works in conjunction with the distal radioulnar joint at the wrist to achieve forearm pronation and supination.

The movements of the elbow complex, produced by muscle action (Tables 6-1 and 6-2), include flexion and extension of the elbow, and pronation and supination of the forearm. Stability of the elbow complex during these movements is provided by the osseous relationships and by medial and lateral ligament complexes (Table 6-3).

The elbow region also has complex innervation (Tables 6-1 and 6-2).

⬤ Clinical Pearl

- The median nerve crosses the elbow medially and passes through the two heads of the pronator teres, which is a potential site of entrapment.
- The ulnar nerve passes along the medial arm and posterior to the medial epicondyle through the cubital tunnel, a likely site of compression.

- The radial nerve descends the arm laterally. It divides into the superficial (sensory) branch and the deep (motor, or posterior interosseous) branch. The deep branch must then pass through the arcade of Fröhse, a fibrous arch formed by the proximal margin of the superficial head of the supinator muscle, where it is most susceptible to injury.

Examination

Most elbow conditions can be correctly diagnosed with a sound knowledge of elbow and forearm anatomy and differential diagnosis, coupled with good history taking.

History

The clinician must determine the chief complaint, its chronicity, and whether there was a specific mechanism of injury.

Clinical Pearl

- Acute pain and swelling after an injury can be caused by a fracture, dislocation, or tendon/ligament rupture.
- Most chronic conditions of the elbow represent overuse injuries from work or sport.
- Loose bodies often develop in arthritic elbows and may produce catching or locking.

In addition to information regarding a specific mechanism, the clinician should seek information about recreational and occupational activities involving a repetitive load that could initiate a cycle of microtrauma, chronic inflammation, tissue degeneration, necrosis, and ultimately tendon rupture (Table 6-4).[1] Hand dominance and alleviating or aggravating factors are also important to establish.

If the injury is traumatic in origin, a mechanism should be determined.

- Flexion-based mechanisms include potential injury to the biceps brachii, brachialis, and brachioradialis, medial collateral ligament (MCL), lateral collateral ligament, joint capsule, and/or ulnar nerve.
- Extension-based mechanisms include potential injury to the triceps, lateral collateral ligament, joint capsule, and median nerve.

Table 6-1 Muscle Compartments of the Forearm

Compartment	Principal Muscles	Action	Peripheral Nerve Innervation	Nerve Root Derivation
Anterior	Pronator teres	Pronation of the forearm	Median	C6–C7
	Flexor carpi radialis	Pronation of the forearm	Median	C6–C7
	Flexor digitorum superficialis	Flexion of the fingers	Ulnar: medial two digits	C7–C8, T1
	Flexor digitorum profundus	Flexion of the fingers	Anterior interosseous (median)	C8, T1
	Flexor pollicis longus	Flexion of the thumb	Superficial head: median (lateral terminal branch)	C8, T1
	Flexor carpi ulnaris	Ulnar deviation of the wrist	Ulnar	C7–C8
	Pronator quadratus	Pronation of the forearm	Anterior interosseous (median)	C8, T1
Posterior	Abductor pollicis longus	Extension of the thumb	Posterior interosseous (radial)	C7–C8
	Extensor pollicis brevis	Extension of the thumb	Posterior interosseous (radial)	C7–C8
	Extensor pollicis longus	Extension of the thumb	Posterior interosseous (radial)	C7–C8
	Extensor digitorum communis	Extension of the fingers	Posterior interosseous (radial)	C7–C8
	Extensor digiti minimi	Extension of the little finger	Posterior interosseous (radial)	C7–C8
	Extensor digiti indicis	Extension of the index finger	Posterior interosseous (radial)	C7–C8
	Extensor carpi ulnaris	Extension of the wrist	Posterior interosseous (radial)	C7–C8
Mobile wad	Brachioradialis	Elbow flexion	Radial	C5–C6, (C7)
	ECRL	Extension of the wrist	Radial	C6–C7
	ECRB	Extension of the wrist	Posterior interosseous (radial)	C7–C8

ECRL = extensor carpi radialis longus; ECRB = extensor carpi radialis brevis.

Table 6-2 Muscles of the Elbow and Forearm: Their Actions, Nerve Supply, and Nerve Root Derivation

Action	Muscles Acting	Peripheral Nerve Supply	Nerve Root Deviation
Elbow flexion	Brachialis	Musculocutaneous	C5–C6, (C7)
	Biceps brachii	Musculocutaneous	C5–C6
	Brachioradialis	Radial	C5–C6, (C7)
	Pronator teres	Median	C6–C7
	Flexor carpi ulnaris	Ulnar	C7–C8
Elbow extension	Triceps	Radial	C7–C8
	Anconeus	Radial	C7–C8, (T1)
Forearm supination	Supinator	Posterior interosseous (radial)	C5–C6
	Biceps brachii	Musculocutaneous	C5–C6
Forearm pronation	Pronator quadratus	Anterior interosseous (median)	C8, T1
	Pronator teres	Median	C6–C7
	Flexor carpi radialis	Median	C6–C7

Table 6-3 Articular and Ligamentous Contributions to Elbow Stability

Stabilization	Elbow Extended	Elbow Flexed to 90 Degrees
Valgus stability	Anterior capsule	MCL
	MCL	Anterior capsule
	Bony articulation	Bony articulation
Varus stability	Anterior capsule	Joint articulation
	Joint articulation	Anterior capsule
	LCL	LCL
Distraction	Anterior capsule	LCL
	LCL	MCL
	MCL	Joint capsule
	Triceps, biceps, brachialis, brachioradialis, and forearm muscles	

LCL = lateral collateral ligament; MCL = medial collateral ligament.

Table 6-4 Sports Associated With Overuse Elbow Injuries

Activity	Injuries
Bowling	Biceps tendinosis, radial neuritis
Boxing	Triceps tendinosis
Football, wrestling, or basketball	Olecranon bursitis
Golf	Golfer elbow, radial neuritis
Gymnastics	Biceps tendinosis, triceps tendinosis
Racquet sports	Pronator teres syndrome, triceps tendinosis, olecranon stress fracture, lateral tennis elbow, radial neuritis, Golfer elbow, ulnar nerve entrapment
Rowing	Radial neuritis
Skiing	Ulnar nerve entrapment
Swimming	Radial neuritis
Throwing	Pronator syndrome, triceps tendinosis, olecranon impingement, olecranon stress fracture, ulnar collateral ligament sprain, Golfer elbow, ulnar nerve entrapment, little Leaguer elbow
Weight lifting	Biceps tendinosis, triceps tendinosis, anterior capsule strain, radial neuritis, ulnar nerve entrapment

- Pronation-based mechanisms include potential injury to the lateral epicondyle structures, radial tunnel, posterior interosseous nerve, pronator teres, brachioradialis, and lateral collateral ligament.
- Supination-based mechanisms include potential injury to the medial epicondyle structures, supinator, brachioradialis, and biceps brachii, and may be associated with supinator syndrome and radial tunnel syndrome.

● Clinical Pearl

One of the most common traumatic injuries to the elbow is the FOOSH (Fall On the Out Stretched Hand) (Table 6-5).

Table 6-5 FOOSH Injury History

Description	Possible Injury
Fell forward and landed on outstretched hand	Distal radial fracture
Fell forward on hand, and sprained my wrist	Scaphoid fracture
Landed on hand with arm outstretched behind	Distal humerus fracture
Landed on outstretched hand with elbow locked	Supracondylar fracture

Data from Dent S. Befuddled by a FOOSH? FR Report. 2000; 6:9.

Pain is the most common presenting symptom. It is also important to determine the location of the symptoms (Table 6-6 and Figure 6-1) as this may assist in the diagnosis:[1]

• Posterior elbow pain.

  • Triceps tendinosis—history of repetitive elbow extension with tenderness of the triceps tendon just superior to its attachment on the olecranon.

Table 6-6 The Location of Elbow Pain and Possible Causes

Anterior Elbow	Lateral Elbow
Biceps tendinosis—Further confirmation may be provided if resisted elbow flexion and forearm supination increase the symptoms	Lateral epicondylitis (tennis elbow)—worsens with grasping activities, forearm supination, and resisted wrist extension
Pronator syndrome (anterior interosseous branch of the median)—pain is associated with distal paresthesias, and resisted forearm pronation increases the symptoms. Further confirmation may be provided if there is weakness of the index and middle FDP, the FPL, and the pronator quadratus	Radial tunnel syndrome—tends to worsen with activities involving repetitive pronation and supination
Anterior capsule strain—Reports of repetitive hyperextension	Radiocapitellar chondromalacia—associated with a history of a repetitive valgus loading of the elbow
Torn brachialis—Reports of repetitive hyperextension	Posterolateral rotary instability

FDP = flexor digitorum profundus; FPL = flexor pollicis longus.

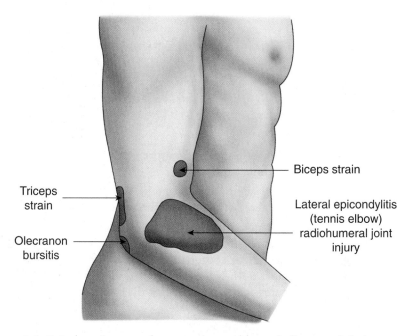

Figure 6-1 Pain locations on the posterior and lateral elbow and their possible causes.

- Olecranon impingement or an olecranon stress fracture—associated with clicking or locking of the elbow with terminal extension. An olecranon stress fracture is often associated with increased pain upon resisted elbow extension.
- Olecranon bursitis—often associated with a localized swelling and tenderness over the posterior aspect of the elbow.
- Medial elbow pain. The most common causes of medial elbow pain include the following:
- Medial epicondylitis (golfer's elbow), a tendinosis of the elbow flexor/ forearm pronator group associated with complaints with activities that require rapid wrist flexion and forearm pronation. The pain can be increased with wrist flexion or forearm pronation against resistance.
- Ulnar collateral ligament (UCL) sprain, characterized by an insidious onset of medial elbow pain that becomes worse with activity.
- Ulnar nerve entrapment, medial elbow pain accompanied with distal paresthesias along the ulnar aspect of the forearm and hand and weakness of the grip. The Tinel sign at the elbow will be positive.

Clinical Pearl

Lateral elbow pain that is exacerbated by forearm pronation/ supination is probably caused by arthritis in the radiohumeral articulation.

The severity, duration, timing, and nature of the pain (intermittent or constant) should be ascertained:

- Severity. The severity of symptoms can be judged by whether they occur only after activity (chronic), with activity (subacute), or at rest (acute).

- Duration. Symptoms that have been present for weeks or months point to overuse, once the more insidious reasons for prolonged pain are ruled out. Information about the patient's occupational and recreational activities can help differentiate (Table 6-4). It is important to identify the specific musculotendinous structures that are at risk for overuse or have been injured through overuse.

- Timing. The timing of the onset of symptoms can often be helpful in identifying the offending activity and thus the tissues at risk for overuse.

- Nature. Mechanical symptoms, such as clicking with motion, locking in extension, and catching are indicative of intra-articular pathology.

 Clinical Pearl

Sharply localized pain is often due to extra-articular pathology, such as tennis elbow.[2] Pain arising from the elbow itself is frequently of a "deep" nature and can extend into the extensor compartment.[2] Referred pain is more often described as being diffuse.

In addition to pain, reported decreases in function can be due to weakness or stiffness. It is particularly important to identify symptoms that are the result of neurological compromise:

- History of neck pain and previous neck injury, and questions that attempt to establish a relationship between head and neck movements and symptom reproduction.

Clinical Pearl

Symptoms that originate from the neck and radiate below the elbow are suggestive of a cervical spine disorder, although weakness or paresthesias can also be clues to peripheral nerve entrapment syndromes.[3]

It is worth remembering that the reported loss of function may only occur with vigorous activity, either at work or during sports, and may therefore be difficult to reproduce.[4]

Finally, adaptations to dysfunction should be noted because disability can be compensated for by enlisting the other extremity or by increasing motion at adjacent joints.[4]

Systems Review

Given its location, a thorough investigation of elbow pain requires ruling out referred symptoms from the neck, shoulder, wrist, and hand. In addition, cardiac referral can occur in the medial elbow region.

Tests and Measures

A systematic examination of the elbow includes observation, palpation, range of motion (ROM) testing, neurological assessment, the use of pertinent special tests, and the assessment of related areas.[1] These related areas include, but are not limited to, the neck, the shoulder, and the wrist/hand.

Observation and Palpation

At the elbow joint complex, observation and palpation are extremely important, as much of the structures are subcutaneous.

 Clinical Pearl

Bony structures feel hard, whereas ligamentous structures feel firm.

For an accurate and thorough examination of the elbow, the clinician must be able to visualize both arms. The involved elbow should be inspected for scars, redness, nodules, atrophy, deformities, and swelling.

Clinical Pearl

The earliest sign of elbow effusion is a loss of the elbow dimples. Sudden swelling of the elbow in the absence of trauma suggests infection, inflammation, or gout. Anterior joint effusion is evidence of significant swelling. Gradual swelling over the posterior tip of the elbow, which can sometimes be golf ball sized, but may not be tender to palpation, could be caused by an inflammation or infection of the olecranon bursa, or by a traction spur of the olecranon.[4] Intraarticular causes of acute synovitis of the elbow include septic arthritis, rheumatoid arthritis, or crystalline deposition diseases (gout, pseudogout).

Observation of the elbow should be from all views. To ensure this, the observation should be systematically divided into anterior, lateral, posterior, and medial aspects.[2,4]

Anterior Aspect

The axial alignment of the elbow should be assessed. With the elbow extended and the forearm positioned in supination, the humerus and forearm should normally be in valgus.[4] This angle is referred to as the *carrying angle.*

 Clinical Pearl

The carrying angle of the elbow varies from 5 to 16 degrees for females, and 5 to 14 degrees for males,[5,6] with a mean value of 10 degrees for men and 13 degrees for women.[7] Any difference in the carrying angle of the elbow is obvious when the elbow is in extension.

Clinical Pearl

The bony congruency of the ulna and humerus makes the forearm flex with respect to the humerus at a fixed angle called the carry angle of the arm.[7]

The carrying angle of the involved elbow should be compared with the other side before any conclusions are drawn.

Clinical Pearl

It is important to note that an accurate assessment of the carrying angle is difficult if a significant fixed flexion deformity of the elbow joint is present.

The most common cause of an altered carrying angle is past trauma, or epiphyseal growth disturbances. A valgus deformity is typically caused by nonunion of a fractured lateral condyle and may be associated with tardy ulnar nerve palsy.[2] A varus deformity (Gunstock) can follow malunion of a supracondylar fracture.[2]

 Clinical Pearl

- The biceps tendon can be easily palpated in the middle of the antecubital fossa, especially when the patient flexes the elbow against resistance with the forearm supinated.
- The brachial artery is deep and medial to the biceps tendon.
- The median nerve is medial to the brachial artery.

Posterior Aspect

The olecranon tip is normally visible subcutaneously (Figure 6-2). Sudden swelling over this area accompanied with a history of trauma is more likely the result of an olecranon fracture, a posterior ulnar subluxation, or a rupture of the triceps tendon (palpable defect).[4] A diminished tip of the olecranon could result from a prior partial olecranon excision or an anterior elbow subluxation or dislocation.[4] Midway between the olecranon and the lateral epicondyle, one palpates the anconeus muscle.

 Clinical Pearl

The triangular relationship of the epicondyles and the olecranon at 90 degrees of elbow flexion and full extension is often disrupted in the presence of a fracture, dislocation, or degeneration. At 90 degrees of flexion the three bony landmarks form an isosceles triangle, and when the arm is extended, they form a straight line.[8,9]

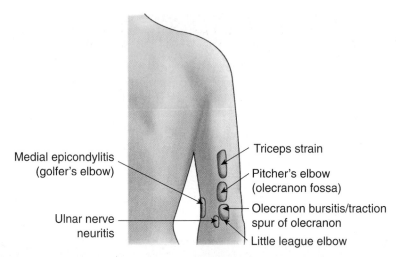

Medial epicondylitis
(golfer's elbow)

Ulnar nerve
neuritis

Triceps strain

Pitcher's elbow
(olecranon fossa)

Olecranon bursitis/traction
spur of olecranon

Little league elbow

Figure 6-2 Pain locations on the posterior and medial elbow and their possible causes.

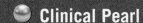

Clinical Pearl

Nodules on the extensor surface of the elbow may indicate the presence of a rheumatoid disease, gout, or other systemic processes.[4]

Medial Aspect

The medial epicondyle is usually visible on the medial aspect of the elbow. Tenderness of the medial epicondyle is a common finding with medial epicondylitis (golfer's elbow) (Figure 6-2). Just posterior to the medial epicondyle is the ulnar nerve groove, which is palpable (Figure 6-3). In certain cases of ulnar neuritis, the ulnar nerve may appear enlarged.[2] Ulnar nerve involvement can be determined using the Tinel test (see Special Tests) or motion and joint play tests. Just anterior and distal to the medial epicondyle one can palpate from proximal to distal the muscle origins of the pronator teres, flexor carpi radialis, palmaris longus, flexor digitorum superficialis, and flexor carpi ulnaris.[10]

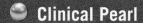

Clinical Pearl

Cubital tunnel syndrome is a form of mononeuropathy caused by compression, stretch, entrapment, ischemia, infection, or inflammation of the ulnar nerve in the cubital tunnel or surrounding tissue. With the exception of carpal tunnel syndrome, cubital tunnel syndrome is the most common nerve compression in the upper extremity. The patient initially complained of pain, tenderness, and swelling at the medial aspect of the elbow, which progresses to numbness and tingling in the medial distal third of the forearm and the little and ring fingers. A combination of sustained flexion (elbow flexion test) and a restriction in joint play decreases the overall volume within the cubital tunnel, which can increase the symptoms.[11,12] The differential diagnoses include cervical spine dysfunction, medial epicondylitis, thoracic outlet syndrome, brachial plexus injury, rheumatoid arthritis, and tumors.

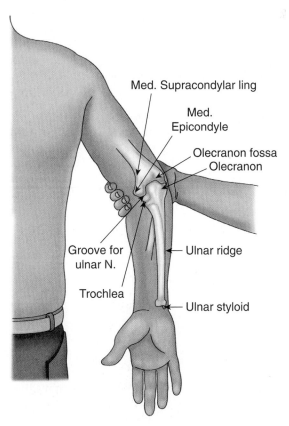

Figure 6-3 Palpation points on the medial and posterior aspect of elbow.

Lateral Aspect

The lateral epicondyle is covered by a large mass of extensor muscle, called the extensor bundle or wad. Tenderness of the lateral epicondyle is commonly found with lateral epicondylitis (tennis elbow) (Figure 6-4), especially over the origin of the extensor carpi radialis brevis (ECRB). Moving from the lateral supracondylar ridge, to the lateral epicondyle one palpates a number of muscles including, from proximal to distal, the brachioradialis, extensor carpi radialis longus (ECRL), ECRB, and extensor digitorum communis.

 Clinical Pearl

- Most swelling of the elbow appears in an area at the center of the triangle bounded by the lateral epicondyle, the tip of the olecranon, and the radial head.

- Fullness in the region of the lateral infracondylar process indicates synovial proliferation if on palpation the swelling has a boggy consistency.[2] If the swelling can be completely obliterated with pressure, and particularly if cross-fluctuation occurs, an increase in synovial fluid is present.[2]

The annular ligament is located distal to the lateral epicondyle, and applying passive supination and pronation of the forearm can facilitate its palpation. To palpate the radial head (Figure 6-4) at the humeroradial joint, the clinician places the index finger on the lateral humeral epicondyle. From here, the index finger slides posteriorly and distally to the capitellum and a further 2 cm distal to the radial head.[9] Bony hard swelling in this region is often associated with radial head pathology, such as a previous fracture or posterior subluxation.[2] Tenderness and crepitus along with limited forearm pronation/supination suggest a radial head fracture (if acute) or arthritis (if chronic).

 Clinical Pearl

The types of fracture of the elbow include supracondylar, medial epicondyle, lateral epicondyle, radial neck or radial head, olecranon, and coranoid. Signs and symptoms associated with a fractured elbow include pain, point tenderness, edema, ecchymosis, restricted motion, deformity, and weakness.

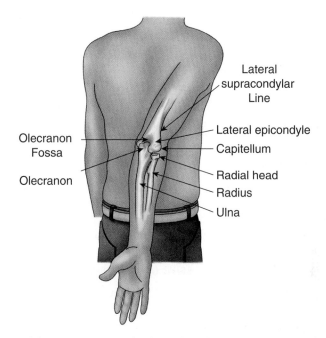

Lateral
supracondylar
Line

Lateral epicondyle

Capitellum

Radial head

Radius

Ulna

Olecranon
Fossa

Olecranon

Figure 6-4 Palpation points on the lateral and posterior aspect of elbow.

Muscles

- Biceps. The short head of the biceps is located at the coracoid process (together with the coracobrachialis muscle).[9] The long head of the biceps cannot be palpated at its origin, but it is palpable in the intertubercular groove. The muscle belly of the biceps is easily identifiable, especially with resisted elbow flexion and forearm supination.

- Brachialis. The origin of the brachialis can be palpated posterior to the deltoid tuberosity. Its insertion can be palpated at a point medial to the musculotendinous junction of the biceps, at the proximal border of the bicipital aponeurosis.[9]

- Brachioradialis. The brachioradialis can be palpated from the radial border of the cubital fossa distally to the radial styloid process.

- The common flexor origin is at the medial epicondyle and the flexor pronator mass is at the medial aspect of the elbow.

- The common extensor origin is at the lateral epicondyle.

- Supinator. The borders of the supinator within the cubital fossa are formed by the brachioradialis (radially), pronator teres (ulnarly), and tendon of the biceps (proximally).[9]

- Triceps. Palpation of the triceps can be simplified by having the patient abduct the arm to 90 degrees. The lateral head of the triceps borders directly on the brachial muscle, whereas the medial head runs underneath both the long and lateral heads of the triceps. These two heads of the triceps can be palpated until their common insertion at the olecranon.[9]
- Anconeus. This small muscular triangle can be palpated between the olecranon, the posterior border of the ulna, and the lateral epicondyle.

Neurovascular Structures

If the radial tuberosity is palpable, the posterior interosseous nerve is usually located no closer than 2 cm from the tuberosity in a posterior direction with the forearm pronated. The brachial artery can be palpated anteriorly to the elbow and the pulse palpated and compared bilaterally.

Active Range of Motion With Passive Overpressure

The patient with elbow pain should have a detailed assessment of his or her motion (Figures 6-5 and 6-6).

 Clinical Pearl

It is important to determine how much ROM is necessary for the patient to perform his or her job and recreational activities. Most activities of daily living may be accomplished with a functional arc of 100 degrees from 30 degrees to 130 degrees, and 50 degrees each of pronation and supination.[13]

In addition to assessing elbow and forearm motions, the various motions that occur at the wrist (flexion, extension, radial deviation, and ulnar deviation) must also be assessed.

 Clinical Pearl

Pain with elbow flexion/extension suggests involvement of the ulnohumeral articulation, whereas pain with forearm's pronation/supination should direct attention to the radiohumeral and proximal radioulnar joints.

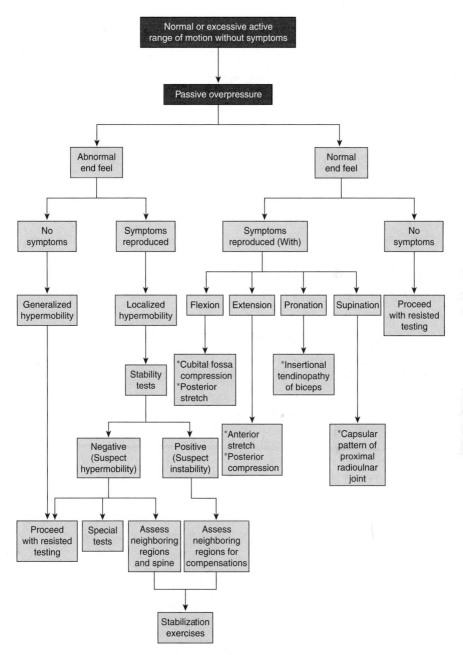

Figure 6-5 Examination sequence in the presence of symptoms with normal or excessive active ROM at the elbow.

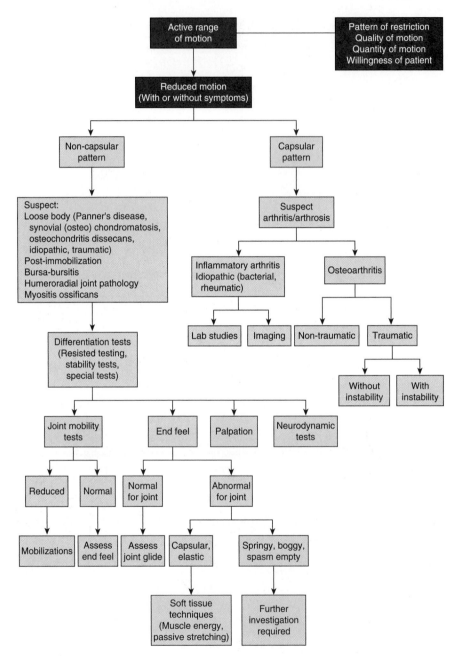

Figure 6-6 Examination sequence in the presence of painful flexion and/or extension at the elbow.

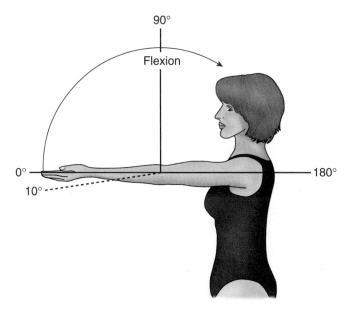

Figure 6-7 Elbow flexion and extension.

ROM of the elbow and forearm can be assessed with the patient seated, although elbow extension is better evaluated with the patient standing. The patient is asked to perform active flexion, extension (Figure 6-7), pronation, and supination (Figure 6-8) of the elbow and forearm and the ranges are recorded. Supination and pronation should be tested with the elbow flexed to 90 degrees (Figure 6-8).

Clinical Pearl

Normal ranges of motion at the elbow complex are 150 degrees of flexion, 0 degrees to 10 degrees of extension/hyperextension, 85 degrees of supination, and 75 degrees of pronation.

Young children commonly hyperextend the elbow by 10 degrees to 15 degrees, but adults show minimal, if any, elbow hyperextension.

If symptoms are not reproduced with the single plane motions, combined motions of the elbow are tested (see following section).

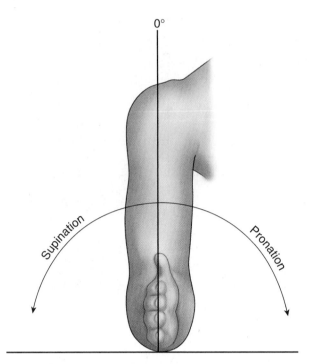

0°

Supination

Pronation

Figure 6-8 Forearm pronation and supination.

Clinical Pearl

The elbow has a particular predisposition to develop stiffness with arthritis, trauma, or immobilization.

Capsular or noncapsular patterns should be determined. The capsular patterns at the elbow are depicted in Table 6-7. Active movement often accentuates any crepitus during motion, which can be due to articular surface damage, a loose body, or an osteophyte.[2]

Clinical Pearl

Nerve injury decreases active but not passive motion.[4]

Table 6-7 Capsular Patterns of Restriction at the Elbow

Joint	Limitation of Motion (Passive Angular Motion)
Humeroulnar	Flexion > extension (±4:1)
Humeroradial	No true capsular pattern. Possible equal limitation of pronation and supination
Superior radioulnar	No true capsular pattern. Possible equal limitation of pronation and supination with pain at end ranges
Inferior radioulnar	No true capsular pattern. Possible equal limitation of pronation and supination with pain at end ranges

The end feels of elbow motion should be classified as either compliant, suggesting soft tissue restriction, or rigid, suggesting a mechanical bony limit. Passive elbow flexion (Figure 6-9) should have an end feel of soft tissue approximation.

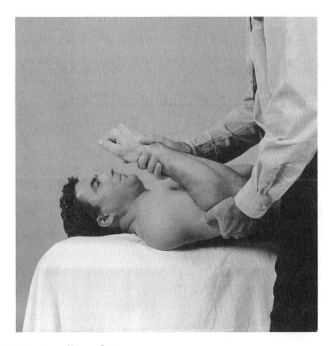

Figure 6-9 Passive elbow flexion.

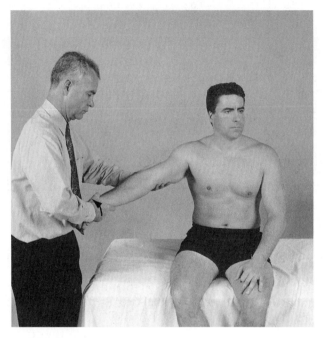

Figure 6-10 Passive elbow extension.

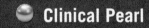

🔵 Clinical Pearl

Passive elbow flexion may aggravate an ulnar nerve neuropathy.[14]

Passive elbow extension (Figure 6-10) should have a bony end feel. A springy end feel with passive elbow flexion may indicate a loose body.

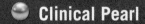

🔵 Clinical Pearl

Elbow extension is usually the first motion to be limited, and the last to be restored with intrinsic joint problems.[14] Thus, it serves as the most sensitive barometer of injury and recovery of the elbow.[4]

Even minor swelling or effusion prevents full extension of the elbow. The clinician should be particularly careful with an elbow that has lost a gross amount of extension post trauma, especially if accompanied by a painful weakness of elbow extension, as this may indicate an olecranon fracture. A significant loss of motion, with no accompanying weakness, could indicate myositis ossificans. Pain that occurs at the limit(s) of motion suggests bony impingement.

 Clinical Pearl

Pain throughout the central arc of flexion and extension, or pronation and supination, implies degeneration of the ulnotrochlear or proximal radioulnar joints, respectively. The predominant cause of fixed flexion contractures can be determined by applying passive overpressure into extension and noting the site of pain. Posterior pain indicates that posterior impingement is the likely culprit, whereas anterior pain indicates that anterior capsule adaptive shortening is the principal cause.[2]

Passive pronation and supination are applied by grasping the proximal aspect of the forearm. Passive overpressure is superimposed at the end of the available ranges.

 Clinical Pearl

A decrease in pronation or supination can represent pathology at either the proximal or distal radioulnar joint, bony deformity of the radius or ulna, or contractures of the interosseous membrane.[4] For example, decreased supination and pronation are frequent sequelae of a Colles fracture, advanced degenerative changes, dislocations, and fractures of the forearm and elbow.

Of particular interest is the acute limitation of supination and extension in children, which likely results from a "pulled elbow."

 Clinical Pearl

The elbow is the second most commonly dislocated joint in the adult and the most common of all dislocations in the child. An elbow dislocation involves a complete loss of continuity of the ulnohumeral articulation with associated radiocapitellar disruption. The most common type of elbow dislocation is posterior displacement of the olecranon in relation to the humerus. Two less common dislocations include anterior and divergent displacements. The most common mechanism for a posterior elbow dislocation is the FOOSH injury. Signs and symptoms include pain and increased swelling to the elbow joint, elbow held in 90 degrees of flexion, and possible neurovascular symptoms.

Combined Motions

Combined movement testing is used to assess the patient who has full ROM, but still has complaints of pain. The following combinations are assessed:

- Elbow flexion, adduction, and forearm pronation.
- Elbow flexion, abduction, and forearm supination.
- Elbow extension, abduction, and forearm pronation.
- Elbow extension, adduction, and forearm supination.

 Clinical Pearl

Elbow flexion combined with supination should have a capsular end feel, whereas elbow flexion combined with pronation should have a bony end feel.

Resistive Testing

In addition to all of the shoulder muscles that insert at or near the elbow (biceps, brachialis, and triceps), the clinician must also test the other muscles responsible for elbow flexion and extension, in addition to the muscles involved with forearm supination, pronation, and wrist flexion and extension (Table 6-1).

 Clinical Pearl

Elbow flexion strength is normally 70% greater than extension strength.[2] Supination strength is normally 15% greater than pronation strength.[2]

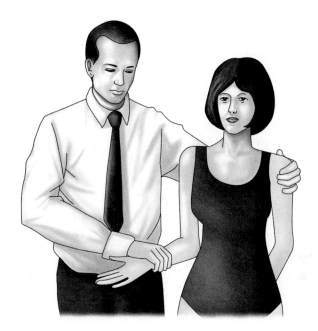

Figure 6-11 Resisted elbow flexion.

Elbow Flexion

Resisted elbow flexion is tested with the forearm in pronation, then supination (Figure 6-11) and then neutral rotation. Pain with resisted elbow flexion most frequently implicates the biceps, especially if resisted supination is also painful. The brachialis is implicated if resisted elbow flexion with the forearm in full pronation is painful. The brachioradialis is rarely involved. Weakness of elbow flexion could suggest median nerve, or C5–C8 nerve root compromise. Both sides are tested for comparison.

Elbow Extension

Resisted elbow extension is tested (Figure 6-12). Both sides are tested for comparison. Pain with resisted elbow extension implicates the triceps muscle, although the anconeus muscle could also be involved. Weakness of elbow extension could suggest radial nerve or C7–C8 nerve root compromise.

Forearm Pronation/Supination

The clinician should test the strength of the forearm muscles by grasping the patient's hand in a handshake. The patient should be asked to exert maximum pressure to turn the palm first up (using supinators) then down (using pronators).

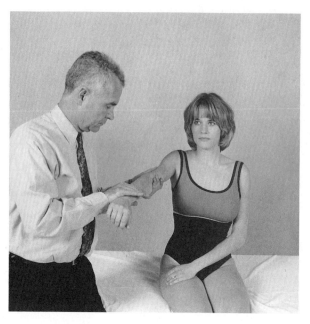

Figure 6-12 Resisted elbow extension.

Clinical Pearl

Weakness in the supinators may indicate tendonitis, a rupture, or a subluxation of the biceps tendon at the shoulder. It may also indicate a C5–C6 nerve root lesion, radial nerve lesion (supinator), or musculocutaneous nerve (C5–C6) lesion (biceps).

Clinical Pearl

Pronator weakness is associated with rupture of the pronator teres from the medial epicondyle, fracture of the medial elbow, and lesions of the C6–C7 or median nerve roots.

Pronator quadratus weakness, which is tested with the elbow held in a flexed position to neutralize the humeral head of the pronator teres muscle, could indicate a lesion of the anterior interosseous nerve.

> ### ⬤ Clinical Pearl
>
> The supinator, pronator teres, or quadratus muscles are rarely injured.

Individuals with medial or lateral epicondylitis will also find the afore-mentioned maneuvers painful, and resisted wrist flexion and extension can be used to help differentiate the former and latter, respectively.

Wrist Flexion
The flexor carpi ulnaris is the strongest wrist flexor. To test the flexors, the clinician stabilizes the patient's mid-forearm with one hand while placing the fingers of the other hand in the patient's palm, with the palm facing the patient. The patient's attempt to flex the wrist with the elbow flexed must be resisted. Weakness is evident in rupture of the muscle origin, lesions involving the ulnar (C8, T1) or median nerve (C6, C7), or tendonitis at the medial elbow.

Wrist Extension
The most powerful wrist extensor is the extensor carpi ulnaris. To test the extensors, the clinician's hands are placed in the same position as in the preceding test, with the patient's palm facing the clinician. The patient is asked to extend the wrist with the elbow flexed. Rupture of the extensor origin, lesions of the C6–C8 nerve root, or lateral tennis elbow can cause weakness.

Radial Deviation
Resisted radial deviation is tested with the elbow at 90 degrees of elbow flexion and at full elbow extension. Pain with resisted radial deviation is usually the result of a tennis elbow.

Ulnar Deviation
Resisted ulnar deviation, although rarely affected, is tested with the fingers in full flexion, and then in full extension.

Extension of Fingers 2-5
For resisted extension of the fingers 2-5, the elbow is positioned in full extension, the wrist in neutral, and the metacarpophalangeal (MCP) joints at 90 degrees of flexion. Pain here is usually the result of extensor digitorum tendonitis or tennis elbow.

Extension of Fingers 2-3

For resisted extension of the fingers 2-3, the patient is positioned as above. Pain with resistance implicates tennis elbow.

Functional Assessment

The elbow, like the shoulder, serves to position the hand for functional activities.

 Clinical Pearl

The essential arc of motion required for daily activities is 30 degrees to 130 degrees of total motions in the sagittal plane (flexion–extension), and 100 degrees of total motion in the transverse plane (50 degrees pronation to 50 degrees supination).[2]

Passive Physiological Articular Motion Testing

The accessory motions can be used for examination and intervention purposes, with the latter incorporating graded glides.

 Clinical Pearl

The open-packed positions and close-packed position of the joints of the elbow complex are as follows:

- Ulnohumeral: open packed—70 degrees elbow flexion, 10 degrees supination. Close packed—elbow extension with supination.

- Radiohumeral: open packed—full elbow extension and full supination. Close packed—elbow flexed to 90 degrees, forearm supinated to 5 degrees.

- Superior radioulnar joint: open packed—35 degrees supination, 70 degrees elbow flexion. Close packed—5 degrees supination.

Ulnohumeral Joint

The patient is positioned supine with their head supported. The clinician sits or stands facing the patient.

Distraction/compression

The clinician interlaces the fingers and wraps them around the proximal one third of the forearm (Figure 6-13). The clinician applies a longitudinal force

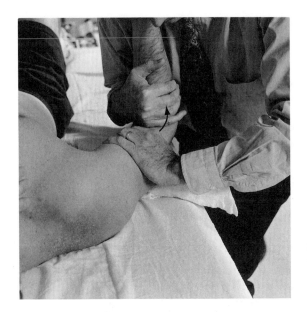

Figure 6-13 Ulnohumeral distraction.

through the proximal forearm and along the line of the humerus to distract the ulnohumeral joint. The quality and quantity of motion are noted. The test is repeated on the opposite extremity and the findings are compared.

Medial glide
The clinician, using the medial aspect of the MCP joint of the index finger of the medial hand, palpates and stabilizes the medial aspect of the distal humerus. Using the other hand, the clinician palpates the lateral aspect of the olecranon with the medial aspect of the MCP joint of the index finger (Figure 6-14). The elbow is extended to the limit of physiological ROM. From this position, the clinician glides the ulna medially on the fixed humerus along the medial–lateral plane of the joint line. The quality and quantity of motion are noted. The test is repeated on the opposite extremity and the findings are compared.

Lateral glide
The clinician, using the medial aspect of the MCP joint of the index finger of the medial hand, palpates and stabilizes the lateral aspect of the distal humerus. Using the other hand, the clinician palpates the medial aspect of the olecranon with the MCP joint of the index finger. The elbow is flexed to the limit of physiological ROM. From this position, the clinician glides the

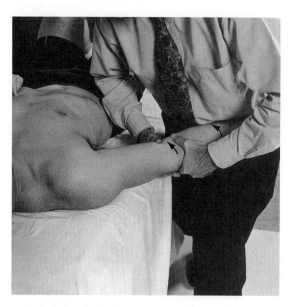

Figure 6-14 Medial glide of ulnohumeral joint.

ulna laterally on the fixed humerus along the medial–lateral plane of the joint line. The quality and quantity of motion are noted. The test is repeated on the opposite extremity and the findings are compared.

Radiohumeral Joint
The joint glides for the radiohumeral joint are performed with elbow positioned in 70 degrees flexion and 35 degrees of supination. The patient is positioned supine. The following tests are performed:

Distraction
The clinician places a thumb of the stabilizing hand between the radial head and the lateral epicondyle. With the other hand, the clinician grasps the radius and applies a longitudinal distraction force along the length of the radius (Figure 6-15). A longitudinal compression force can be applied using the same patient–clinician position.

Motion testing of the radial head
Once located, the clinician grasps the radial head between the thumb and index finger. The radial head is moved in an anterior and posterior direction, and any restriction of motion is noted. The posterior glide of the radius is coupled with pronation/extension, and anterior glide is coupled

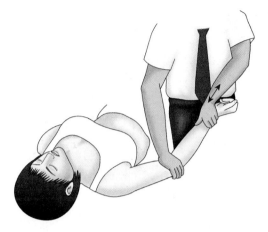

Figure 6-15 Distraction of radius.

with supination/flexion. The most common dysfunction of the radial head is a posterior radial head, which is accompanied with a loss of the anterior glide.

Proximal Radioulnar Joint

Anterior–posterior glide
The clinician palpates and stabilizes the proximal one third of the ulna with one hand. With a pinch grip of the index finger and thumb, the clinician palpates the head of the radius in a posterior–lateral plane with the other hand (Figure 6-16). From this position, the clinician glides the head of the radius anteriorly–posteriorly at the proximal radioulnar joint, in an obliquely anterior–medial/posterior–lateral direction. The quality and quantity of motion are noted. The test is repeated on the opposite extremity and the findings are compared.

Distal Radioulnar Joint

Anterior–posterior glide
The patient is positioned supine with their head resting on a pillow. The clinician palpates and stabilizes the distal one third of the ulna with one hand. With a pinch grip of the fingers and thenar eminence of the other hand, the clinician palpates the distal one third of the radius (Figure 6-17). From this position, the clinician glides the radius anteriorly/posteriorly at the distal radioulnar joint, in an obliquely anterior–medial/posterior–lateral direction. The quality and quantity of motion are noted. The test is repeated on the opposite extremity and the findings are compared.

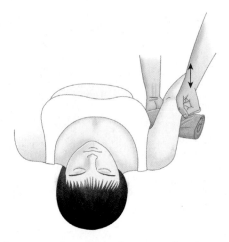

Figure 6-16 Anterior–posterior glide of proximal radioulnar joint.

Stress Tests

Medial (Ulnar) Collateral Ligament (Valgus Test)

The clinician stabilizes the distal humerus with one hand and palpates the distal forearm with the other. The anterior band of the MCL tightens in the ranges of 0 degrees to 90 degrees of flexion, becoming lax in full extension, before tightening again in hyperextension to about 20 degrees

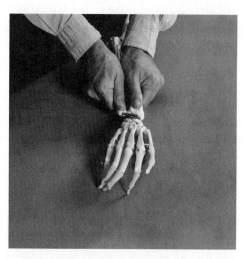

Figure 6-17 Anterior–posterior glide of distal radioulnar joint.

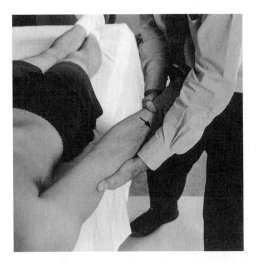

Figure 6-18 MCL stress test.

to 30 degrees of flexion. The posterior bundle is taut in flexion beyond 90 degrees.[15–18]

The anterior band is tested with the sustained application of a valgus stress while flexing the elbow to between 15 degrees and 30 degrees (Figure 6-18).[19,20]

The posterior band is best tested using a "milking" maneuver. The patient is seated and their arm is positioned in shoulder flexion, elbow flexion beyond 90 degrees, and forearm supination. The clinician pulls downward on the patient's thumb.[19] This maneuver generates a valgus stress on the flexed elbow. A positive sign is indicated by the reproduction of pain.

The tests are repeated on the opposite extremity and the findings compared.

 Clinical Pearl

There are no studies in the literature that discuss the sensitivity, specificity, positive predictive value, or negative predictive value of the valgus stress test.

Lateral Pivot-Shift Apprehension Test

The lateral pivot-shift test is used in the diagnosis of posterolateral rotatory instability. The patient is positioned supine with the involved extremity overhead. The clinician grasps the patient's wrist and elbow. The elbow is supinated with a mild force at the wrist, and a valgus moment and compressive force are applied to the elbow during flexion.[21] This results in a typical apprehension response with reproduction of the patient's symptoms and a sense that the elbow is about to dislocate. Reproducing the actual subluxation, and the clunk that occurs with reduction, usually can only be accomplished with the patient under general anesthesia or occasionally after injecting local anesthetic into the elbow.

Lateral (Radial) Collateral Ligament (Varus Test)

The lateral collateral ligament is tested with the elbow positioned in 15 degrees to 30 degrees short of full extension. The clinician stabilizes the humerus and adducts the ulnar, producing a varus force at the elbow (Figure 6-19). The end feel is noted and compared with the results from the same test on the other elbow.

⬤ Clinical Pearl

There are no studies in the literature that discuss the sensitivity, specificity, positive predictive value, or negative predictive value of the varus stress test.

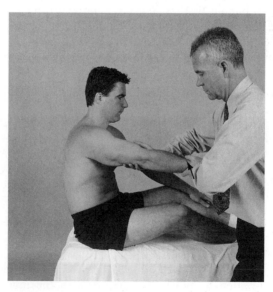

Figure 6-19 Lateral collateral ligament stress test.

Special Tests

Tennis Elbow

A number of tests exist for tennis elbow (lateral epicondylitis). Two are described here.

Cozen test

The clinician stabilizes the patient's elbow with one hand and the patient is asked to pronate the forearm, extend, and radially deviate the wrist against the manual resistance of the clinician (Figure 6-20). A reproduction of pain in the area of the lateral epicondyle indicates a positive test. There are no studies in the literature that discuss the sensitivity, specificity, positive predictive value, or negative predictive value of this maneuver.

Mill test

The clinician palpates the patient's lateral epicondyle with one hand, while pronating the patient's forearm, fully flexing the wrist, and extending the elbow. A reproduction of pain in the area of the lateral epicondyle indicates a positive test. There are no studies in the literature that discuss the sensitivity, specificity, positive predictive value, or negative predictive value of this maneuver.

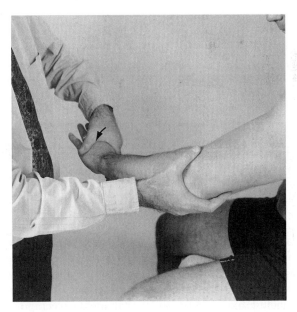

Figure 6-20 Cozen test.

Golfer's Elbow (Medial Epicondylitis)

The clinician palpates the medial epicondyle with one hand, while supinating the forearm, and extending the wrist and elbow with the other hand. A reproduction of pain in the area of the medial epicondyle indicates a positive test.

Elbow Flexion Test for Cubital Tunnel Syndrome

The patient is positioned in sitting. The patient is asked to depress both shoulders, flex both elbows maximally, supinate the forearms, and extend the wrists.[22] This position is maintained for 3 to 5 minutes. Tingling or paresthesia in the ulnar distribution of the forearm and hand indicates a positive test. There are no studies in the literature that discuss the sensitivity, specificity, positive predictive value, or negative predictive value of this maneuver.

Pressure Provocative Test for Cubital Tunnel Syndrome

With the elbow held in 20 degrees of flexion and the forearm in supination, the clinician applies pressure proximal to the cubital tunnel.[23] The test is positive if pain or paresthesia is elicited

Tinel Sign (at the Elbow)

The clinician locates the groove between the olecranon process and the medial epicondyle through which the ulnar nerve passes. This groove is tapped by the index finger of the clinician. A positive sign is indicated by a tingling sensation in the ulnar distribution of the forearm and hand distal to the tapping point.

Imaging Studies

Radiographs will confirm a fracture or dislocation, although some radial head or other articular surface fractures can be easily missed. Standard radiographs of the elbow consist of an anteroposterior (AP) view of the extended elbow and a lateral view with the elbow flexed to 90 degrees and with the forearm supinated.

 Clinical Pearl

Oblique views can be helpful in identifying subtle fractures and when the elbow cannot be extended enough to obtain an AP view.

The radial head normally articulates with the capitellum, and a line bisecting the proximal radial shaft should always pass through the capitellum on any radiographic view. Subtle radiographic signs such as bony avulsions or soft tissue swelling seen with a fat-pad sign can signal important bony injury. Special views include axial projections to evaluate the olecranon fossa, oblique views to assess the radial head, and stress views to evaluate joint stability.[24]

Clinical Pearl

When radiographs are normal, a tendon or ligament rupture, such as of the distal biceps or triceps, is possible.

 Clinical Pearl

Bone scanning is sensitive but not specific for detecting stress fractures, healing fractures, infections, and tumors.

Computed tomographic scanning is useful for delineating complex osseous anatomy. For example, these tests are useful in demonstrating if impingement from the olecranon or coranoid process is present, and are also useful in determining the presence of loose bodies.[2]

Magnetic resonance imaging (MRI) can be helpful in identifying soft tissue masses, articular cartilage anatomy, ligament ruptures, and chondral defects.

Arthrography may be useful for defining articular surfaces and identifying loose bodies or capsular defects.[25]

Electromyography and nerve conduction studies are used to evaluate suspected nerve compression syndromes.

Examination Conclusions—The Evaluation

Following the examination, and once the clinical findings have been recorded, the clinician must determine a specific diagnosis or a working hypothesis, based on a summary of all of the findings. This diagnosis can be structure related (medical diagnosis) (Table 6-8), or a diagnosis based on the preferred practice patterns as described in the "Guide to physical therapist practice."[26]

INTERVENTION

The rehabilitation procedures chosen to progress the patient will depend on the type of tissue involved, the extent of the damage, and the stage of healing (see Chapter 3). The intervention must be related to the signs and symptoms present rather than the actual diagnosis.

Table 6-8 Differential Diagnosis for Common Causes of Elbow Pain

Condition	Patient Age	Mechanism of Injury	Area of Symptoms	Symptoms Aggravated By	Observation	AROM	PROM	End Feel	Resisted	Special tests	Tenderness With Palpation
Bicipital tendonitis	20–50	Repetitive hyperextension of the elbow with pronation, or repetitive stressful pronation–supination	Anterior aspect of the distal part of the arm	Elbow extension and shoulder extension	Unremarkable	Possible pain with elbow flexion	Pain with passive shoulder and elbow extension		Pain on elbow flexion and supination		Distal biceps belly The musculotendinous portion of the biceps Bicipital insertion of the radial tuberosity
Triceps tendonitis	20–50	Overuse of the upper arm and elbow, especially in activities such as throwing and hammering	Posterior aspect of elbow	Activities involving elbow extension or full elbow flexion	Possible swelling near the point of the elbow	Elbow extension Possible pain with extreme elbow flexion	Pain with passive shoulder and elbow flexion		Pain on elbow extension		Posterior aspect of elbow
Lateral epicondylitis	35–55	Gradual overuse	Lateral aspect of elbow	Activities involving wrist extension/grasping	Possible swelling (over lateral elbow)	Possible pain on wrist flexion with elbow extension	Pain on wrist flexion with the forearm pronated and the elbow extended		Pain on resisted wrist extension and radial deviation, with the elbow extended Pain on finger extension	Cozen Mill	Lateral elbow (over the ECRB and ECRL)

(continued on following page)

Condition	Patient Age	Mechanism of Injury	Area of Symptoms	Symptoms Aggravated By	Observation	AROM	PROM	End Feel	Resisted	Special tests	Tenderness With Palpation
Medial epicondylitis	35–55	Gradual overuse	Anteromedial aspect of elbow	Activities involving wrist flexion	Possible swelling (over medial elbow)	Pain on wrist extension	Pain on combined wrist extension and forearm supination		Pain on pronation with wrist flexion	Passive supination of the forearm, and extension of the wrist and elbow	Anteromedial elbow
Olecanon bursitis	20–50	Trauma	Posterior aspect of elbow	Contact with posterior elbow	Swelling over posterior elbow	Possible pain with extreme elbow flexion	Pain on full elbow flexion		Strong and pain free		Posterior elbow
Ulnar collateral ligament Injury	20–45	Excessive valgus force to medial compartment of the elbow	Ulnar aspect of the elbow	Valgus stress of the elbow, throwing, pitching	May have ecchymosis over ulnar aspect	Pain with full extension possible	Passive extension of the elbow, valgus stress	Depends on severity	Usually unremarkable	Valgus stress with elbow flexed at approx 25 degrees and humerus in external rotation	Ulnar aspect of elbow
Ulnar nerve entrapment	20–40	Gradual overuse Trauma	Medial elbow, forearm, and hand Medial 11/2 fingers	Activities involving elbow and wrist extension	Atrophy of hand muscles if chronic	Inability to fully close hand	Full and pain free		Weakness of grip	Elbow flexion and pressure provocative test Tinel at elbow Wartenberg sign Froment sign	Anteromedial elbow

(continued on following page)

Table 6-8 *(continued from previous page)*

Condition	Patient Age	Mechanism of Injury	Area of Symptoms	Symptoms Aggravated By	Observation	AROM	PROM	End Feel	Resisted	Special tests	Tenderness With Palpation
Radial nerve entrapment	Varies	Can be overuse, direct trauma	Lateral elbow	Varies	Usually unremarkable	Usually unremarkable	Usually unremarkable		Pain with resisted forearm supination, resisted extension of middle finger	Tinel sign or tenderness along the course of the radial nerve	Maximal tenderness is usually elicited over the radial tunnel if radial tunnel syndrome
Median nerve entrapment	20–40	Gradual overuse	Anterior forearm Lateral 31/2 fingers	Activities involving full elbow extension or pronation of the forearm	Atrophy of anterior forearm and hand muscles if chronic	Pain on forearm pronation	Full and pain free		Weakness on pronation, wrist flexion, and thumb opposition	Benediction sign Inability to perform 'OK' sign (anterior interosseous syndrome) Resisted supination (compression of the lacertus fibrosis)	Over the pronator teres 4 cm distal to the cubital crease with concurrent resistance against pronation, elbow flexion, and wrist flexion - Pronator syndrome

ECRB = extensor carpi radialis brevis; ECRL = extensor carpi radialis longus.

COMMON ORTHOPEDIC CONDITIONS

ARTHRITIS OF THE ELBOW

Diagnosis

Arthritis of the elbow—ICD-9: 715.12.1 (osteoarthrosis, localized, primary, of the elbow), 714.02 (rheumatoid arthritis of the elbow), 274.02 (gouty arthropathy of the elbow), and 711.02 (pyogenic arthritis of the elbow).

Description

Arthritis of the elbow may result from numerous conditions including trauma, rheumatoid arthritis, crystalline diseases (gout, pseudogout), infection (septic arthritis), and osteoarthritis.

 Clinical Pearl

Osteoarthritis of the elbow is most common in men ages 40 to 60 years old with a history of strenuous work, throwing sports, or trauma.

Subjective Findings

The subjective findings vary according to the cause:

- Rheumatoid arthritis: pain and swelling. In advanced cases there may be complaints of instability.
- Nonrheumatoid inflammatory arthritis: acute pain, swelling, effusion, loss of motion, and warmth.
- Posttraumatic arthritis: pain or stiffness.
- Osteoarthritis: pain, stiffness, mechanical locking, and occasionally deformity.
- Septic arthritis: acute and severe pain, stiffness, warmth, swelling, effusion, constitutional symptoms of fever, chills, and malaise.

Objective Findings

The objective findings vary according to the cause:

- Rheumatoid arthritis: joint swelling, rheumatoid nodules over the olecranon and extensor surface of the forearm (on occasion), *tenderness*, joint instability (in advanced cases).

- Nonrheumatoid inflammatory and septic arthritis: severely painful and restricted ROM in the presence of significant effusion and warmth.
- Posttraumatic arthritis and osteoarthritis: minimum effusion, joint line tenderness.

Confirmatory/Special Tests

- Valgus/varus stability tests to help rule out/rule in joint instability.
- Cozen test to help rule out/rule in lateral epicondylitis.

Medical/Imaging Studies

If an effusion is present, aspiration and inspection of the joint fluid may be helpful.

AP and lateral radiographs of the elbow often are sufficient for diagnosis.

 Clinical Pearl

Rheumatoid arthritis produces the typical picture of osteopenia, symmetric joint narrowing, and periarticular erosions, or may show gross joint destruction.

Differential Diagnosis

- Elbow fracture (distal humerus or radial head).
- Elbow dislocation.
- Osteochondritis dissecans.
- Elbow instability.
- Medial or lateral epicondylitis.
- Synovial chondromatosis.

Intervention

The planned intervention varies according to the cause and severity:

- Osteoarthritis: rest, nonsteroidal anti-inflammatory drugs (NSAIDs), gentle stretching to preserve motion, and activity modification.
- Rheumatoid arthritis: intra-articular corticosteroid injection, gentle physical therapy, static/hinged splints.
- Nonrheumatoid inflammatory arthritis: treated medically to address the underlying pathology.

Prognosis

Arthroscopic debridement and removal of loose bodies can be quite helpful in cases of posttraumatic arthritis and osteoarthritis.

Synovectomy with or without radial head excision can provide pain relief in early stages of rheumatoid arthritis that is resistant to conservative intervention.

Total elbow arthroplasty is the best option for patients with rheumatoid arthritis who have advanced joint destruction.

FRACTURE OF THE RADIAL HEAD–NECK

Diagnosis

Fracture of the radial head–neck—ICD-9: 813.05 (fracture of head of radius), 813.06 (fracture of neck of radius).

Description

Radial head fractures are the result of trauma, usually from a FOOSH, with the force of impact transmitted up the hand through the wrist and forearm to the radial head, which is forced into the capitellum. Blunt or penetrating trauma rarely causes radial head injury. The wrist, especially the distal radioulnar joint, may be damaged simultaneously, and the presence of wrist pain, grinding, or swelling should be determined.

 Clinical Pearl

Radial head fractures are traumatic injuries that require adequate treatment to prevent disability from stiffness, deformity, posttraumatic arthritis, nerve damage, or other serious complications.

 Clinical Pearl

The Mason Johnston classification system is commonly used to separate radial fractures into four types:

• Type I: a nondisplaced or minimally displaced fracture.

- Type II: includes radial head fractures that are displaced more than 2 mm at the articular surface or angulated neck fractures that produce articular incongruity or a mechanical block.
- Type III: fractures that are severely comminuted fractures of the radial head and neck.
- Type IV: associated with ulnohumeral dislocation.

Subjective Findings

The subjective findings typically include the following:

- Complaints of pain and swelling over the lateral aspect of the elbow.
- Loss of elbow motion—related to pain inhibition and joint diffusion, but may also be related to a mechanical block.

● Clinical Pearl

The presence of bleeding, even with small puncture wounds, should alert the clinician to the possibility of open injury.

Neurovascular symptoms of numbness, tingling, or loss of sensation should be identified to rule out nerve or vascular injury.

The presence of severe pain should alert the clinician to the possibility of compartment syndrome.

Objective Findings

The clinician should palpate the elbow, especially the radial head, feeling for deformity, and the wrist should be examined, especially feeling for stability of the distal radioulnar joint. All three major nerves of the forearm are in danger with elbow fractures, so the clinician should also carefully assess neurovascular function for all of the nerves of the forearm and hand. The physical examination typically reveals the following findings:

- Tenderness to palpation over the lateral aspect of the elbow joint.
- Passive forearm pronation/supination is typically limited and may be associated with palpable crepitus.
- Active/passive elbow flexion and extension also may be limited by pain.

Clinical Pearl

Fractures of the radial head may rarely be associated with an Essex-Lopresti fracture—a fracture of the radial head with proximal radius migration and disruption of the distal radioulnar joint and interosseous membrane.

Confirmatory/Special Tests

Fractures of the radial head are diagnosed on the basis of patient history, physical examination, and results from imaging studies.

Medical/Imaging Studies

- Type I fractures may be difficult to visualize radiographically.
- Type II and III fractures are usually obvious on AP and lateral radiographs.

Differential Diagnosis

- Elbow dislocation.
- Supracondylar fracture of the humerus.
- Fracture of the olecranon.
- Hemarthrosis of the elbow.

Intervention

The intervention varies according to the type of fracture:

- Type I: initially placed in a sling or splint with early active motion as soon as pain allows. As much early mobilization as the patient can tolerate is the key to a favorable outcome. Strengthening, initially involving isometric exercises, begins at 3 weeks and progresses to concentric exercises at 5 to 6 weeks. Heavy resistance is not performed until after 8 weeks, or when adequate healing is demonstrated on radiographs.
- Type II: The rule of threes is used. Nonsurgical treatment is considered if the fracture involves less than one third of the articular surface, less than 30 degrees of angulation, and if the displacement is less than 3 mm. Type III fractures usually require operative intervention but may occasionally be treated closed with early motion if the radial head is not reconstructible. If a mechanical block to motion is present, then nonsurgical treatment cannot be used.
- Type III: best treated by early excision of the bone fragments.

Rehabilitation following elbow fractures that undergo internal fixation usually lasts for 12 weeks. Immediately following the immobilization of elbow fractures, active and passive motion exercises for flexion/extension are initiated. The goal is to achieve 15 to 105 degrees of motion by the end of week 2. Isometric exercises for elbow flexion and extension, and forearm pronation/supination are started within the first week. Active assistive pronation/supination exercises do not begin until week 6. Concentric exercises are given for the shoulder and the wrist and hand. Joint mobilizations, which begin if needed in the second week, are used to help regain elbow extension.

By the third week, the patient should be performing lightweight concentric exercises for elbow flexion and extension, and beginning at week 7, eccentric and plyometric exercises are prescribed. At about the same time, neuromuscular reeducation exercises and functional training exercises are added.

 Clinical Pearl

Radial head fractures present several challenges during the rehabilitative process, as the radial head is a secondary stabilizer for valgus forces at the elbow, and resists longitudinal forces along the forearm.

Prognosis

A successful outcome for this condition correlates directly with accuracy of anatomic reduction, restoration of mechanical stability that allows early motion, and attention to the soft tissues.

LATERAL EPICONDYLITIS

Diagnosis

Lateral epicondylitis—ICD-9: 726.32. More commonly known as tennis elbow.

Clinical Pearl

Although the terms *epicondylitis* and *tendonitis* are commonly used to describe tennis elbow, histopathological studies have demonstrated that tennis elbow is often not an inflammatory condition; rather, it is a degenerative condition, a tendonosis.

Description

A pathological condition of the common extensor muscles at their origin on the lateral humeral epicondyle. Specifically, the condition involves the tendons of the muscles that control wrist extension and radial deviation resulting in pain on the lateral side of the elbow with use of these muscles.

 Clinical Pearl

Tennis elbow affects between 1 and 3% of the population, occurs most commonly between the ages 35 and 50 years of age with a mean age of 45, is seldom seen in those less than 20 years of age, and usually affects the dominant arm.

Subjective Findings

An accurate history includes the description of the onset of symptoms, duration and progression of pain, history of a traumatic event, activities that worsen the pain, and previous treatments and outcomes.

• Complaints of diffuse achiness and morning stiffness of the elbow.

• Reports of localized tenderness over the lateral aspect of the elbow.

 Clinical Pearl

Repetitive grasping, with the wrist positioned in extension, places the elbow particularly at risk as it is the wrist extensors that must contract during grasping activities to stabilize the wrist. Participants of tennis, baseball, javelin, golf, squash, racquetball, swimming, and weight lifting are all predisposed to this risk.

Objective Findings

• Tenderness is usually found over the ECRB and ECRL, especially at the lateral epicondyle.

• Active motions are usually painless, although there may be pain with wrist flexion if combined with elbow extension.

• Passive motion can produce pain, especially passive wrist flexion with the forearm pronated and the elbow extended.

- The resisted tests typically reproduce symptoms especially resisted wrist extension and radial deviation with the elbow extended.

Confirmatory/Special Tests

- Cozen test—The clinician stabilizes the patient's elbow with one hand and the patient is asked to pronate the forearm, and extend and radially deviate the wrist against the manual resistance of the clinician (Figure 6-20). A reproduction of pain in the area of the lateral epicondyle indicates a positive test.
- Mill test—The clinician palpates the patient's lateral epicondyle with one hand, while pronating the patient's forearm, fully flexing the wrist, and extending the elbow. A reproduction of pain in the area of the lateral epicondyle indicates a positive test.

Medical Studies

Radiographs, which are typically used to rule out other diagnoses, will occasionally show soft tissue calcification at the origin of the ECRB.

Differential Diagnosis

- Radiocapitellar arthritis.
- Posterior interosseous nerve compression (radial tunnel syndrome).
- Osteochondritis dissecans of the capitellum.

Intervention

The ultimate treatment decision is based on a variety of factors, including the patient's overall medical condition, severity, and duration of symptoms, expectations, associated shoulder pathology, and surgeon preference. The intervention is directed at decreasing specific activities that cause pain, a progression of wrist extension strengthening exercises, and patient education. Cyriax recommends the Mill manipulation to treat true tennis elbow (the same procedure as the Mill test but with forcible elbow extension applied at the end), a thrust technique that is intended to maximally stretch the ECRB tendon to try to pull apart the two surfaces of the painful scar.

 Clinical Pearl

The benefit of tennis elbow braces remains unproven, although counterforce braces may reduce acceleration forces.

Corticosteroid injections have good results initially but high recurrence rates after 6 weeks.

Studies comparing the effects of phonophoresis versus ultrasound have shown that both treatment options result in decreased pain and increased pressure tolerance in selective soft tissue injuries.

Prognosis

Tennis elbow is normally a self-limiting complaint. Surgery is indicated in recalcitrant cases; several approaches are helpful but all include release of the common extensor tendon.

MEDIAL EPICONDYLITIS

Diagnosis

Medial epicondylitis—ICD-9: 726.31. Also referred to as golfer's elbow, medial tennis elbow, or bowler's elbow.

Description

Medial epicondylitis is a tendinopathy at the attachment of the flexor/pronator muscles at their origin. The mechanism for medial epicondylitis is not usually related to direct trauma, but rather to overuse. The overuse results in a strain on the small origin of the common tendon at the medial epicondyle that creates a high load per unit area.

 Clinical Pearl

Medial epicondylitis is only one third as common as lateral epicondylitis.[10]

Subjective Findings

An accurate history includes the description of the onset of symptoms, duration and progression of pain, history of a traumatic event, activities that worsen the pain, and previous treatments and outcomes. The following are typical findings:

• Complaints of pain along the medial elbow.

- History of unaccustomed or repetitive lifting, tooling, hammering, or sports activities involving tight gripping.
- Reports of increased pain with active wrist flexion and forearm pronation.

Objective Findings

- Tenderness with palpation at about 5 mm distal and anterior to the midpoint of the medial epicondyle.
- Pain elicited on resisted wrist flexion (with the elbow straight) and pronation.
- Pain at extremes of passive wrist extension with forearm supination (and elbow extension) and ulnar deviation.

Confirmatory/Special Tests

An increase in symptoms while pronating the forearm and flexing the wrist against resistance. Otherwise, the diagnosis is based on a history of medial epicondyle pain and on an examination showing local tenderness and pain aggravated by isometric wrist flexion, pronation, or both.

Medical Studies

Radiographs are not typically helpful, except to rule out other causes of medial elbow pain (arthritis or osteochondral loose bodies).

Differential Diagnosis

- MCL disruption.
- Synovitis of the elbow: swelling, palpable effusion.
- Fracture of the radial head: radiographs should differentiate.
- Medial compartment elbow arthritis.
- Osteochondral lesions of the trochlea and olecranon: medial joint line pain, symptoms of locking.
- Ulnar nerve neuropraxia (cubital tunnel syndrome): paresthesias in little and ring fingers.
- Osteoarthritis of the radiocapitellar portion of the elbow joint: radiographs should differentiate.
- Cervical spine disease.

Intervention

The ultimate treatment decision is based on a variety of factors, including the patient's overall medical condition, severity, and duration of symptoms, expectations, associated shoulder pathology, and surgeon preference. Conservative intervention for medial epicondylitis has been shown to have success rates as high as 90%.[10] The conservative intervention for this condition initially involves rest, activity modification, and local modalities. Complete immobilization is not recommended, even in the acute phase, as it eliminates the stresses necessary for maturation of new collagen tissue, resulting in healed tissue that is not strong enough to withstand the stresses associated with a return to activity. Once the acute phase has passed, the focus is to restore the ROM, and correct imbalances of flexibility and strength. The strengthening program is progressed to include concentric and eccentric exercises of the flexor pronator muscles.

Prognosis

Surgical debridement may be helpful in recalcitrant cases, the common tendon should not be released or should be reattached, if released.

OLECRANON BURSITIS

Diagnosis

Olecranon bursitis—ICD-9: 726.33. Also referred to as draftsman's elbow and student's elbow.

Description

Olecranon bursitis is inflammation of the bursa located between the olecranon process of the ulna and the overlying skin. Olecranon bursitis is common in students and wrestlers, as well as in those athletes who play basketball, football, indoor soccer, and hockey, in which the potential for falling and striking an elbow on hard playing surfaces is high.

 Clinical Pearl

Because of its location, the olecranon bursa is easily bruised through direct trauma or is irritated through repetitive grazing and weight bearing.

Subjective Findings

The subjective findings typically include the following:

- Complaints of pain and swelling that can be gradual as in chronic cases, or sudden as in acute injury or an infection.

- Patients often note a decreased ROM or an inability to don a long-sleeved shirt.

Objective Findings

The physical examination typically reveals the following findings:

- Swelling over the olecranon process (posterior aspect of the elbow) that can vary in size from a slight distension to a mass as large as 6 cm in diameter.
- No loss of active ROM at the elbow.

 Clinical Pearl

Redness and heat suggest infection, whereas exquisite tenderness indicates trauma or infection as the underlying cause.

Confirmatory/Special Tests

The definitive diagnosis is based on the laboratory evaluation of the bursal aspirate. Aspiration also helps to reduce the level of discomfort and restriction of movement.

 Clinical Pearl

Every patient with acute bursitis must undergo aspiration and laboratory testing to determine the definitive cause accurately.

Medical Studies

The intervention rarely is influenced by radiographic studies. Cell count, Gram stain, and crystal analysis help to differentiate acute traumatic bursitis from the inflammatory reaction of gout and infection.

Differential Diagnosis

- Septic bursitis
- Triceps tendonitis
- Acute fractures
- Rheumatoid arthritis
- Gout

- Synovial cysts
- Diabetes mellitus

Intervention

Although the simple posttraumatic bursitis can be treated with the principles of Protection, rest, ice, compression, elevation, manual therapy, early motion, and medications (PRICEMEM), the infected bursa needs prompt medical attention.

 Clinical Pearl

If the patient is experiencing significant pain or discomfort with movement of the elbow, a sling helps to reduce these symptoms and quiet the joint.

Prognosis

The success of the intervention depends on accurate diagnosis, appropriate therapy based on the laboratory studies, complete aspiration of the contents of the bursa, and protective padding to prevent recurrence.

 Clinical Pearl

Bursitis that recurs despite three or more repeated aspirations, or infection that does not respond to antibiotics, requires evaluation for surgical excision.

MEDIAL COLLATERAL LIGAMENT TEAR

Diagnosis

MCL tear—ICD-9: 841.1 (sprains and strains of elbow and forearm, MCL). Also referred to as UCL tears

Description

The MCL is the primary structure resisting valgus stress at the elbow. Associated injuries after trauma may include fractures of the radial head, olecranon, or medial humeral epicondyle. MCL injury also can be iatrogenic, secondary to excessive medial epicondylectomy for cubital tunnel syndrome. Irritation of the ulnar nerve, with symptoms of ulnar neuritis, may be present secondary to inflammation of the ligamentous complex.

 Clinical Pearl

The most common mechanisms of MCL insufficiency are a chronic attenuation of valgus and external rotation forces, as seen in the tennis serve or in the baseball throwing pitch, and posttraumatic, usually after a FOOSH injury.

Subjective Findings

The subjective findings typically include the following:

- Complaints of medial elbow pain at the ligament's origin, or at the insertion site if there is an acute avulsion.

Objective Findings

The physical examination typically reveals the following findings:

- Tenderness with palpation along the course of the MCL. Tenderness over the ulnar nerve and a positive Tinel sign are common.
- Possible loss of terminal elbow extension.
- Valgus stress test is positive.

Confirmatory/Special Tests

Valgus stress test.

Medical/Imaging Studies

- AP and lateral radiographs are necessary to rule out fracture.
- MRI with intra-articular contrast is the gold standard to image and diagnose pathology of the UCL.

Differential Diagnosis

- Cubital tunnel syndrome.
- Medial epicondyle avulsion.
- Medial epicondylitis.

Intervention

The intervention for early symptoms of MCL injury in the throwing athlete includes rest and activity modification or restriction for about 2 to 4 weeks, ROM exercises, physical therapy modalities, and nonsteroidal anti-inflammatory medications.

- Strengthening and stretching of the flexor carpi ulnaris, pronator teres, and flexor digitorum superficialis are initiated once the acute inflammatory stage has subsided, and are performed in the pain-free mid-ROM.

- Initial emphasis is placed on isometric exercises of the forearm flexors, ulnar deviators, and pronators to enhance their role as secondary stabilizers of the medial joint.

- Strengthening of the shoulder and elbow muscles may help prevent or minimize injury and may facilitate rehabilitation.

Prognosis

Operative repair of the MCL typically is required only in competitive throwing athletes or those involved in heavy manual labor, as valgus laxity has been shown to cause minimal functional impairment with normal activities of daily living. The surgical repair or reconstruction can be performed with or without ulnar nerve transposition.

REHABILITATION LADDER

ELBOW

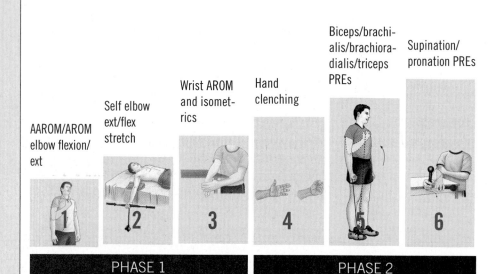

Biceps/brachi-
alis/brachiora-
dialis/triceps
PREs

Supination/
pronation PREs

Wrist AROM
and isomet-
rics

Hand
clenching

Self elbow
ext/flex
stretch

AAROM/AROM
elbow flexion/
ext

1 **2** **3** **4** **5** **6**

| PHASE 1 | PHASE 2 |

The purpose of these training ladders is to provide the clinician with a safe and progressive framework of exercises that are designed to allow the patient to improve in an efficient manner. The patient begins at the appropriate step, which is based on the stage of healing and the goal of the intervention.

- Phase 1: Acute—pain management, restoration of full passive range of motion, and restoration of normal accessory motion.

- Phase 2: Subacute—active range of motion exercises and early strengthening.

- Phase 3: Chronic—specific strengthening with a strong emphasis on enhancing dynamic stability.

The degree of movement and the speed of progression both are guided by the signs and symptoms. Once the patient is able to perform an exercise for

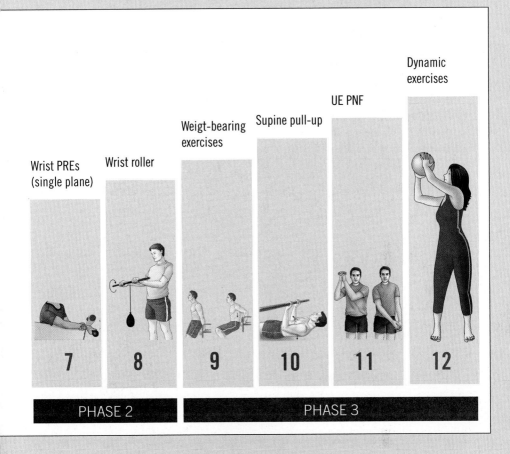

Wrist PREs (single plane) — 7

Wrist roller — 8

Weigt-bearing exercises — 9

Supine pull-up — 10

UE PNF — 11

Dynamic exercises — 12

PHASE 2 | PHASE 3

8–12 reps without pain, he or she progresses up to the next exercise step. This continues until the patient attempts an exercise that reproduces the pain. At this point, the patient returns to the last exercise that he or she was able to perform without pain and performs that exercise five times per day for 1 to 2 days before attempting to progress again. The patient is advanced through the training ladders to the appropriate point, with particular attention paid to patient response to treatment in terms of changes in symptoms, swelling, degree of irritability, or motion. In addition, muscle imbalances are addressed with appropriate flexibility exercises.

Once the patient is able to perform the last exercise of Phase 3 (Step 12 of the ladder), he or she can move on to functional and sport-specific training (Phase 4) as appropriate, which focus on power and higher-speed exercises similar to sport-specific demands.

1. Active Assisted Range of Motion (AAROM)/Active Range of Motion (AROM) of the elbow

The patient is positioned in sitting or standing. Using the hand of the uninvolved arm, the patient grips the wrist of the involved arm and moves the involved arm into elbow flexion and extension. The same method can be used for pronation and supination. Once able, the patient then performs the exercise actively (without help from the uninvolved arm) (1).

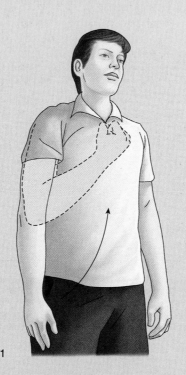

1

2. Passive elbow stretching

2a. To increase elbow flexion, the patient is positioned in sitting or standing and a towel roll is placed in the cubital fossa. Using the uninvolved arm, the patient flexes the elbow as far as can be tolerated using the towel as a fulcrum.

2b. To increase elbow extension, the patient is positioned supine with a weight attached to the wrist or grasped in the hand. The elbow is positioned in extension and the forearm is positioned in pronation. With the proximal humor stabilized the patient places the remainder of the arm over the side of the table allowing the elbow and shoulder to extend as far as possible as tolerated.

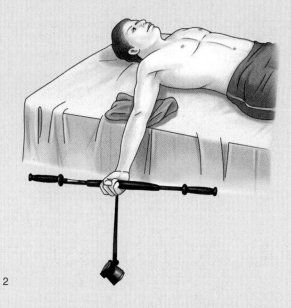

2

3. Wrist AROM with passive overpressure and isometrics

3a and 3b—The patient is positioned in sitting with the wrist and hand over the edge of the table. The patient is asked to actively flex/extend the wrist. At the end point in the active range, the patient is then asked to apply passive overpressure for 5 to 10 seconds and then to perform an isometric contraction in the opposite direction to the desired motion. For example, to increase wrist flexion, the patient first actively flexes the wrist, then applies passive overpressure into further wrist flexion, holds this position for 5 to 10 seconds, and then attempts to extend the wrist against an isometric block.

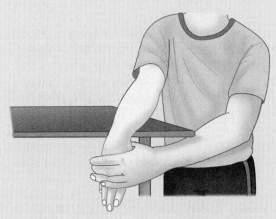

3a

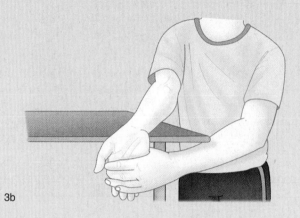

3b

4. Hand clenching

The patient is positioned in sitting or standing. Using a variety of wrist positions, the patient is asked to open and close the hand, holding the end range of each motion for 5 to 10 seconds.

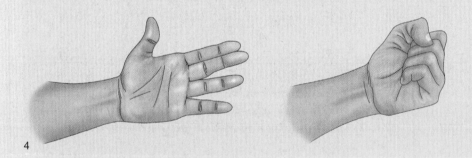

4

5. Biceps and triceps Progressive Resistive Exercises (PREs)

5a. The patient is positioned in sitting or standing with the arm by the side. The patient is asked to grasp the elastic tubing and to flex and extend the elbow, thereby concentrically and eccentrically strengthening the elbow flexors throughout the available range of motion. This motion is then performed with the forearm supinated, pronated, and in the midposition.

5b. The patient is positioned in sitting or standing with the arm held overhead and the elbow flexed so that the elastic tubing is near the shoulder. The patient is asked to pull the tubing while raising the arm toward the ceiling and then to lower it back to the opposition, thereby concentrically and eccentrically strengthening the elbow extensors. This motion is then performed with the forearm supinated, pronated, and in the midposition.

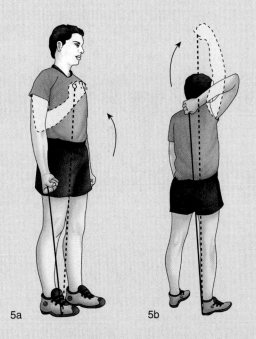

5a   5b

6. Pronation and supination PREs

The patient is positioned in sitting with the hand and wrist over the edge of a table. The patient is asked to grasp one end of the dumbbell and then to move the forearm into pronation (6a) or supination (6b), or both.

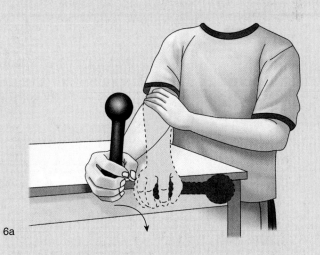

6a

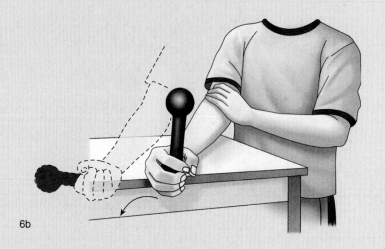

6b

7. Wrist PREs

The patient is positioned in sitting with the forearm supported by the table and the hand and wrist over the edge of the table, holding a small weight. When the forearm is pronated, resistance is against the wrist extensors (7a); when supinated, the resistance is against the wrist flexors (7b). Exercises for the radial and ulnar deviators can be performed by placing the forearm in the midposition between pronation and supination (7c).

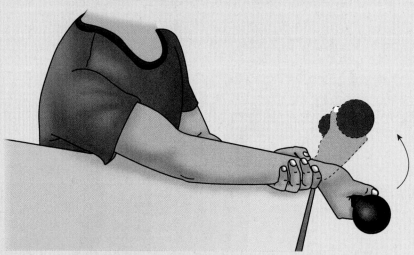

7a

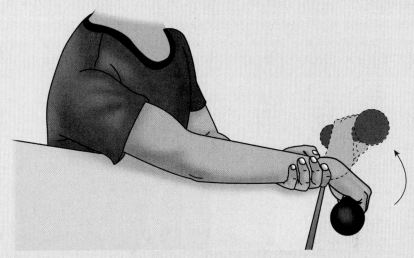

7b

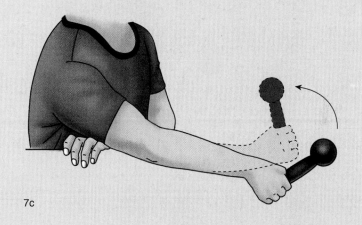

7c

8. Wrist roller exercise

The patient is positioned in sitting or standing, with the elbows flexed or extended and the forearms pronated or supinated. The patient holds each end of the rod (8) and, with alternating wrist action, turns the rod, causing the cord to wind around the rod and elevate the weight. The weight is then lowered with the reverse action.

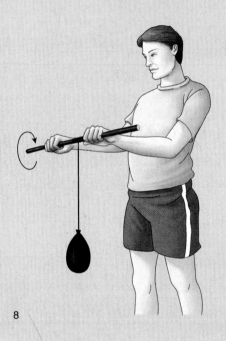

8

9. Weight-bearing exercises.

These exercises incorporate closed chain activities while using bodyweight as the resistance. Examples of these exercises include the triceps dip (9a), prone weight-bearing (9b), and the chair push-up (9c).

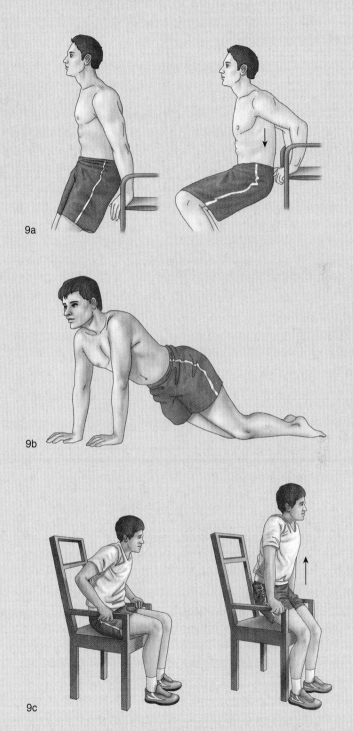

9a

9b

9c

10. Supine pull-up

The patient is positioned in supine. The patient is asked to grasp an overhead bar or trapeze and to perform a modified pull-up (10).

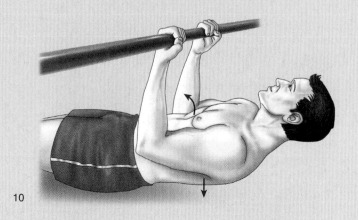

10

11. Upper extremity Proprioceptive Neuromuscular Facilitation (PNF)

Refer to Chapter 5 for full description.

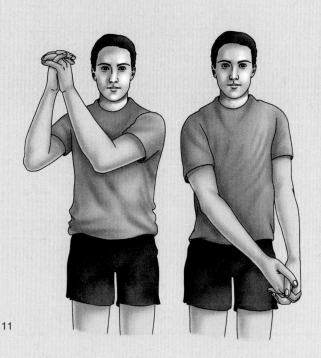

11

12. Dynamic strengthening
A variety of techniques can be used to dynamically strengthen the muscles of the upper quadrant using different types of resistance, including medicine balls (12), a Bodyblade, and a ProFitter.

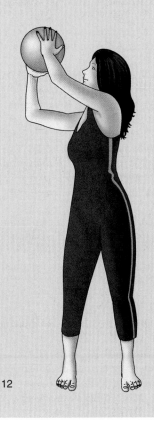

12

REFERENCES

1. Chumbley EM, O'Connor FG, Nirschl RP. Evaluation of overuse elbow injuries. *Am Fam Physician.* 2000;61:691–700.
2. Bell S. Examination of the elbow. *Aust Fam Physician.* 1988;17:391–392.
3. Woodward TW, Best TM. The painful shoulder: part I. Clinical evaluation. *Am Fam Physician.* 2000;61:3079–3088.
4. Colman WW, Strauch RJ. Physical examination of the elbow. *Orthop Clin North Am.* 1999;30:15–20.
5. An KN, Morrey BF. Biomechanics of the elbow. In: Morrey BF, ed. *The Elbow and Its Disorders.* 2nd ed. Philadelphia, PA: WB Saunders Co; 1993:53–73.

6. An KN, Morrey BF, Chao EY. The carrying angle of the human elbow joint. *J Orthop Res.* 1984;1:369–378.
7. Beals RK. The normal carrying angle of the elbow. A radiographic study of 422 patients. *Clin Orthop Relat Res.* 1976;119:194–196.
8. American Academy of Orthopaedic Surgeons. *Orthopedic Knowledge Update 4: Home Study Syllabus.* Rosemont, IL: The Academy; 1992.
9. Winkel D, Matthijs O, Phelps V. *Examination of the Elbow, Diagnosis and Treatment of the Upper Extremities.* Maryland, MD: Aspen; 1997:207–233.
10. Jobe FW, Ciccotti MG. Lateral and medial epicondylitis of the elbow. *J Am Acad Orthop Surg.* 1994;2:1–8.
11. Pecina MM, Krmpotic-Nemanic J, Markiewitz AD. *Tunnel Syndromes.* Boca Raton, FL: CRC Press; 1991.
12. Vennix MJ, Werstsch JJ. Entrapment neuropathies about the elbow. *J Back Musculoskel Rehabil.* 1994;4:31–43.
13. Morrey BF, Askew LJ, Chao EYS. A biomechanical study of normal functional elbow motion. *J Bone Joint Surg Am.* 1981;63:872–877.
14. Hammer WI. *Functional Soft Tissue Examination and Treatment by Manual Methods.* Gaithersburg, MD: Aspen; 1991
15. Morrey BF. Applied anatomy and biomechanics of the elbow joint. *Instr Course Lect.* 1986;35:59–68.
16. Morrey BF, An KN, Chao EYS. Functional evaluation of the elbow. In: Morrey BF, ed. The *Elbow and Its Disorders.* 2nd ed. Philadelphia, PA: WB Saunders; 1993:86–97.
17. Morrey BF, An KN. Articular and ligamentous contributions to the stability of the elbow joint. *Am J Sports Med.* 1983;11:315–319
18. Morrey BF, An KN. Functional anatomy of the ligaments of the elbow. *Clin Orthop Relat Res.* 1985;201:84–90.
19. Jobe FW, Kvitne RS. Elbow instability in the athlete. *Instr Course Lect.* 1991;40:17–23.
20. Conway JE, Jobe FW, Glousman RE, et al. Medial instability of the elbow in throwing athletes: treatment by repair or reconstruction of the ulnar collateral ligament. *J Bone Joint Surg Am.* 1992;74:67–83.
21. O'Driscoll SW, Bell DF, Morrey BF. Posterolateral rotatory instability of the elbow. *J Bone Joint Surg.* 1991;73:440–446.
22. Buehler MJ, Thayer DT. The elbow flexion test. A clinical test for cubital tunnel syndrome. *Clin Orthop Relat Res.* 1988;233:213–216.
23. Novak CB, Lee GW, Mackinnon SE, et al. Provocative testing for cubital tunnel syndrome. *J Hand Surg Am.* 1994;19:817–820.
24. Tamisiea DF. Radiologic aspects of orthopedic diseases. In: Mercer LR, ed. *Practical Orthopedics.* 4th ed. St Louis, MO: Mosby; 1995: 327–418.
25. Tung GA, Brody JM. Contemporary imaging of athletic injuries. *Clin Sports Med.* 1997;16:393–417.
26. American Physical Therapy Association. Guide to physical therapist practice. *Phys Ther.* 2001;81:9–746.

QUESTIONS

1. What are the three articulations that make up the elbow complex?
2. What is the normal carrying angle of the elbow?
3. What are the three primary stabilizers of the elbow?
4. Which muscle is considered the "workhorse" of elbow flexion?
5. Which nerve of the brachial plexus innervates the triceps muscle?
6. Which nerve of the brachial plexus innervates the brachialis?
7. Which peripheral nerve is vulnerable to compression on the posterior aspect of the elbow?
8. Which peripheral nerve can be compressed at the arcade of Fröhse?
9. What two elbow conditions are associated with clicking or locking of the elbow with terminal extension?
10. Which wrist and forearm motions tend to aggravate medial epicondylitis of the elbow?
11. What is Little League elbow?
12. What is the medical term for tennis elbow?
13. What is a Granger?
14. What is a Laugier fracture?
15. What is the most common type of elbow dislocation?
16. Which nerve is compressed in pronator teres syndrome?
17. The anterior interosseous nerve is a branch of which nerve?
18. What is the common name given to a compression injury in the portion of the radial nerve between the radiospiral groove and the lateral intramuscular septum?
19. What is the normal range of motion for forearm pronation?
20. What is the capsular pattern of the elbow (humeroulnar joint)?
21. What is the open-packed position of the superior radioulnar joint?

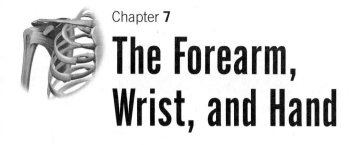

Chapter **7**

The Forearm,
Wrist, and Hand

OVERVIEW

Although the shoulder, elbow, and wrist serve to position the hand, it is only the hand that is capable of producing a remarkable level of dexterity and precision.

 Clinical Pearl

The hand accounts for about 90% of upper limb function.[1]

The thumb, which is involved in 40% to 50% of hand function, is the most functionally important of the digits.[1]

The index finger, involved in about 20% of hand function, is the second most important, and the ring finger the least important.

The middle finger, which accounts for about 20% of all hand function, is the strongest finger, and is important for both precision and power functions.[1]

ANATOMY

An understanding of the forearm, wrist, and hand requires an intimate knowledge of the respective bones, joints, soft tissues, and nerves of the hand and wrist, detailing both their individual and collective functions.

The open-packed, close-packed, and capsular patterns of the wrist and hand are outlined in Table 7-1.

439

Table 7-1 The Open-pack and Close-pack Positions, and Capsular Patterns for the Articulations of the Wrist and Hand

Joint	Open Pack	Close Pack	Capsular Pattern
Distal radioulnar	10 degree of supination	5 degree of supination	Minimal to no limitation with pain at the end ranges of pronation and supination
Radiocarpal (wrist)	Neutral with slight ulnar deviation	Extension	Equal limitation of flexion and extension
Intercarpal	Neutral or slight flexion	Extension	None
Midcarpal	Neutral or slight flexion with ulnar deviation	Extension with ulnar deviation	Equal limitation of flexion and extension
Carpometacarpal	Thumb—Midway between abduction and adduction and mid way between flexion and extension	Thumb—Full opposition	Thumb—Abduction then extension
	Fingers—Midway between flexion and extension	Fingers—Full flexion	Fingers—Equal limitation in all directions
Metacarpophalangeal	Slight flexion	Thumb—Full opposition Fingers—Full flexion	Flexion then extension
Interphalangeal	Slight flexion	Full extension	Flexion, extension

 Clinical Pearl

Proper diagnosis and management of wrist and hand injuries are vital to maintaining proper function of the hand and preventing permanent disability.

EXAMINATION

The examination of the wrist and hand requires a sound knowledge of surface anatomy and differential diagnosis, and must include an examination of the entire upper kinetic chain, and the cervical and thoracic spine.

Clinical Pearl

Most hand and wrist problems can be diagnosed by carefully consider-
ing three factors: anatomy, mechanism of injury, and epidemiology.

History

All relevant information must be gathered about the site, nature, behavior,
and onset of the current symptoms. This should include information about the
patient's age, hand dominance, avocational activities, and occupation.

 Clinical Pearl

Activities or occupations that involve sustained non-neutral positions of the hand and wrist subject nerves to prolonged stretch and
periods of high pressure.[2] In addition, these positions place muscles
at inefficient length–tension relationships,[3] resulting in decreased
transmission of contractile forces to the fingers.[3,4]

The history should include questions about the following:

- When and how did the injury occur? If the problem is trauma related, the
  clinician should ascertain the following:
  - The forces applied. If the patient describes the mechanism of injury as a
    Fall On an Out Stretched Hand (FOOSH) injury, the history can provide
    some important clues (Table 6-5).[5]
  - Where and when did the injury occur?
  - The position of the wrist and hand at the time of the trauma.
  - Whether the environmental conditions at the time of injury were clean or
    dirty. The environment in which the injury took place as well as the inflict-
    ing instrument help determines the level of contamination, and therefore
    the risk of infection.[6] In cases of potential contamination, it is well worth
    checking the patient's tetanus status.
  - Whether there was an accompanying "pop" or "click." The presence of pops
    and clicks at the time of injury could indicate a fracture or ligamentous tear.
  - Whether swelling occurred and if so, how and where. Refer to
    Observation.
- If the problem is nontrauma related, the onset of pain or sensory change,
  swelling, or contracture should be ascertained.

- Are there any local areas of tenderness? Determining the location of the pain can provide some clues as to the cause (Figure 7-1).
  - Radial pain: posttraumatic tenderness and pain over the radial aspect of the wrist may suggest a fracture of the scaphoid. In the absence of trauma, pain associated with tenderness over the radial styloid is most likely de

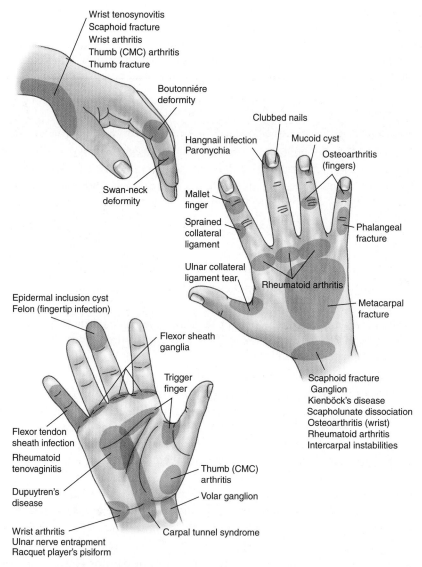

Figure 7-1 Pain locations of the wrist and hand and possible causes.

Quervain tenosynovitis. Pain that is posterior (dorsal) and slightly more proximal may be caused by intersection syndrome (tenosynovitis of the radial wrist extensors) or superficial radial neuritis.

- Posterior pain: generalized posterior wrist pain may be associated with radial carpal arthritis. Pain associated with a defined mass over the posterior-radial aspect of the wrist is usually the result of a ganglion cyst.
- Ulnar pain: pain in this region following trauma can be caused by a tear of the triangular fibrocartilage complex (TFCC).
- Anterior (palmar) pain: the most common causes of anterior wrist pain are carpal tunnel syndrome, ganglion cyst formation, and tenosynovitis.
- Are they any associated medical factors? Factors such as medications, malnutrition, diabetes, Raynaud's and immunosuppression may inhibit the healing process.[6]
- The sequence of symptoms, the level of functional impairment, the progression of symptoms, the time of day the symptoms are worse, and whether the symptoms appear to be posture, or work-related.
- The past behavior of previous wrist, hand and finger disorders, and their interventions

Clinical Pearl

In addition to pain, patients with chronic wrist and hand injuries typically have one or more of the following symptoms:

- Stiffness: morning stiffness is a common symptom of arthritis or tenosynovitis.
- Swelling: swelling in the joints of the hand and wrist is caused by synovitis, which can be secondary to osteoarthritis, infection, or a systemic inflammatory disease (such as rheumatoid arthritis (RA) or gout). Pain and swelling around the wrist flexor or extensor tendons suggest tendonitis.
- Instability: typical symptoms include sensations of clicking, popping, or clunking with certain wrist motions after an injury. Chronic ligamentous instability commonly occurs in the metacarpophalangeal (MCP) joint of the thumb.
- Weakness: weakness in the hand may be secondary to pain. Weakness in the absence of pain suggests possible peripheral nerve entrapment.
- Numbness: numbness/paresthesia is commonly associated with entrapment neuropathy.

> • A mass/growth: the most common mass in the hand and wrist is a ganglion cyst.

The patient's goals should be ascertained. Dysfunction of the hand can be very disabling, so inquiries concerning the functional demands of the patient must be made, and the intervention tailored accordingly.

Systems Review

Elucidating the cause of forearm, wrist, and hand pain can be challenging. The examination must include all regions that may contribute to the symptoms of forearm wrist and hand symptoms to determine the suitability of the patient for physical therapy. This requires a sound knowledge of differential diagnosis, and often incorporates an examination of the entire upper kinetic chain, including the cervical and thoracic spine.

 Clinical Pearl

All inflammatory conditions, whether infectious or not, are accompanied by diffuse pain or tenderness with movement. RA often affects this region with more severity and frequency than elsewhere. Therefore, questions concerning other joint involvement and general debility must be asked. The presence of carpal tunnel syndrome, which is usually felt at night, may also indicate RA.

Tests and Measures

Observation

The physical examination of the wrist and hand should begin with a general observation of the patient's posture, especially the cervical and thoracic spine, and the position of hand in relation to the body. For example, the clinician should note whether the arm is held against the chest in a protective manner, or whether the arm swings normally during gait, or whether it just hangs loosely.

 Clinical Pearl

Dupuytren contracture is a benign, slowly progressive fibroproliferative disease of the palmar fascia. The etiology of Dupuytren disease is thought to be multifactorial. There is a higher incidence in the alcoholic population, the diabetic population, and the epileptic population.[7-9] Although not usually related to hand trauma, Dupuytren disease occasionally develops after significant hand injuries, including surgery.[10] The diagnosis of Dupuytren disease in its early stages may be difficult and is based on the palpable nodule, characteristic skin changes, changes in the fascia, and progressive joint contracture. The skin changes are caused by a retraction of the skin, resulting in dimples or pits.

The clinician inspects the wrist and hands for evidence of lacerations, surgical scars, masses, localized swelling, or erythema.

- Scars should be examined for their degree of adherence, degree of maturation, hypertrophy (excess collagen within boundary of wound), and keloid (excess collagen that no longer conforms to wound boundaries).
- A determination is made as to whether the swelling is generalized or localized, hard or soft. Localized swellings can suggest the presence of a ganglion. Localized swelling, accompanied with redness and tenderness may indicate an infection.
- The location and type of edema should be noted.
  - Swellings on the posterior aspect can be highlighted by passively flexing the wrist.
  - Anterior effusion over the flexor tendons at the wrist may indicate rheumatoid tenovaginitis.

Clinical Pearl

Rings and other jewelry should be removed if swelling has the potential to turn these objects into a tourniquet, even if the swelling appears to be remote.[6]

Clinical Pearl

Swelling following trauma for more than a few days probably suggests a carpal fracture.

The posture and alignment of the wrist and hand is examined:

- Wrist angulation into ulnar deviation increases shearing in the first posterior (dorsal) compartment. This angulation can predispose the patient to

De Quervain syndrome.[11] A prominence of the distal ulna may indicate distal radioulnar joint instability.[12]

- The normal resting hand exhibits progressively increasing digital flexion as one progresses from the index to little fingers. An alteration in this normal cascade is often present in tendon injuries.[6]

- The contour of the anterior surface, including the arches, should be examined. If a finger is involved, its attitude should be observed. Digital deformities are the hallmark of RA.[13] Atrophy of the thenar muscles is indicative

 Clinical Pearl

An indirect method of assessing the integrity of the flexor tendons is to apply digital pressure over the ulnar anterior aspect of the forearm at the junction of the middle and distal thirds of the forearm. If the tendons are intact, the fingers will flex, especially the ulnar three.[6] Pressure over the radial aspect causes flexion of the thumb if the flexor pollicis longus tendon is intact.[6]

of a median nerve injury, whereas atrophy of the hypothenar muscles is indicative of an ulnar injury. Pain elicited by pressure over the thumb MCP joint suggests arthritis or instability of this joint.

- Any wrist and finger deformities should be noted. For example, a wrist deformity of radial deviation with a prominent ulna could suggest a Colles fracture. Finger deformities include mallet finger, swan-neck deformity (PIP joint hyperextension with concurrent distal interphalangeal [DIP] joint flexion), and boutonniere, in addition to those caused by fractures and dislocations (Table 7-2).[14–16]

The nails should be inspected to see if they are healthy, and pink. Local trauma to the nails seldom involves more than one or two digits. The nails should be checked for hangnail infection, or whether they appear ridged, which could indicate a RA dysfunction. Clubbed nails are an indication of hypertrophy of underlying structures.

 Clinical Pearl

The presence of a paronychia or a paleparonychia should prompt the clinician to probe the axilla and neck lymph nodes for tenderness and swelling.

Table 7-2 Hand and Finger Deformities and Their Possible Causes

Deformity	Possible Cause
MCP joint flexion	Rupture of the extensor tendon just proximal to the MCP joint
Mallet finger: resting DIP flexion due to a loss of active extension at the DIP joint	The result of excessive stretching or tearing of the extensor tendon mechanism at or near the DIP joint
Hyperextension of the MCP joint	Paralysis of the interossei
Deepening of the palmar gutter, and an inability to fully stretch out the palm	Tightness of the palmar aponeurosis
Wasting of the hypothenar eminence and a clawed hand with flexion of the fourth and fifth digits (hand of benediction)	Ulnar nerve palsy
Wrist drop with increased flexion of the wrist, flexion of the MCP joint, and extension of the DIP joints	Radial nerve lesion
Isolated thenar atrophy	Arthritis of the carpometacarpal joint Median nerve lesion C8 or the T1 nerve root lesion
Ape-hand deformity with a wasting of the thenar eminence, and an inability to oppose or flex the thumb or abduct it in its own plane[*]	Median nerve palsy
Z-deformity of the wrist	Pattern of deformity in the rheumatoid hand[†]
Atrophy of the hand intrinsics	Pancoast tumor
Claw hand deformity	Loss of the ulnar nerve motor innervation to the hand, with resultant paralysis of the interosseous muscles, and muscle atrophy of the hypothenar eminence. This deformity is more severe in lesions distal to innervation of the FDP muscle, as this muscle adds to the flexion force upon the IP joints[‡]
PIP hyperextension and slight flexion of the DIP	Rupture or paralysis of the FDS
A fixed flexion deformity of the MCP and proximal interphalangeal joints, especially in the ring or little finger	Dupuytren contracture
A hook-like contracture of the flexor muscles, which is worse with wrist extension as compared to flexion	Volkmann ischemic contracture

(continued on following page)

Table 7-2 *(continued from previous page)*

Deformity	Possible Cause
PIP joint flexion and DIP joint and MCP joint hyperextension of the finger (boutonnière deformity)	Flexion of the PIP joint is caused by disruption of the common extensor tendon (central slip) that inserts on the base of the middle phalanx. The disruption results in the lateral bands migrating anteriorly to the PIP joint as the head of the proximal phalanx moves posteriorly through the gap created by the central slip rupture

Data from references *, 14; †, 15; ‡, 16.

Beau lines are transverse furrows that begin at the lunula (the crescent-shaped whitish area of the bed of the fingernail) and progress distally as the nail grows. They result from a temporary arrest of growth of the nail matrix caused by trauma or systemic stress.[17] Spoon nails (koilonychias) may occur in a form of iron deficiency anemia, coronary disease, and with the use of strong detergents.[17] Clubbing of the nails, characterized by a bulbous enlargement of the distal portion of the digits, may occur in association with cardiovascular disease, subacute endocarditis, advanced cor pulmonale, and pulmonary disease.[17]

Finger color should be observed. Fingers that are white in appearance might indicate Raynaud disease. Blotchy or red fingers might indicate liver disease. Blue fingers may indicate a circulatory problem.

 Clinical Pearl

Muscle atrophy in the hand likely indicates a nerve compression syndrome. Atrophy of the thenar eminence suggests median nerve involvement, whereas atrophy of the hypothenar eminence suggests ulnar nerve involvement.

Active Range of Motion (AROM), Then Passive Range of Motion (PROM) With Overpressure

The gross motions of wrist, hand, finger, and thumb flexion, extension, and radial and ulnar deviation are tested, first actively and then passively (Table 7-3). Palpation may be performed with the range of motion tests or separately (refer to Palpation).

Table 7-3 Active Range of Motion Norms for the Forearm, Wrist, and Hand

Motion	Degrees
Forearm pronation	85–90
Forearm supination	85–90
Radial deviation	15
Ulnar deviation	30–45
Wrist flexion	80–90
Wrist extension	70–90
Finger flexion	MCP: 85–90; PIP: 100–115; DIP: 80–90
Finger extension	MCP: 30–45; PIP: 0; DIP: 20
Finger abduction	20–30
Finger adduction	0
Thumb flexion	CMC: 45–50; MCP: 50–55; IP: 85–90
Thumb extension	MCP: 0; IP: 0–5
Thumb adduction	30
Thumb abduction	60–70

Clinical Pearl

During flexion of the fingers, the overall area of the fingers should converge to a point on the wrist corresponding to the radial pulse. This can only occur if the index finger flexes in a sagittal plane and all the others in an increasing oblique plane. Malrotation is a rotary malalignment that can be seen in phalangeal or metacarpal fractures with this maneuver, as the involved finger will not converge with the others.[6] A skyline view of the knuckles is made. In full flexion, a posteriorly subluxed capitate may be seen as a local swelling on the back and middle of the flexed wrist.

Clinical Pearl

During measurement of motion, one must be aware that finger joint positions may affect wrist joint ranges (and vice versa) due to the constant length of the extrinsic tendons that cross multiple joints. For example, greater wrist flexion occurs with finger extension than with finger flexion because the extensor digitorum tendons are not stretched maximally. Thus, during the examination, the clinician should maintain all joints in a consistent position (usually neutral), except the one being measured. In addition, the clinician should identify wrist and finger joint position when measuring the strength of related muscles.

Fanning and folding of the hand is performed by palpating the anterior surface of the pisiform, scaphoid, hamate, and trapezium with the index and middle fingers, and the posterior surface of the capitate with the thumbs as the hand is alternately fanned and folded. During these motions, the clinician should note the quantity and quality of the conjunct rotations.

 Clinical Pearl

During active and passive testing, the presence of crepitus must be determined. The presence of crepitus with motion may indicate a tendon sheath synovitis or vaginitis.

Wrist

Pronation and supination of the wrist on the forearm will provisionally test the TFCC, and the proximal and distal radioulnar (PRUJ and DRUJ) joints.

 Clinical Pearl

Full forced pronation–supination without evoking pain, essentially eliminates the DRUJ and the TFCC as potential sources of the patient's complaints.[18]

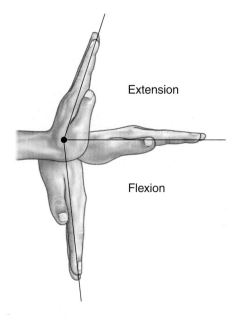

Figure 7-2 Wrist flexion and extension.

Wrist flexion, extension, (Figure 7-2) ulnar deviation, and radial deviation (Figure 7-3) are assessed. Wrist extension can be tested bilaterally by asking the patient to place the palms together and then to lift up the elbows.

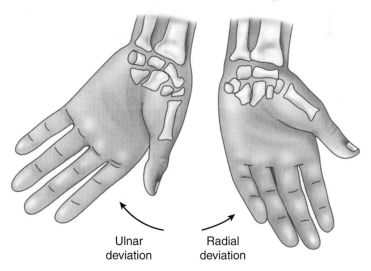

Figure 7-3 Radial and ulnar deviation.

Wrist flexion is tested bilaterally by asking the patient to place the posterior aspect of the hands together and then dropping the elbows. Radial and ulnar deviations are also assessed. Radial deviation should be tested in three positions: forearm pronation, forearm supination, and neutral.

 Clinical Pearl

If the single plane motions do not provoke symptoms, combined motions can be used. These include combining wrist extension with ulnar and then radial deviation, and combining wrist flexion with ulnar and radial deviation.

Thumb

The following motions are tested in varying degrees of wrist flexion and extension:

- First CMC abduction, adduction, flexion, extension, opposition. During opposition (Figure 7-4), the clinician should observe for the conjunct rotation component of the motion.
- First MCP (Figure 7-5), and IP flexion and extension (Figure 7-6)

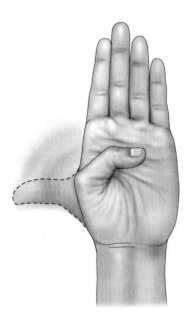

Figure 7-4 Thumb opposition.

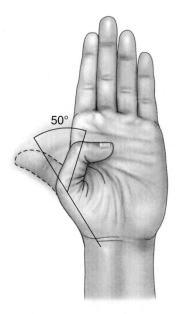

Figure 7-5 Flexion and extension of the first MCP joint.

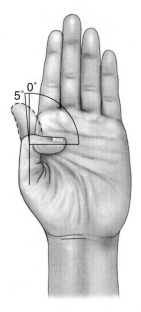

Figure 7-6 Flexion and extension of the first IP joint.

Fingers

Total active motion of the fingers is the sum of all angles formed by the MP, PIP, and DIP joints in simultaneous maximum active flexion, minus the total extension deficit at the MP, PIP, and DIP joints (including hyperextension at the IP joints) in maximum active extension.

 Clinical Pearl

It should never be assumed that lack of full active flexion or extension of the PIP is merely secondary to joint pain or fusion, because a closed rupture of the middle slip of the extensor hood is easily missed until the appearance of a boutonniere deformity.[19]

A comparison of active and passive motion indicates the efficiency of flexor and extensor excursion and/or degree of muscle strength within the available passive range of motion.[20] Instances of greater passive than active motion may indicate a limited tendon glide due to adherence of the tendon to surrounding structures, relative lengthening of the tendon due to injury or surgery, weakness or pain.[20]

 Clinical Pearl

A normal value for total active range of motion in the absence of a normal contralateral digit for comparison is 260 degree, based on 85 degree of MP flexion, 110 degree of PIP motion, and 65 degree of DIP motion.[20]

Due to the multitude of joints and multiarticular muscles found in the hand, the clinician may need to differentiate between various structures to determine the cause of a motion restriction. The soft tissue structures that may contribute to a motion restriction include the following[20]:

• Hand intrinsics. The Bunnell–Littler test (also known as the intrinsic-plus test) is used to determine whether flexion restriction of the PIP is due to tightness of the intrinsic muscles, or to a restriction of the MCP joint capsule. The MCP joint is held by the clinician in a few degrees of extension with one hand, whereas the other hand attempts to flex the PIP joint. If the joint cannot flex, tightness of the intrinsics or a joint capsular contraction should be suspected.[21] From this position, the clinician now slightly flexes the MCP joint, thereby relaxing the intrinsics, and attempts to flex the PIP joint. If the joint can now flex, the intrinsics are tight. If the joint still cannot flex, then restriction is probably due to a capsular contraction of the joint.

- Oblique retinacular (Landsmeer) ligament. The Haines–Zancolli test is used to determine whether restricted flexion in the DIP joints is due to a restriction of the proximal interphalangeal (PIP) joint capsule, or tightness of the oblique retinacular ligament. The test for a contracture of this ligament is the same as the Bunnell–Littler test, only at the PIP and DIP joints. The clinician positions and holds the PIP joint in a neutral position with one hand, and attempts to flex the DIP joint with the other hand. If no flexion is possible, it can be due to either a tight retinacular ligament or capsular contraction. The PIP joint is then slightly flexed to relax the retinacular ligament. If the DIP can now flex, the restriction is due to tightness in the retinacular ligament. If the DIP cannot flex, then the restriction is due to a capsular contraction.

- Extrinsic flexor and extensor tendons. Adherence of the extrinsic flexors is tested by passively maintaining the fingers and thumb in full extension while passively extending the wrist. In the presence of flexor tightness, the increasing flexor tension that develops as the wrist is passively extended will pull the fingers into flexion. Adherence of the extensor tendons is simply a reverse process. The digits are passively maintained in full flexion while the wrist is passively flexed. If tension pulling the fingers into extension is detected by the clinician's hand as the wrist is brought into flexion, extrinsic extensor tightness exists.

Functional Screen

A number of motions can be used to quickly assess hand function, including the following:

- Opposition of the thumb and little finger.
- Pad to pad mobility of thumb and other fingers. The majority of the functional activities of the hand require at least 5 cm of opening of the fingers and thumb.[22]
- The ability to make three different fists include the following:
  - The hook fist (placing fingertips onto MCP joint).
  - Standard fist.
  - Straight fist (placing fingertips on the thenar and hypothenar eminences). The ability to flex the fingers to within 1– to 2 cm of the distal palmar crease is an indication of functional range of motion for many hand activities.[22]

Palpation

Palpation of the following muscles, tendon, insertions, ligaments, capsules, bones should occur as indicated, and be compared with the uninvolved side. Clinically important information about the course of the hand nerves can be provided using the cardinal line, which is an imaginary line drawn from the apex of the thumb–index web space across the palm parallel to the proximal palmar crease[6,23]:

- The radial borderline is drawn along the radial border of the long finger and intersects the cardinal line at the point where the motor branch of the median nerve enters the thenar musculature.

- The point where the thenar crease intersects the cardinal line is approximately over the point where the motor branch emerges from the median nerve.

- A line drawn between the two points of intersection described above approximates the course of the superficial nerve.

- A line drawn from the intersection of the cardinal line and the radial border of the index finger palmar digital crease approximates the course of the radial digital nerve to the index finger.

- The ulnar borderline is drawn along the ulnar border of the ring finger. It intersects the cardinal line over the hook of the hamate. A line drawn from this intersection to the ulnar border of the little finger palmar digital crease overlies the course of the ulnar digital nerve to the little finger.

Radial Styloid Process

The radial styloid process (Figure 7-7) is located at the most proximal point of the anatomic snuff box (see below), during radial abduction of the thumb. With simultaneous radial deviation of the wrist, this prominence becomes visible.

 Clinical Pearl

Tenderness over the styloid, especially with radial deviation, may indicate contusion, fracture, or radioscaphoid arthritis.[24]

Scaphoid

The scaphoid (Figure 7-7) is palpated just distal to the radial styloid in the anatomic snuffbox. The neck of the scaphoid is located on the floor of the anatomic snuffbox. Palpation can be made easier by positioning the wrist in

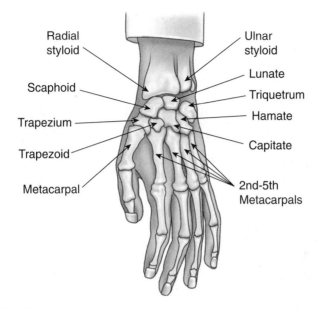

Figure 7-7 Palpation points.

ulnar deviation. The scaphoid may be grasped and moved passively, by firm pressure between an opposed index finger and thumb applied to the anterior surface and anatomic snuffbox simultaneously.

🌑 Clinical Pearl

In most individuals, the scaphoid is mildly tender to palpation, but those with scaphoid fracture, nonunion, or scaphoid instability have severe discomfort (see Special Tests).[18,25]

🌑 Clinical Pearl

The scaphoid receives its blood supply through its ligaments. The main arterial supply enters around the waist (midpoint) of the scaphoid, with additional vessels entering distally. The scaphoid has a high incidence of avascular necrosis.

Trapezium

The trapezium is located immediately proximal to the base of the first metacarpal bone, just distal to the scaphoid (Figure 7-7). The tubercle of the trapezium lies anteriorly at the base of the thenar eminence. It can be made more prominent by opposing the thumb to the little finger, and ulnarly deviating the wrist.

 Clinical Pearl

Tenderness over this carpal may indicate scaphotrapezial arthritis secondary to scaphoid instability.[26]

Thumb Carpometacarpal (CMC) Joint

To examine the thumb CMC joint, the clinician palpates carefully along the shaft of the thumb metacarpal down to its proximal flare. Just proximal to this flare is a small depression where the CMC joint is located. By applying direct radial and ulnar stresses to the joint, the clinician can determine the overall stability of the joint, as compared to the other thumb.

Extensor Pollicis Brevis and Abductor Pollicis Longus Tendons

The extensor pollicis brevis (EPB) and abductor pollicis longus (APL) tendons make up the first extensor compartment on the dorsum of the wrist, and together form the radial border of the anatomic snuffbox. Extending and radially abducting the thumb can enhance prominence of these tendons.

 Clinical Pearl

Tenderness at the CMC joint is usually indicative of degenerative arthritis.

Tenderness over the EPB and APL tendons may indicate De Quervain tenosynovitis.

Lister Tubercle

This is a small bony prominence on the posterior and distal end of radius. It is found by sliding a finger proximally from a point between the index and middle finger. Just distal to the Lister tubercle is the joint line of the scaphoid and radius. The extensor carpi radialis longus (ECRL) and extensor carpi radialis brevis (ECRB) tendons travel radial to the Lister tubercle, and insert on the base of the second and third metacarpals. The extensor digitorum communis (EDC) tendon travels ulnar to the Lister tubercle.

Lunate

The lunate is located just distal and ulnar to the Lister tubercle with the wrist flexed, and is immediately proximal to, and in line with, the capitate (Figure 7-7). The mobile lunate can be felt to glide posteriorly with extension. It is the most commonly dislocated carpal and the scapho–lunate articulation is the most common area for carpal instability. Scapholunate synovitis (posterior wrist syndrome) or a scapholunate ligament injury presents with tenderness or fullness in this region.[18]

 Clinical Pearl

Tenderness specific to the lunate can indicate Kienböck disease (avascular necrosis of the lunate).[27,28]

Capitate

The capitate (Figure 7-7) is palpated proximally over the posterior aspect of the third metacarpal until a small depression is felt. While palpating in this depression as the wrist is flexed, the clinician should feel the capitate, the central bone of the carpus, move posteriorly.

 Clinical Pearl

Tenderness in this depression may indicate scapholunate or lunotriquetral instability, or capitolunate degenerative joint disease.

Second and Third Metacarpals

The base of the second and third metacarpals and the CMC joints are localized by palpating proximally along the posterior surfaces of the index and long metacarpals to their respective bases.[12] A bony prominence found at the base of the second or third metacarpal may be a carpal boss, a variation found in some individuals due to hypertrophic changes of traumatic origin.[12]

Ulnar Head and Styloid Process

The ulnar head forms a rounded prominence on the ulnar side of the wrist, which is easily palpated with the forearm in pronation (Figure 7-7).[12] The ulnar styloid process is ulnar, and distal, to the head of the ulna. It is best located with the forearm in supination.

Triangular Fibrocartilage Complex

The TFCC is located distal to the ulnar styloid, and proximal to the triquetrum. Tenderness over this structure indicates an injury to the TFCC.[29]

Hamate

The hook of the hamate is palpated just distal and radial (in the direction of the thumb web space) to the pisiform on the anterior aspect (Figure 7-7). Locating the hamate can be made easier if the clinician places the middle of the distal phalanx of the thumb on the pisiform, with the thumb pointing between the web space between the index and long finger.

 Clinical Pearl

> Tenderness over the hamate is common, and so the clinician should compare findings with the other side. Severe tenderness could indicate a fracture of the hamate, especially if associated with a FOOSH injury or a missed hit swing of a racket or bat.[30]

Triquetrum

The triquetrum is located by radially deviating the wrist while palpating just distal to the ulnar styloid (Figure 7-7). With ulnar deviation, the triquetrum articulates with the TFCC, which functions as a buffer between the styloid and the triquetrum.

 Clinical Pearl

> Tenderness and swelling in the triquetral-hamate region are often present with midcarpal instability, which occurs when the anterior (palmar) triquetral-hamate-capitate ligament is ruptured or sprained.[31]

Pisiform

The pisiform is located on the flexor aspect of the palm, on top of the triquetrum, at the distal crease (Figure 7-8).

 Clinical Pearl

> Tenderness of the pisiform indicates pisotriquetral arthritis or inflammation of the flexor carpi ulnaris tendon.[29]

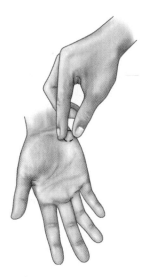

Figure 7-8 Palpating the pisiform.

Tunnel of Guyon
The tunnel of Guyon is located in the space between the hamate and pisiform.[16] This tunnel serves as a passageway for the ulnar nerve and artery into the hand. The flexor carpi ulnaris tendon lies outside the tunnel.

Carpal Tunnel
The distal wrist crease marks the proximal edge of the carpal tunnel. The boundaries of the carpal tunnel are as follows:

- Radial: anterior scaphoid tubercle and trapezium
- Ulnar: pisiform and hamate
- Posterior: the carpal bones
- Anterior : transverse carpal ligament
- Proximal: anterior antebrachial fascia
- Distal: distal edge of retinaculum at CMC level, FCR, and scaphoid tubercle.

🌑 Clinical Pearl

The 10 structures that pass through the carpal tunnel include the following:
- The eight tendons of the FDS, and FDP

- FPL

- Median nerve

NB: the FCR tendon is not considered to occupy the tunnel because it passes through its own compartment.

Flexor Retinaculum

The flexor retinaculum transforms the carpal arch into the carpal tunnel. It is attached laterally to the tubercle of the scaphoid and tubercle of the trapezium, and attached medially to the pisiform and hook of the hamate. Its proximal edge is at the distal crease of the wrist.

Metacarpophalangeal Joint

The MCP joint lies distal to the palmar digital crease over the proximal phalanx in an imaginary line connecting the radial aspect of the proximal palmar crease to the ulnar aspect of the distal palmar crease.

 Clinical Pearl

The MCP joints should be splinted in some degree of flexion and not in extension as the extended position places the collateral ligaments in a shortened position.

Proximal Interphalangeal Joints

The PIP crease approximates the level of the PIP joint. Palpation of the PIP joint offers important information. Palpation of the joint over four planes (posterior, anterior, medial, lateral) allows assessment of point tenderness over ligamentous origins and insertions that is highly suggestive of underlying soft-tissue disruption.[19]

 Clinical Pearl

In cases in which the PIP joint is grossly swollen and tender, palpation may provide more accurate information when performed several days after the injury.[19]

Distal Interphalangeal Joint

The DIP crease is just proximal to the level of the PIP joint.

> ### 🌑 Clinical Pearl
>
> The six posterior compartments of the hand contain the following (from radial to ulnar):
>
> 1. (APL) and (EPB).
> 2. Extensor carpi radialis longus and brevis.
> 3. Extensor pollicis longus (EPL).
> 4. Extensor digitorum (four tendons) and extensor indicis.
> 5. Extensor digiti minimi.
> 6. Extensor carpi ulnaris.

Strength Testing

The muscles of the forearm, wrist, and hand are detailed in Table 7-4.[32] Isometric tests are carried out in the extreme range, and if positive, in the neutral range. These isometric tests must include the interossei and lumbricales. The straight plane motions of wrist flexion, extension, ulnar, and radial deviation are tested initially. Pain with any of these tests requires a more thorough examination of the individual muscles.

Wrist

Flexor carpi radialis/flexor carpi ulnaris
During the testing of these muscles, substitution by the finger flexors should be avoided by having patient not make a fist. The clinician applies the resistive force into extension and radial deviation for the FCU, and extension and ulnar deviation for the FCR

Extensor carpi radialis longus/brevis
Any action of the EDC should be ruled out by having the patient make a fist while extending the wrist. The clinician applies the resistive force on the dorsum of the second and third metacarpals with the force directed into flexion and ulnar deviation.

Extensor carpi ulnaris
Having patient make a fist in wrist extension, and the clinician applying the resistance on the ulnar dorsum of hand, with the force directed into flexion and radial deviation, tests the ECU.

Table 7-4 Muscles of the Forearm, Wrist, and Hand: Their Motions and Peripheral Nerve Supply

Motion	Involved Muscles	Peripheral Nerve Supply
Forearm supination	Supinator	Posterior interosseous
	Biceps brachii	Musculocutaneous
Forearm pronation	Pronator quadratus	Anterior interosseous
	Pronator teres	Median
	Flexor carpi radialis	Median
Wrist extension	Extensor carpi radialis longus	Radial
	Extensor carpi radialis brevis	Posterior interosseous
	Extensor carpi ulnaris	Posterior interosseous
Wrist flexion	Flexor carpi radialis	Median
	Flexor carpi ulnaris	Ulnar
Ulnar deviation of wrist	Flexor carpi ulnaris	Ulnar
	Extensor carpi ulnaris	Posterior interosseous
Radial deviation of wrist	Flexor carpi radialis	Median
	Extensor carpi radialis longus	Radial
	Abductor pollicis longus	Posterior interosseous
	Extensor pollicis brevis	Posterior interosseous
Finger extension	Extensor digitorum communis	Posterior interosseous
	Extensor indices	Posterior interosseous
	Extensor digiti minimi	Posterior interosseous
Finger flexion	Flexor digitorum profundus	Anterior interosseous: lateral two digits
		Ulnar: medial two digits
	Flexor digitorum superficialis	Median
	Lumbricals	First and second: median
		Third and fourth: Ulnar
	Interossei	Ulnar
	Flexor digiti minimi	Ulnar
Abduction of fingers	Dorsal interossei	Ulnar
	Abductor digiti minimi	Ulnar
Adduction of fingers	Palmar interossei	Ulnar

(continued on following page)

Motion	Involved Muscles	Peripheral Nerve Supply
Thumb extension	Extensor pollicis longus	Posterior interosseous
	Extensor pollicis brevis	Posterior interosseous
	Abductor pollicis longus	Posterior interosseous
Thumb flexion	Flexor pollicis brevis	Superficial head: median
		Deep head ulnar
	Flexor pollicis longus	Anterior interosseous
	Opponens pollicis	Median
Abduction of thumb	Abductor pollicis longus	Posterior interosseous
	Abductor pollicis brevis	Median
Adduction of thumb	Adductor pollicis	Ulnar
Opposition of thumb and little finger	Opponens pollicis	Median
	Flexor pollicis brevis	Superficial head: median
	Abductor pollicis brevis	Median
	Opponens digiti minimi	Ulnar

Data from reference 32.

Thumb

Abductor pollicis longus/brevis

The forearm is positioned midway between pronation and supination, or in maximal supination. The MCP and IP joints are positioned in flexion. The muscles are tested with palmar abduction of the thumb in the frontal plane for the longus and in the sagittal plane for the brevis.

Opponens pollicis

The forearm is positioned in supination and the posterior aspect of the hand rests on the table. The patient is asked to touch the finger pads of the thumb and little finger together. Using one hand, the clinician stabilizes the first and fifth metacarpals and palm of the hand. With the other hand, the clinician applies a force in the opposite direction of opposition to the distal end of the first metacarpal.

Flexor pollicis longus/brevis

The forearm is positioned in supination and supported by the table, and the hand is positioned so that the posterior aspect rests on a table. The thumb is adducted. Applying resistance to the distal phalanx tests the longus, whereas resistance applied to the proximal phalanx tests both heads of the brevis.

Adductor pollicis

This muscle is tested by having the patient hold a piece of card between the thumb and radial aspect of the index finger's proximal phalanx while the clinician attempts to remove it. If weak or nonfunctioning, the IP joint of thumb flexes during this maneuver due to substitution by the flexor digitorum profundus (FDP) (Froment sign).

Extensor pollicis longus/brevis

Both of these muscles can be tested with the patient's hand flat on the table, palm down, and asking the patient to lift only the thumb off the table. To test each individually, resistance is applied to the posterior aspect of the distal phalanx for the EPL, while stabilizing the proximal phalanx and metacarpal, and to the posterior aspect of the proximal phalanx for the EPB while stabilizing the first metacarpal.

Intrinsics

Lumbricals

The four lumbricals are tested by applying resistance to the posterior surface of the middle and distal phalanges, while stabilizing under the proximal phalanx of the finger being tested.

Anterior interossei

The anterior and posterior interossei act with the lumbricals to achieve MCP flexion coupled with PIP and DIP extension. The three anterior interossei also adduct the second, fourth, and fifth fingers to midline. Resistance is applied by the clinician to the radial aspect of the distal end of the proximal phalanx of the second, fourth, and fifth fingers, after first stabilizing the hand and fingers not being tested.

Posterior interossei/abductor digiti minimi

The four posterior interossei abduct the second, third, and fourth fingers from midline. The abductor digiti minimi abducts the fifth finger from midline.

The intrinsic muscles are tested in the frontal plane to avoid substitution by the extrinsic flexors and extensors. Resistance is applied by the clinician to the ulnar aspect of the distal end of the proximal phalanx of each of the four fingers, after first stabilizing the hand and fingers not being tested.

Fingers

Flexor digitorum profundus

This muscle is tested with DIP flexion of each digit, while the MCP and PIP are stabilized in extension and wrist neutral. Due to the variability of nerve innervation for this muscle group, each of the fingers can be tested to determine whether a peripheral nerve lesion is present. The anterior interosseous nerve provides the nerve supply to the index finger; the main branch of the median nerve serves the middle finger; and the ulnar nerve serves the ring and little finger.

 Clinical Pearl

The quadriga effect, demonstrated by an inability to flex, especially the DIP joints of the fingers adjacent to the injured finger, occurs because of the shared muscle belly of the FDP. For this reason it is very important to check the FDP glide of each digit, not just the injured digit, and to promote active DIP flexion of the adjacent digits during treatment.

Flexor digitorum superficialis
There is normally one muscle tendon unit for each finger, however, an absent flexor digitorum superficialis (FDS) to the little finger is common. The clinician should only allow the finger to be tested to flex, by firmly blocking all joints of the non-tested fingers, and wrist in neutral.

Extensor digitorum/extensor indices proprius/EDM
There is only one muscle belly for this 4-tendon unit. These three muscles are the sole MP joint extensors. With the wrist in neutral, the strength is tested with the metacarpals in extension and the PIP/DIP flexed. The EIP is isolated by positioning the index finger and hand, in the "number one" position— the index finger in extension with other fingers clenched in a fist. The EDM muscle is tested with resistance of little finger extension with the other fingers maintained in a fist.

To isolate intrinsic muscle function, the patient is asked to actively extend the MP joint and then to attempt to actively extend the PIP joint. Because the ED, EI, and EDM tendons are "anchored" at the MP joint by active extension, only the intrinsic muscles can now extend the PIP joint.[33] To test the terminal extensor tendon function, the clinician stabilizes the middle phalanx and asks the patient to extend the DIP joint.[33]

Flexor digiti minimi
The forearm is positioned in supination and the posterior aspect of the hand rests on the table. The clinician stabilizes the fifth metacarpal and the palm with one hand, and then applies resistance to the anterior surface of the proximal phalanx of the fifth digit with the other hand.

Opponens digit minimi

The forearm is positioned in supination and the posterior aspect of the hand rests on the table. The patient is asked to touch the finger pads of the thumb and little finger together. Using one hand, the clinician stabilizes the first and fifth metacarpals and palm of the hand. With the other hand, the clinician applies a force in the opposite direction of opposition to the distal end of the fifth metacarpal.

Grip Strength

A patient's grip strength is commonly used to assess hand function.

 Clinical Pearl

The position of maximal power grip is achieved with 35 degrees of wrist extension and 7 degrees of ulnar deviation

A number of protocols using a sealed hydraulic dynamometer, such as the Jamar dynamometer (Asimow Engineering Co. Santa Monica, California), have been shown to be accurate, reliable and valid in measuring grip strength.[34]

It is wise to combine the results of different grip strength tests before making any decisions.[35]

The assessment of pinch strength is also used to assess function of the hand, using a pinch meter.

 Clinical Pearl

In full wrist flexion, only 25% of full grip strength can be achieved.

Functional Assessment

The *functional position* of the wrist is the position in which optimal function is likely to occur.[36,37] This position involves wrist extension of between 20 degree and 35 degrees, ulnar deviation of 10 degrees to 15 degrees, slight flexion of all of the finger joints, midrange thumb opposition, and slight flexion of the thumb MCP and IP joints.[36] In this position, which minimizes the restraining action of the long extensor tendons, the pulps of the index finger and thumb are in contact.

The *functional range of motion* for the hand is the range in which the hand can perform most of its grip and other functional activities.

Hand Disability Index[38]
The patient is asked to rate the following seven questions on a 0 to 3 scale, with 3 being the most difficult.

Unable to perform task = 0

Able to complete task partially = 1

Able to complete task but with difficulty = 2

Able to perform task normally = 3

Are you able to:

1. Dress yourself, including tying shoelaces and doing buttons?
2. Cut your meat?
3. Lift a full cup or glass to your mouth?
4. Prepare your own meal?
5. Open car doors?
6. Open jars that have previously been opened?
7. Turn taps on and off?

Dexterity tests include the following:

Minnesota Rate of Manipulation Test (MRMT)
This test, which primarily measures gross coordination and dexterity, consists of five functions:

1. Placing
2. Turning
3. Displacing
4. One hand turning and placing
5. Two-hand turning and placing

The activities are timed and compared with the time taken by the other hand, and then compared with normal values.[22,39]

Jebsen–Taylor Hand-function test[40]
This test, which requires the least amount of extremity coordination, measures prehension and manipulative skills, consists of seven subtests:

1. Writing
2. Card turning
3. Picking up small objects

4. Simulated feeding
5. Stacking
6. Picking up large, light objects
7. Picking up large, heavy objects

The subtests are timed and compared with the time taken by the other hand. The results are compared with normal values.[22,39]

Nine–Hole Peg Test

This test was designed to assess the finger dexterity of each hand.[41] The patient is asked to use one hand to place nine 3.2-cm (1.3 inch) pegs in a 12.7 cm × 12.7 cm (5 in. × 5 in.) board, and is then asked to remove them. The task is timed and compared with the time taken by the other hand. The results are compared with normal values.[22,39]

Purdue Pegboard Test[42,43]

This test evaluates finer coordination, requiring prehension of small objects, with measurement categories divided into the following:

1. Right hand
2. Left hand
3. Both hands
4. Right, left, and both hands
5. Assembly

The subtests are timed and compared with normal values based on gender and occupation.[22,39]

Crawford Small Parts Dexterity (CSPD) Test[44]

The CSPD test involves the use of tweezers and a screwdriver, and requires patients to control not only their hands, but also small tools. This test correlates positively with vocational activities that demand fine coordination skills.[22]

The problem with most of these tests and others is that the critical measure of function used is time, even though time is not an accurate measure of function.

Although not standardized, a few other simple tests can be used to assess hand dexterity. These include writing in a straight line, buttoning and unbuttoning different sized buttons, zipping and unzipping using a variety of zip sizes. The following scale can be used to grade these activities:

Unable to perform task = 0

Able to complete task partially = 1

Able to complete task but with difficulty = 2

Able to perform task normally = 3

Passive Physiological Mobility Testing

In the following tests, the patient is positioned in sitting, and the clinician is standing/sitting, facing the patient. In each of the tests, the clinician notes the quantity of motion as well as the joint reaction. The tests are always repeated on, and compared to, the same joint in the opposite extremity.

The Wrist

Using one hand, the clinician palpates and stabilizes the distal aspect of the forearm, while using the other hand to grasp the patient's hand, distal to the wrist.

Flexion/extension

The carpal bones are flexed and extended about the appropriate coronal axis through the midcarpal and radiocarpal joints.

Radial/ulnar deviation

The clinician radially and ulnarly deviates the carpal bones about the appropriate sagittal axis through the midcarpal and radiocarpal joints.

Fanning/folding—metacarpal

Using both hands, the clinician grasps the anterior and posterior aspects of the thenar and hypothenar eminence, and then fans and folds the metacarpal bones about a longitudinal axis. This technique can also be used as a passive/active mobilization technique.

Phalanges

Using one hand, the clinician palpates and stabilizes the distal end of the metacarpal/phalanx close to the joint line, while using the other hand to palpate the proximal end of the adjacent phalanx.

Flexion/extension

The clinician flexes and then extends the phalanx about the appropriate coronal axis through the MCP/interphalangeal joint.

Abduction/adduction

The clinician abducts, and then adducts the phalanx about the appropriate sagittal axis through the MCP joint.

Passive Accessory Mobility Tests

In the following tests, the patient is positioned in sitting, and the clinician is standing/sitting, facing the patient. In each of the tests, the joint being tested is placed in its open packed position and the clinician notes the quantity of joint motion as well as the joint reaction to the test. The tests are always repeated on, and compared to, the same joint in the opposite extremity.

Radiocarpal Joint

Posterior–anterior glide: The patient's hand rests on the table with the wrist supported with a towel (Figure 7-9). Using one hand to stabilize the patient's distal forearm, the clinician grasps the patient's hand with the other hand using the styloid processes and pisiform for landmarks. The proximal row of carpals is then moved posteriorly and anteriorly. The posterior glide tests the joint's ability to extend, whereas the anterior glide assesses the ability of the joint to flex.

Ulnar and radial glide: The patient's hand rests on the table with the wrist supported with a towel (Figure 7-10). Using one hand to stabilize the patient's distal forearm, the clinician grasps the patient's hand with the other hand using the styloid processes and pisiform for landmarks. The proximal row of carpals is then moved posteriorly and anteriorly. The posterior glide tests the joint's ability to extend, whereas the anterior glide assesses the ability of the joint to flex.

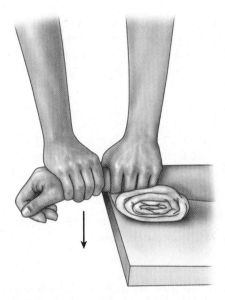

Figure 7-9 Anterior glide of the radiocarpal (wrist) joint.

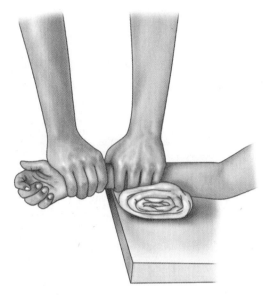

Figure 7-10 Ulnar glide of the radiocarpal (wrist) joint.

Intercarpal Joints

Example—Anterior glide of the scaphoid on the radius. The patient's hand rests on the table or is held forward by the clinician (Figure 7-11). The clinician grasps the patient's hand with both hands, with the index fingers placed on the proximal anterior surface of the radius, and the thumbs contacting the scaphoid posteriorly (Figure 7-11). The scaphoid is moved anteriorly relative to the radius.

Carpal Motion Assessment

The Atkinson method

Lateral column

The clinician assesses the motion of the scaphoid in relation to the following:

- *Radius*
- *Capitate*
- *Lunate*
- *Trapezium*
- *Trapezoid*

Central column

The clinician assesses the motion of the lunate in relation to the following:

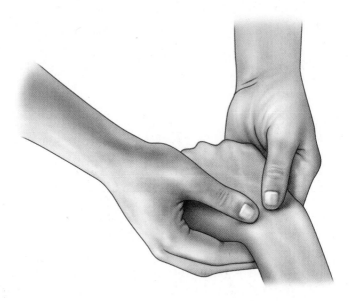

Figure 7-11 Anterior glide of the scaphoid on the radius.

- *Radius*
- *Capitate*

Medial column
The clinician assesses the motion of the hamate in relation to the following:
- *Ulna*
- *Lunate*
- *Triquetrum*

Carpometacarpal Joints
Using one hand, the clinician uses a pinch grip of the index finger and thumb to palpate and stabilize the carpal bone that articulates with the metacarpal bone being tested. With a pinch grip of the index finger and thumb of the other hand, the clinician palpates the metacarpal.

The first through fifth carpometacarpal joints are tested. The carpal bone is stabilized and the metacarpal is distracted (Figure 7-12) and glided posterior-anteriorly along the plane of the carpometacarpal joint. At the first carpometacarpal joint, radial and ulnar glides are also performed:

Ulnar glide. The ulnar glide is used to assess the flexion glide of the joint. Using the thumb and index finger of one hand the clinician stabilizes the trapezium and trapezoid as a unit (Figure 7-13). The thenar eminence of

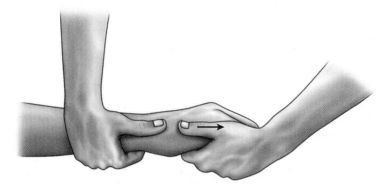

Figure 7-12 Distraction of the carpometacarpal joint.

the other hand is placed on the first metacarpal of the patient's thumb, and the fingers wrap around the thumb to assist in maintaining the open packed position. The clinician applies a glide in an ulnar direction through the thenar eminence toward the radial aspect of the patient's metacarpal (Figure 7-13).

Radial glide. The radial glide is used to assess the extension glide of the joint. Using the thumb and index finger of one hand the clinician

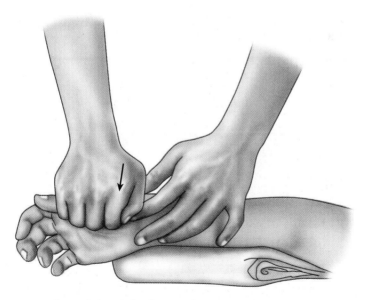

Figure 7-13 Ulnar glide of the first carpometacarpal joint.

stabilizes the trapezium and trapezoid as a unit. The thenar eminence of the other hand is placed on the first metacarpal of the patient's thumb, and the fingers wrap around the thumb to assist in maintaining the open packed position. The clinician applies a glide in a radial direction through the thenar eminence.

Intermetacarpal Joints

Although these joints between the metacarpal heads are not true synovial joints, motion does occur here during tasks involving grasping and releasing. The following example describes the technique to test the third and fourth intermetacarpal joint.

Using one hand the clinician stabilizes the head and neck of the third metacarpal, while the other hand grasps the fourth metacarpal in a similar fashion (Figure 7-14). The head of the fourth metacarpal is then glided anteriorly or posteriorly with respect to the third metacarpal. The other metacarpals are tested similarly, with the third metacarpal always being the one stabilized as the third metacarpal serves as the center of movement during fanning and folding motions of the hand.

Metacarpophalangeal/Interphalangeal Joints

Using a pinch grip of the index finger and thumb of one hand, the clinician palpates and stabilizes the metacarpal/phalanx. With a pinch grip of the index finger and thumb of the other hand, the clinician palpates the adjacent phalanx.

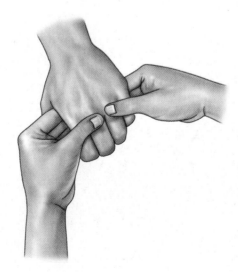

Figure 7-14 Mobility testing of the third and fourth intermetacarpal joint.

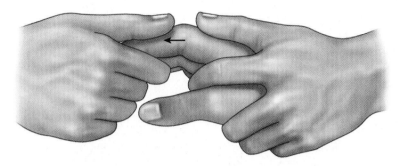

Figure 7-15 Long axis distraction of the MCP or interphalangeal joints.

Distraction
The clinician stabilizes the proximal bone, and then applies a long axis distraction (Figure 7-15)

Posterior–anterior glide
The clinician stabilizes the proximal bone, and then glides the phalanx posterior-anteriorly along the plane of the joint (Figure 7-16) and anterior-posteriorly (Figure 7-17).

Medial–lateral (radial–ulnar glide)
The clinician stabilizes the proximal bone, and then glides the phalanx medial-laterally along the plane of the joint (Figure 7-18).

Ligament Stability

The major ligaments of the wrist and hand are detailed in Table 7-5. A number of tests are available to evaluate the ligamentous stability of the forearm,

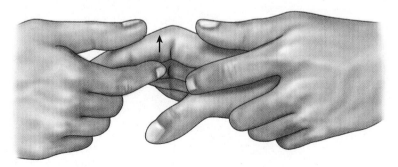

Figure 7-16 Posterior (dorsal) glide of the MCP or interphalangeal joints.

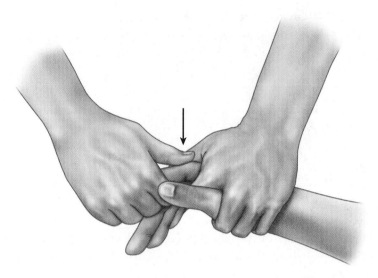

Figure 7-17 Anterior (ventral) glide of the MCP or interphalangeal joints

wrist, hand, and finger joints—see Special Tests. A nonspecific screening test for pseudo instability involves holding the patient's hand with one hand and the patient's forearm in the other, while passively flexing and extending the patient's wrist. The presence of palpable clunks or shifts with this maneuver could suggest instability.

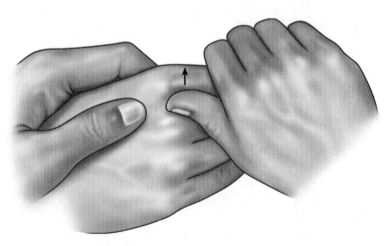

Figure 7-18 Radial glide of the MCP or interphalangeal joints.

Table 7-5 Ligaments of the Wrist and Hand

Intrinsic		Extrinsic
Interosseous	**Midcarpal**	**Radiocarpal/Ulnocarpal**
Distal row	*Dorsal*	*Dorsal*
Trapezium-trapezoid	Scaphotriquetral	Dorsal radiocarpal
Trapezoid-capitate	Dorsal intercarpal	
Capitohamate		
Proximal row	*Palmar*	*Palmar*
Scapholunate	Scaphotrapeziotrapezoid	Radioscaphocapitate
Lunotriquetral	Scaphocapitate	Lond radiolunate
	Triquetrocapitate	Short radiolunate
	Triquetrohamate	Radioscapholunate
		Ulnolunate
		Ulnotriquetral
		Ulnocapitate
		Carpometacarpal

Neurovascular Status

A number of tests can be used to document the neurovascular status of the wrist and hand—See Special Tests.

Sensibility Testing

Sensation is the conscious perception of basic sensory input. Sensibility describes the neural events occurring at the periphery, nerve fibers, and nerve receptors. Sensation is what clinicians re-educate, whereas sensibility is what clinicians assess.[45]

The assessment of sensibility of the hand is an important component of every hand examination because sensation is essential for precision movements and object manipulation. Altered sensory perceptions can result from injuries to peripheral nerves or from spinal nerve root compression. The sensory system is described in chapter 2. Two types of sensibility can be assessed[46]:

- Protective: this is evidenced by the ability to perceive pinprick, touch, and temperature.

- Functional: this is evidenced by a return of sensibility to a level that enables the hand to engage in full activities of daily living.

There exists a hierarchy of sensibility capacity[46,47]:

- Detection: this is the simplest level of function and requires that the patient be able to distinguish a single point stimulus from normally occurring atmospheric background stimulation.

- Innervation density or discrimination: this represents the ability to perceive that stimulus A differs from stimulus B.

- Quantification: this involves organizing tactile stimuli according to degree, texture etc.

- Recognition: this is the most complicated level of function and involves the identification of objects with the vision occluded.

Special Tests

Ligament Stability Tests
In the following specific tests, the patient is positioned in sitting, and the clinician is standing/sitting, facing the patient. The clinician must remember to perform these tests on the uninvolved sides to provide a basis for comparison.

Piano key test
The piano key test evaluates the stability of the distal radioulnar joint.[29] The clinician firmly stabilizes the distal radius with one hand and grasps the head of the ulna between the thumb and index fingers of the other hand. The ulnar head is depressed in an anterior direction (as in depressing a key on a piano).[48] The test is positive if there is excessive movement in an anterior direction, or if, upon release of the ulna, the bone springs back into its high posterior position. There may also be discomfort reported during the test.[12]

The lunotriquetral ballottment (Reagan) test
The lunotriquetral shear maneuver[49] assesses the stability of the lunotriquetral interosseous ligament.[29] The lunate is moved posteriorly with the thumb of one hand, while the triquetrum is pushed anteriorly by the index finger of the other hand. The wrist is placed in either radial or ulnar deviation. Stress is created between these two bones in the anterior–posterior plane (Figure 7-19). Crepitation, clicks, or discomfort in this area suggests injury to the ligament.[14,48]

 Clinical Pearl

Marx et al.[50] found the sensitivity of the lunotriquetral shear maneuver to be 64% and the specificity to be 44% making it difficult at best to base a diagnosis of instability primarily on a positive test.

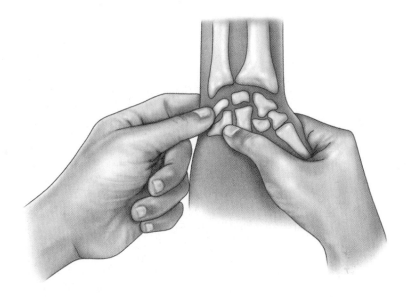

Figure 7-19 The lunotriquetral shear maneuver, or Reagan test.

The pisotriquetral shear test

The pisotriquetral shear test assesses the integrity of the pisotriquetral articulation.[48] The clinician stabilizes the wrist with the fingers posterior to the triquetrum, and the thumb over the pisiform. The pisiform is rocked back and forth in a medial and lateral direction (Figure 7-20). A positive test is manifested with pain during this maneuver.

Pivot shift test of the midcarpal joint

The patient is positioned in sitting with the elbow flexed to 90 degrees, resting on a firm surface, and the forearm supinated. The clinician uses one hand to stabilize the forearm, while using the other hand to take the patient's hand into full radial deviation while maintaining the wrist in neutral with regard to flexion and extension. The patient's hand is then taken into full ulnar deviation. A positive test results if the capitate is felt to shift away from the lunate and indicates an injury to the anterior capsule and interosseous ligaments.[51]

Triangular fibrocartilage complex (TFCC) load test

This test can be used to detect an injury to the TFCC. It is performed by ulnarly deviating and axially loading the wrist and moving it posteriorly and anteriorly, or by rotating the forearm. A positive test elicits pain, clicking, or crepitus.[12]

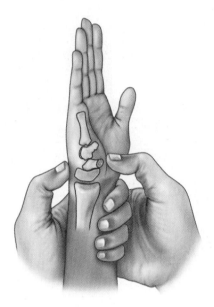

Figure 7-20 The pisotriquetral shear test.

Neurovascular Stress Tests
Stress tests are those that combine the use of sensory tests with activities that provoke the symptoms of nerve compression. These tests are helpful in cases of patient reports of mild nerve compression when no abnormalities are detected by baseline sensory testing. Examples of stress tests include the Phalen test, the Reverse Phalen test, and the Hand Elevation test.

Phalen test for carpal tunnel syndrome
For Phalen[52,53] test, the patient sits comfortably with the wrists and elbows flexed. The test is positive if the patient experiences numbness or tingling within 45 seconds. For some patients, performance of this test recreates their wrist, thumb, or forearm ache.[54]

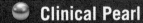

Clinical Pearl

Phalen sign has a sensitivity of 75% and a specificity of 47%. The reliability and validity of Phalen test is moderately acceptable for use in clinical practice.[55-57]

Reverse Phalen test for carpal tunnel syndrome
For the reverse Phalen test, the patient sits comfortably with the wrists extended and elbows flexed.[58] Wrist extension has demonstrated a larger increase in intracarpal canal pressure when compared to wrist flexion.[59,60]

Clinical Pearl

De Krom et al.[61] found only 45% of hands with electrodiagnostically confirmed carpal tunnel syndrome had a positive reverse Phalen test. In addition, they found the reverse Phalen positive in 49% of hands with negative electrodiagnostic testing for carpal tunnel syndrome.

Hand elevation test for carpal tunnel syndrome
The patient is seated or standing and is asked to elevate both arms above the head, and maintain them in this position for 2 minutes, or until the patient feels paresthesia or numbness in the hands.[62]

Clinical Pearl

In one study, the hand elevation test was found to be more specific than Phalen and Tinel tests in detecting carpal tunnel.[62]

Innervation Density Tests
These are a class of sensory tests that test the ability to discriminate between two identical stimuli placed close together on the skin. These tests are helpful in assessing sensibility after nerve repair and during nerve regeneration.[63]

Weber (Moberg) two-point discrimination test
Weber first introduced the two-point discrimination tests in 1953, using calipers, which were subsequently modified by Moberg for use with a paper clip in 1958.[63]

The clinician repeats the tests in an attempt to find the minimal distance at which the patient can distinguish between the two stimuli, decreasing or increasing the distance between the points depending on the response by the patient.[51] This distance is called the *threshold for discrimination*. Normal discrimination distance is less than 6mm, although this can vary between individuals and in the area of the hand, with normal fingertip scores occurring between 2 and 5 mm, and the finger surfaces scores between 3 and 7mm.[64]

Allen Test

The Allen test is used to determine the patency of the vessels supplying the hand. The clinician compresses both the radial and ulnar arteries at the wrist, and then asks the patient to open and clench the respective fist three to four times to drain the venous blood from the hand. The patient is then asked to hold the hand open while the clinician releases the pressure on the ulnar artery, and then the radial artery. The fingers and palm should be seen to regain their normal pink color. This procedure is repeated with the radial artery released and compression on the ulnar artery maintained. Normal filling time is usually less than 5 seconds. A distinct difference in the filling time suggests the dominance of one artery filling the hand.[14]

 Clinical Pearl

Kohonen et al.[65] found the sensitivity of the Allen test to be 73.2% and the specificity to be 97.1%, whereas others have had more disappointing results.[66]

Tinel Test for Carpal Tunnel Syndrome

The Tinel test is used to assist in the diagnosis of carpal tunnel syndrome. The area over the median nerve is tapped gently at the anterior surface of the wrist. If this produces tingling in the median distribution, then the test is positive.[60]

 Clinical Pearl

Tinel sign has a sensitivity of 60% and a specificity of 67%.[67] The reliability and validity of the Tinel test is minimally to moderately acceptable for use in clinical practice.[55-57,68]

Wartenberg Sign

Wartenberg sign is characterized by a position of abduction assumed by the little finger as a result of ulnar nerve paralysis.

Carpal Shake Test

This test is used if intercarpal synovitis is suspected.[48] The clinician grasps the patient's distal forearm. The patient is asked to relax and the clinician shakes the wrist. Pain or resistance to this test indicates a positive test.

Sit to Stand Test

This test is used if synovitis of the wrist is suspected.[48] The patient is instructed to place both hands on the armrest of a chair and attempt to lift their body slightly off the chair. Pain or resistance to this test indicates a positive test.

Ulnar Impaction (Ulnocarpal Stress) Test

This test is used to assess the articulation between the ulnar carpus and the triangular fibrocartilage.[48] The patient is positioned in sitting, with the elbow flexed to about 90 degrees and the wrist positioned in ulnar deviation, and the fingers positioned in a slight fist. The clinician loads the wrist by applying a compressive force through the ring and small metacarpals. Pain with this test indicates a possible tear of the triangular fibrocartilage or ulnar impaction syndrome. There are no studies in the literature that discuss the sensitivity, specificity, positive predictive value, or negative predictive value of this maneuver.

Finkelstein Test[69]

This test is used to detect stenosing tenosynovitis of the APL and EPB. The clinician grasps the patient's thumb, stabilizes the forearm with one hand, and then deviates the wrist to the ulnar side with the other hand (Figure 7-21). There are no studies in the literature that discuss the sensitivity, specificity, positive predictive value, or negative predictive value of this maneuver.

Flexor Digitorum Superficialis Test

This test is used to test the integrity of the FDS tendon. The clinician holds the patient's fingers in extension except for the finger being tested (this isolates the FDS tendon). The patient is instructed to flex the finger at the PIP joint. If this is possible, the FDS tendon is intact. As this tendon can act independently because of the position of the finger, it is the only functioning tendon at the PIP joint. The DIP joint, motored by the FDP, has no power of flexion when the other fingers are held in extension.

Flexor Digitorum Profundus Test

These tendons work only in unison. To test the FDP, stabilize the PIP joint and the MCP joint in extension. Instruct the patient to flex this finger at the DIP joint. If flexion occurs, the FDP is intact. If no flexion is possible the tendon is severed or the muscle denervated.

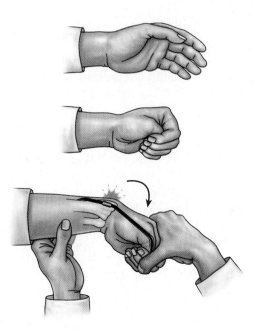

Figure 7-21 Finkelstein' test.

Extensor Hood Rupture

Elson[70] describes a test in which, from 90 degree of PIP flexion, the patient tries to extend the PIP joint against resistance. The absence of extension force at the PIP joint, and fixed extension at the distal joint, indicate complete rupture of the central slip.[19]

Froment Sign

This is more of a sign than a test and may present as a complaint from the patient who reports an inability to pinch between the index finger and thumb without flexion at the DIP joint occurring.[71] A positive Froment sign, which results from a weakness in the adductor pollicis and short head of the FPB muscles, indicates an ulnar nerve entrapment at the elbow or at the wrist.

Murphy Sign

The patient is asked to make a fist. If the head of the third metacarpal is level with the second and fourth metacarpals, the sign is positive for the presence of a lunate dislocation.[72]

Wartenberg Test

The Wartenberg test is used with patients who complain of pain over the distal radial forearm associated with paresthesias over the posterior radial hand

(Wartenberg syndrome). These patients frequently report increased symptoms with wrist movement or when tightly pinching the thumb and index digit together. The Wartenberg test involves tapping the index finger over the superficial radial nerve (similar to the Tinel test for carpal tunnel syndrome). A positive test is indicated by local tenderness and paresthesia with this maneuver. Hyperpronation of the forearm can also cause a positive Tinel sign.

Pain Provocation Tests

Radioulnar ballottement test
The radioulnar ballottement test is used to assess distal radioulnar joint instability. The patient's elbow is flexed and the clinician uses their thumb and index finger to stabilize the radius radially and the ulnar head ulnarly (Figure 7-22). Stress is applied in an anterior–posterior direction. Normally there is no movement in the anterior or posterior direction in maximum supination or pronation. Pain or mobility with this test is suggestive of radioulnar instability.

Pain with wrist flexion
To determine whether a painful wrist flexion is due to a problem between the scaphoid and radius, or scaphoid and the trapezium and trapezoid, the wrist is placed in full flexion, with the posterior surface of the hand resting on the treatment table. The clinician pushes on the scaphoid and second metacarpal in a posterior direction. An increase in pain with this maneuver may indicate a problem at the scaphoid-radius articulation.

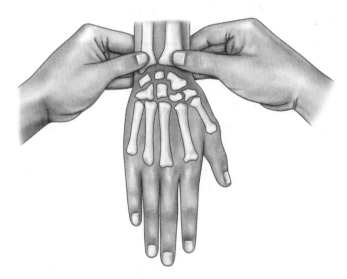

Figure 7-22 Radioulnar ballottement test.

If there is no increase in pain with this maneuver, the wrist is placed in a neutral position with regard to flexion and extension. The clinician stabilizes the trapezium and trapezoid and pushes the scaphoid posteriorly. An increase in pain with this maneuver may indicate a problem at the trapezium/trapezoid–scaphoid articulation.

To determine whether the painful wrist flexion is due to a problem between the capitate and the lunate, or the lunate and the radius, the wrist is placed in full flexion. The clinician pushes the lunate in anterior direction. An increase in pain with this maneuver may indicate a problem at the capitate–lunate articulation. If the pain is not increased with this maneuver, the wrist is placed in full flexion and the clinician pushes the lunate in a posterior direction. An increase in pain with this maneuver may indicate a problem at the lunate-radius articulation. A decrease in pain with this maneuver may indicate a problem at the capitate–lunate articulation.

Pain with wrist extension

To determine whether the pain with wrist extension is due to a problem between the scaphoid and the radius, or the scaphoid and the trapezium/trapezoid, the wrist is positioned in full extension with the palm positioned on the table. The clinician pushes on the radius in an anterior direction thus increasing the amount of wrist extension. An increase in pain with this maneuver may indicate a problem at the scaphoid-radius articulation. If this maneuver does not increase pain, the wrist is positioned as before. The clinician now pushes on the radius in a posterior direction. A decrease in pain with this maneuver may indicate a problem at the scaphoid-radius articulation. An increase in pain with this maneuver may indicate a problem at the scaphoid and trapezium/trapezoid articulation.

Placing the wrist as before in full extension and pushing on the scaphoid in a posterior direction confirm this. A decrease in pain with this maneuver indicates a problem between the scaphoid and radius, whereas an increase in pain with this maneuver indicates the problem is between the scaphoid and the trapezium/trapezoid.

The clinician fixes the scaphoid and pushes the trapezium/trapezoid in an anterior direction. A decrease in pain with this maneuver may indicate a problem at the scaphoid-trapezium/trapezoid articulation. If the pain remains unchanged with this maneuver, the problem is likely to be at the scaphoid-radius articulation. To confirm this hypothesis, the scaphoid can be pushed in an anterior direction while the wrist is maintained in the position of full extension. This should increase the pain if the hypothesis is correct.

To determine whether pain is due to a problem between the capitate and lunate, or the lunate and radius, the wrist is positioned in full extension, with the palm of the hand on the table. The clinician pushes on the radius in an anterior direction. An increase in pain with this maneuver indicates a problem at the capitate–lunate articulation.

If pushing the lunate and capitate in an anterior direction increases the pain, this may indicate a problem at the lunate-radius articulation.

If fixing the lunate and pushing the capitate in an anterior direction (a relative motion of the lunate posteriorly in relation to the capitate) increases the pain, the problem is likely at the capitate–lunate articulation.

Thumb CMC grind test

The grind test is used to assess the integrity of the thumb CMC joint by axially loading the thumb metacarpal into the trapezium.[48,73] The clinician grasps the thumb metacarpal using the thumb and index finger on one hand, and the proximal aspect of the thumb CMC joint with the other hand. An axial compressive force, combined with rotation, is applied to the thumb CMC joint. Reproduction of the patient's pain, and crepitus, is a positive test for arthrosis and synovitis. There are no studies in the literature that discuss the sensitivity, specificity, positive predictive value, or negative predictive value of this maneuver.

Lichtman test

The Lichtman test is a provocative test for midcarpal instability.[48] The patient's forearm is positioned in pronation and the hand is held relaxed and supported by the clinician. The clinician gently moves the patient's hand from radial to ulnar deviation while compressing the carpus into the radius. A positive test is when the midcarpal row appears to "jump" or "snap" from an anteriorly subluxed position to the height of the proximal row.[48]

Linscheid test

The Linscheid test is used to detect ligamentous injury and instability of the second and third CMC joints. The metacarpal shafts are supported and the metacarpal heads are then pressed distally in an anterior and posterior direction.[12] A positive test produces pain localized to the CMC joints.[74]

Scapholunate provocation tests

Scapholunate Shear Test

The patient is positioned in sitting with their forearm pronated. With one hand, the clinician places an index finger on the scaphoid tuberosity and the thumb on the posterior aspect of the scaphoid (Figure 7-23). With the other hand, the clinician grasps the lunate between the thumb and index finger. The lunate and scaphoid are then sheared in an anterior and then posterior direction.[18] Laxity and reproduction of the patient's pain are positive signs for this test.[48]

Watson Test (Scaphoid Shift) for Carpal Instability

As the scaphoid plays a critical role in coordinating and stabilizing movements between the proximal and distal rows of the carpals, damage to the intrinsic and extrinsic ligaments that support the scaphoid can result in persistent pain and dysfunction with loading activities.[26,75,76]

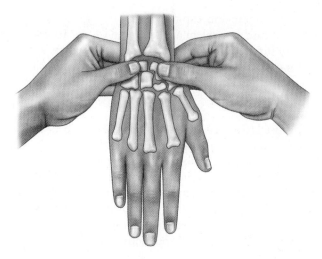

Figure 7-23 Scapholunate Shear (Ballottment) test.

The scaphoid shift maneuver examines the dynamic stability of the wrist, in particular the integrity of the scapholunate ligament.[26]

The patient is positioned with their elbow resting in their lap in approximately 90 degree of flexion. The forearm slightly pronated, and the wrist ulnarly deviated. The clinician stabilizes the scaphoid tubercle with the thumb (Figure 7-24). As the wrist is brought passively into radial deviation, the normal flexion of the proximal row forces the scaphoid tubercle into an anterior direction (into the clinician's thumb). The clinician attempts to prevent the anterior motion of the scaphoid (Figure 7-24). When the scaphoid is unstable its proximal pole is forced to sublux posteriorly.[48] Pain at the posterior wrist or a clunk suggests instability.[77,78] The results are compared with the other hand.

 Clinical Pearl

The results from the scaphoid shift test should be used with caution as the test can be positive in up to one third of uninjured individuals,[75] and has been found to have a sensitivity of 69%, and a specificity of between 64% and 68%.[79,80]

Finger extension test
This test is used to demonstrate posterior wrist syndrome, a localized scapholunate synovitis.[26] The clinician instructs the patient to fully flex the

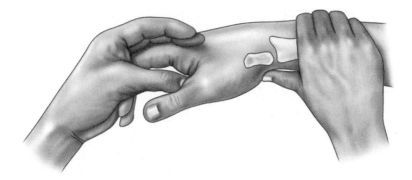

Figure 7-24 Watson' test.

wrist, and then actively extend the digits at both the IP and MCP joints. The clinician then applies pressure on the fingers into flexion at the MCP joints while the patient continues to actively extend (Figure 7-25). A positive test occurs when there is production of central posterior wrist pain and indicates the possibility of Kienböck disease, carpal instability, joint degeneration or synovitis.[48]

Diagnostic and Imaging Testing

Diagnostic testing of the forearm, wrist, and hand is limited to plain radiographs for most patients. Bony tenderness with a history of trauma or a suspicion of bone or joint disruption indicates a need for radiographs. Standard projections for the wrist are the posteroanterior, lateral, and oblique. For the patient with a suspicion of a scaphoid injury, a scaphoid view should be added.[29] Wrist conditions rarely require computed tomography (CT) scans and magnetic resonance imaging (MRI) scans.[14]

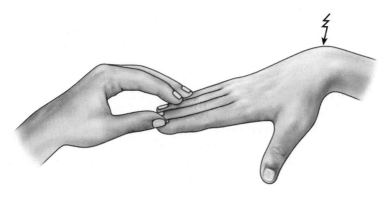

Figure 7-25 Finger extension test.

Clinical Pearl

Fractures of the distal radius are classified according to the direction of angulation of the radius and whether the radiocarpal joint, radioulnar joint, or both are involved.

- Colles' fracture: involves the distal 2cm of the radius, is angled posteriorly and laterally, resulting in the characteristic dinner-fork deformity. The most common mechanism of injury is a FOOSH.

- Smith fracture: identical to Colles' fracture except for the anterior displacement in relationship to the proximal forearm. The most common mechanism of injury is a FOOSH.

- Barton fracture: a fracture/dislocation of the distal radius that is often accompanied by a fracture of the styloid of the ulnar. Unlike Smith and Colles' fractures, which are extra-articular, a Barton fracture involves the intra-articular joint of the radius and its adjoining carpal bones. There are two types of Barton fracture: posterior (dorsal) and anterior (palmar). The most common mechanism of injury is a FOOSH.

- Chauffeur fracture: an avulsion fracture of the distal end of the radial styloid process that typically results from a FOOSH.

Examination Conclusions: The Evaluation

Following the examination, and once the clinical findings have been recorded, the clinician must determine a specific diagnosis or a working hypothesis, based on a summary of all of the findings. This diagnosis can be structure related (medical diagnosis) (Table 7-6), or a diagnosis based on the preferred practice patterns as described in the Guide to Physical Therapist Practice.[81]

INTERVENTION

The rehabilitation procedures chosen to progress the patient will depend on the type of tissue involved, the extent of the damage, and the stage of healing (see Chapter 3). The intervention must be related to the signs and symptoms present rather than the actual diagnosis.

Table 7-6 Differential Diagnosis for Common Causes of Wrist and Hand Pain

Condition	Patient Age	Mechanism of injury	Symptoms Aggravated By	Observation	AROM	PROM	End Feel	Resisted	Special Tests	Tenderness With Palpation
Carpal tunnel syndrome	35-55	Gradual overuse Wide-variety of factors	Repetitive activities of wrist Sustained positioning of wrist in flexion	Thenar muscle atrophy (later stages)	Full and pain free			Weakness of grip on radial side (chronic) Strong and pain free (acute)	Tinel's Phalen's	Reproduction of symptoms with compression applied on anterior aspect of wrist
Wrist extensor tendonitis	20-50	Repetitive or prolonged activities, forceful exertion, awkward and static postures, vibration, and localized mechanical stress		Unremarkable		Wrist pain with finger flexion combined with radial/ulnar deviation		Pain with wrist extension		Anterior carpus
Wrist flexor tendonitis	20-50	Forceful gripping, rapid wrist movements, moving the wrist and fingers to the extremes of range	Activities involving wrist extension	Unremarkable	Wrist extension	Pain with combined wrist extension and elbow extension		Pain with wrist flexion		Pisiform In palm over base of 2nd metacarpal

(continued on following page)

Table 7-6 *(continued from previous page)*

Condition	Patient Age	Mechanism of injury	Symptoms Aggravated By	Observation	AROM	PROM	End Feel	Resisted	Special Tests	Tenderness With Palpation
OA of 1st CMC Joint	40-60	Repetitive trauma Degeneration	Repetitive use of thumb Strong gripping	Soft tissue thickening at base of thumb	Mid-limitation of all thumb movements	Pain with thumb rotation Pain on thumb extension and abduction		Weakness of grip on radial side (chronic)		Anatomic snuff box
Trigger finger	50+	Disproportion between the flexor tendon and its tendon sheath		Thickening/ puckering of skin in palm	Decreased finger extension Clicing or jerking with movements	Full and pain free	Soft tissue resistance to finger extension	Strong and pain free		No pain, but snapping of flexor tendon felt with finger extension
De Quervains tenosynovitis	50+	Repetitive finger-thumb gripping combined with radial deviation	Overuse, repetitive tasks which involve overexertion of the thumb	Swelling over lateral wrist/ thumb	Decreased ulnar deviation Decreased thumb flexion	Pain on thumb flexion combined with ulnar deviation of wrist		Pain with abduction and extension of thumb	Finkelstein's	Lateral wrist and thumb

Duputryens contracture	40+	Multifactorial (alcohol, diabetes, epilepsy, smoking, trauma)		Thickening/ puckering of skin in palm	Decreased finger extension	Soft tissue resistance to finger extension	Strong and pain free	Inability to place the palm of the hand completely flat on a hard surface	No tenderness, but thickening of soft tissues evident
Thumb ulnar collateral ligament injury	Varies	Forced hyperabduction and/or hyperextension stress of the thumb MCP joint	Extension of the thumb	Swelling at the ulnar side of the MCP joint	Usually unremarkable	Pain with passive hyperextension/ hyperabduction	Usually unremarkable	Stress testing of the UCL	Ulnar side of the MCP joint of the thumb
Wrist sprain	20-40	Trauma (FOOSH injury)	Taking weight through the hand	Possible swelling around wrist joint	Extremes of all ranges	Wrist pain with ulnar or radial deviation	Pain with strong resistance in any direction		Medial or lateral joint line

COMMON ORTHOPEDIC CONDITIONS

CARPAL TUNNEL SYNDROME

Diagnosis

Carpal tunnel syndrome—ICD-9: 354.0.

Description

- A compression neuropathy of the median nerve that occurs under the transverse carpal ligament at the wrist.
- Often idiopathic but may be associated with pregnancy, hypothyroidism, diabetes, overuse phenomena, trauma, and tumors in the carpal tunnel.

 Clinical Pearl

The carpal tunnel is a space on the palmar aspect of the wrist bounded by the scaphoid, trapezium, capitate, hook of hamate, pisiform, and transverse carpal ligament.

Subjective Findings

- Complaints of numbness in the median nerve distribution, primarily in the tips of the first three fingers.
- Complaints of pain in the forearm and wrist.
- Symptoms may awaken patient from sleep.
- Activities involving wrist flexion are uncomfortable.

Objective Findings

- Thenar atrophy may be present (sign of advanced disease).

 Clinical Pearl

Check the sensation on the two sides of the pulp of the ring finger. The ulnar nerve innervates the ulnar side and the median nerve, the radial side.

Confirmatory/Special Tests

- Phalen.
- Tinel.
- Carpal compression test.
- ULTT 1 (median nerve bias).

Medical Studies

Plain radiographs (carpal tunnel view) can be used to rule out bony causes of CTS. EMG/NCS can help differentiate CTS from other entities.

 Clinical Pearl

> A negative result on nerve conduction studies (NCS) does not totally exclude the presence of median nerve compression.

Differential Diagnosis

- Cervical radiculopathy
- Peripheral neuropathy
- Proximal median nerve compression syndromes—pronator syndrome, anterior interosseus syndrome

Intervention

Initiated with splinting in slight extension.

Prognosis

Surgery (release of the transverse carpal ligament) is indicated for persistent or slow the progressive nerve function or motor loss.

DE QUERVAIN TENOSYNOVITIS

Diagnosis

De Quervain tenosynovitis—ICD-9: 727.0.

Description

An inflammation of the extensor and abductor tendons of the thumb (extensor pollicis longus, extensor pollicis brevis, and abductor pollicis longus) caused by repetitive or unaccustomed use of the thumb.

> ### ● Clinical Pearl
>
> If left untreated, this friction induced tenosynovitis can progress to stenosis tenosynovitis—fibrosis and a loss of flexibility of the thumb in flexion.

Subjective Findings

- Wrist pain on the radial side
- Difficulty with grasping and gripping

Objective Findings

- Possible swelling at the radial styloid process.
- Palpation elicits pain at the site of the retinaculum at the radial styloid.

Confirmatory/Special Tests

Finkelstein test—thumb is put in the palm and enclosed by the fingers; the wrist is then abruptly deviated ulnarly; positive tests indicated by pain at the radial side of the wrist.

Medical Studies

Imaging studies are rarely used with this condition.

Differential Diagnosis

- Scaphoid fracture
- Tendon rupture
- Radial nerve neuritis
- Basal joint arthritis (CMC joint of the thumb)
- Rheumatoid arthritis

Intervention

The goals of the intervention are to reduce the inflammation, to prevent adhesions from forming, and to prevent recurrent tendonitis.
- Symptomatic relief through splinting—thumb spica splint.
- Steroid injections made directly into the fibrous sheath of the first dorsal compartment.
- Electrotherapeutic and thermal modalities to help decrease inflammation.

- Gentle active range of motion exercises for short periods. These are progress to isometric exercises and then concentric exercises.
- Grasping and releasing of small objects emphasizing a wide variety of prehensile patterns.

Prognosis

Patients who receive treatment within 6 months of developing the condition have an excellent prognosis—90% of nonsevere cases may expect relief with conservative management.

FRACTURE OF THE DISTAL RADIUS

Diagnosis

Fracture of the distal radius—ICD-9: 813.41 (Colles fracture, Smith fracture, Barton fracture); 813.42 (other fractures of distal end of radius).

Description

Fracture of the distal radius is the most common wrist injury for all age groups. The older patient usually sustains an extra-articular metaphyseal fracture, whereas the younger patient experiences the more complicated intra-articular fracture.

Clinical Pearl

- Colles fracture: The most common type of distal radius fracture: the distal radius fracture fragment is tilted upward, or dorsally.
- Smith fracture: the opposite of the Colles fracture: the distal fragment is tilted downward, or volarly.
- Barton fracture: an intra-articular fracture associated with subluxation of the carpus, either dorsally or volarly, along with the displaced articular fragment of the radius.
- Chauffeurs fracture: an oblique fracture through the base of the radial styloid.
- Die-punch fracture: a depressed fracture of the articular surface opposite the lunate or scaphoid bone.

Subjective Findings

The subjective findings typically include the following:

- Acute pain, tenderness, swelling, and deformity of the wrist.
- History of falling onto an outstretched arm or hand.

Objective Findings

The physical examination typically reveals the following findings:

- Swelling, deformity, and discoloration around the wrist and distal radius.
- May have associated skin injury and bleeding.
- May have decreased sensation in the median, radial, or ulnar nerve distribution.
- May have decreased circulation to the hand.

Confirmatory/Special Tests

The diagnosis of a fracture of the distal radius is made based on the subjective history, physical examination, and confirmation through imaging studies.

Medical/Imaging Studies

AP and lateral radiographs of the forearm, including the wrist, are necessary.

 Clinical Pearl

A Colles fracture has the characteristic dorsiflexion or "silver fork" deformity. Radiographs of the anteroposterior view show the usual comminuted fracture.

Differential Diagnosis

- Carpal fracture-dislocation.
- Scaphoid fracture.
- Tenosynovitis of the wrist.

Intervention

Successful treatment of a fracture of the distal radius must take into account the integrity of the soft tissues by not relying on tight casts or restricting the gliding structures that control the hand, while restoring anatomic alignment of the bones. Conservative intervention can begin while the fracture is immobilized, and involves AROM of the shoulder in all planes, elbow flexion and extension, and finger flexion and extension. The finger exercises must include isolated MCP flexion, composite flexion (full fist), and intrinsic minus fisting

(MCP extension with IP flexion). If a fixator or pins are present, pin site care should be performed according to physician preference.

Following the period of immobilization, an immobilization capsular pattern will initially be present. Extension and supination are commonly limited and need to be mobilized. AROM exercises of wrist flexion and extension and ulnar and radial deviation are initiated. Wrist extension exercises are performed with the fingers flexed, especially at the MCP joints. PROM is performed according to physician preference, either immediately or after 1 to 2 weeks.

The AROM exercises of the wrist and forearm are progressed to strengthening exercises, using light weights and tubing. Putty can be used to increase grip strength if necessary.

Plyometrics and neuromuscular reeducation exercises are next, followed by return to function or sports activities.

Prognosis

These fractures typically run an uncomplicated course. On occasion, malunion, posttraumatic wrist arthritis, compartment syndrome, or nerve injury can occur.

FRACTURE OF THE SCAPHOID

Diagnosis

Fracture of the scaphoid—ICD-9: 814.01. Also referred to as navicular fracture.

 Clinical Pearl

The scaphoid is the most commonly fractured carpal bone with young male adults being the most commonly affected.

Description

Fractures of the scaphoid are important both because of their frequency and because their diagnosis is often delayed or missed. Although a fracture can occur in any part of the scaphoid, the common areas are at the waist and at the proximal pole.

 Clinical Pearl

The scaphoid spans the distal and proximal rows of the carpals and consequently is vulnerable to FOOSH injuries.

Subjective Findings

The subjective findings typically include the following:
- History of a FOOSH type injury.
- Complaints of dorsal wrist pain, especially with any type of wrist motion or activity, such as gripping.
- Tenderness over the anatomic snuffbox.

Objective Findings

The physical examination typically reveals the following findings:
- Palpation over the anatomic snuffbox, defined by the abductor and long thumb extensor tendons just distal to the radial styloid, reveals marked tenderness.
- Decreased active range of motion of the wrist.
- Decreased grip strength.
- Normal neurologic examination.

⚫ Clinical Pearl

When wrist pain is severe, snuff box or dorsal wrist tendonitis is dramatic, and the range of motion of the wrist has been decreased by 50%, the clinician should suspect a scaphoid fracture, lunate dislocation, or carpal avascular necrosis.

Confirmatory/Special Tests

Many investigators feel a reliable test for scaphoid injury is axial compression of the thumb along its longitudinal axis, which translates force directly across the scaphoid and elicits pain if there is a fracture.

Medical Studies

At the time of initial injury, scaphoid fractures may not be visible on PA and lateral radiographs of the wrist. In these cases, it is necessary to obtain a scaphoid view of the wrist (a clenched fist view with the wrist held in ulnar deviation) and an oblique view to help visualize the fracture. If the radiographs remain normal but pain persists, a bone scan is the next step.

Differential Diagnosis

- De Quervain tenosynovitis.
- Fracture of the distal radius.
- Scapholunate dissociation.

- Wrist osteoarthritis.
- Intersection syndrome.
- Intercarpal instabilities
- Superficial radial neuritis
- C6 cervical radiculitis/radiculopathy.

Intervention

Conservative management of a scaphoid fracture is controversial. There is no agreement on the optimum position for immobilization. Current management is immobilization in a long-arm or short-arm thumb spica cast, with the wrist position and length of immobilization dependent on the location of the fracture.

For the patient with pain over the anatomic snuffbox but normal initial radiographs, application of a thumb spica cast for 3 weeks followed by repeat radiographs is indicated.

 Clinical Pearl

Following the removal of the splint, a capsular pattern of the wrist will dominate. In addition, there will be a painful weakness of thumb and/or wrist extension/radial deviation and compression of the first metacarpal on the scaphoid will be painful.

AROM exercises for wrist flexion and extension, and radial and ulnar deviation are initiated as early as possible after the splint removal, with PROM to the same motions beginning after 2 weeks.

 Clinical Pearl

A wrist and thumb immobilization splint can be fabricated to wear between exercises and at night for comfort and protection.

At about the same time as the PROM exercises, gentle strengthening exercises are begun with 1- to 2-lb weights or putty. Over a period of several weeks, the exercise program is progressed to include weight-bearing activities, plyometrics, open and closed chain exercises, and neuromuscular reeducation, before finally progressing to functional and sport-specific exercises and activities.

Prognosis

Accurate early diagnosis of scaphoid fracture is critical as the morbidity associated with a missed or delayed diagnosis is significant, and can result in long-term pain, loss of mobility, and decreased function.

FLEXOR DIGITORUM PROFUNDUS AVULSION

Diagnosis

Flexor digitorum profundus avulsion—ICD-9: 842.13 (sprain of interphalangeal joint). Also referred to as Jersey finger.

Description

Avulsion of the FDP can occur in any digit, but is most common in the ring finger. This injury usually occurs when a hyperextension stress is applied to a flexed finger such as when an athlete grabs an opponent's jersey. Three types are recognized:

- In Type I the tendon retracts into the palm with or without a bony fragment.
- Type II is the most common. The tendon retracts to the proximal interphalangeal joint and the long vinculum remains intact. As in type I, type II injuries may have a small bony avulsion.
- Type III injuries involve a large bony fragment.

 Clinical Pearl

An FDP avulsion is often misdiagnosed as a sprained or "jammed" finger, as there is no characteristic deformity associated with it.

 Clinical Pearl

The FDP insertion into the ring finger is anatomically weaker than in the middle finger.

Subjective Findings

The subjective findings typically include the following:
- History of trauma involving the digit.

- History of rheumatoid arthritis or other inflammatory arthritis conditions.

Objective Findings

The physical examination typically reveals the following findings:

- Specific testing of the isolated DIP joint flexion in all digits will reveal the involved digit—the inability to flex the DIP joint is pathognomic of a Jersey finger.
- Tenderness along the flexor tendon sheath or in the palm may indicate the level of tendon retraction.

 Clinical Pearl

Flexion of the FDP is assessed by asking the patient to flex the fingertip at the DIP joint, while the PIP joint is held in extension.

Confirmatory/Special Tests

No specific test exists for this condition.

Medical Studies

Anteroposterior and lateral radiographs of the finger (not hand) may show a small avulsed fragment from the distal phalanx.

 Clinical Pearl

Fracture patterns are not reliable in predicting the level of tendon retraction.

Differential Diagnosis

- Distal phalanx fracture.
- Mallet finger.
- Anterior interosseous nerve paralysis.
- Partial tendon laceration.
- Stenosing tenosynovitis (trigger finger).

Intervention

The treatment of FDP avulsion is primarily surgical.

Prognosis

The success of the treatment depends on the acuteness of the diagnosis, rapidity of surgical intervention, and level of tendon retraction.

 Clinical Pearl

If left untreated, loss of flexion and of grip and pinch strength in the involved and adjacent fingers is possible.

GAMEKEEPER'S THUMB

Diagnosis

Gamekeeper's thumb (ulnar collateral joint ligament sprain)—ICD-9: 842.12. Also referred to as skier's thumb or break dancer's thumb.

Description

Gamekeeper's thumb involves an injury to the ulnar collateral ligament of the thumb (the MCP joint). Whether by injury or repetitive use, the disrupted ligament leads to instability of the MCP joint, and decreased functioning in both pinching and opposition involving the thumb.

 Clinical Pearl

The ulnar collateral ligament of the thumb MCP joint is an important stabilizer of the thumb.

Subjective Findings

The subjective findings typically include the following:
- Pain and swelling along the ulnar side of the MCP joint (in the acute phase).
- Complaints of pain, weakness, or loss of stability (in the chronic phase).

Objective Findings

The physical examination typically reveals the following findings:
- Local tenderness and swelling with palpation along the ulnar side of the MCP joint.

- Pain or excessive motion with valgus stress testing of the ulnar collateral ligament (see Confirmatory/Special Tests).
- Impaired MCP joint flexion and extension, especially when acute and swollen.
- Decreased pinching strength resulting from instability or acute pain.

Confirmatory/Special Tests

The stability of the MCP joint is tested in full extension, and at 30 degrees of flexion, which stress the accessory collateral ligament and the ulnar collateral ligament, respectively.

 Clinical Pearl

An angulation of greater than 35 degrees or 15 degrees greater than the uninvolved side indicates instability (Grade III) and the need for surgical intervention. Grades I and II are typically treated conservatively.

Medical Studies

AP and lateral radiographs are necessary to rule out a fracture or a fracture-dislocation.

Differential Diagnosis

The diagnosis for this condition can be made based on the pain and swelling of the first MCP joint, the localized tenderness along the ulnar side of the MCP joint, and the characteristic aggravation of symptoms with valgus stress applied across the joint. Other conditions to consider include the following:

- Extensor tendon rupture (boutonniere deformity).
- Fracture.

Intervention

The intervention for Grade I and II tears is immobilization in a thumb spica cast for 3 weeks, with additional protective splinting for 2 weeks. The splint is worn at all times except for removal for hygiene and exercise. AROM of flexion and extension begins at 3 weeks, and progresses to strengthening exercises by 8 weeks, taking care not to apply any abduction stress to the MCP joint during the first 2 to 6 weeks.

Grade III tears and displaced bony avulsions are treated with surgery and immobilization. Postsurgical rehabilitation involves wearing a thumb spica cast or splint for 3 weeks with an additional 2 weeks of splinting, except during the exercises of active flexion and extension. Otherwise the exercise progression is the same as for the Grade I and II sprains.

 Clinical Pearl

Thumb spica splints, which are a forearm-based splint fabricated from a palmar or radial approach, are designed to immobilize the wrist, carpometacarpal, and MCP joints of the thumb, thereby permitting the radial wrist extensors and the proximal thumb to rest. Thumb spicas can be used for the intervention of a number of conditions including de Quervain disease and CMC arthritis. When applying these splints, it is very important to ensure that the superficial radial nerve and the ulnar digital nerve of the thumb are not compromised.

Prognosis

The outcome of the intervention is related directly to the severity of the initial injury and whether or not injury to the underlying articular cartilage has occurred concomitantly. The principal indication for surgery is instability or in cases where symptoms persist over months.

OSTEOARTHRITIS OF THE THUMB CARPOMETACARPAL (CMC) JOINT

Diagnosis

Osteoarthritis of the thumb carpometacarpal (CMC) joint—ICD-9: 715.14 (osteoarthritis, primary, localized to the hand). Also known as basal joint arthritis.

Description

Osteoarthritis of the thumb CMC joint is caused by anatomic factors (joint configuration and ligamentous laxity) that predispose the joint to instability, shear forces, and subsequent degenerative change.

Clinical Pearl

First CMC arthritis is more common in women than men and is typically found in those 45 years and older.

Subjective Findings

Patients with first CMC joint arthritis typically present with joint pain at
the base of the thumb, which is increased with usage, restricted ROM in a
capsular pattern, and joint crepitus. The patient may also report difficulty
performing tip to tip pinching, lateral pinching, and twisting motion (starting
a car) and heavy gripping.

Objective Findings

The physical examination typically reveals the following findings:

- Tenderness over the palmar and radial aspects of the thumb in the region of
  the base of the thumb.
- Positive grind test at the CMC joint.

Confirmatory/Special Tests

The diagnosis of arthritis of the thumb carpometacarpal joint is made based on
patient history, physical examination, and confirmation through imaging studies.

Medical/Imaging Studies

PA and lateral radiographs of the thumb show joint space narrowing, subchondral sclerosis, and varying degrees of subluxation or dislocation at the
CMC joint.

Differential Diagnosis

- Fracture of the scaphoid.
- De Quervain tenosynovitis.
- Arthritis of the wrist.
- Carpal tunnel syndrome.
- Flexor carpi radialis tendonitis.

Intervention

Conservative intervention includes splinting, thermal modalities (moist heat
or paraffin), and patient education.

- Splinting. The thumb spica splint should position the CMC joint in palmar abduction, to maximize the stability and anatomic alignment of the joint, with the IP joint free. The splint is typically worn for 3 weeks.
- Patient education. The patient should be advised to
  - minimize or avoid mechanical stresses including sustained pinching.
  - avoid sleeping on the hands as this forces the thumb into adduction.
  - use self-help devices such as jar lid openers and ergonomic scissors.

Prognosis

If symptoms recur, intermittent splinting that immobilizes the entire thumb should be continued. If splinting fails, a corticosteroid preparation may be injected into the joint. Surgical options include joint fusion, osteotomy, trapeziectomy, and joint replacement.

TRIGGER FINGER

Diagnosis

Trigger finger—ICD-9: 727.03. Also known as locked finger, or stenosing tenosynovitis, of the flexor tendons.

 Clinical Pearl

A higher prevalence of trigger finger is observed in patients with carpal tunnels syndrome and de Quervain stenosing tenosynovitis.

Description

Trigger finger is an inflammation of the two flexor tendons of the finger, which become thickened and narrowed as they cross the MCP head in the palm causing a painful snapping phenomenon. The thumb, long and ring fingers are most commonly affected. Trigger finger maybe idiopathic (often observed in middle-aged women) or associated with rheumatoid arthritis or diabetes mellitus.

 Clinical Pearl

The flexor tendons of the fingers glide back and forth under four annular and three cruciform pulleys that keep the tendons from bowstringing.

Subjective Findings

The subjective findings typically include the following:

- Complaints of a painful finger or loss of smooth motion (catching) of the finger when gripping or pinching.
- There may be complaints of a painful nodule in the distal palm usually at the level of the distal flexion crease.

Objective Findings

The physical examination typically reveals the following findings:

- Local tenderness is elicited with palpation at the base of the finger, directly over the tendon as it courses over the metacarpal head.
- The clinician may palpate crepitus or a moving nodular mass in the vicinity of, or slightly proximal to, the A1 pulley.
- Pain is typically aggravated by stretching the tendon into extension or by resisting the action of flexion isometrically.
- Clicking or locking with active flexion may or may not be present.
- Full flexion of the finger may not be possible.

 Clinical Pearl

To induce a triggering during examination, it is necessary to have the patient make a full fist and then completely extend the fingers.

Confirmatory/Special Tests

No confirmatory/special tests are indicated.

Medical Studies

This is a clinical diagnosis; radiographs are not needed.

Differential Diagnosis

- Diabetes mellitus
- Dupuytren disease.
- Ganglion of the tendon sheath.
- Rheumatoid arthritis

Intervention

The goals of the intervention are to reduce swelling and inflammation in the flexor tendon sheath, and to promote smooth movement of the tendon under the A1 pulley. Historically, conservative treatment included immobilization using buddy taping, or a hand-based MP flexion block splint for the involved digit only, with the MP joint only immobilized in full extension, but this has been abandoned because of stiffening and poor results. Corticosteroid injection into the flexor sheet is now considered the treatment of choice.

Prognosis

Spontaneous long-term resolution of trigger finger is rare. Patients with recurrent tenosynovitis or mechanical locking need to evaluate their work and recreational habits (repetitive grasping or the use of tools that apply pressure over the area). Surgical release of the trigger finger, a relatively simple outpatient procedure, is reserved for the recalcitrant cases.

ULNAR NERVE ENTRAPMENT

Diagnosis

Ulnar nerve entrapment—ICD-9: 354.2 (lesion of the ulnar nerve). Also known as ulnar tunnel syndrome.

 Clinical Pearl

Entrapment of the ulnar nerve at the wrist can occur at the Guyon canal. Typically caused by repetitive trauma or a space occupying lesion such as a lipoma, ganglion, ulnar artery aneurysm, or muscle anomaly.

Description

Peripheral nerve entrapments are common in the forearm and wrist. Neurogenic syndromes are usually incomplete, indicating the absence of severe motor or sensory deficits, but in the typical case they are accompanied by a history of pain or vague sensory disturbances. As a result, nerve injuries are frequently overlooked as a source of acute, or more commonly chronic, symptomatology.

Subjective Findings

The subjective findings typically include the following:

• May or may not have pain.

• Reports of weakness and numbness in the ulnar the distribution of the hand.

Objective Findings

The clinical features of an ulnar nerve entrapment at the wrist include the following:

- Claw hand (in advanced cases) resulting from unopposed action of the extensor digitorum communis in the fourth and fifth digits.
- An inability to extend the second and distal phalanges of any of the fingers.
- An inability to adduct or abduct the fingers, or to oppose all the fingertips, as in making a cone with the fingers and thumb.
- An inability to adduct the thumb.
- Positive Froment sign.
- Atrophy of the interosseous spaces (especially the first) and of the hypothenar eminence.
- A loss of sensation on the ulnar side of the hand, the ring finger, and most markedly over the entire little finger. The dorsal ulnar aspect of the hand should be normal as that is innervated by the dorsal cutaneous branch.

Confirmatory/Special Tests

- Nerve conduction studies may be performed, focusing on the sites of interest.
- Froment sign.

Medical/Imaging Studies

Imaging studies are not typically ordered unless there is a history of trauma.

Differential Diagnosis

- Peripheral neuropathy—diabetes, with its associated neuropathies or cheiroarthropathy, may be an underlying cause of chronic wrist pain.
- Carpal tunnel syndrome.
- Thoracic outlet syndrome.
- Arthritis of the wrist.
- Ulnar neuropathy at the elbow.
- Cervical radiculopathy (C 7–8).

Intervention

The intervention for ulnar nerve compression can be surgical or conservative depending on the severity. Indications for surgical intervention include preventing deformity and increasing functional use of the hand. Conservative intervention for mild compression involves the application of a protective splint and patient education to avoid positions and postures that could compromise the nerve.

Prognosis

Loss of intrinsic muscle function causes decreased grip strength and pinch. If the cause of the ulnar nerve entrapment at the wrist is due to extrinsic compression, treatment is usually surgical.

REHABILITATION LADDER

WRIST AND HAND

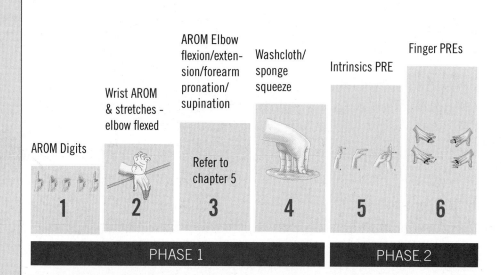

The purpose of these training ladders is to provide the clinician with a safe and progressive framework of exercises that are designed to allow the patient to improve in an efficient manner. The patient begins at the appropriate step, which is based on the stage of healing and the goal of the intervention.

- Phase 1: Acute - pain management, restoration of full passive range of motion, and restoration of normal accessory motion.

- Phase 2: Subacute - active range of motion exercises and early strengthening.

- Phase 3: Chronic - specific strengthening with a strong emphasis on enhancing dynamic stability.

The degree of movement and the speed of progression are both guided by the signs and symptoms. Once the patient is able to perform an exercise for

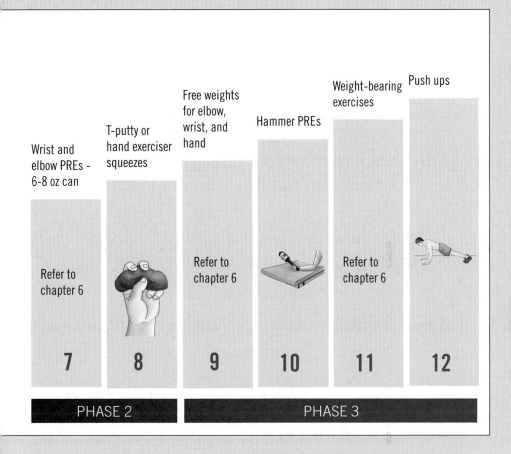

8–12 reps without pain, he/she progresses up to the next exercise step. This continues until the patient attempts an exercise that reproduces the pain. At this point, the patient returns to the last exercise that he/she was able to perform without pain and performs that exercise 5 times/day for 1-2 days before attempting to progress again. The patient is advanced through the training ladders to the appropriate point, with particular attention paid to patient response to treatment in terms of changes in symptoms, swelling, degree of irritability or motion. In addition, muscle imbalances are addressed with appropriate flexibility exercises.

Once the patient is able to perform the last exercise of Phase 3 (Step 12 of the ladder), he or she can move on to functional and sport-specific training (Phase 4) as appropriate, which focus on power and higher-speed exercises similar to sport specific demands.

1. AROM of the digits

The patient is positioned in sitting with the involved hand held out in front. The patient is asked to move each digit individually throughout its entire range of motion (1a). A more extensive exercise involves having the patient sit next to a table with the forearm supported on the table in a position of pronation or supination. To increase extension at anyone joint, the patient's forearm is supinated; to increase flexion the forearm is pronated, and the phalanx to be stretched is at the edge of the table. Other active range of motion exercises to include are fingertip to fingertip exercises (1b), thumb opposition (1c), and pinching activities (1d).

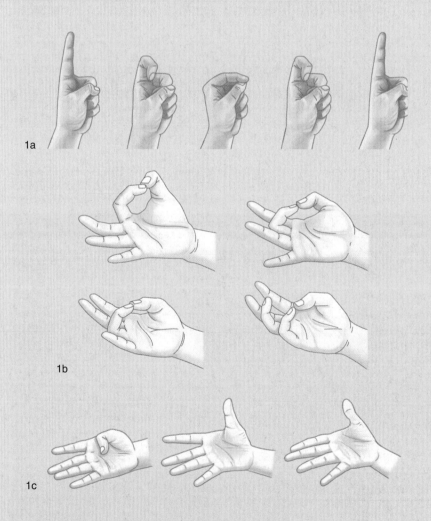

1a

1b

1c

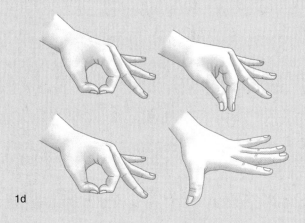

1d

2. Wrist active range of motion

The patient is positioned in sitting next to a table with the forearm supported on the table and the wrist and hand over the edge of the table. The patient is asked to move the hand and wrist actively into flexion/extension (2a). At the end range of motion the patient applies passive overpressure to move the joint further into the range. The wrist must also be moved into radial and ulnar deviation (2b). The prayer position (2c) can be used to increase wrist extension. The patient places the palms and fingers of the hands together and then slowly raises both elbows towards the ceiling while keeping the hands together.

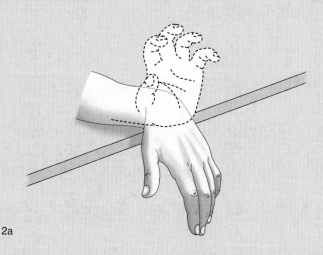

2a

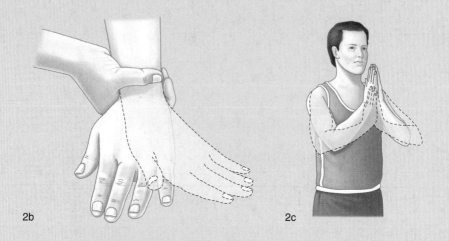

2b   2c

3. AROM Elbow flexion/extension/forearm pronation/supination
See chapter 6 for full description.

4. Washcloth/sponge squeeze
The patient is positioned in sitting or standing next to a table on which is placed a washcloth or sponge. Using the fingers only, the patient is asked to squeeze and release the washcloth or sponge (4).

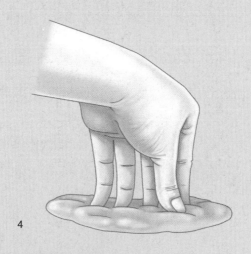

4

5. Intrinsics PRE

To strengthen the intrinsic muscles of the hand for motions that require a combination of MCP flexion and IP extension, The patient is asked to start with the MCP joints extended and the PIP joints flexed, and then to actively push the fingertips outward, performing the desired combined motion (5a and b). Isometric resistance can be added by pushing the fingertips against the palm of the other hand (5c).

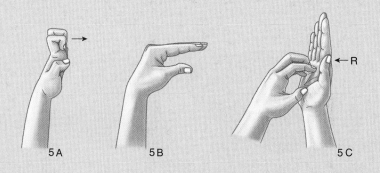

6. Finger PREs

Resistance can be applied to digits using a variety of techniques (6a-b).

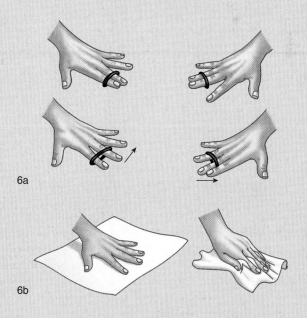

7. Wrist and elbow PREs
See chapter 6 for full description.

8. Theraputty or hand exerciser squeezes
Resistance for the muscles of the hand and fingers can be applied using Thera-putty (8) or a hand exerciser, emphasizing the gripping motions throughout a variety of wrist positions.

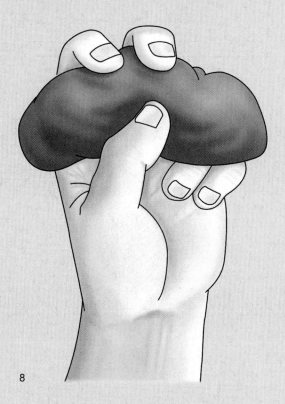

8

9. Free weight exercises for elbow, wrist and hand
See chapter 6 for full description.

10. Hammer PREs
The patient is positioned in sitting and is asked to grasp a hammer or an asym-metrically weighted bar. The patient moves the bar into supination (10a) and pronation (10b). Radial and ulnar deviation can also be exercised in a similar manner by having the patient stand with the arms by the side and holding the hammer with the palm facing the body. The hammer is raised in front of

the patient using only wrist motion to increase radial deviation strength, and behind the patient to increase ulnar deviation strength.

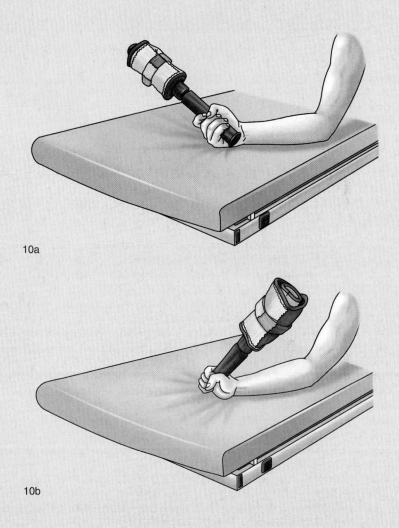

10a

10b

11. Weight-bearing exercises
See chapter 6 for full description.

12. Push-ups
A full push-up (12) or a modified push-up can be used as appropriate.

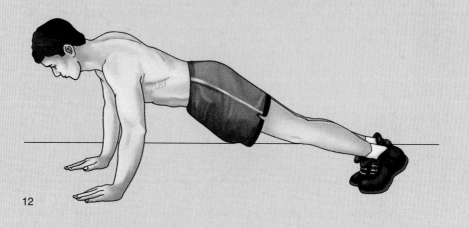

12

REFERENCES

1. Hume MC, Gellman H, McKellop H, et al. Functional range of motion of the joints of the hand. *J Hand Surg.* 1990;15A:240–243.
2. Butler DS. *Mobilization of the Nervous Sysytem.* New York, NY: Churchill Livingstone; 1992.
3. Kiser DM. Physiological and biomechanical factors for understanding repetitive motion injuries. *Semin Occup Med.* 1987;2:11–17.
4. Keller K, Corbett J, Nichols D. Repetitive strain injury in computer keyboard users: Pathomechanics and treatment principles in individual and group intervention. *J Hand Ther.* 1998;11:9–26.
5. Dent S. *Befuddled by a FOOSH?* FR Report. 2002;6:9.
6. Overton DT, Uehara DT. Evaluation of the injured hand. *Emerg Med Clin North Am.* 1993;11:585–600.
7. Noble J, Arafa M, Royle SG, et al. The association between alcohol, hepatic pathology and Dupuytren's disease. *J Hand Surg* (Br). 1992;17:71–74.
8. Saar JD, Grothaus PC. Dupuytren's disease: an overview. *Plast Reconstr Surg.* 2000;106:125–136.
9. Yi IS, Johnson G, Moneim MS. Etiology of Dupuytren's disease. *Hand Clin.* 1999;15:43–51.
10. Lanzetta M, Morrison WA. Dupuytren's disease occurring after a surgical injury to the hand. *J Hand Surg* (Br). 1996;21:481–483.
11. Muckart RD. Stenosing tendovaginitis of abductor pollicis brevis at the radial styloid (de Quervain's disease). *Clin Orthop.* 1964;33:201–208.
12. Skirven T. Clinical examination of the wrist. *J Hand Ther.* 1996;9:96–107.
13. Nalebuff EA. The rheumatoid swan-neck deformity. *Hand Clin.* 1989;5:203–214.
14. Onieal M-E. The hand: examination and diagnosis. In: *American Society for Surgery of the Hand.* 3rd ed. New York, NY: Churchill Livingstone; 1990.

15. Feldon P, Millender LH, Nalebuff EA. Rheumatoid arthritis in the hand and wrist. In: Green DP, ed. *Operative Hand Surgery,* 3rd ed. New York, NY: Churchill Livingstone; 1993:1587–1690.
16. Wadsworth CT. Anatomy of the hand and wrist. In: *Manual Examination and Treatment of the Spine and Extremities.* Baltimore, MD: Williams & Wilkins; 1988:128–138.
17. Judge RD, Zuidema GD, Fitzgerald FT. General appearance. In: Judge RD, Zuidema GD, Fitzgerald FT, eds. *Clinical Diagnosis,.* 4th ed. Boston, MA: Little, Brown and Company; 1982: 29–47.
18. Watson HK, Weinzweig J. Physical examination of the wrist. *Hand Clin.* 1997; 13:17–34.
19. Freiberg A, Pollard BA, Macdonald MR, et al. Management of proximal interphalangeal joint injuries. *J Trauma Inj Inf Crit Care.* 1999;46:523–528.
20. Nicholson B. Clinical evaluation. In: Stanley BG, Tribuzi SM, eds. *Concepts in Hand Rehabilitation.* Philadelphia, PA: FA Davis; 1992:59–91.
21. Hoppenfeld S. *Physical Examination of the Spine and Extremities.* East Norwalk, CT: Appleton-Century-Crofts; 1976.
22. Blair SJ, McCormick E, Bear-Lehman J, et al. Evaluation of impairment of the upper extremity. *Clin Orthop.* 1987;221:42–58.
23. Riordan DC, Kaplan EB. *Kaplan's Functional and Surgical Anatomy of the Hand,.* 3rd ed. Philadelphia, PA: JB Lippincott; 1984.
24. Whipple TL. Preoperative evaluation and imaging. In: Whipple TL, ed. *Athroscopic Surgery: The Wrist.* Philadelphia, PA: JB Lippincott; 1992:11–36.
25. Osterman AL, Mikulics M. Scaphoid nonunion. *Hand Clin.* 1988;14:437–455.
26. Watson HK, Ashmead D, Makhlouf MV. Examination of the scaphoid. *J Hand Surg.* 1988;13A:657–660.
27. Alexander AH, Lichtman DM. Kienbock's disease. In: Lichtman DM, ed. *The Wrist and its Disorders.* Philadelphia, PA: WB Saunders; 1988.
28. Kienböck R. Concerning traumatic malacia of the lunate and its consequences: Degeneration and compression fractures. *Clin Orthop Relat Res.* 1980;149:4–5.
29. Onieal M-E. Common wrist and elbow injuries in primary care. Lippincott's Primary Care Practice. *Musculosk Cond.* 1999;3:441–450.
30. Polivy KD, Millender LH, Newberg A, et al. Fractures of the hook of the hamate—a failure of clinical diagnosis. *J Hand Surg.* 1985;10A:101–104.
31. Rao SB, Culver JE. Triquetralhamate arthrodesis for midcarpal instability. *J Hand Surg.* 1995;20A:583–589.
32. Magee DJ, ed. *Orthopedic Physical Assessment.* Philadelphia, PA: WB Saunders; 2002.
33. Wadsworth C. Wrist and hand. In: Wadsworth C, ed. *Current Concepts of Orthopedic Physical Therapy—Home Study Course.* La Crosse, WI: Orthopaedic Section, APTA; 2001.
34. Mathiowetz V, Weber K, Volland G, et al. Reliability and validity of grip and pinch strength evaluations. *J Hand Surg.* 1984;9A:222–226.
35. Stokes HM, Landrieu KW, Domangue B, et al. Identification of low effort patients through dynamometry. *J Hand Surg.* 1995;20A:1047–1056.
36. Kapandji IA. *The Physiology of the Joints, Upper Limb.* New York, NY: Churchill Livingstone; 1991.

37. Norkin C, Levangie P. *Joint Structure and Function: A Comprehensive Analysis.* Philadelphia, PA: FA Davis Company; 1992.
38. Eberhardt K, Malcus Johnson P, Rydgren L. The occurrence and significance of hand deformities in early rheumatoid arthritis. *Br J Rheum.* 1991;30:211–213.
39. Fess EE. The need for reliability and validity in hand assessment instruments [editorial]. *J Hand Surg.* 1986;11A:621–623.
40. Jebsen RH, Taylor N, Triegchmann R, et al. An objective and standardized test for hand function. *Arch Phys Med Rehab.* 1969;50:311.
41. Beckenbaugh RD, Shives TC, Dobyns JH, et al. Kienböck's disease: The natural history of Kienböck's disease and consideration of lunate fractures. *Clin Orthop.* 1980;149:98–106.
42. *Purdue Pegboard Test of Manipulative Dexterity.* Chicago, MA: Service Research Associates; 1968.
43. Tiffin J, Asker E. The Purdue pegboard: Norms and studies of reliability and validity. *J Appl Psychol.* 1948;32:324
44. Crawford J. *Crawford Small Parts Dexterity Test (CSPDT), Psychological Corp (Catalog): Tests, Products and Services for Business, Industry, and Government.* Cleveland, OH: Harcourt Brace Jovanovich; 1985:32.
45. Mackinnon SE, Dellon AL. Sensory rehabilitation after nerve injury. In: Mackinnon SE, Dellon AL, eds. *Surgery of the Peripheral Nerve.* New York, NY: Thieme Medical Publishers; 1988:521.
46. Anthony MS. Wounds. In Clark GL, Shaw Wilgis EF, Aiello B, et al. eds. *Hand Rehabilitation: A Practical Guide,* 2nd ed. Philadelphia, PA: Churchill Livingstone, 1998:1–15.
47. Fess EE. Documentation: essential elements of an upper extremity assessment battery. In: Hunter JM, Mackin EJ, Callahan AD (eds). *Rehabilitation of the Hand: Surgery and Therapy,* 4th ed.. St Louis, MO: Mosby; 1995:185.
48. Waggy C. Disorders of the wrist. In: Wadsworth C, ed. *Orthopaedic Physical Therapy Home Study Course—The Elbow, Forearm, and Wrist.* La Crosse, WI: Orthopaedic Section, APTA, Inc.; 1997.
49. Reagan DS, Linscheid RL, Dobyns JH. Lunotriquetral sprains. *J Hand Surg.* 1984;9A:502–514.
50. Marx RG, Bombardier C, Wright JG. What we know about the reliability and validity of physical examination tests used to examine the upper extremity. *J Hand Surg.* 1999;24A:185–193.
51. Tubiana R, Thomine J-M, Mackin E. *Examination of the Hand and Wrist.* London: Mosby; 1996.
52. Phalen GS. The carpal tunnel syndrome: clinical evaluation of 598 hands. *Clin Orthop.* 1972;83:29–40.
53. Phalen GS. Spontaneous compression of the median nerve at the wrist. *J Am Med Assoc.* 1951;145:1128–1133.
54. Onieal M-E. *Essentials of Musculoskeletal Care,* 1st ed. Rosemont, IL: American Academy of Orthopaedic Surgeons; 1997.
55. Marx RG, Hudak PL, Bombardier C, et al. The reliability of physical examination for carpal tunnel syndrome. *J Hand Surg.* 1998;23B:499–502.
56. Golding DN, Rose DM, Selvarajah K. Clinical tests for carpal tunnel syndrome: An evaluation. *Br J Rheum.* 1986;25:388–390.

57. Heller L, Ring H, Costeff H, et al. Evaluation of Tinel's and Phalen's signs in diagnosis of the carpal tunnel syndrome. *Eur Neurol.* 1986;25:40–42.
58. Robert AW, Cynthia B, Thomas JA. Reverse Phalen's maneuver as an aid in diagnosing carpal tunnel syndrome. *Arch Phys Med Rehab.* 1994;75:783–786.
59. Brain WR, Wright AD, Wilkinson M. Spontaneous compression of both median nerves in the carpal tunnel: six cases treated surgically. *Lancet.* 1947;1:277–282.
60. Werner CO, Elmqvist D, Ohlin P. Pressure and nerve lesion in the carpal tunnel. *Acta Orthop Scand.* 1983;54:312–316.
61. de Krom MC, Knipschild PG, Kester AD, et al. Efficacy of provocative tests for diagnosis of carpal tunnel syndrome. *Lancet.* 1990;335:393–395.
62. Duck-Sun A. Hand elevation: a new test for carpal tunnel syndrome. *Ann Plast Surg.* 2001;46:120–124.
63. Moberg E. Objective methods for determining the functional value of sensibility in the hand. *J Bone Joint Surg.* 1958;40A:454–476.
64. Omer GE. Report of committee for evaluation of the clinical result in peripheral nerve injury. *J Hand Surg.* 1983;8:754–759.
65. Kohonen M, Teerenhovi O, Terho T, et al. Is the Allen test reliable enough? *Eur J Cardiothorac Surg.* 2007;32:902–905.
66. McGregor AD. The Allen test—an investigation of its accuracy by fluorescein angiography. *J Hand Surg Br.* 1987;12:82–85.
67. Stewart JD, Eisen A. Tinel's sign and the carpal tunnel syndrome. *Br Med J.* 1978;2:1125–1126.
68. Gellman H, Gelberman RH, Tan AM, et al. Carpal tunnel syndrome. An evaluation of the provocative diagnostic tests. *J Bone Joint Surg.* 1986;68A:735–737.
69. Finkelstein H. Stenosing tenovaginitis at the radial styloid process. *J Bone Joint Surg.* 1930;12A:509–540.
70. Elson RA. Rupture of the central slip of the extensor hood of the finger: a test for early diagnosis. *J Bone Joint Surg Br.* 1986;68:229–231.
71. Preston D, Shapiro B. Electromyography and neuromuscular disorders. In: *Clinical Electrophysiologic Correlations.* Boston, MA: Butterworth-Heinemann; 1998.
72. Booher JM, Thibodeau GA. *Athletic Injury Assessment.* St Louis, MO: CV Mosby; 1989.
73. Swanson A. Disabling arthritis at the base of the thumb: treatment by resection of the trapezium and flexible implant arthroplasty. *J Bone Joint Surg.* 1972;54A:456.
74. Beckenbaugh RD. Accurate evaluation and management of the painful wrist following injury. *Orthop Clin North Am.* 1984;15:289–306.
75. Wolfe SW, Gupta A, Crisco JJ, III. Kinematics of the scaphoid shift test. *J Hand Surg.* 1997;22A:801–806.
76. Taleisnik J. Scapholunate dissociation. In: Taleisnik J, ed. *The Wrist.* New York, NY: Churchill Livingstone; 1985: 239–278.
77. Burton RI, Eaton RG. Common hand injuries in the athlete. *Orthop Clin North Am.* 1973;4:809–838.
78. Taleisnik J. Classification of carpal instability. In: Taleisnik J, ed. *The Wrist.* New York, NY: Churchill Livingstone; 1985: 229–238.
79. LaStayo P, Howell J. Clinical provocative tests used in evaluating wrist pain: a descriptive study. *J Hand Surg.* 1995;8:10–17.

80. Easterling KJ, Wolfe SW. Scaphoid shift in the uninjured wrist. *J Hand Surg.* 1994;19A:604–606.

81. Guide to physical therapist practice. *Phys Ther.* 2001;81:S13–S95.

QUESTIONS

1. Which tendon is in the third dorsal compartment of the hand?
2. Of the hand digits, which is the more functionally important?
3. Which two structures passed through Guyon canal?
4. Starting radially, name the four proximal carpal bones.
5. What areas of the hand typically have autonomous innervation?
6. What is the open-packed position of the distal radioulnar joint?
7. Which special test is used to assess intrinsic muscle tightness?
8. What is the name given to an injury of the extensor mechanism at the DIP joint?
9. What is the closed-pack position of the radiocarpal (wrist) joint?
10. What is the name of the disease characterized by inflammation of the abductor pollicis longus and extensor pollicis brevis tendons?
11. What is the capsular pattern of the interphalangeal joints?
12. Define a jersey finger.
13. What is the name given to an injury of the ulnar collateral ligament of the thumb MP joint?
14. What is the difference between a Colles fracture and a Barton fracture?
15. Which nerve is involved with Wartenberg disease?
16. Froment sign is used to detect a lesion of which nerve?
17. What are the three different kinds of Colles fractures?
18. What is a Galleazzi fracture?
19. What is the differential diagnosis for Raynaud syndrome?
20. What is the differential diagnosis for a patient reporting pain and tenderness in the snuffbox?
21. What is the differential diagnosis for carpal tunnel syndrome?
22. Name two special tests used to help diagnose carpal tunnel syndrome.
23. What does the acronym FOOSH stand for?
24. What is a Dupuytren contracture?
25. Describe what is involved with a swan-neck deformity?
26. What are Beau lines?
27. Which nerve may be involved with atrophy of the thenar eminence?

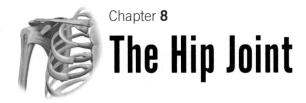

Chapter **8**

The Hip Joint

OVERVIEW

Due to its location, design, and function, the hip joint transmits truly impressive loads, both tensile and compressive. Loads of up to eight times body weight have been demonstrated in the hip joint during jogging, with potentially greater loads present during vigorous athletic competition.[1] In addition to providing stability, the hip joint permits a great deal of mobility. Any imbalance between these two variables can leave the hip joint and surrounding tissues prone to soft tissue injuries, impingement syndromes, and joint dysfunction.

ANATOMY

The hip joint consists of the articulation between the femoral head and the horseshoe shaped articulating surface of the pelvic acetabulum.

🔘 Clinical Pearl

The acetabulum is formed from three bones: the ilium, ischium, and pubis.

A number of structures about the hip are uniquely adapted to transfer forces:

- Labrum: The acetabular labrum deepens the acetabulum and increases articular congruence.
- Ligaments: The major ligaments of the pelvis and hip are known to be the strongest in the body and are well adapted to the forces transferred between the spine and the lower extremities.
- Muscles (Table 8-1): The abdominal musculature and the erector muscles of the spine provide further stabilization of the hip region and must be considered in conditions that affect pelvic tilt and the hip joint.

Table 8-1 Muscles Acting Across the Hip Joint

Muscle	Origin	Insertion	Innervation
Adductor brevis	External aspect of the body and inferior ramus of the pubis	By an aponeurosis to the line from the greater trochanter of the linea aspera of the femur	Obturator nerve, L3
Adductor longus	Pubic crest and symphysis	By an aponeurosis to the middle third of the linea aspera of the femur	Obturator nerve, L3
Adductor magnus	Inferior ramus of pubis, ramus of ischium and the inferolateral aspect of the ischial tuberosity	By an aponeurosis to the linea aspera and adductor tubercle of the femur	Obturator nerve and tibial portion of the sciatic nerve, L2–L4
Biceps femoris (long head)	Arises from the sacrotuberous ligament and posterior aspect of the ischial tuberosity	By way of a tendon, on the lateral aspect of the head of the fibula, the lateral condyle of the tibial tuberosity, the lateral collateral ligament, and the deep fascia of the leg	Tibial portion of the sciatic nerve, S1
Gemelli (superior and inferior)	Superior-dorsal surface of the spine of the ischium, inferior-upper part of the tuberosity of the ischium.	Superior and inferior-medial surface of the greater trochanter	Sacral plexus, L5–S1
Gluteus maximus	Posterior gluteal line of the ilium, iliac crest, aponeurosis of the erector spinae, dorsal surface of the lower part of the sacrum, side of the coccyx, sacrotuberous ligament, and intermuscular fascia	Iliotibial tract of the fascia latae, gluteal tuberosity of the femur	Inferior gluteal nerve, S1–S2
Gluteus medius	Outer surface of the ilium between the iliac crest and the posterior gluteal line, anterior gluteal line and fascia	Lateral surface of the greater trochanter	Superior gluteal nerve, L5
Gluteus minimus	Outer surface of the ilium between the anterior and inferior gluteal lines, and the margin of the greater sciatic notch	A ridge laterally situated on the anterior surface of the greater trochanter	Superior gluteal nerve, L5

(continued on following page)

Muscle	Origin	Insertion	Innervation
Gracilis	The body and inferior ramus of the pubis	The anterior-medial aspect of the shaft of the proximal tibia, just proximal to the tendon of the semitendinosus	Obturator nerve, L2
Iliacus	Super two-thirds of the iliac fossa, upper surface of the lateral part of the sacrum	Fibers converge with tendon of the psoas major to lesser trochanter	Femoral nerve, L2
Obturator externus	Rami of the pubis, ramus of the ischium, medial two-thirds of the outer surface of the obturator membrane	Trochanteric fossa of the femur	Obturator nerve, L4
Obturator internus	Internal surface of the anterolateral wall of the pelvis, and obturator membrane	Medial surface of the greater trochanter	Sacral plexus, S1
Pectineus	Pecten pubis	Along a line leading from the lesser trochanter to the linea aspera	Femoral or obturator or accessory obturator nerves, L2
Piriformis	Front of the sacrum, gluteal surface of the ilium, capsule of the sacroiliac joint, and sacrotuberous ligament	Upper border of the greater trochanter of femur	Sacral plexus, S1
Psoas major	Transverse processes of all the lumbar vertebrae, bodies, and intervertebral discs of the lumbar vertebrae	Lesser trochanter of the femur	Lumbar plexus, L2–L3
Quadratus femoris	Ischial body next to the ischial tuberosity	Quadrate tubercle on femur	Nerve to quadratus femoris
Rectus femoris	By two heads, from the anterior inferior iliac spine, and a reflected head from the groove above the acetabulum	Base of the patella	Femoral nerve, L3–L4
Sartorius	Anterior superior iliac spine and notch below it	Upper part of the medial surface of the tibia in front of the gracilis	Femoral nerve, L2–L3
Semimembranosus	Ischial tuberosity	The posterior–medial aspect of the medial condyle of the tibia	Tibial nerve, L5–S1

(continued on following page)

Table 8-1 *(continued from previous page)*

Muscle	Origin	Insertion	Innervation
Semitendinosus	Ischial tuberosity	Upper part of the medial surface of the tibia behind the attachment of the sartorus and below that of the gracilis	Tibial nerve, L5–S1
Tensor Fasciae Latae	Outer lip of the iliac crest and the lateral surface of the anterior superior iliac spine	Iliotibial tract	Superior gluteal nerve, L4–L5

 Clinical Pearl

Given that the hip region is also a common source of symptom referral from other regions, the examination of the hip rarely occurs in isolation, and almost always involves an assessment of the lumbar spine, pelvis, and knee joint complex.

EXAMINATION

History

The history should determine the patient's chief complaint and the mechanism of injury, if any. To aid the clinician as to the source of the symptoms, the patient should complete a pain diagram and a medical history questionnaire. The patient should also be encouraged to describe the location and type of pain (Table 8-2 to 8-5 and Figure 8-1 and 8-2).

 Clinical Pearl

Pain arising from the hip joints may be secondary to osteoarthritis, osteonecrosis, inflammatory conditions (such as rheumatoid arthritis), septic arthritis, fractures of the proximal femur or pelvis, or dislocations of the femoral head.

Symptoms including prolonged morning stiffness (greater than 1 hour) should raise suspicion for an inflammatory arthritis (Table 8-6).

Table 8-2 Differential Diagnosis for Pain in the Hip or Buttock Area

Pain Distribution	Potential Cause
Groin area	Stress fractures of the pelvis and femur
	Crystal-induced synovitis (gout)
	An inguinal/femoral hernia
	Hip adductor strain
	Iliopectineal bursitis
	Iliopsoas strain
	Osteoarthritis of the hip/osteonecrosis of the femoral head
	Femoral neck fracture
	Sacroiliac joint lesion
	Tumor
	Hernia
	Inflammatory synovitis (e.g., rheumatoid arthritis, ankylosing spondylitis, systemic lupus)
	Subluxation
	Transient synovitis
	Loosened prosthesis
	Inflamed lymph nodes
	Referred pain—viscera or spinal nerve
Pubic area	Pubic symphysis dysfunction
	• Osteitis pubis
	• Osteomyelitis pubis
	• Pyogenic arthritis
	• Pubic fracture
	• Pubic osteolysis
	• Post-partum symphyseal pain
	Abdominal muscle strain
	Bladder infection
Lateral buttock area	Trochanteric bursitis
	Tendonitis of abductors or external rotators
	Apophysitis of greater trochanter
	Referred pain from mid or lower lumbar spine
	Thrombosis of gluteal arteries

(continued on following page)

Table 8-2 *(continued from previous page)*

Pain Distribution	Potential Cause
Anterior and lateral thigh	Strain of quadriceps
	Meralgia paresthetica
	Entrapment of femoral nerve
	Thrombosis of femoral artery or great saphenous vein
	Stress fracture of femur
	Referred pain from hip or mid lumbar spine
Medial thigh	Strain of adductor muscles
	Entrapment of obturator nerve
	Referred pain from hip or knee
ASIS	Apophysitis or sartorius or rectus femoris
Iliac crest	Strain of gluteal, oblique abdominals, tensor fasciae latae, quadratus lumborum
	Entrapment of iliohypogastric nerve
	Referred pain from upper lumbar spine

A careful history should be obtained to pinpoint other joint involvement, enthesopathy (tendinous pain and inflammation at the site of muscle insertion), associated skin disease, systemic symptoms, eye problems, sexually transmitted diseases, inflammatory bowel disease, and a family history of inflammatory disease.

 Clinical Pearl

Conditions involving both the hip joint and bony pelvis often manifest as pain in the groin, buttock, or lateral thigh.

The location of the symptoms can provide the clinician with some useful information.

 Clinical Pearl

Anterior hip pain usually indicates pathology of the hip joint (i.e., degenerative arthritis), hip flexor muscle strains or tendonitis, and iliopsoas bursitis.

Table 8-3 Clinical Findings, Differential Diagnosis, and Special Tests for Some Hip Conditions

Diagnosis	History	Physical Findings	Special Tests	Differential Diagnosis
Legg–Calvé–Perthes disease	Insidious onset (1–3 months) of limp with hip or knee pain	Limited hip abduction, flexion, and internal rotation	Normal CBC and ESR, plain films positive (early with changes in the epiphysis, later with flattening of the femoral head)	Juvenile arthritis, other inflammatory conditions of the hip
Slipped capital femoral piphysis	Acute (<1 month) or chronic (up to 6 months) presentation, pain may be referred to knee or anterior thigh	Pain and limited internal rotation, leg more comfortable in external rotation; chronic presentation may have leg length discrepancy	Plain films show widening of epiphysis early, later slippage of femur under epiphysis	Muscle strain, avulsion fracture
Avulsion fracture	Sudden, violent muscle contraction; may hear or feel a "pop"	Pain on passive stretch and active contraction of involved muscle; pain on palpation of involved apophysis	Plain films; if these are negative, CT or MRI	Muscle strain, slipped capital femoral epiphysis
Hip pointer	Direct trauma to iliac crest	Tenderness over iliac crest, may have pain on ambulation and active abduction of hip.	Plain films if suspect fracture	Contusion, fracture
Contusion	Direct trauma to soft tissue	Pain on palpation and motion, ecchymosis	Plain films negative	Hip pointer, fracture, myositis ossificans
Myositis ossificans	Contusion with hematoma approximately 2 to 4 weeks earlier	Pain on palpation, firm mass may be palpable	Radiograph or ultrasound examination reveals typical calcified, intramuscular hematoma	Contusion, soft tissue tumors, callus formation from prior fracture

(continued on following page)

Table 8-3 *(continued from previous page)*

Diagnosis	History	Physical Findings	Special Tests	Differential Diagnosis
Femoral neck stress fracture	Persistent groin discomfort increasing with activity, history of endurance exercise, female athlete triad (eating disorder, amenorrhea, osteoporosis)	ROM may be painful, pain on palpation of greater trochanter	Plain films may show cortical defects in femoral neck (superior or inferior surface); bone scan, MRI, CT may also be used if plain films are negative and diagnosis is suspected	Trochanteric bursitis, osteoid osteoma, muscle strain
Osteoid osteoma	Vague hip pain present at night and increased with activities	Restricted motion, quadriceps atrophy	Plain films, if these are negative and symptoms persist, MRI or CT	Femoral neck stress fracture, trochanteric bursitis
Iliotibial band syndrome	Lateral hip, thigh or knee pain, snapping as iliotibial band passes over the greater trochanter	Positive Ober's test	Positive Ober's test	Trochanteric bursitis
Trochanteric bursitis	Pain over greater trochanter on palpation, pain during transitions from standing to lying down to standing	Pain on palpation of greater trochanter	Plain films, bone scan, MRI negative for bony involvement	Iliotibial band syndrome; femoral neck stress fracture

Avascular necrosis of the femoral head	Dull ache or throbbing pain in groin, lateral hip or buttock, history of prolonged steroid use, prior fracture, slipped femoral capital epiphysis	Pain on ambulation, abduction, internal and external rotation	Plain films, MRI	Early degenerative joint disease
Piriformis syndrome	Dull posterior pain, may radiate down the leg mimicking radicular symptoms, history of track competition or prolonged sitting	Pain on active external rotation, passive internal rotation of hip and palpation of sciatic notch	EMG studies may be helpful, MRI of lumbar spine if nerve root compression is suspected	Nerve root compression, stress fractures
Iliopsoas bursitis	Pain and snapping in medial groin or thigh	Reproduce symptoms with active and passive flexion/extension of hip	Plain films are negative	Avulsion fracture
Meralgia paresthetica	Pain or paresthesia of anterior or lateral groin and thigh	Abnormal distribution of lateral femoral cutaneous nerve on sensory examination	Nerve conduction velocity testing may be helpful	Other causes of peripheral neuropathy
Degenerative arthritis	Progressive pain and stiffness	Reduction in internal rotation early, in all motion later, pain on ambulation	Plain films help with diagnosis and prognosis	Inflammatory arthritis

PPB = prepubescent; CBC = complete blood count; ESR = erythrocyte sedimentation rate; ROM = range of motion; CT = computed tomography; MRI = magnetic resonance imaging; NSAIDs = nonsteroidal anti-inflammatory drugs; PT = physical therapy; ORIF = open reduction internal fixation; EMG = electromyelography.

Table 8-4 Differentiation Between Hip Strains and Tendonitis

Condition	Presentation	Examination Findings	Imaging and Diagnostic Studies	Basis of Diagnosis
Muscle and tendon strains	Acute mechanism; localized pain occurring immediately	Local swelling and tenderness, ecchymosis, weakness	MRI or ultrasonography	Clinical findings with imaging if needed
Tendonitis	Overuse; delayed onset, pain localized, and worsening with activity	Local swelling and tenderness, crepitus "snapping," weakness	MRI or ultrasonography	Clinical findings with imaging if needed

- Groin pain is a common complaint in this region and can result from local and referred sources (Table 8-7).
- Lateral hip pain is usually associated with greater trochanteric pain syndrome, iliotibial band (ITB) syndrome, or meralgia paresthetica (Table 8-8).

Table 8-5 Differentiation Between Occult Hernia and Nerve Entrapment

Condition	Presentation	Examination Findings	Imaging and Diagnostic Studies	Basis of Diagnosis
Sports hernia (occult hernia or tear of oblique aponeurosis)	Chronic groin pain (i.e., particularly common in soccer, and ice hockey); pain worse with "cutting" and sprinting	Tenderness at superficial inguinal ring	Herniography may identify occult hernia	Clinical findings
Obturator or ilioinguinal nerve entrapment	Same as for sports hernia but with adductor weakness or spasm	Adductor tenderness; decreased sensation	Electromyelography Obturator nerve block	Clinical findings and diagnostic tests

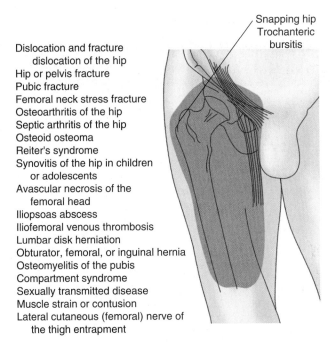

Snapping hip
Trochanteric
bursitis

Dislocation and fracture
    dislocation of the hip
Hip or pelvis fracture
Pubic fracture
Femoral neck stress fracture
Osteoarthritis of the hip
Septic arthritis of the hip
Osteoid osteoma
Reiter's syndrome
Synovitis of the hip in children
    or adolescents
Avascular necrosis of the
    femoral head
Iliopsoas abscess
Iliofemoral venous thrombosis
Lumbar disk herniation
Obturator, femoral, or inguinal hernia
Osteomyelitis of the pubis
Compartment syndrome
Sexually transmitted disease
Muscle strain or contusion
Lateral cutaneous (femoral) nerve of
    the thigh entrapment

Figure 8-1 Potential causes of trochanteric, pubic, and anterior thigh pain.

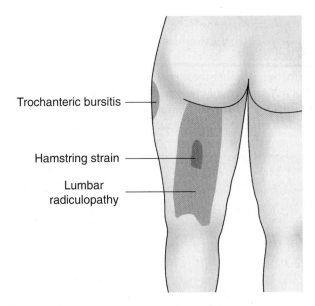

Trochanteric bursitis

Hamstring strain

Lumbar
radiculopathy

Figure 8-2 Potential causes of posterior thigh pain.

Table 8-6 Differentiation Between OA and RA of the Hip

Condition	Presentation	Examination Findings	Imaging and Diagnostic Studies	Basis of Diagnosis
OA	Groin pain on activity; gradual worsening of pain; limp	Pain and decreased range of motion on internal rotation and extension	Radiographs: joint space narrowing, sclerosis, osteophytes	Clinical findings, confirmed with radiographs
RA	Pain in the morning; activity limitation; systemic involvement	Generalized joint involvement; enthesopathy; skin or bowel symptoms	Elevated erythrocyte sedimentation rate and C-reactive protein level. Arthrocentesis: white blood cell count in joint fluid of 2500 to 50,000 per mm^3 Radiographs: erosions, osteopenia	Clinical and laboratory findings Significant improvement with NSAIDs

- Posterior hip pain is the least common pain pattern, and it usually suggests a source outside the hip joint. Posterior pain is typically referred from such disorders of the lumbar spine as degenerative disc disease, facet arthropathy, and spinal stenosis. Posterior hip pain is also caused by disorders of the sacroiliac joint (seronegative arthritides or traumatic arthritis), hip extensor and external rotator muscles, or, rarely, aortoiliac vascular occlusive disease.

After identifying whether the pain is anterior, lateral, or posterior, the clinician should focus on other characteristics of the pain—sudden versus insidious onset, movements, and positions that reproduce the pain, predisposing activities, and the effect of ambulation or weight-bearing activity on the pain.

 Clinical Pearl

Hip joint pathology is often associated with difficulty in weight-bearing, and functional activities such as donning shoes.

As the hip is a weight bearing joint, it is very important to gather information concerning the role of weight bearing in pain activities, particularly whether the patient has pain at rest as well as during weight bearing, or

Table 8-7 Differentiation of Hip Pathologies that have the Potential to Produce Groin Pain

Factor	Congenital Hip Dislocation	Septic Arthritis	Legg–Calvé–Perthes	Transient Synovitis	Slipped Femoral Capital Epiphysis	Avascular Necrosis	Degenerative Joint Disease	Fracture
Age	Birth	Less than 2 years; rare in adults	2–13 years	2–12 years	Males 10–17 years; Females 8–15 years	30–50 years	>40 years	Older adults
Incidence Male: female	Female>male; Left>right; Blacks<whites	Variable	Male>female; Rare in blacks; 15% bilateral	Male>female; Unilateral	Male>female; Blacks>whites	Male>female	Women>men	Women > men
Observation	Short limb, associated with torticollis	Irritable child; motionless hip; prominent greater trochanter, mild illness	Short limb; high greater trochanter; quad atrophy; adductor spasm	Decreased flexion; abduction; external rotation; thigh atrophy; muscle spasm	Short limb; obese; quadriceps atrophy; adductor spasm	Antalgic gait	Frequently obese, joint crepitus, atrophy of gluteal muscles	Ecchymosis, may be swelling, short limb
Position	Flexed and abducted	Flexed; abducted; externally rotated	Externally rotated and adducted	Antalgic gait, capsular pattern	Flexion, abduction, external rotation	Capsular pattern	Capsular pattern	External rotation
Pain	Variable	Mild pain with palpation and passive motion; often referred to knee	Gradual onset; aching in hip, thigh and knee; tenderness	Acute: severe pain in knee, Moderate: pain in thigh and knee; tenderness over hip	Vague pain in knee, suprapatellar area, thigh and hip; also in extreme motion	50% sharp pain, 50% insidious and intermittent pain in extreme ends of range	Insidious onset, pain with fall in barometric pressure	Severe pain in groin area

(continued on following page)

Table 8-7 *(continued from previous page)*

Factor	Congenital Hip Dislocation	Septic Arthritis	Legg–Calvé–Perthes	Transient Synovitis	Slipped Femoral Capital Epiphysis	Avascular Necrosis	Degenerative Joint Disease	Fracture
History	May be breech birth	Steroid therapy Fever	20%–25% familial; low birth weight; growth delay	Low grade fever	May be trauma		May be prolonged trauma, faulty body mechanics	May be trauma, fall
Range of motion	Limited abduction	Decreased	Limited abduction, extension	Decreased flexion; limited extension, internal rotation	Limited internal rotation, abduction, flexion, increased external adductor spasm	Decreased range of motion	Decreased motion external, internal rotation, and extreme flexion	Limited
Special tests	Galeazzi sign Ortolani sign Barlow sign Piston sign	Joint aspiration						
Gait	Refused to walk	Refused to walk	Antalgic gait after activity	Refused to walk; antalgic limp	Acute: antalgic Chronic: Trendelenberg External rotation	Coxalgic limp	Limp	Unable to weight bear
Radiological findings	Upward and lateral displacement, delayed development of acetabulum	CT scan: localized abscess; increased separation of ossification center from the lateral pelvic tear drop margin	In stages: increased density, fragmentation, flattening of epiphysis	Normal at first, widened medial joint space	Displacement of upper femoral epiphysis; especially in frog position	Flattening followed by collapse of femoral head	Increased bone density, osteophytes, subarticular cysts; degenerated articular cartilage	Fracture line, possible displace-ment; short femoral neck

Table 8-8 Differential Diagnosis of Pain in the Greater Trochanter Region

Pathology	Clinical Examination
Gluteus maximus/gluteus medius insertional tendopathy	Local tenderness over the posterior aspect of the greater trochanter (tender area is slightly more proximal on the posterior aspect of the greater trochanter for gluteus medius). May have pain with resisted hip extension, external rotation or abduction in severe cases
Calcification at the insertion of the gluteus maximus	Same clinical findings as for gluteus maximus insertional tendopathy
Subtendinous/intertendinous trochanteric bursitis	Same clinical findings as for gluteus maximus insertional tendopathy. Often passive hip flexion, external rotation, and/or adduction are also painful Positive FABER test Pain with combined motion of passive flexion, external rotation, and adduction
Snapping hip (coxa saltans)	Snapping occurs during flexion of the hip from a position of extension or in alternating internal and external rotation from a position of hip flexion. Usually no associated pain
Lateral compartment syndrome of the thigh	Pain and local swelling over the tensor fascia latae muscle in the area over the greater trochanter. Pain with sitting and activities
Stress fracture of the greater trochanter	Local pain with percussion/ultrasound
Referred pain from L4 or L5	Positive findings in lower quarter scanning examination

whether specific weight bearing activities (e.g., stair climbing and walking) are the cause of increased pain.[2]

Information must be gathered with regard to the activities or times of day that appear to change the pain for better or worse.

 Clinical Pearl

With any adult who has acute hip pain, the clinician should be alert for "red flags" that may indicate a more serious medical condition as the source of pain.

Systems Review

Pain may be referred to the hip region from a number of sources. These include the lumbar spine, peripheral nerve entrapments, the sacroiliac joint and the abdominal viscera.

- Anterior thigh pain and knee pain may be indicative of lumbar radiculopathy.
- Pain that is decreased with walking up stairs may indicate the patient has lumbar spine stenosis, especially if the pain is increased when walking on the level.
- Pain with sitting could indicate a lumbar disc lesion, or ischial bursitis (weaver's bottom).
- Night pain, that is unaffected by movement or positional changes is strongly suggestive of cancer.
- Constitutional symptoms such as fever, chills, and weight loss.

 Clinical Pearl

Fever, malaise, night sweats, weight loss, night pain, intravenous drug abuse, a history of cancer, or known immuno-compromised state should prompt you to consider such conditions as tumor, infection (i.e., septic arthritis or osteomyelitis), or an inflammatory arthritis.

Intense inflammation on examination suggests infectious or microcrystalline processes such as gout or pseudogout.

 Clinical Pearl

Weight loss, fatigue, fever, and loss of appetite should be sought out because these are clues to a systemic illness such as polymyalgia rheumatica, rheumatoid arthritis, lupus, or sepsis.

Clinical Pearl

Pediatric patients presenting with an antalgic gait, pain, and loss of range at the hip joint should always alert the clinician to the possibility of transient synovitis, Legg–Calvé–Perthes disease, or a slipped femoral capital epiphysis.

Tests and Measures

Observation

The clinician observes the hip region noting any scars, bruising, swelling, and so on. The patient is observed from the front, back, and sides for general alignment of the hip, pelvis, spine, and lower extremities.

- Atrophy of one buttock cheek compared with the other side may indicate superior or inferior gluteal nerve palsy.
- A balling-up of the gluteal muscle typically indicates a grade III tear of the gluteal muscles.
- Buttock swelling occurs with the sign of the buttock.[3]
- Swelling over the greater trochanter could indicate trochanteric bursitis.
- Adaptive shortening of the short hip adductors is indicated by a distinct bulk in the muscles of upper third of the thigh.[4] The bulk of the tensor fascia latae should not be distinct.
- A visible groove passing down the lateral aspect of the thigh may indicate that the tensor fascia latae (TFL) is overused, and both it and the iliotibial band (ITB) are adaptively shortened.[4]

Screening tests

Screening tests for the hip joint include gait analysis and tests that apply a load of the joint.

Gait Analysis

Analysis of both the stance and swing phases of gait is essential to determine the problems that must be dealt with during the intervention. Determinants of stance-phase gait involve interaction between the pelvis and hip and distal limb joints (knee and ankle).[5,6] An abducted or gluteus medius lurch (Trendelenburg sign), manifested by a lateral shift of the body to the weight-bearing side of ambulation (see Chapter 3), often occurs in patients with osteoarthritis, inflammatory arthritis, or osteonecrosis of the hip.

 Clinical Pearl

Patients who report a popping or snapping sensation in the hip while ambulating most likely have a thickened iliotibial band snapping over the greater trochanter.

Joint Loading Tests

Pain on weight bearing is a common complaint in some patients with hip joint pathology including rheumatoid arthritis and osteoarthritis.[7] Depending on the capability of the patient, the following weight bearing tests may produce pain.

High step: The patient places one foot on a chair, and then leans onto it. The test is repeated on the other side. This test moves the hip joint through its full range of motion in the sagittal plane (flexion and extension). In addition, the pelvic innominates are also rotated in both directions (anterior and posterior).

Unilateral standing: The patient stands on one leg. An inability to maintain the pelvis in a horizontal position during unilateral standing is called a positive Trendelenburg (see Special tests).

Palpation

Palpation must be systematic and focus on specific anatomical structures. The optimal methods of palpating occur in regions where there is the least amount of overlying soft tissue.[8] The hip area should be palpated for warmth, tenderness, deformity, and crepitus. Palpation should include examination of the following structures.

Anterior Aspect of Hip and Groin

Anterior superior iliac spine
The anterior iliac spine serves as the origin for the sartorius muscle and the TFL.

Anterior inferior iliac spine
The anterior inferior iliac spine (AIIS) can be palpated in the space formed by the sartorius and the TFL during passive flexion of the hip in the space known as the *lateral femoral triangle*. The lateral femoral cutaneous nerve of the thigh passes through this triangle. Compression of this nerve produces a condition called *meralgia paresthetica*.

 Clinical Pearl

The AIIS serves as the origin for the rectus femoris tendon.

Pubic tubercle
Finding the groin crease and then traveling in an inferior–medial direction, or by following the tendon of the adductor longus proximally locate the pubic tubercle. Inguinal hernias are usually found cranial and medial to the tubercle, while femoral hernias are located lateral to the tubercle.

Adductor magnus
The adductor magnus is palpable in a small triangle in the distal thigh, posterior to the gracilis muscle, and anterior to the semimembranosus.

Rectus femoris
The rectus femoris has its origin at the AIIS, which is located just distal to the anterior superior iliac spine (ASIS), between the TFL and sartorius.

Iliopsoas bursa
To palpate this bursa, the patient is positioned in supine with their hip positioned in approximately 40 degrees of flexion and external rotation, and resting on a pillow. At the proximal end of the femur, the clinician palpates the adductor tubercle and then moves to the ASIS. From there, the clinician proceeds to the inguinal ligament, under the fold of the external oblique (this area is more tender in men due to the proximity of the spermatic cord and tends to be the area for inguinal hernias in men), and into the femoral triangle. The psoas bursa is located under the floor of the triangle, close to the pubic ramus.

Femoral triangle
The femoral artery lies superficial and medial to the iliopsoas muscle and is easily located by palpation of the pulse. The femoral nerve is the most lateral structure in the femoral triangle. To examine the femoral triangle the patient is positioned in supine and, if it is possible for the patient to do this, the heel of the leg resting upon the opposite knee. This places the patient in a position of flexion-abduction and external rotation.

Inguinal ligament
The inguinal ligament is located in the fold of the groin, running from the ASIS to the pubic tubercle. It can be located by using transverse palpation.

Adductor longus
Together with the gracilis, the adductor longus forms the medial border of the femoral triangle. The gracilis is located medial and posterior to the adductor longus. The adductor longus is best viewed during resisted adduction when it forms a cord like structure just distal to the pubic tubercle, before crossing under the sartorius.

Lateral Aspect of the Hip
The patient is positioned in side lying.

Iliac crest
The iliac crest is easy to locate (Figure 8-3). The cluneal nerves are superficial structures and can be located just superior to the crest.

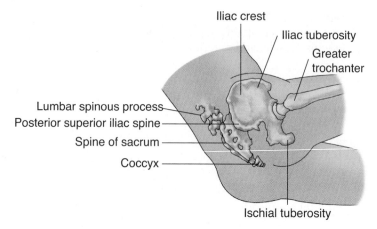

Figure 8-3 Bony landmarks—posterior and lateral view.

Greater trochanter
The superior border of the greater trochanter represents the transverse axis of hip, and when the leg is abducted, an obvious depression appears above the greater trochanter. Palpation of the greater trochanter (Figure 8-3) is important because of the possibility of trochanteric bursitis. A number of muscles attach to the greater trochanter (Table 8-9). The gluteus medius inserts into the upper portion of the trochanter and can be palpated on the lateral aspect.[2]

 Clinical Pearl

Tenderness directly over the greater trochanter reproduces pain with greater trochanteric bursitis.

Tenderness at the proximal tip of the greater trochanter may indicate gluteus medius tendonitis.

Tenderness at the posterior margin of the greater trochanter may indicate external rotator tendonitis.

Lesser trochanter
The lesser trochanter, covered as it is with the iliopsoas and adductor magnus, is very difficult to palpate directly, but it can be located on the posterior aspect if the hip is placed in extension and internal rotation, and the palpation is performed deeply lateral to the ischial tuberosity.

Table 8-9 Muscles that Attach to the Greater Trochanter

Piriformis

Gluteus medius

Gluteus minimus

Obturator internus

Gemellus superior

Gemellus inferior

Piriformis attachment

The origin of the piriformis can be found on the medial aspect of the superior point of the greater trochanter. Moving inferiorly from this point and the quadratus femoris, on the quadrate tubercle, the following tendon insertions can be palpated: superior gemelli, obturator internus, and inferior gemelli.

Psoas

The insertion for the psoas is located on the inferior aspect of the greater trochanter, and can be found by placing the patient's leg in maximum internal rotation of the hip. Once the superior aspect of the greater trochanter is located, the clinician moves in a posterior/medial/inferior direction to locate the inferior aspect of the greater trochanter.

Posterior Aspect of the Hip

The patient is positioned in side lying.

Quadratus lumborum

Palpation of the quadratus lumborum is best accomplished with the patient in side lying with the arm abducted overhead to open the space between the iliac crest and the 12th rib.

Ischial tuberosity

The ischial tuberosity is best palpated in the side lying position with the hip flexed to 90 degrees (Figure 8-3). This position moves the gluteus maximus upwards so permitting direct palpation at the tuberosity. A number of structures have their attachments on the ischial tuberosity (Table 8-10). These include the ischial bursa, the semimembranosus tendon, the long head of the biceps femoris and semitendinosus tendon, the sacrotuberous ligament, and the tendons of the quadratus femoris, adductor magnus, and inferior gemellus. The *ischial bursa* is located on the inferior and medial aspect of the ischial tuberosity.

Table 8-10 Muscles that Attach to the Ischial Tuberosity

Semimembranosus
Semitendinosus
Long head of the biceps femoris
Adductor magnus
Quadratus femoris
Gemellus inferior

Sciatic nerve
The sciatic nerve can be palpated at a point half way between the greater trochanter and the ischial tuberosity. Tenderness of this nerve can be produced by a piriformis muscle spasm, or by direct trauma.

Active, Passive, and Resistive Tests

During the examination of the range of motion, the clinician should note which portions of the range of motion are pain-free, and which portion causes the patient to feel pain. At the end of available active range of motion passive overpressure is applied to determine the end-feel. The normal ranges and end-feels for the various hip motions are outlined in Table 8-11. Abnormal end-feels common in the hip are firm capsular end-feel before expected end range, empty end-feel from severe pain, as in the Sign of the Buttock, and bony block in cases of advanced osteoarthritis (Figure 8-4).[9] Horizontal abduction and adduction of the femur occur when the hip is in 90 degrees of flexion. Because

Table 8-11 Normal Ranges and End-feels at the Hip

Motion	Range of Motion (Degrees)	End-feel
Flexion	110–120	Tissue approximation or tissue stretch
Extension	10–15	Tissue stretch
Abduction	30–50	Tissue stretch
Adduction	25–30	Tissue approximation or tissue stretch
External rotation	40–60	Tissue stretch
Internal rotation	30–40	Tissue stretch

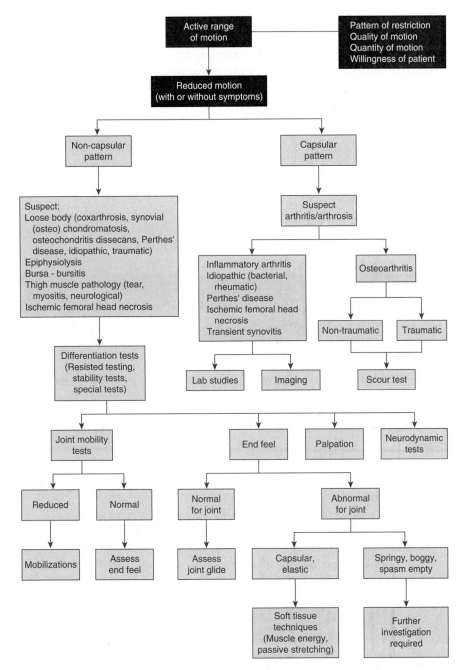

Figure 8-4 Examination sequence in the presence of symptom-free or incomplete active range of motion at the hip.

these actions require simultaneous, coordinated actions of several muscles, they can be used to assess the overall strength of the hip muscles.

Resisted testing is performed to provide the clinician with information about the integrity of the neuromuscular unit, and to highlight the presence of muscle strains (Table 8-12).[10]

If the history indicates that repetitive motions or sustained positions cause the symptoms, the clinician should have the patient reproduce these motions or positions.[11]

In addition to reports of pain and overall range of motion, the clinician also notes information about weakness, joint end-feel, palpation of the moving joint, and muscle tightness.

Flexion

The six muscles primarily responsible for hip flexion are the iliacus, psoas major, pectineus, rectus femoris, sartorius, and TFL (Table 8-12).

 Clinical Pearl

The primary hip flexor is the iliopsoas muscle.

Hip flexion motion can be tested in sitting or supine first with the knee flexed (Figure 8-5), and then with the knee extended. With the hip flexed, the range of motion should be approximately 110 degrees to 120 degrees. More hip flexion should be available with the knee flexed. Passive overpressure is applied.

Resisted tests are then performed.

• To test the strength of the iliopsoas, the patient is supine with the thigh raised off the bed and the clinician applies resistance.

• Asking the patient to bring the plantar aspect of the foot toward the opposite knee tests the action of the sartorius muscle, which flexes, abducts, and externally rotates the hip. The clinician applies resistance at the medial mallelous and at the lateral aspect of the thigh to resist flexion, abduction, and external rotation.

 Clinical Pearl

A painless weakness of hip flexion is rarely a good sign. Theoretically, it could indicate a disc protrusion at the L1 or L2 level.

Table 8-12 Muscle Actions at the Hip

Hip flexion	Psoas Iliacus Rectus femoris Sartorius Pectineus Adductor longus Adductor brevis Gracilis
Hip extension	Biceps femoris Semimembranosus Semitendinosus Gluteus maximus Gluteus medius (posterior fibers) Adductor magnus (ischiocondylar portion)
Hip adduction	Adductor longus Adductor brevis Adductor magnus (ischiofemoral portion) Gracilis Pectineus
Hip abduction	Tensor fascia latae Gluteus medius Gluteus minimus Gluteus maximus Sartorius
Hip internal rotation	Adductor longus Adductor brevis Adductor magnus Gluteus medius (anterior fibers) Gluteus minimus (anterior fibers) Tensor fascia latae Pectineus Gracilis
Hip external rotation	Gluteus maximus Obturator internus Obturator externus Quadratus femoris Piriformis Gemellus superior Gamellus inferior Sartorius Gluteus medius (posterior fibers)

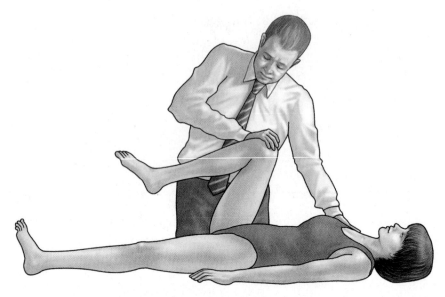

Figure 8-5 Active hip flexion with passive overpressure.

However, protrusions at these levels are not common. A more likely scenario is compression of the nerves by a neurofibroma or a metastatic invasion.

Pain with the active motion or resisted tests, should prompt the clinician to examine the contractile tissues individually. Passive stretching can also produce pain in a contractile structure.

Extension

The patient is positioned in prone or over the end of the table (Figure 8-6). As the clinician palpates the buttock mass, and stabilizes the sacrum to prevent the lumbar spine from extending, the patient is asked to lift the thigh toward the ceiling.

 Clinical Pearl

The primary hip extensor is the gluteus maximus. The hamstrings also serve as hip extensors. Hip extension also involves assistance from

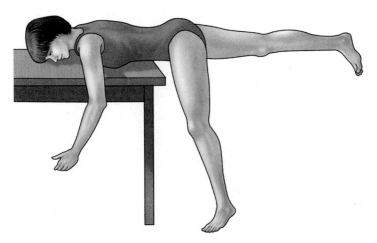

Figure 8-6 Position for testing hip extension range of motion and strength.

the adductor magnus, gluteus medius and minimus, and indirect assistance from the abdominals and the erector spinae.[12]

The normal range of motion for hip extension is approximately 10 degrees to 15 degrees. Reduced hip extension can be the result of a number of reasons including adaptive shortening of the iliopsoas or a hip flexion contracture.

To test the strength of the gluteus maximus the patient is positioned in prone, with their knee flexed. As before, the sacrum is stabilized and the patient is asked to raise the thigh off the table. The clinician then applies resistance. The hamstrings can be tested in supine with the knee extended. A strong and painful finding with resisted hip extension may indicate a grade I muscle strain of the gluteus maximus or hamstrings. It may also indicate a gluteal bursitis, or a lumbosacral strain.

Abduction/Adduction

Hip adduction and abduction range of motion can be tested in supine, making sure that both ASISs are level, and the legs are perpendicular to a line joining the ASISs (Figure 8-7).

Abduction

The patient is supine. The clinician monitors the ipsilateral ASIS, and the patient is asked to abduct the leg (Figure 8-7). The abduction motion is

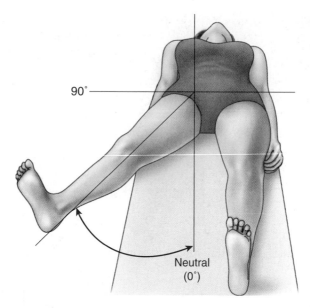

Figure 8-7 Active hip abduction.

stopped when the ASIS is felt to move. The prime movers for this movement are the gluteus medius/minimus and the TFL. The quadratus lumborum functions as the stabilizer of the pelvis. The strength of the gluteus medius and minimus is tested with the patient in side lying. The patient is asked to perform hip abduction, without any flexion or external rotation occurring. The clinician applies resistance to the distal thigh.

Adduction
Hip adduction is tested with the patient supine, and with the uninvolved leg adducted over the other leg, or held in flexion. As before, the ASIS is monitored for motion, indicating the end of range for adduction.

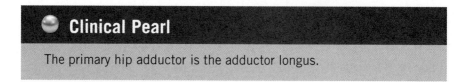

Clinical Pearl

The primary hip adductor is the adductor longus.

Adaptive shortening of the hip adductors can theoretically result in inhibition of the gluteus medius, a decrease in frontal stability, Iliotibial band (ITB) tendonitis, and anterior knee pain. Pain can be referred from the hip adductors into the anterior–lateral hip, groin, medial thigh, the anterior knee, and medial tibia. Pain in these regions with passive abduction, or active adduction, may indicate a strain of one of the adductors. The cause of the pain can be differentiated between the two-joint gracilis and the other hip adductors (longus, brevis, and pectineus) in the following manner. The patient is positioned in side lying with the tested leg supported by the clinician. The clinician places the hip into the fully abducted position and the knee is flexed. If no pain is reproduced with this maneuver, the patient is asked to extend the knee, thereby bringing in the gracilis, and implicating it if the pain is now reproduced. This can be confirmed with resisted hip adduction and knee flexion. If the other adductors are implicated, this can be confirmed with resisted adduction (longus and brevis) or resisted hip adduction and hip flexion (pectineus).

The strength of the hip adductor muscle group is tested in side lying, by flexing the uninvolved leg over the tested leg, or by supporting the upper leg and then applying resistance. This position also stretches the hip abductors, and can be a source of pain in the case of an iliotibial band syndrome.

🔵 Clinical Pearl

A strong and painful finding with resisted adduction is usually the result of an adductor longus lesion, whereas a painless weakness with resisted abduction is often found in a palsy of the fifth lumbar root due to a disc herniation of the same level.

Internal and External Rotation

Although a number of muscles contribute to external rotation of the femur (Table 8-12), six muscles function solely as external rotators.[13] These are the piriformis, gemellus superior, gemellus inferior, obturator internus, obturator externus, and quadratus femoris. Normal range of motion for hip external rotation is approximately 40 degrees to 60 degrees. Excessive external rotation of the hip may indicate hip retroversion.

🔵 Clinical Pearl

The major internal rotator of the femur is the gluteus minimus, assisted by the gluteus medius, TFL, semitendinosus, and semimembranosus.

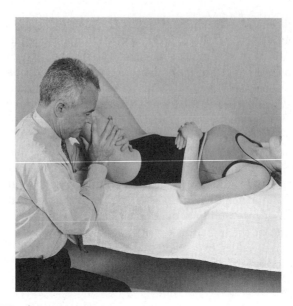

Figure 8-8 Hip distraction.

The internal rotators of the femur are estimated to be only approximately one-third the strength of the external rotators.[14] Normal range of motion for hip internal rotation is approximately 30 degrees to 40 degrees. Excessive internal rotation of the hip may indicate hip anteversion.

To assess the range of motion of the hip rotators, the patient is positioned in supine with the leg in 90 degrees of hip flexion, and 90 degrees of knee flexion. Alternatively, the patient can be positioned in prone, with the knee flexed to 90 degrees and the hip in neutral.

Functional Assessment

An assessment of the patient's functional status can also be made through observation or through use of a self-report measure, which allow a patient to rate his or her capacity to perform.

Passive Accessory Movements

Due to the extreme congruency of the joint partners at the hip joint, this is a difficult area to assess with any degree of accuracy, especially as the glides that occur are very slight. Thus, only one accessory motion, lateral distraction, is examined.

The patient is positioned in supine with the hip and knee flexed (Figure 8-8). The clinician places one hand over the lateral thigh and the other close to the superior aspect of the medial thigh (Figure 8-8). A distraction force and then a compression force are applied in line with the femoral neck. The test is positive if excessive movement or pain is detected.

Special Tests

Special tests are merely confirmatory tests and should not be used alone to form a diagnosis. The results from these tests are used in conjunction with the other clinical findings to help guide the clinician. To assure accuracy with these tests, both sides should be tested for comparison.

Quadrant (Scour) Test

The quadrant or scour test is a dynamic test of the inner quadrant and outer quadrant of the hip joint surface.[15]

The patient is positioned in supine, close to the edge of the bed, with their hip flexed and foot resting on the bed. The clinician wraps the fingers of one hand over the top of the patient's knee. The patient's hip is placed in 90 degrees of flexion with the knee allowed to flex comfortably. From this point, the clinician adducts the hip to the point when the patient's pelvis begins to lift on the bed to assess the inner quadrant (Figure 8-9). At the end range of flexion and adduction, a compression force is applied at the knee along the longitudinal

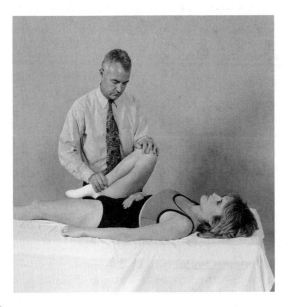

Figure 8-9 Scour test.

axis of the femur. From this point, the clinician moves the hip into a position of flexion and abduction to examine the outer quadrant. Throughout the entire movement, the femur is held midway between internal and external rotation, and the movement at the hip joint should follow the smooth arc of a circle. An abnormal finding is resistance felt anywhere during the arc. The resistance may be caused by capsular tightness, an adhesion, a myofascial restriction, or a loss of joint congruity. Despite its widespread use, there are no studies in the literature that discuss the diagnostic value of this maneuver.

FABER (Flexion, Abduction, External Rotation) or Patrick's Test

The FABER test (flexion, abduction, and external rotation) test is a screening test for hip, lumbar, or sacroiliac joint dysfunction, or an iliopsoas spasm. A positive test results in pain and/or loss of motion as compared with the uninvolved side. Despite its widespread use, there are no studies in the literature that discuss the sensitivity, specificity, positive predictive value, or negative predictive value of this maneuver. Having the patient demonstrate where the pain is with this test may assist with the interpretation of this test.

Stinchfield Test

The patient is positioned in supine with the knee extended. The clinician resists the patient's hip flexion at 20 degrees to 30 degrees. Reproduction of groin pain is considered a positive test indicating hip intra-articular dysfunction. There are no studies in the literature that discuss the sensitivity, specificity, positive predictive value, or negative predictive value of this maneuver.

Squeeze Test[16]

A pain provocation test used to assess chronic groin pain in athletes. The patient is positioned supine with the hips and knees flexed (45 degrees and 90 degrees, respectively) and the feet flat on the bed. The clinician places his clenched fist between the patient's knees and asks the patient to perform a maximal adduction contraction of the hips. A positive test is indicated by signs of weakness and pain.

Bilateral Hip Adduction Test[16,17]

A pain provocation test used to assess chronic groin pain in athletes. The patient is positioned in supine with the legs extended. The patient is asked to perform a maximal adduction contraction against the clinician's resistance. A positive test is indicated by signs of weakness and pain.

Single Adductor Test[16]

A pain provocation test used to assess chronic groin pain in athletes. The patient is positioned with one hip flexed to 30 degrees with the other lower extremity resting on the table. The patient is asked to apply a maximal adduc-

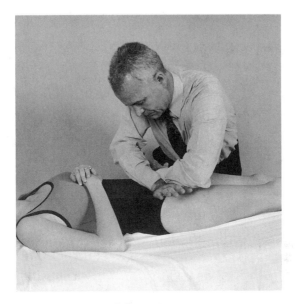

Figure 8-10 Anterior gapping of the SI joint.

tion contraction using the flexed leg against the clinician's resistance. Both legs are tested. A positive test is indicated by pain and weakness on the tested leg or pain in the contralateral leg.

SI Provocation Tests

Unless the patient history or the physical examination highlights the presence of a sacroiliac dysfunction, the clinician relies on two simple stress tests to rule out sacroiliac pathology, the anterior gapping (Figure 8-10) and posterior gapping (Figure 8-11) tests.

In addition to the provocative tests, the passive motions of the hip can be examined with the innominate stabilized. The hip motions and their respective innominate motions, in parenthesis, are outlined in Table 8-13.

Craig Test

The Craig test is used to assess femoral anteversion/retroversion. The patient is positioned in prone with the knee flexed to 90 degrees. The clinician rotates the hip through the full ranges of hip internal and external rotation while palpating the greater trochanter and determining the point in the range at which the greater trochanter is the most prominent laterally. If the angle is greater than 8 degrees to 15 degrees in the direction of internal rotation when measured from the vertical and long axis of the tibia, the femur is considered to be in anteversion.[18–21]

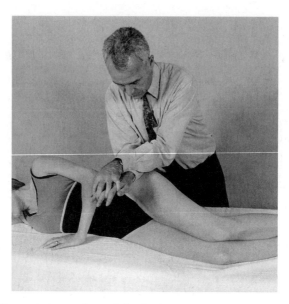

Figure 8-11 Posterior gapping of the SI joint.

Flexion–Adduction Test

This test is used as a screening test for early hip pathology.[22] The patient is positioned in supine and the hip is passively flexed to 90 degrees and in neutral rotation. From this position, the clinician stabilizes the pelvis and the hip is passively adducted. The resultant end-feel, restriction, discomfort, or pain is noted and compared with the normal side.

Trendelenburg Sign

The Trendelenburg sign indicates weakness of the gluteus medius muscle during unilateral weight bearing. This position requires a strong contraction of the gluteus medius, which is powerfully assisted by the gluteus minimus and

Table 8-13 Hip Motions and Their Associated Innominate Motions

Extension (anterior rotation)
Abduction (upward)
Adduction (downward)
Internal rotation (IR)
External rotation (ER)

TFL, in order to keep the pelvis horizontal. For example, when the right foot supports the body weight, the right hip abductors contract isometrically, and eccentrically, to prevent the left side of the pelvis from being pulled downward.

 Clinical Pearl

Bird et al. found the Trendelenberg sign to have the sensitivity of 72.7% and a specificity of 76.9% and an intraobserver κ of 0.676 when assessing for a gluteus medius tear.

The clinician crouches or kneels behind the patient with their eyes level with the patient's pelvis, and ensures that the patient does not lean to one side during the testing. The patient is asked to stand on one limb for approximately 30 seconds and the clinician notes whether the pelvis remains level. If the hip remains level, the test is negative. A positive Trendelenburg sign is indicated when, during unilateral weight bearing, the pelvis drops toward the unsupported limb.

 Clinical Pearl

A number of dysfunctions can produce the Trendelenburg sign. These include superior gluteal nerve palsy, a lumbar disc herniation, weakness of the gluteus medius, and advanced degeneration of the hip.

Pelvic Drop Test[23]
The patient is asked to place one foot on a 20 cm (8 inch) stool or step and to stand up straight. The patient then lowers the nonweight bearing leg to the floor. On lowering the leg there should be no arm abduction, anterior or pelvic motion or trunk flexion. Nor should there be any hip adduction or internal rotation of the weight bearing hip. These compensations are indications of an unstable hip or weak external rotators.

Sign of the Buttock
To test for the presence of this syndrome the patient is positioned in supine. The clinician performs a passive unilateral straight leg raise. If there is a unilateral restriction, the clinician flexes the knee and notes whether the hip flexion

increases. If the restriction was due to the lumbar spine or hamstrings, hip flexion increases. If the hip flexion does not increase when the knee is flexed, it is a positive sign of the buttock test. If the sign of the buttock is encountered, the patient must be immediately returned to the physician for further investigation.

Fulcrum Test

The fulcrum test[24] is used to test for the presence of a stress fracture of the femoral shaft. The patient is positioned in sitting with their knees bent over the edge of the bed, and feet dangling. A firm towel roll is placed under the involved thigh, and is moved proximal to distal as gentle pressure is applied posterior to the knee with the clinician's hand. A positive test is when the patient reports sharp pain or expresses apprehension when the fulcrum arm is placed under the fracture site. There are no studies in the literature that discuss the sensitivity, specificity, positive predictive value, or negative predictive value of this maneuver.

Auscultatory Patellar-pubic Percussion Test

The ausculatory patellar-pubic percussion test[25-27] is used when there is a suspicion of occult hip fracture. The patient is positioned in supine, and the clinician places the head of the stethoscope over the pubic symphysis. With the lower extremities extended and positioned symmetrically, the clinician taps (percusses) each patella and compares the generated sound. The percussion note should have symmetrical quality and intensity of sound. Any bony disruption along the conduction path (femur) will result in a diminished or muffled sound intensity and sound of a duller quality.

 Clinical Pearl

> Reliability and validity of the ausculatory patellar-pubic percussion test has been demonstrated.[25] Tiru et al.[28] noted a positive predictive value of 0.98, sensitivity over 0.96, and specificity of 0.76.

A positive patellar-pubic percussion test should prompt diagnostic imaging, including bone scan or magnetic resonance imaging (MRI), even if the initial hip radiographs are negative.[25]

Muscle Length Tests

Thomas test and modified thomas test

The original Thomas test was designed to test the flexibility of the iliopsoas complex, but has since been modified and expanded to assess a number of other soft tissue structures.

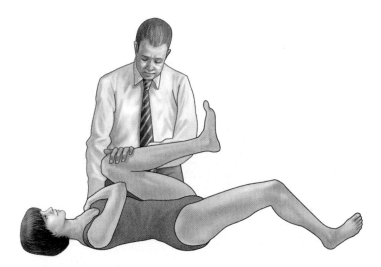

Figure 8-12 Thomas test.

The original test involved positioning the patient in supine, with one knee held to the chest at the point when the lumbar spine begins to flex (Figure 8-12). The clinician assesses whether the thigh of the extended leg maintains full contact with the surface of the bed. If the thigh is raised off the surface of the treatment table (Figure 8-12), the test is positive. A positive test indicates a decrease in flexibility in the rectus femoris or iliopsoas muscles or both. There is a lack of studies in the literature to provide definitive reliability and validity of this maneuver.

A modified version to this test is commonly used. For the modified version, the patient is positioned in sitting at the end of the bed (Figure 8-13). From this position, the patient is asked to lie down, while bringing both knees against the chest. Once in this position, the patient is asked to perform a posterior pelvic tilt. While the contralateral hip is held in maximum hip flexion with the arms, the tested limb is lowered over the end of the bed, towards the floor. In this position, the thigh should be parallel with the bed, in neutral rotation, and neither abducted nor adducted, with the lower leg perpendicular to the thigh and in neutral rotation. 100 degrees to 110 degrees of knee flexion should be present with the thigh in full contact with the table.

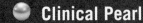

Clinical Pearl

Harvey found the modified Thomas test to have an intraclass coefficient reliability of 0.91.[29]

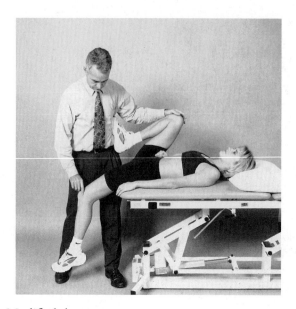

Figure 8-13 Modified thomas test.

Rectus femoris contracture test

The rectus femoris contracture test is similar to the modified version of the Thomas test. The patient is positioned in supine with the knees bent over the end of the edge of the examining table. The patient flexes one knee onto the chest. The angle of the test knee should remain at 90 degrees. A contracture may be present if the test knee extends slightly.

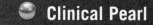

Clinical Pearl

The rectus femoris contracture test has been found to have an intra-class coefficient reliability of 0.94.[29]

Ely test

This is a test to assess the flexibility of the rectus femoris. The patient is positioned in prone lying and the knee is flexed. If the rectus is tight, the pelvis is observed to anteriorly rotate early in the range of knee flexion, and the hip flexes. There are no studies in the literature that discuss the sensitivity, specificity, positive predictive value, or negative predictive value of this maneuver.

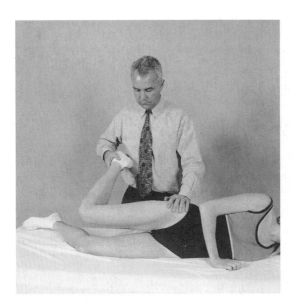

Figure 8-14 Ober test.

Ober test
The Ober test is used to evaluate tightness of the iliotibial band and tensor fascia latae (see Thomas test also).[30] The patient is placed in the side lying position, and, with the hip extended and abducted and the knee flexed, the proximal part of the leg is allowed to drop passively onto the contralateral limb (Figure 8-14). The test is considered positive when the leg fails to lower.

🌑 Clinical Pearl

There have been some doubts expressed as to the reliability of the Ober test as a measure for ITB tightness.[31]

Creak test
The patient stands on the involved leg. As the patient flexes the knee to approximately 30 degrees, a "creak" will occur over the lateral femoral condyle if ITB friction syndrome is present.[32]

Noble's compression test[33]
The patient is positioned supine, with the affected knee flexed to 90 degrees. Pressure is applied over the proximal, prominent part of the lateral femoral condyle

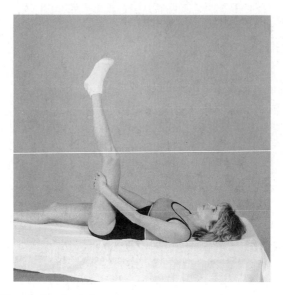

Figure 8-15 Hamstring length.

as the knee is gradually extended. A positive test is indicated when pain is reproduced at 30 degrees to 40 degrees and is indicative of ITB friction syndrome.

Straight leg raise test for hamstring length
The patient is positioned in supine with the legs together and extended. The clinician stands on the side of the leg to be tested and grasps the patient's ankle with one hand, while using the other hand to stabilize the opposite thigh. With the patient's knee extended, the clinician lifts the patient's leg, flexing the hip, until motion is seen to occur at the opposite ASIS. The angle of flexion from the treatment table is measured. The clinician returns the leg to the table and repeats the maneuver from the other side of the table with the other leg. The hamstrings are considered shortened if a straight leg cannot be raised to an angle of 80 degree from the horizontal, while the other leg is straight.[4] Any limitation of flexion is interpreted as being caused by contracted hamstring muscles.

 Clinical Pearl

The straight leg raise test may also be used as a screen for adverse neural tension, particularly of the sciatic nerve.

90–90 straight leg raise

The hamstring length can also be assessed with the patient positioned in supine and the tested leg flexed at the hip and knee to 90 degrees. From this position, the patient is asked to extend the knee of the involved side without extending the hip (Figure 8-15). The measurement is taken at the first resistance barrier.

Piriformis

The patient is positioned in sidelying. The clinician flexes the involved hip to 60 degrees. After stabilizing the patient's pelvis, the clinician applies a downward pressure through the femur, and maximally adducts the involved hip. From this position, the hip is moved into internal rotation and then external rotation. Internal rotation stresses the superior fibers, while external rotation stresses the inferior fibers. Normal range of motion should be 45 degrees into either rotation. Pain is elicited in the muscle if the piriformis is adaptively shortened. There are no studies in the literature that discuss the sensitivity, specificity, positive predictive value, or negative predictive value of this maneuver.

Hip adductors

The patient is positioned supine with the leg to be tested close to the edge of the table. The leg not to be tested is 15 degrees to 25 degrees abducted at the hip joint with the heel over the end of the table. Maintaining the tested knee in extension, the clinician passively abducts the tested leg. The normal range is 40 degrees. When the full range is reached, the knee of the tested leg is passively flexed and the leg abducted further. If the maximum range does not increase when the knee is flexed, the one-joint adductors (pectineus, adductor magnus, adductor longus, adductor brevis) are shortened. If the range does increase with the knee passively flexed, the two joint adductors (gracilis, biceps femoris, semimebranosus, and semitendinosus) are shortened.

Leg Length Discrepancy

The test for a leg length discrepancy is best performed radiographically. However, the following clinical test can be used to highlight the more significant discrepancies.

The patient is positioned in supine and the clinician palpates the ASIS. From this point, the clinician slides distally into the depression and then measures from this point to the tip of the medial malleolus making sure that the course of the tape follows the same route for both legs. The average of two measurements between the ASIS and medial malleolus may have acceptable validity and reliability when used as a screening tool.[34]

Pediatric Screening Tests for Congenital (CHD), or Developmental Dysplasia (DDH), of the Hip

The value of the neonatal hip screening examination remains controversial.[35] At present, the Ortolani and Barlow tests are currently used to examine the infant. Both tests are designed to detect motion between the femoral head and the acetabulum.[35] The reproducibility of these tests is dependent on ligamentous or capsular laxity, which usually disappears by 10 to 12 weeks of age.[35]

In addition to the special tests, the clinician looks for asymmetry between the lower extremities. Asymmetric thigh folds, a short leg appearance, or a prominent greater trochanter may be significant findings.[35]

In addition to the clinical tests, both CHD and DDH can be detected with radiographs or ultrasound.

Neurovascular Assessment

Manual muscle testing and sensation testing may be used to assess the integrity of the neurological structures. In addition, neurodynamic mobility tests including the straight leg raise and the prone knee bending tests may be used. In order to gain the most from these tests, the clinician should be aware of the dermatomal pattern as well as the areas supplied by the peripheral nerves (inferior femoral cutaneous, lateral femoral cutaneous, and posterior femoral cutaneous nerves).

 Clinical Pearl

It is very important to remember, that reports of paresthesia in the 'saddle' region is indicative of cauda equina compression and constitutes a medical emergency.

Imaging Studies

Imaging studies continue to be developed and refined to help clinicians diagnose more accurately, and these often provide prognostic information. These imaging studies are most effective when selected on the basis of a thorough history and physical examination.

Radiographs

Plain anteroposterior (AP) radiographs of the pelvis will clearly show a hip dislocation in most patients but lateral views may be required to confirm the diagnosis and to show the direction if the signs are subtle. AP and lateral views are also used to demonstrate most fractures. For patients in whom femoral neck fracture is strongly suspected but standard x-ray findings are negative, an AP view with hip internally rotated provides a better view of the femoral neck.

Clinical Pearl

Early avascular necrosis in patients of any age and fractures in patients with osteopenia are especially problematic. Avascular necrosis may not show significant radiographic changes until it has advanced.

Magnetic Resonance Imaging

When plain radiographs show no apparent fracture in an elderly patient who has osteoarthritic as well as osteoporotic changes in the hips, but the physical examination findings strongly suggest one, MRI can more accurately assess these subtle occult fractures because it is very sensitive to marrow edema.

 Clinical Pearl

MRI is superior to radiographs in the early detection of avascular necrosis, enabling institution of appropriate intervention. MRI can also be used to assess for abdominal aortic dissection, aneurysms, vascular anomalies, and coarctation.

In the athletic population, there is increasing use of MRI to diagnose pelvic and hip fractures, muscle contusion and strain, tendon injuries, acetabular labral tears, bursitis, and osteitis pubis and chronic symphyseal injury.[36]

Computed Tomography

A computed tomography (CT) scan may be required to confirm the diagnosis of a hip dislocation if the signs are subtle. Associated acetabular wall fractures and femoral head fractures also may be identified by CT scans. CT is also more sensitive in detecting osteochondral fragments.

Ultrasonography

Ultrasonography provides visualization of the cartilage, hip stability, and features of the acetabulum, and has been identified as the technique of choice for clarifying a physical finding suggestive of developmental dysplasia of the hip (DDH), both for assessing a high-risk infant and for monitoring the condition.

Examination Conclusions—The Evaluation

Following the examination, and once the clinical findings have been recorded, the clinician must determine a specific diagnosis or a working hypothesis, based

Table 8-14 Correlating the History, Examination and Diagnostic Studies

Category	History	Physical Examination Findings	Laboratory Studies	Radiology
Traumatic	Fall	Localized pain, swelling, loss of motion	None unless infection is possible	Plain films, bone scan
Infectious	Fever, chills, erythema, pain	Rigid guarding, warmth, erythema	CBC, ESR, CRP, joint aspirate	Plain films, MRI, bone scan
Neoplastic	Night pain, pain unrelated to activity	Mass	CBC, ESR, CRP, alkaline phosphatase, calcium, electrolytes, joint aspirate	Plain films, MRI/ CT, bone scan, staging work-up
Congenital	Problem since birth	Deformity, leg-length discrepancy, loss of ROM	None	Plain films
Neurologic	Ataxia, loss of balance, disorganized gait	High/low muscle tone, increased/ decreased deep tendon reflexes, cavus foot or claw toes	Creatine kinase (if DMD is in differential diagnosis)	Plain films
Inflammatory	Pain >6 months, family history of rheumatoid arthritis	Warmth/erythema, one or more joints	CBC, ESR, CRP, joint aspiration	Plain films
Developmental	Painless limp (LCP disease) Knee pain (LCP disease, SCFE)	Loss of ROM in joints, asymmetric ROM, pain with ROM	None	Plain films

CBC = complete blood count; ESR = erythrocyte sedimentation rate; CRP = C-reactive protein; MRI = magnetic resonance imaging; CT = computed tomography; ROM = range of motion; DMD = Duchenne's muscular dystrophy; LCP = Legg–Calvé–Perthes; SCFE = slipped capital femoral epiphysis.

on a summary of all of the findings (Table 8-14). This diagnosis can be structure related (medical diagnosis) (Table 8-15), or a diagnosis based on the preferred practice patterns as described in the Guide to Physical Therapist Practice.[37]

Table 8-15 Differential Diagnosis for Common Causes of Hip Pain

Condition	Patient Age	Mechanism of Injury/ Onset	Area of Symptoms	Symptoms Aggravated By	Observation	AROM	PROM	Resisted	Tenderness with Palpation
Trochanteric bursitis	15-45	Direct trauma Microtrauma	Lateral aspect of hip/thigh	Lying on involved side	Unremarkable	Painful hip abduction with rotation	Pain at end range hip ER Pain with hip ER with abduction	Pain with resisted hip abduction Pain with resisted hip IR	Lateral thigh over greater trochanter
Groin strain	20-40	Sudden overload	Anteromedial thigh Medial thigh	Running	Possible bruising around medial thigh	Hip extension only limited movement Hip ER limited and painful	Pain at end range hip extension Pain at end range hip abduction Pain at end range hip flexion	Pain with resisted hip adduction	Proximal medial thigh
Hamstring muscle tear	15-45	Sudden overload	Buttock and posterior thigh	Running	Possible bruising around posterior thigh	SLR limited and painful	Pain at end range hip extension Pain with passive SLR	Pain with resisted hip extension Pain with resisted knee flexion	Posterior thigh
Piriformis syndrome	25-55	Gradual	Buttock and posterior thigh Back of leg	Prolonged sitting	Unremarkable	SLR limited and painful	Pain at end range hip ER Pain with passive SLR	Pain with resisted hip ER	Buttock

(continued on following page)

Table 8-15 *(continued from previous page)*

Condition	Patient Age	Mechanism of Injury/ Onset	Area of Symptoms	Symptoms Aggravated By	Observation	AROM	PROM	Resisted	Tenderness with Palpation
Hip OA	50+	Gradual	Anterior thigh Anteromedial thigh	Weight bearing	Possible atrophy of thigh muscles Altered gait	Limited hip IR and extension Painful hip IR Painful hip extension	Pain at end range hip IR All movements feel stiff	Weak hip abduction General weakness of hip muscles	Anterior hip
Iliotibial band syndrome	25-55	Overuse	Lateral aspect of thigh Lateral aspect of knee		Unremarkable	Pain on moving from knee extension to flexion	Pain at end range hip ER with abduction	All resistive tests negative	Lateral epicondyle of femur Lateral aspect of knee
Psoas bursitis	20-40	Overuse	Anteromedial thigh		Unremarkable	Hip extension only limited movement	Pain at end range hip extension	Pain with resisted hip flexion	Anterior hip
Lumbar/ thoracic disc pathology	20-50	Gradual Sudden overload	Varies according to spinal nerve root involved but occurs in dermatomal distribution	Lumbar/ thoracic flexion (bending/ sitting) activities that increase intrathecal pressure	May have associated deviation of trunk	Increased symptoms with trunk flexion Increased symptoms with hip flexion with knee extended (SLR)	Symptoms invariably increased with passive SLR	Fatiguable weakness of associated myotome	Possible tenderness over involved spinal segment

INTERVENTION

The rehabilitation procedures chosen to progress the patient will depend on the type of tissue involved, the extent of the damage, and the stage of healing (See Chapter 3). The intervention must be related to the signs and symptoms present rather than the actual diagnosis.

COMMON ORTHOPEDIC CONDITIONS

AVASCULAR NECROSIS OF THE FEMORAL HEAD

Diagnosis

Osteonecrosis of the femoral head—ICD-9: 733.42 (aseptic necrosis of femoral head and neck). Also referred to as aseptic necrosis of the hip or avascular necrosis of the hip.

Description

Avascular necrosis of the femoral head is characterized by variable areas of dead trabecular bone and bone marrow, extending to and including the subchondral plate. The anterolateral region of the femoral head is characteristically affected but no area is necessarily spared. Most reports on the natural history of the disease demonstrate an ineffective healing response, with resorption of bone predominating over formation of bone. The lack of repair at the center of the lesion and the incomplete repair at the periphery lead to partial resorption of dead bone and replacement with fibrous and granulation tissue.

 Clinical Pearl

Avascular necrosis of the femoral head is a debilitating disease that usually leads to destruction of the hip joint in patients who are in the third, fourth, or fifth decade of life.

Clinical Pearl

Common risk factors associated with AVN include
• Cumulative corticosteroid total dose rather than the daily dose
• Alcohol use
• Systemic lupus
• Sickle cell disease
• Gaucher disease
• Trauma
• Cancer

Subjective Findings

The subjective findings typically include the following:

• Pain in the groin, although symptoms can also radiate to the lateral hip, knee, or buttocks. The pain, usually described as throbbing and deep, is most often intermittent and of gradual onset; occasionally, it appears suddenly.

Objective Findings

The physical examination typically reveals the following findings:

• Usually a painful range of motion, especially on forced internal rotation.
• Patients have pain with attempted straight leg raising
• Antalgic gait.

 Clinical Pearl

There must be a high index of suspicion of avascular necrosis in anyone who has pain in the hip, negative radiographic findings, and any of the risk factors.

Confirmatory/Special Tests

The diagnosis osteonecrosis of the hip is based on subjective history, physical examination findings, and the results from medical/imaging studies.

Medical/Imaging Studies

An AP view of the pelvis and AP and frog lateral radiographs of the hip should be obtained. Although negative in the earliest stages of the disease, AP radiographs usually demonstrate the principal area of involvement. However, because the anterior and posterior acetabular margins overlap the superior portion of the femoral head, subtle evidence of osteosclerotic or cystic changes in the subchondral regions may be missed. Therefore, it is imperative that good-quality frog-leg lateral radiographs of the femoral head also be made.

Other diagnostic modalities that are currently available include scintigraphy, functional evaluation of bone, magnetic resonance imaging (in those patients in whom osteonecrosis is suspected but radiographic findings are normal or equivocal), computer-assisted tomography, and histological study.

Differential Diagnosis

- Femoral neck fracture
- Lumbar disc herniation
- Muscle strain
- Osteoarthritis of the hip
- Septic arthritis of the hip
- Transient osteoporosis of the hip
- Ankylosing spondylitis
- Visceral pathology

Intervention

Most studies have shown that nonoperative treatment yields poor results. The only condition for which protected weight bearing might be effective is in those cases involving of the medial aspect of the femoral head.

Prognosis

The success of the treatment of avascular necrosis of the femoral head is related to the stage at which the care is initiated. Complications of AVN include incomplete fracture and superimposed degenerative arthritis.

HAMSTRING STRAIN

Diagnosis

Hamstring strain—ICD-9: 848.9.

 Clinical Pearl

The hamstrings are the most commonly strained muscles in the body. The most commonly injured hamstring muscle is the biceps femoris.

Description

A hamstring injury involves a strain/rupture of one or more of the three hamstring muscles. The muscle tear is typically partial and commonly takes place during the eccentric phase of muscle usage when the muscle develops tension while lengthening. Most strain injuries of a muscle/tendon occur near the musculotendinous junction.

Subjective Findings

An accurate history includes the description of the onset of symptoms, duration and progression of pain, history of a traumatic event, activities that worsen the pain, and previous treatments and outcomes.

- Patient reports a distinctive mechanism of injury with immediate pain during full stride running or while decelerating quickly.
- In acute cases, the patient may report a "pop" or a tearing sensation.
- Posterior thigh pain, often approximately near the buttock, which is worsened with activities that involve resisted knee flexion.

Objective Findings

- Tenderness reported with passive stretching of the hamstrings.
- Tenderness to palpation generally is located at the origin at the ischial tuberosity but also may be present in the muscle belly and distal insertions.

 Clinical Pearl

Examination of the lumbar spine is important, because muscle injury may be related to referred pain with subsequent muscle inhibition and weakness

Confirmatory/Special Tests

A hamstring strain is diagnosed on the basis of patient history, pain with straight leg raise with the hip and knee flexed to 90 degrees and pain with resisted knee flexion.

Medical Studies

Radiographs or other specialized imaging studies usually are not needed in patients with a typical history and physical examination except in cases where there is suspicion of a fracture or bony avulsion injury.

Differential Diagnosis

The differential diagnosis for posterior thigh pain includes neoplasms, overt disc protrusions with definite signs of nerve root impingement, ischial tuberosity apophysitis, or an avulsion fracture.

Intervention

The ultimate treatment decision is based upon a variety of factors, including the patient's overall medical condition, severity, and duration of symptoms, expectations, associated pathology, and surgeon preference. Patients with a grade I strain may continue activities as much as possible. A grade II strain typically requires 5 to 21 days for rehabilitation, whereas a patient with a grade III strain might require 3 to 12 weeks of rehabilitation.

 Clinical Pearl

Muscle imbalances of strength and flexibility must be addressed, and proper techniques to stretch and strengthen the hamstrings should be taught. Special emphasis should be placed on eccentric loading. Where possible the biomechanical factors, including excessive anterior tilt of the pelvis, lumbar spine and sacroiliac joint dysfunction, and leg length discrepancies, should be corrected.

Prognosis

Because there is a great deal of variability in the rehabilitation time, anywhere from 2 to 3 weeks to 2 to 6 months, an athlete should not be permitted to return to full participation in sports until flexibility and strength ratios have been restored, and before plyometric and functional exercises are able to be performed pain free.

HIP ADDUCTOR TENDINOPATHY

Diagnosis

Hip adductor tendinopathy. ICD-9: 762.5 (enthesopathy of hip region), 726.9 (unspecified enthesopathy).

Description

Adductor tendinopathy most commonly refers to proximal adductor tendon pathology. The hip adductor muscles, including the gracilis, pectineus, and adductor longus; brevis; and magnus are the most frequent cause of groin region pain, with the adductor longus being the most commonly injured. Adductor strains, thought to result from constant exposure to repetitive loading with activities that involve twisting and turning, have been known to cause long-standing problems. In addition, a number of causative factors for an adductor strain exist, including a muscular imbalance of the combined action of the muscles stabilizing the hip joint, resulting from fatigue or an abduction overload.

Subjective Findings

The subjective findings typically include the following:

- Twinging or stabbing pain in the groin area with quick starts and stops.
- Edema or echemosis several days postinjury.
- Symptoms aggravated with running, especially with direction changes, kicking, single leg exercises, cutting, and lunges.

Objective Findings

The physical examination typically reveals the following findings:

- Pain with passive abduction or manual resistance to hip adduction when tested in different degrees of hip flexion (0 degree [gracilis], 45 degrees [adductor longus and brevis], and 90 degrees [if combined with adduction, pectineus]).
- Possibly a palpable defect in severe ruptures.
- Muscle guarding.

Confirmatory/Special Tests

The diagnosis for his condition is made based on the subjective and objective findings.

Medical/Imaging Studies

Medical/imaging studies are not typically required with this condition unless an avulsion is suspected.

Differential Diagnosis

- Osteitis pubis
- Hip joint pathology
- Inguinal, femoral, or sports related hernia
- Lumbosacral joint pathology
- Peripheral nerve entrapment
- Visceral pathology

Intervention

Conservative intervention involves the principles of PRICEMEM in the acute stage. This is followed by heat applications, hip adductor isometrics, and gentle stretching during the subacute phase, progressing to a graded resistive program, including concentric and eccentric exercises, PNF diagonal motions to promote balance strength and flexibility around the joint, and then a gradual return to full activity. As part of the rehabilitation program, any imbalance between the adductors and the abdominals needs to be addressed. In addition, the clinician should examine the patient's technique in their required activity, as poor technique can overload and fatigue the adductors.

Prognosis

Most patients recover fully or have minimal pain with high intensity activities only.

ILIOTIBIAL BAND SYNDROME

Diagnosis

Iliotibial band syndrome ICD-9: 726.60. Synonyms include iliotibial band friction syndrome (ITBFS).

Description

Iliotibial band syndrome is a common repetitive stress injury that results from friction of the iliotibial band as it slides over the prominent lateral femoral condyle at approximately 30 degrees of knee flexion.

 Clinical Pearl

Iliotibial band syndrome is the most common overuse syndrome of the knee, being particularly common in long-distance runners (20–40 miles/week) who train on hilly terrain, graded slopes, or road cambers and cyclists.

Subjective Findings

• Reports of lateral knee pain, which is diffuse and hard to localize, with the repetitive motions of the knee.
• Rarely a history of trauma.

- Climbing or descending stairs often aggravates the pain.
- History of changes in training surfaces, increased mileage, or training on crowned roads.

Objective Findings

- Localized tenderness to palpation at the lateral femoral condyle or Gerdy's tubercle on the anterolateral portion of the proximal tibia.
- The resisted tests are likely to be negative for pain.
- The special tests for the iliotibial band should be positive for pain, or crepitus or both, especially at 30 degrees of weight-bearing knee flexion.

 Clinical Pearl

The following findings have all been associated with iliotibial band friction problems, although they have yet to be substantiated: cavus foot (calcaneal varus) structure, leg-length difference (with the syndrome developing on the shorter side), fatigue, internal tibial torsion (increased lateral retinaculum tension), anatomically prominent lateral femoral epicondyle, and genu varum.

Confirmatory/Special Tests

- Ober's test (see text)
- Noble compression test (see text)
- Creak test (see text)

Medical Studies

Radiographs are negative.

Differential Diagnosis

- Lateral meniscus tear
- Lateral compartment degenerative joint disease
- Popliteal tenosynovitis

Intervention

Conservative intervention consists of activity modification to reduce the irritating stress (decreasing mileage, changing the bike seat position, and changing the training surfaces), using new running shoes, heat or ice applications, strengthening of the hip abductors, and stretching of the iliotibial band.

Prognosis

Surgical intervention, which is reserved for the more recalcitrant cases, consists of a resection of the posterior half of the iliotibial band at the level that passes over the lateral femoral condyle.

LEGG–CALVÉ–PERTHES DISEASE

Diagnosis

Legg–Calvé–Perthes disease—ICD-9: 732.1. The condition is also referred to as aseptic necrosis of the femoral head, avascular necrosis of the femoral head, or idiopathic osteonecrosis of the femoral head.

Description

Legg–Calvé–Perthes disease is idiopathic osteonecrosis of the femoral head in children aged 4 to 10 years. Although the definitive cause of Legg–Calvé–Perthes disease remains unknown, there is considerable epidemiologic, histologic, and radiographic evidence to support the theory that Legg–Calvé–Perthes disease is probably a localized manifestation of a generalized disorder of epiphyseal cartilage manifested in the proximal femur because of its unusual and precarious blood supply.

 Clinical Pearl

Legg–Calvé–Perthes disease is unilateral in 90% of patients, four times more common in boys, and uncommon in African–Americans.

Subjective Findings

The subjective findings typically include the following:

- The patient complains of a vague ache in the groin that radiates to the medial thigh and inner aspect of the knee.
- Muscle spasm is another common complaint in the early stages of the disease.

Objective Findings

The physical examination typically reveals the following findings:

- The initial sign is a limp. There may also be a slight dragging of the leg and slight atrophy of the thigh muscles.
- The child may be small for his/her age.

- A positive Trendelenburg sign is often seen.
- There may be some out-toeing of the involved extremity.
- There is usually decreased abduction and internal rotation.
- There may be contracture in hip flexion (0 degree to 30 degrees).

 Clinical Pearl

Limited hip abduction may not be apparent unless movement of the pelvis is recognized. Hip abduction should be examined by placing one hand on the opposite pelvis and using the other hand to abduct the hip. The point at which the pelvis starts to move or tilt indicates the degree of abduction.

Confirmatory/Special Tests

The diagnosis of Legg–Calvé–Perthes disease is based on the subjective history, findings from the physical examination, and confirmation with imaging studies.

Medical/Imaging Studies

AP and frog-lateral radiographs of the pelvis should be obtained. Although radiographs are normal early in the disease course, progressive fragmentation, irregularity, and eventual collapse of the femoral head is seen as the disease progresses.

Differential Diagnosis

- Gaucher disease
- Multiple epiphyseal dysplasia
- A typical septic arthritis
- Sickle cell anemia
- Transient synovitis
- Hypothyroidism

Intervention

The intervention for Legg–Calvé–Perthes disease remains controversial.

Children who are less than 6 years of age (possibly 5 years in girls) and those with minimal capital femoral epiphysis involvement and normal range of motion are often followed with intermittent physical exams and radiographs approximately every 2 months.

In the more severe cases, there is lack of agreement regarding whether operative or nonoperative intervention is beneficial.[1] In reviewing long-term studies, most patients (70%–90%) are active and pain free regardless of intervention.

Prognosis

The prognosis is much improved if there is no collapse of the femoral head. Treatment has no effect on outcome if the patient has a chronologic age ≥8 years at onset of the disease.

MERALGIA PARESTHETICA

Diagnosis

Meralgia paresthetica—ICD-9: 355.1.

Description

Meralgia paresthetica is a syndrome of pain and/or dysesthesia caused by entrapment or neurinoma formation of the lateral cutaneous (lateral femoral cutaneous) nerve of the thigh. Neuropathy of this nerve may cause pain, numbness, and dysesthesia in the anterolateral aspect of the thigh that is most marked on walking, standing, and sleeping in the prone position. Common causes include

- Obesity
- Direct trauma
- Surgical scarring
- Abdominal distention including pregnancy
- Tight clothing around the waist

Subjective Findings

Subjective findings with this condition are typically vague and include the following:

 Clinical Pearl

The lateral cutaneous nerve of the thigh is primarily a sensory nerve but also includes efferent sympathetic fibers carrying vasomotor, pilomotor, and sudomotor impulses.

- Numbness/tingling/burning pain in the front and lateral thigh area that can vary in intensity.
- No history of trauma.

Objective Findings

Most of the physical examination is normally negative. However, there may be decreased sensation to light touch and pinprick over the anterolateral skin of the thigh. Hip extension or ambulation may aggravate the condition.

 Clinical Pearl

Motor nerve dysfunction does not occur because the lateral femoral cutaneous nerve of the thigh is a sensory nerve.

Confirmatory/Special Tests

There may be a positive inverse Lasegue sign (prone knee bend with hip placed in extension), or a leg length discrepancy. The femoral nerve stretch test, with the hip placed in adduction, may also be positive.

Medical Studies

Abdominal and pelvic examinations may be needed to exclude intra-abdominal pathology. An AP radiograph of the pelvis may be used to rule out any bony abnormality, and AP and lateral radiographs of the hip may be appropriate when the patient has restricted internal rotation of the hip and groin pain. CT or MRI is appropriate to investigate a suspected intrapelvic mass.

Differential Diagnosis

Differential diagnosis includes back (disc herniation), hip (arthritis, trochanteric bursitis), and groin pathology, and peripheral neuropathy.

 Clinical Pearl

Meralgia paresthetica symptoms may be confused with more frequently seen symptoms produced by entrapment of the upper lumbar nerve roots.

Intervention

Intervention is dependent on the cause and can include any of the following:

- Weight reduction.
- Removal of constricting corsets and loosening of tight belts.
- Insertion of heel lifts (creates an anterior pelvic tilt, which approximates the pelvis to the lower extremity).

Prognosis

If conservative management yields no relief, then neurolysis or nerve resection may be performed.

OSTEOARTHRITIS OF THE HIP

Diagnosis

Osteoarthritis of the hip—ICD-9: 721.5. Also known as hip degenerative joint disease and hip arthritis.

Description

The development of osteoarthritis at any joint site depends upon a generalized predisposition to the condition, and abnormalities of biomechanical loading which act at specific joints.

Subjective Findings

It is important to identify patients with symptomatic OA correctly and to exclude conditions that may be mistaken for or coexist with OA. Osteoarthritis of the hip joint generally presents with fairly steady pain that becomes more severe as the disease advances.

- Insidious onset of pain: The pain may be felt in the area of the buttock, groin, thigh, or knee and varies in character from a dull ache to sharp stabbing pains. Progressively worsening pain with activity and exercise is common, and a painful, limping gait generally develops.
  - Pain is worse initially with full internal rotation and extension of the hip, and hip range of motion is progressively lost.
  - The distribution of painful joints is helpful to distinguish OA from other types of arthritis because MCP, wrist, elbow, ankle, and shoulder arthritis are unlikely locations for OA except after trauma.
  - Physical activity may induce bouts of pain that last for several hours.

- Depending on the level of disease progression, the patient may report having difficulty climbing stairs with the involved leg, and may have difficulty in putting on socks or stockings.

 Clinical Pearl

Periarticular pain that is not reproduced by passive motion and direct joint palpation suggests an alternate etiology such as bursitis, tendonitis, or periostitis.

Objective Findings

- Early physical signs include restriction of internal rotation and abduction or flexion of the affected hip, with pain at the end of the range.

 Clinical Pearl

Patients with hip osteoarthritis typically have the following history and/or symptoms:

- Pain along the front and/or side of the hip when putting weight on the leg.
- Age over 50.
- Morning stiffness lasting less than 1 hour (gets better with movement).
- Hip motions that are limited include internal rotation and flexion. Comparisons should be made between the involved side with the other nonpainful side. More than a 15-degree difference is significant.
- Decreased weight bearing in stance phase of gait.
- Painfully resisted hip flexion and resisted hip adduction

Confirmatory/Special Tests

- Scour test
- FABER test

Medical Studies

The diagnosis can usually be confirmed by radiography; joint space width of 2.5 mm or less indicates substantial loss of cartilage in the hip joint, and osteophytes, subchondral bone sclerosis, or cysts are usually present.

Differential Diagnosis

- Avascular necrosis of the femoral head
- Rheumatoid arthritis, psoriatic arthritis, reactive arthritis, ankylosing spondylitis, infection, and crystal induced disorders
- Stress fracture of the femur
- Aneurysm of the aorta
- Pelvic inflammatory disease
- Lumbar radiculopathy
- Hernia
- Bursitis

Intervention

The intervention goals for hip OA include relieving symptoms, minimizing disability and handicap, and reducing the risk of disease progression. Intervention in the earlier stages includes:

- Education and empowerment: Giving advice about what patients can do for themselves is of immense value. Modification of activities of daily living and self-care is one of the most important components. Contact sports and activities, such as jogging, which can cause repetitive high impact loading of the hip, are probably best avoided.
- Modalities for muscle relaxation, pain relief, and anti-inflammation.
- In addition to specific exercises for hip range of motion, recreations such as swimming or cycling may help.
- A reduction in weight can significantly improve a patient's symptoms, increase mobility, and improve health status.
- A simple walking stick can make a big difference, reducing loading on a hip by 20%–30%.
- Manual techniques to mobilize the joint, and passive stretches of the capsule, particularly distractive techniques, are helpful to maintain mobility.
- Strengthening exercises are performed for the trunk stabilizers and the major muscle groups of the hip region, especially the gluteus medius.

Prognosis

Various factors predict the progress of osteoarthritis. Increasing age is a general factor for increased osteoarthritis, as is finding calcium apatite crystals in joint fluid. In addition, obesity, a greater number of joints involved, worsening symptoms, the presence of Heberden's nodes, and abnormal 99mTc bone scan are all associated with progressive osteoarthritis.

PIRIFORMIS SYNDROME

Diagnosis

Piriformis syndrome—ICD-9: 355.0 (lesion of sciatic nerve), 724.3 (sciatica).

Description

The "piriformis syndrome," an uncommon and often undiagnosed cause of buttock and leg pain, has been described as an anatomic abnormality of the piriformis muscle and the sciatic nerve which can result in irritation of the sciatic nerve by the piriformis muscle causing buttock and hamstring pain. Common causes include:

- Hypertrophy of the piriformis muscle.
- Trauma.
- Inflammation and spasm of the piriformis muscle.
- Anatomical anomalies.

Subjective Findings

- A history of trauma to the sacroiliac and gluteal regions.
- Pain in the region of the sacroiliac joint, greater sciatic notch, and piriformis muscle that usually causes difficulty with walking.
- Acute exacerbation of pain caused by stooping or lifting

Objective Findings

An examination of the hip and lower leg usually demonstrates restricted external rotation of the hip and lumbosacral muscle tightness.

- Positive FABER test.
- Weak gluteus maximus, gluteus medius, and biceps femoris.
- Neurologic symptoms in the posterior lower limb if the fibular nerve is involved.
- Ipsilateral short leg.

Confirmatory/Special Tests

Pace and Nagle[1] described a diagnostic maneuver that is now referred to as Pace's sign:

- pain and weakness in association with resisted abduction and external rotation of the involved thigh.

---

[1]Pace JB, Nagle D. Piriformis syndrome. *Western J Med.* 1976;124:435-439.

- Positive straight leg raise test.

Medical Studies

The piriformis syndrome is usually a diagnosis of exclusion.

Differential Diagnosis

- Lumbar radiculopathy
- Spinal stenosis
- Diabetic neuropathy
- Fibular (peroneal) nerve injury
- Bursitis
- Sacroiliac joint dysfunction

Intervention

Conservative intervention for this condition includes gentle, pain-free static stretching of the piriformis muscle, strain–counterstrain techniques, soft tissue therapy (longitudinal gliding combined with passive internal hip rotation, as well as transverse gliding and sustain longitudinal release with the patient lying on one side), ice massage to the gluteal region, and spray and stretch techniques. Local corticosteroid or botox injections may be useful in more acute cases.

Prognosis

Piriformis syndrome typically responds well to conservative management. Patients who experience no significant relief of symptoms after several months of treatment may undergo surgery in which the entrapped nerve is freed by sectioning one of the heads of origin of the piriformis muscle.

PUBALGIA-OSTEITIS PUBIS

Diagnosis

Pubalgia/osteitis pubis—ICD-9: 848.5 (pelvic sprain).

Description

Pubalgia is a collective term for all disorders that cause chronic pain in the region of the pubic tubercle and the structures attached to the pubic bone (inguinal region), including osteitis pubis, a chronic inflammatory and overuse condition of the pubic symphysis and adjacent ischial rami.

Clinical Pearl

Although the exact etiology of osteitis pubis is unknown, it is most likely caused by repetitive microtrauma or shearing forces to the pubic symphysis. A number of abnormalities in joints and muslces around the groin may increase the mechanical stress placed on the pubic region:

- Limited hip range of motion
- Increased adductor muscle tone
- Increased rectus abdominis tone
- Iliopsoas muscle shortening often associated with hypomobility of the upper lumbar spine
- Lumbar spine/SIJ dysfunction
- Decreased lumbopelvic stability

Subjective Findings

An accurate history includes the description of the onset of symptoms, duration, and progression of pain, history of a traumatic event, activities that worsen the pain, and previous treatments and outcomes.

- Complaints of lower abdominal pain with exertion, minimal to no pain at rest, and increased pain with sit-ups and activities that involve resisted hip adduction (running, kicking, or pushing off to change direction).

Objective Findings

- Pain may be elicited with passive hip flexion, when combined with hip adduction, or with passive abduction with a straight or bent knee. However, in some cases, range of motion may appear normal.
- Point tenderness at the pubic tubercles, rectus abdominis insertion, adductor origin, and inferior pubic rami.

Confirmatory/Special Tests

The diagnosis for this condition is made on the basis of the patient history and the results of the physical examination. Special tests that may help with the diagnosis include:

- Squeeze test (see chapter text; not specific for osteitis pubis)
- Bilateral hip adduction test (see chapter text; not specific for osteitis pubis)
- Single adductor test (see chapter text; not specific for osteitis pubis)
- Active straight leg raise (ASLR) test (see Chapter 13; not specific for osteitis pubis)

Medical Studies

Radiographs are often negative early in osteitis pubis (it takes approximately 1 month after the initial injury or onset of symptoms for radiographic changes to manifest, although radiographic signs tend to persist even after symptoms have receded following resolution):

- After a few weeks, some widening of the pubic symphysis may be seen on anteroposterior (AP) films.
- As osteitis pubis progresses, sclerosis, and osteolysis of the pubic symphysis can be seen.
- If pelvic inequity is suspected as a cause, flamingo views (with the patient in single leg stance) can expose a pubic instability.

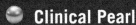 **Clinical Pearl**

In the case of osteomyelitis, bone erosions can be seen on plain films.

Bone scans (technetium-99m [^{99m}Tc]) or single-photon emission computerized tomography (SPECT) scans are often positive early in the disease. Computed tomography provides the earliest detection of traumatic osteitis pubis, and demonstrates hematomas, soft tissue swelling, and small avulsion fractures not discernible on plain radiographs.

MRI is especially useful when fat suppression views are obtained— this imaging modality helps distinguish between muscle, tendon, periosteal, or bony disruption.

Differential Diagnosis

- Inguinal hernia
- Pelvic inflammatory disease (females)
- Abdominal muscle pull
- Adductor strain
- Ankylosing spondylitis (rare)
- Femoral neck fracture
- Inguinal hernia
- Osteomyelitis
- Pelvic inflammatory disease
- Prostatitis
- Pubic stress fracture
- Reiter syndrome (rare)

Clinical Pearl

An adductor strain is easily confused with traumatic osteitis pubis because of the adjacent area of injury and also because of the common mechanism of injury. Although clinical presentation of both types of injury are often identical, adductor tendonitis exhibits groin tenderness maximally at the distal muscle insertion, whereas osteitis pubis is maximally tender at the pubic bone.

Intervention

The ultimate treatment decision is based upon a variety of factors, including the patient's overall medical condition, severity, and duration of symptoms, expectations, associated pathology, and surgeon preference.

- A period of relative rest and anti-inflammatory medications.
- Transverse friction massage (TFM) can be applied locally.
- Ultrasound, electrical stimulation, thermotherapy, and cryotherapy.
- Stretching as tolerated to the muscles surrounding the injured area:
  - The short and long adductors
  - Hip flexors (iliopsoas and rectus femoris)
  - Hip internal rotators
  - Abdominals
  - Gluteal muscles
- Strengthening of the same muscle groups. The strengthening exercises are performed isometrically initially and then concentrically and eccentrically, and finally isokinetically as appropriate.
- Core stability training.
- Proprioception training.

 Clinical Pearl

Effective warm ups and preparation before the sporting activity can play an important preventative role.

Prognosis

In cases of failed conservative intervention, which is common, surgical intervention (pelvic floor repair) or cessation from the offending activity becomes the patient's only choice.

SLIPPED CAPITAL FEMORAL EPIPHYSIS

Diagnosis

Slipped capital femoral epiphysis—ICD-9: 732.2.

Description

Slipped capital femoral epiphysis (SCFE) is displacement of the femoral head through the physis that typically occurs during the adolescent growth spurt. The term slipped capital femoral epiphysis is actually a misnomer in that there is a sudden or gradual anterior displacement of the femoral neck from the capital femoral epiphysis while the femoral head remains in the acetabulum.

 Clinical Pearl

Slipped capital femoral epiphysis is the most common disorder of the hip in adolescents. The average age for girls in whom slipped capital femoral epiphyses develop is 12.1 ± 1 years, and for boys 14.4 ± 1.3 years.

Subjective Findings

The subjective findings typically include the following:

- Pain exacerbated by activity is the most common presenting symptom. Patients with chronic slipped capital femoral epiphysis generally have a history of groin or medial thigh pain. However, approximately 45% of patients report knee or lower thigh pain as their initial symptom. The pain is reported as dull or aching.
- There may be reports of a mild weakness of the leg.
- There may be no history of trauma—the initiating traumatic episode may be as minimal as turning over in bed.

 Clinical Pearl

In the child, complaints of pain and loss of range at the hip joint should always alert the clinician to the possibility of transient synovitis, Legg–Calvé–Perthes disease, or a slipped femoral capital epiphysis.

Objective Findings

The physical examination typically reveals the following findings:

- If the patient can walk, it is with difficulty and with a limp, often with external rotation of the involved foot.
- The hip will often show decreased range of motion, particularly of internal rotation (the most sensitive and specific finding), abduction, and flexion.
- On passive flexion of the hip, the patient will frequently demonstrate obligatory external rotation of the hip.
- The involved extremity may be between 1 and 3 cm shorter than the uninvolved extremity, depending on the severity of the slip.

 Clinical Pearl

Obesity, male gender, and greater involvement with sports activities are predisposing factors.

 Clinical Pearl

SCFE is the only pediatric disorder that causes greater loss of internal rotation when the hip is moved into a flexed position.

Confirmatory/Special Tests

Assessing internal rotation with the hip flexed to 90 degrees is an effective screening maneuver and is usually done on all adolescents who have lower extremity pain.

Medical/Imaging Studies

AP and frog-lateral radiographs of the pelvis confirm the diagnosis as the slip is always posterior. If a Klein line drawn along the lateral femoral neck (AP view) or anterior femoral neck (lateral view) does not intersect any portion of the epiphysis, the child has SCFE.

Most cases are idiopathic, but endocrine abnormalities (e.g. hypothyroidism) should be considered.

 Clinical Pearl

On the basis of the patient's history, physical examination, and radiographs, slipped capital femoral epiphysis can be classified as a stable or unstable hip:

- In the stable hip, weight bearing is possible with or without crutches.
- In the unstable hip, the patient presents more with fracture-like symptoms with pain so severe that weight bearing is impossible.

Differential Diagnosis

- Transient synovitis
- Legg–Calvé–Perthes disease
- Meralgia paresthetica
- Neoplasm

Intervention

The goals of intervention are relief of symptoms, containment of the femoral head, and restoration of range of motion. The current method of choice is in situ surgical fixation. Other treatments are epiphysiodesis, osteotomy, salvage procedure, or spica cast. Conservative intervention includes the use of traction for the relief of symptoms, at home or in the hospital, for periods ranging from 1 or 2 days to several weeks; partial weight bearing with use of crutches in order to rest an inflamed, painful joint; and the use of anti-inflammatory medication. The goal of containment is to maintain the sphericity of the femoral head.

Prognosis

Patients are at risk for recurrent slippage until the physis closes. Progressive arthritis, chondrolysis, and osteonecrosis may occur.

SNAPPING HIP

Diagnosis

Snapping hip—ICD-9: 719.65. Also referred to as coxa saltans, iliopsoas syndrome, and trochanteric syndrome.

Description

Snapping hip is characterized by a snapping or popping sensation that occurs as tendons around the hip move over bony prominences. Multiple etiologies for snapping hip exist. The etiologies are categorized as internal, external, and intra-articular.

- Internal: there are two common internal causes

- The iliopsoas snapping over structures just deep to it, namely the femoral head, proximal lesser trochanter, pectineus fascia, and iliopectineal eminence, which produces a snapping in the anterior groin region.
  - Stenosing tenosynovitis of the iliopsoas insertion.
- External: include snapping of the iliotibial band or gluteus maximus over the greater trochanter. This condition is more common in females with a wide pelvis and prominent trochanters, and is exacerbated with running on banked surfaces.
- Intra-articular: include synovial chondromatosis, loose bodies, fracture fragments, and labral tears. Snapping of the iliofemoral ligament over the anterior femoral head also has been described, as has snapping of the long head of biceps femoris origin over the ischium.

Subjective Findings

The subjective findings typically include the following:

- Complaints of a snapping or popping sensation localized to the greater trochanter area (iliotibial band) that occurs with ambulation, and sometimes when the patient lies with the involved side up and rotates the leg. Snapping caused by subluxation of the iliopsoas tendon usually is felt in the groin as the hip extends from a flexed position, as when rising from a chair.
- There may be complaints of pain associated with the snapping if the trochanteric bursa is inflamed.

 Clinical Pearl

Snapping from an intra-articular cause is more disabling and more likely to cause patients to grab for support.

Objective Findings

The physical examination typically reveals the following findings:

- The iliotibial band can be felt to sublux when asking the patient to stand and then rotate the hip while holding it in an adducted position. Snapping of the iliopsoas tendon may be palpated while asking the patient to extend the hip from a flexed position while palpating over the pectineal eminence of the pelvis.

Confirmatory/Special Tests

- Ober test
- Thomas test

Medical/Imaging Studies

AP radiographs of the pelvis and lateral hip, although typically normal for patients with a snapping hip, can exclude bony pathology or intra-articular hip disease.

Differential Diagnosis

- Tear of the acetabular labrum. MRI with gadolinium may be necessary to rule out such a tear.
- Osteonecrosis of the femoral head.
- Osteoarthritis of the hip.
- Osteochondral loose body.

Intervention

The intervention is based on etiology. If an imbalance of the tensor fascia latae or iliopsoas is producing the symptoms, the intervention is focused on reconditioning and prevention. This includes increasing the flexibility of the soft tissues, and the correction of any strength imbalances. If the iliotibial band is tight, the emphasis is on stretching the iliotibial band.

Prognosis

Snapping hip usually respond very well to conservative management. Surgery is reserved for the uncommon cases that are disabling and fail to resolve.

STRESS FRACTURE OF THE FEMORAL NECK

Diagnosis

Stress fracture of the femoral neck—ICD-9: 820.00 (femoral neck fracture [transcervical]), 821.0 (fracture of shaft or unspecified part of femur closed), 821.2 (fracture of lower end of femur closed).

Description

Stress fractures result from accelerated bone remodeling in response to repeated stress. Stress fractures of the femoral neck occur most commonly in military recruits and athletes, especially runners. The fracture typically occurs on the superior side in older patients (tension-side fractures) or the inferior side (compression-side fractures) of the femoral neck in younger patients.

Clinical Pearl

Because stress fractures are a relatively uncommon etiology of hip pain, they are therefore often misdiagnosed or missed. If not diagnosed in a timely fashion, progression to serious complications can occur.

Subjective Findings

The subjective findings typically include the following:

- An onset of sudden hip pain is the most frequent symptom and is usually associated with a recent change in training (particularly an increase in distance or intensity) or a change in training surface.
- Pain in the deep thigh (inguinal or anterior groin area) is the earliest and most frequent symptom.
- Pain can also occur in the lateral aspect or anteromedial aspect of the thigh.
- The pain usually occurs with weight bearing or at the extremes of hip motion, and can radiate into the knee. Less severe cases may only have pain following a long run.
- Night pain may occur if the fracture progresses.

Objective Findings

The physical examination is often negative, although there may be a noncapsular pattern of the hip, an empty end feel, or pain at the extremes of hip internal (more common) or external rotation, or pain with resisted hip external rotation. Occasionally, the patient will walk with an antalgic gait.

Confirmatory/Special Tests

There are no objective tests in physical therapy that completely rule in or rule out a femoral stress fracture. Therefore, the clinician must rely on a cluster of subjective and objective findings. Special tests that may help with the diagnoses include:

- Resisted straight leg raising maneuver—lifting the heel of the involved side off the examination table within the knee held straight. A positive test is reproduction of the groin or thigh pain.
- Auscultatory patellar-pubic percussion test may be positive (sensitivity: 0.96; specificity: 0.76; positive predictive value: 0.98).
- Fulcrum test (see Special Tests in chapter). A positive test includes an exacerbation of sharp thigh pain and apprehension and is shown to have a high clinical correlation for femoral shaft stress injuries.

Medical/Imaging Studies

Radiographs taken soon after the symptoms begin have been reported to be positive in only 20% of cases. Diagnosis is best confirmed with MRI or bone scintigraphy (scan), although these have also been shown to be prone to false negatives.

Differential Diagnosis

- Osteoarthritis of the hip
- Referred symptoms from the spine
- Trochanteric bursitis
- Septic arthritis
- Muscle strain or groin pull
- Osteonecrosis of the hip
- Pathologic fracture
- Tear of the acetabular labrum

Intervention

All tension-side stress fractures are treated surgically whether the fracture is displaced or nondisplaced. The intervention for compression fractures varies according to the bone scintigraphy findings.

- If there is a positive scan only, or sclerosis and no fracture line on the radiographs, the intervention ranges from modified bed rest to nonweight bearing with crutches until symptoms subside. Once pain free, weight bearing is progressed. When significant partial weight bearing is pain free, cycling, and swimming may be permitted. Weekly radiographs are obtained until the athlete is full weight bearing without pain. Water running and water walking are progressed. If these remain pain free, running on land is commenced, with the initial run being no further than one quarter mile.

- If there is an overt fracture line on the radiographs with no displacement, and provided that only the cortex is involved, an initial period of either bed rest or complete nonweight bearing is necessary. The patient is progressed to partial and then full weight bearing on crutches as symptoms permit. Roentgenograms every 2 to 3 days during the first week are necessary to detect any widening of the fracture line. If healing does not occur, internal fixation with some form of hip pin is indicated.

Prognosis

An overt fracture with radiographic evidence of opening or displacement is significant and requires surgical intervention, usually in the form of a hip screw and plate. Displaced fractures must be treated as an orthopedic emergency.

THIGH CONTUSION

Diagnosis

Thigh contusion—ICD-9: 924.0. The term *charley horse* is synonymous with a contusion of the quadriceps muscle.

Description

The usual cause of the quadriceps contusion is a direct blow to the anterior thigh from an object or another person (e.g., helmet, knee).

 Clinical Pearl

Severe trauma to the thigh and a large contusion can lead to a compartment syndrome. This diagnosis should be considered in patients with crush injuries, in patients with fractures resulting from high-energy trauma, in patients on anticoagulants, in patients with bleeding disorders, and in patients with multiple traumas.

Subjective Findings

• Reports of a blow to the anterior thigh with an object, or contact with another athlete or gear
• Painful anterior thigh
• Painful weight bearing
• Unwillingness to flex the knee because of thigh pain

Objective Findings

• Tense, edematous, and tender anterior thigh.
• Variable swelling. Extreme swelling should alert the clinician to the possibility of an injury to major vessels.
• Negative neurologic exam.

 Clinical Pearl

Quadriceps contusions can be graded according to functional loss:

• *Grade I.* In a mild contusion, the patient has localized tenderness with no alteration of gait. Knee motion can be performed without pain up to at least 90 degrees of flexion.

- **Grade II.** In a moderate contusion, the patient displays swelling and a tender muscle mass. Knee flexion motion is restricted to less than 90 degrees and an antalgic gait is present. The patient is unable to climb stairs or arise from a chair without considerable discomfort.

- **Grade III.** In a severe contusion, the patient cannot bend their knee beyond approximately 45 degrees. The patient is unable to walk unaided. Marked tenderness and swelling are present.

 Clinical Pearl

The anterior compartment contains the femoral nerve, and testing of the lateral, intermediate, and medial cutaneous nerves should be performed if compartment syndrome is suspected.

Confirmatory/Special Tests

The diagnosis is made based on a history of acute or repetitive trauma, and the history and physical examination findings are consistent with these working diagnoses.

Medical Studies

Initially, imaging studies may not be indicated in patients with partial rectus tears, minimally symptomatic quadriceps contusions, and mild quadriceps tendonitis.

Differential Diagnosis

- Soft tissue tumors
- Femur fractures
- Referred pain
- Herniated nucleus pulposus
- Slipped capital femoral epiphysis, avascular necrosis
- Stress fracture—hip, femur, pelvis

Intervention

Conservative intervention involves a gradual progression of range of motion and strengthening exercises.

Prognosis

Surgical intervention is indicated for compartment syndrome (decompressive fasciotomy), hematoma removal, complete quadriceps muscle rupture, and bony avulsion of muscle insertion at the patellar tendon.

TRANSIENT SYNOVITIS

Diagnosis

Transient synovitis of the hip—ICD-9: 719.05 (effusion of joint, pelvic region, and thigh). Transient synovitis is also known as toxic synovitis, irritable hip, and observation hip.

Description

Transient synovitis of the hip is a sterile infusion of the joint that resolves without therapy or sequelae.

 Clinical Pearl

Transient synovitis is the most common cause of hip pain and of limp in preschool and early grade school age children.

Subjective Findings

The subjective findings typically include the following:

• The child usually presents with a limp of acute onset with no history of an inciting episode.

• There is usually unilateral pain at the hip, knee, or thigh.

• The child may refuse to move the affected leg in any direction due to pain.

Objective Findings

The physical examination typically reveals the following findings:

• The hip is typically held in flexion, abduction, and external rotation (position of maximum capacity). If range of motion can be examined, it is usually limited in abduction and internal rotation, although with gentle, slow range of motion it is possible to obtain full passive range of the hip.

• Most children are afebrile.

Confirmatory/Special Tests

Transient synovitis is a diagnosis of exclusion.

Medical/Imaging Studies

Diagnostic studies and radiographs are indicated if the patient has very limited motion or temperature is higher than 99.5°F (37.5°C).

Differential Diagnosis

- Septic arthritis
- Slipped capital femoral epiphysis
- Juvenile rheumatoid arthritis
- Legg–Calvé–Perthes disease

Intervention

The intervention for transient synovitis is decreased weight bearing for 1 to 2 weeks, along with nonsteroidal anti-inflammatory medications.

Prognosis

The condition should be self-limiting unless there is a more serious condition such as septic arthritis or juvenile rheumatoid arthritis present. Recurrence can occur in up to 17% of patients.

TROCHANTERIC BURSITIS

Diagnosis

Trochanteric bursitis—ICD-9: 726.5.

Description

Trochanteric bursitis is the collective name given to inflammation of any one of the trochanteric bursae.

 Clinical Pearl

Trochanteric bursitis is the second most frequent cause of lateral hip pain. Osteoarthritis is the most common.

Subjective Findings

An accurate history includes the description of the onset of symptoms, duration, and progression of pain, history of a traumatic event, activities that worsen the pain, and previous treatments and outcomes. The typical subjective findings include:

- Complaints of lateral thigh, groin, and gluteal pain, especially when lying on the involved side. Although the pain is typically local to the hip region, it can radiate distally to the knee and the lower leg, or proximally into the buttock.

- The pain is typically worse when rising from a seated or recumbent position, feel somewhat better after a few steps, and recurs after walking for half an hour or more.

Objective Findings

Objectively, the clinical findings include:

- The reproduction of pain with palpation, or with stretching of the iliotibial band (ITB) across the trochanter with hip adduction or the extremes of internal or external hip rotation.

- Resisted abduction, extension, or external rotation of the hip are also painful.

- There is often associated tightness of the hip adductors, which cause the patient's feet to cross the midline, resulting in increased stress on the trochanteric bursae.

Confirmatory/Special Tests

- Ober's Test: The Ober's test is used to evaluate tightness of the ITB and tensor fascia latae. The patient is placed in the side lying position, and with the hip extended and abducted and the knee flexed, the proximal part of the leg is allowed to drop passively onto the contralateral limb (see text). The test is considered positive when the leg fails to lower.

- Modified Ober's test: The modified Ober's test is performed in the same fashion as the Ober test except that the knee is extended.

 Clinical Pearl

The use of an inclinometer to measure hip adduction using both the Ober test and the modified Ober test appears to be a reliable method for the measurement of IT band flexibility

Medical Studies

AP radiographs of the pelvis and lateral radiographs of the hip may be necessary to rule out bony abnormalities and intra-articular hip pathology. Bone scans and MRI are rarely needed to make the diagnosis but occasionally may be helpful to rule out uncommon conditions such as occult fractures, tumors, or osteonecrosis of the femoral head.

Differential Diagnosis

- Tendinopathy of the gluteus medius or maximus muscles, with or without calcification
- Inguinal and femoral hernia
- An irritation of the L4 or L5 nerve roots
- Meralgia paresthetica
- A "snapping" hip
- Lower spinal neoplasm
- Pelvic tumor
- Hip infection/septic arthritis
- Avascular necrosis
- Stress fracture of the femur
- Bone or soft tissue tumor

Intervention

The ultimate treatment decision is based upon a variety of factors, including the patient's overall medical condition, severity, and duration of symptoms, expectations, associated hip pathology, and surgeon preference. The intervention for trochanteric bursitis usually consists of

- The removal of the causative factors by stretching the soft tissues of the lateral thigh, especially the tensor fascia latae and ITB.
- Focusing on the flexibility of the external rotators, quadriceps, and hip flexors.
- Strengthening of the hip abductors.
- Establishing muscular balance between the hip adductors and abductors.
- Orthotics may be prescribed if there is a biomechanical fault in the kinetic chain due to an ankle/foot dysfunction.

Prognosis

This condition usually responds well to conservative measures. On occasion, injection of a local anesthetic and corticosteroid preparation into the greater trochanteric bursa can be helpful in relieving symptoms.

REHABILITATION LADDER

HIP

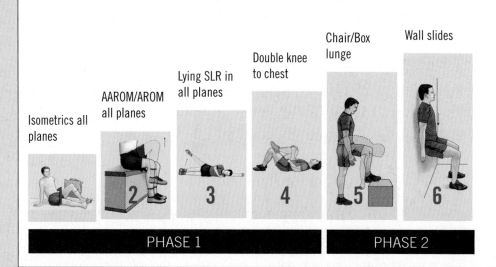

Isometrics all planes

AAROM/AROM all planes 2

Lying SLR in all planes 3

Double knee to chest 4

Chair/Box lunge 5

Wall slides 6

PHASE 1   PHASE 2

The purpose of these training ladders is to provide the clinician with a safe and progressive framework of exercises that are designed to allow the patient to improve in an efficient manner. The patient begins at the appropriate step, which is based on the stage of healing and the goal of the intervention.

• Phase 1: Acute—pain management, restoration of full passive range of motion, and restoration of normal accessory motion.

• Phase 2: Subacute—active range of motion exercises and early strengthening.

• Phase 3: Chronic—specific strengthening with a strong emphasis on enhancing dynamic stability.

The degree of movement and the speed of progression are both guided by the signs and symptoms. Once the patient is able to perform an exercise

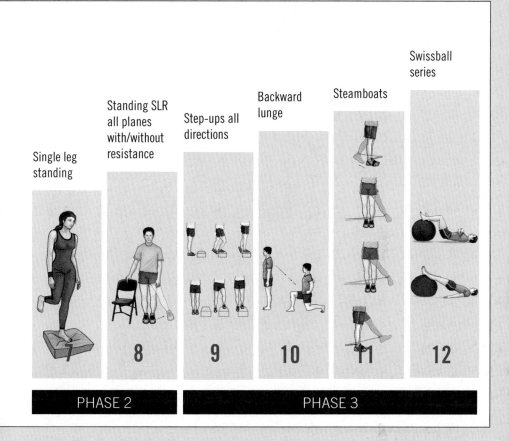

for 8–12 reps without pain, he/she progresses up to the next exercise step. This continues until the patient attempts an exercise that reproduces the pain. At this point, the patient returns to the last exercise that he/she was able to perform without pain and performs that exercise 5 times/day for 1 to 2 days before attempting to progress again. The patient is advanced through the training ladders to the appropriate point, with particular attention paid to patient response to treatment in terms of changes in symptoms, swelling, degree of irritability, or motion. In addition, muscle imbalances are addressed with appropriate flexibility exercises.

Once the patient is able to perform the last exercise of Phase 3 (Step 12 of the ladder), he or she can move onto functional and sport-specific training (Phase 4) as appropriate, which focus on power and higher-speed exercises similar to sport specific demands.

1. Isometrics in all planes
The patient is positioned in supine. Isometric exercises for the hip musculature include gluteal sets (contraction of the buttock muscles), hip abduction (1a), and hip adduction (1b). The isometric contractions should be held for 10 seconds.

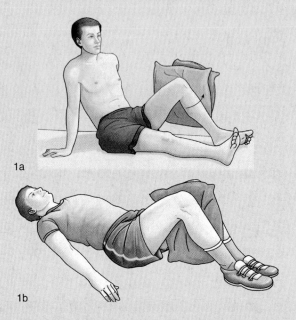

1a

1b

2. Hip AROM
AROM exercises for the hip include seated hip flexion (2a), seated internal rotation (2b), seated external rotation (2c), and heel slides (2d).

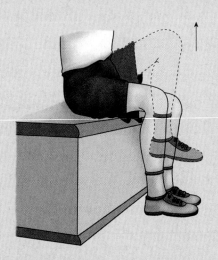

2a

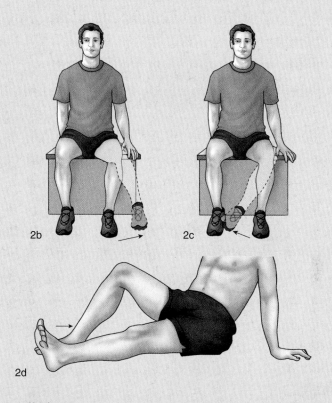

2b   2c

2d

3. SLR in all planes

The SLR can be performed into abduction (3a), adduction (3b), flexion (3c), and extension (3d).

🔵 **Clinical Pearl**

Care must be taken when exercising into hip extension to avoid over-stressing the lumbosacral spine.

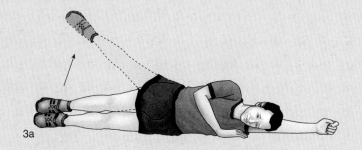

3a

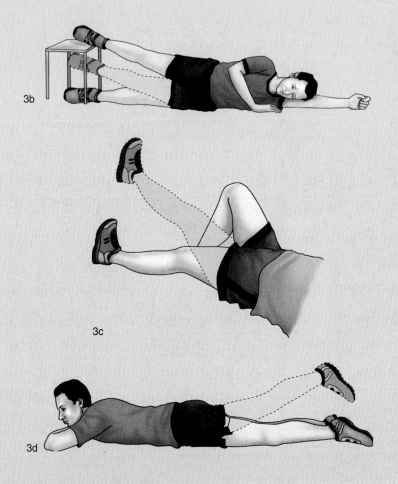

3b

3c

3d

4. Double knees to chest

The patient is positioned in supine and is asked to draw one knee at a time to the chest. When both knees are to the chest (4), the patient holds the position for 10 seconds.

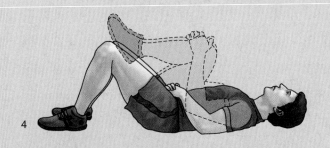

4

5. Chair lunge

The patient stands in front of a chair or high box. Placing one foot on the chair/box, the patient bends forward so that flexion is increased at the hip (5).

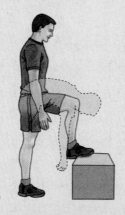

5

6. Wall slide

The patient stands with his/her back against a wall. While maintaining full contact with the back against the wall, the patient slowly bends the legs at the knees into a partial squat (6) and holds the position for 10 seconds.

 Clinical Pearl

Arm motions such as alternating or bilateral shoulder flexion/extension can be superimposed on to the wall slide exercise.

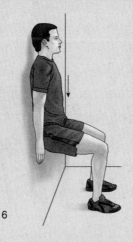

6

7. Single leg standing

The patient attempts to stand on one leg and to hold the position for 30 seconds. The exercises can be made more challenging by altering the standing surface (7).

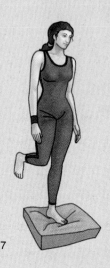

7

8. Standing SLR in all planes

The patient is positioned in standing. The SLR exercise can be performed into hip abduction (8a), hip adduction (8b), hip extension (8c), and hip flexion (8d).

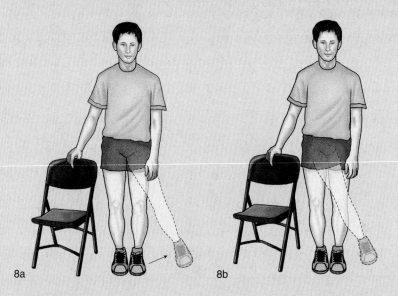

8a   8b

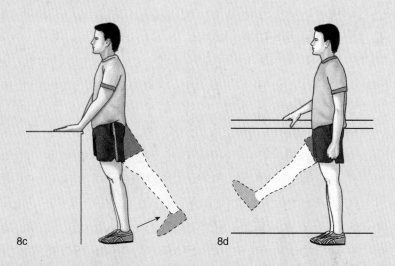

8c   8d

9. Step-ups

Step-ups can be performed in a forward/backward direction (9a), and in a sideways direction (9b).

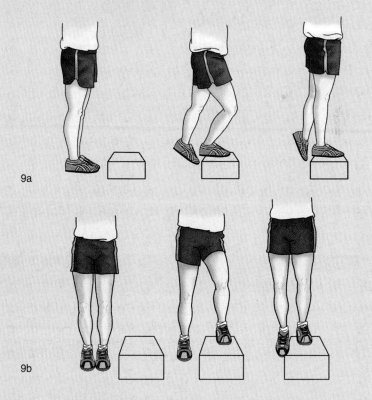

9a

9b

10. Backward lunge

The patient is positioned in standing and is asked to take a step back with one leg while slowly flexing the standing leg (10).

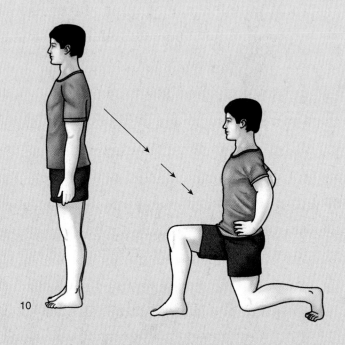

11. Steamboats

Elastic tubing is attached to both of the patient's ankles, or to a stable structure. The patient is positioned in standing—holding onto something for balance if necessary. The patient is asked to move the hip into hip extension (11a), abduction (11b), adduction (11c), and then flexion (11d) using a variety of speeds. The exercise can be made more challenging by altering the standing surface.

● Clinical Pearl

The steamboat exercise can also be performed into diagonals or can be used to focus on the gluteus medius by asking the patient to move the hip into abduction, external rotation, and extension.

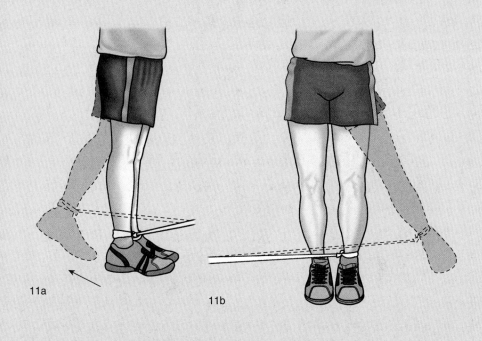

11a

11b

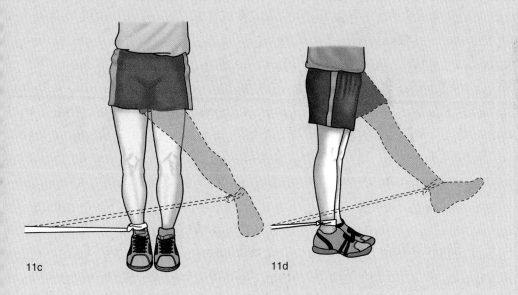

11c

11d

12. Swissball series

A variety of Swissball exercises can be used to challenge the hip muscles (12a and 12b).

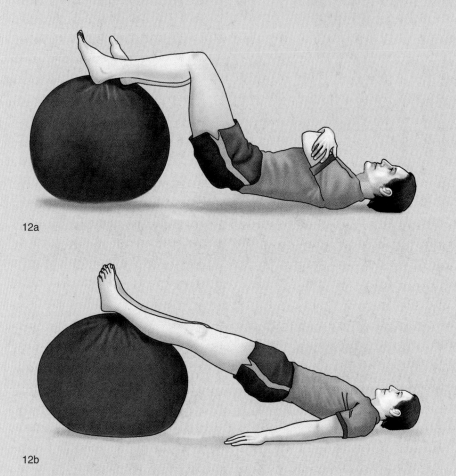

12a

12b

REFERENCES

1. Crowninshield RD, Johnston RC, Andrews JG, et al. A biomechanical investigation of the human hip. *J Biomech*. 1978;11:75–85.
2. Echternach JL. Evaluation of the hip, in Echternach JL, ed. *Physical Therapy of the Hip*. New York: Churchill Livingstone; 1990:17–32.
3. Cyriax J. *Textbook of Orthopaedic Medicine, Diagnosis of Soft Tissue Lesions*. 8th ed.. London: Bailliere Tindall; 1982.

4. Jull GA, Janda V. Muscle and motor control in low back pain. In: Twomey LT, Taylor JR, eds. *Physical Therapy of the Low Back: Clinics in Physical Therapy.* New York: Churchill Livingstone; 1987: 258.

5. Inman VT, Ralston HJ, Todd F. *Human Walking.* Baltimore: Williams & Wilkins; 1981.

6. Lehmkuhl LD, Smith LK. *Brunnstrom's Clinical Kinesiology.* Philadelphia: F.A. Davis; 1983.

7. Yoder E. Physical therapy management of nonsurgical hip problems in adults. In: Echternach JL, ed. *Physical Therapy of the Hip.* New York: Churchill Livingstone; 1990:103–137.

8. Mattingly GE, Mackarey PJ. Optimal methods for shoulder tendon palpation: a cadaver study. *Phys Ther.* 1996;76:166–174.

9. Fagerson TL. Hip. In: Wadsworth C, ed. *Current Concepts of Orthopedic Physical Therapy - Home Study Course.* La Crosse, WI: Orthopaedic Section, APTA; 2001.

10. Hoppenfeld S. Physical examination of the hip and pelvis. In: *Physical Examination of the Spine and Extremities.* East Norwalk, CT: Appleton-Century-Crofts; 1976:143.

11. McKenzie R, May S. History. In: McKenzie R, May S, eds. *The Human Extremities: Mechanical Diagnosis and Therapy.* Waikanae, New Zealand: Spinal Publications New Zealand Ltd; 2000:89–103.

12. Janda V. *Muscle Function Testing.* London: Butterworths; 1983.

13. Hall SJ. The biomechanics of the human lower extremity. In: *Basic Biomechanics.* 3rd ed.. New York: McGraw-Hill; 1999:234–281.

14. Johnston RC. Mechanical considerations of the hip joint. *Arch Surg.* 1973;107:411.

15. Maitland GD. *The Peripheral Joints: Examination and Recording Guide.* Adelaide, Australia: Virgo Press; 1973.

16. Verrall GM, Slavotinek JP, Barnes PG, et al. Description of pain provocation tests used for the diagnosis of sports-related chronic groin pain: relationship of tests to defined clinical (pain and tenderness) and MRI (pubic bone marrow oedema) criteria. *Scand J Med Sci Sports.* 2005;15:36–42.

17. Holmich P.: Adductor related groin pain in athletes. *Sports Med Arth Rev.* 1998;5:285–291.

18. Gelberman RH, Cohen MS, Hekhar S, et al. Femoral anteversion. *J Bone Joint Surg.* 1987;69B:75.

19. Pizzutillo PT, MacEwen GD, Shands AR. Anteversion of the femur. In: Tonzo RG, ed. *Surgery of the Hip Joint.* New York: Springer-Verlag; 1984.

20. Reikeras O, Bjerkreim I, Kolbenstvedt A. Anteversion of the acetabulum and femoral neck in normals and in patients with osteoarthritis of the hip. *Acta Orthop Scandinavica.* 1983;54:18–23.

21. Ruwe PA, Gage JR, Ozonoff MB, et al. Clinical determination of femoral anteversion: a comparison with established techniques. *J Bone and Joint Surg.* 1992;74:820.

22. Woods D, Macnicol M. The flexion-adduction test: an early sign of hip disease. *J Pediatr Orthop.* 2001;10:180–185.

23. Zimney NJ. Clinical reasoning in the evaluation and management of undiagnosed chronic hip pain in young adult. *Phys Ther.* 1998;78:62–73.

24. Johnson AW, Weiss CB, Wheeler DL. Stress fractures of the femoral shaft in athletes - more common than expected: a new clinical test. *Am J Sports Med.* 1994;22:248–256.

25. Adams SL, Yarnold PR. Clinical use of the patellar-pubic percussion sign in hip trauma. *Am J Emerg Med.* 1997;15:173–175.

26. Peltier LF. The diagnosis of fractures of the hip and femur by auscultatory percussion. *Clin Orthop Relat Res.* 1977;123:9–11.

27. Gurney B, Boissonnault WG, Andrews R. Differential diagnosis of a femoral neck/head stress fracture. *J Orthop Sports Phys Ther.* 2006;36:80–88.

28. Tiru M, Goh SH, Low BY. Use of percussion as a screening tool in the diagnosis of occult hip fractures. *Singapore Med J.* 2002;43:467–469.

29. Harvey D. Assessment of the flexibility of elite athletes using the modified Thomas test. *Br J Sports Med.* 1998;32:68–70.

30. Grelsamer RP, McConnell J. *The Patella: A Team Approach.* Gaithersburg, Maryland: Aspen; 1998.

31. Melchione WE, Sullivan MS. Reliability of measurements obtained by the use of an instrument designed to indirectly measure ilio-tibial band length. *J Orthop Sports Phys Ther.* 1993;18:511–515.

32. Lehman WL Jr. Overuse syndromes in runners. *Am Fam Phys.* 1984;29:152–161.

33. Noble HB, Hajek MR, Porter M. Diagnosis and treatment of iliotibial band tightness in runners. *Phys Sports Med.* 1982;10:67–74.

34. Krabak BJ, Jarmain SJ, Prather H. Physical examination of the hip. In: Malanga GA, Nadler SF, eds. *Musculoskeletal Physical Examination—An Evidence-based Approach.* Philadelphia: Elsevier-Mosby; 2006:251–278.

35. Aronsson DD, Goldberg MJ, Kling TF, et al. Developmental dysplasia of the hip. *Pediatrics.* 1994;94:201–208.

36. Kneeland JB. MR imaging of sports injuries of the hip. *Magn Reson Imaging Clin N Am.* 1999;7:105–115.

37. Guide to physical therapist practice. *Phys Ther.* 2001;81:S13–S95.

QUESTIONS

1. Name the three bones that together create the articular surface of the hip joint.

2. What is the angle of inclination of the femur?

3. What is Ober's test?

4. How much force is unloaded from the hip when a cane is used in the opposite hand?

5. Which nerve is involved in meralgia paresthetica?

6. What is a hip pointer?

7. What is one of the more serious complications of a quadriceps contusion?

8. What is piriformis syndrome?
9. What is a Malgaigne fracture?
10. Name three complications that are associated with hip dislocation.
11. Which bursa can become inflamed by running on pronated feet?
12. What is avascular necrosis of the femoral head called when it occurs in 6 to 10 year old males?
13. Pain in the inguinal area with all directions of passive range of motion (with the exception of internal rotation) of the hip especially flexion and adduction, and negative resistive testing, could indicate which condition?
14. Give three potential causes for a Trendelenburg gait.
15. Palpating from superior to inferior on the posterior aspect of the greater trochanter, what are the eight muscle attachments that would be located?
16. With a slipped epiphysis, which of the hip rotations is increased?
17. To increase hip flexion ROM using a Hold-Relax technique, which muscle group would you resist?

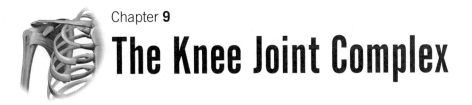

Chapter **9**

The Knee Joint Complex

OVERVIEW

The knee joint complex includes three articulating surfaces, which form two distinct joints contained within a single joint capsule: the patellofemoral and tibiofemoral joint.[1,2] One of the problems facing the knee joint complex is the fact that it was not originally designed for bipedal motion.[3] Evolutionary modifications have allowed the knee to adapt to the major changes placed on it during functional demands.[2] Despite these adaptations, however, the knee is one of the most commonly injured joints in the body.

 Clinical Pearl

Despite its proximity to the tibiofemoral joint, the patellofemoral joint can be considered as its own entity, in much the same way as the craniovertebral joints are when compared to the rest of the cervical spine.

ANATOMY

Tibiofemoral Joint

The tibiofemoral joint is a ginglymoid, or modified hinge joint, which has six degrees of freedom. The bony configuration of the knee joint complex is geometrically incongruous and lends little inherent stability to the joint.

 Clinical Pearl

Joint stability of the knee is dependent upon the static restraints of the joint capsule, ligaments, and menisci, and the dynamic restraints of the quadriceps, hamstrings, and gastrocnemius.[4,5]

Clinical Pearl

The two central intra-articular cruciate ligaments cross each other forming an x-pattern. Both the ACL and PCL lie in the center of the joint, and each are named according to their attachment sites on the tibia.[6] These two ligaments, composed mainly of type I collagen, are the main stabilizing ligaments of the knee and restrain against anterior (ACL) and posterior (PCL) translations of the tibia on the femur. They also restrain against excessive internal and external rotation and varus movement of the tibia.[7]

Patellofemoral Joint

The patellofemoral joint is composed of the articulation of the patella with the femoral condyles of the femur. The patella is a passive component of the knee extensor mechanism, where the static and dynamic relationships of the underlying tibia and femur determine the patellar-tracking pattern.

 Clinical Pearl

To assist in the control of the forces around the patellofemoral joint, there are a number of static and dynamic restraints.

EXAMINATION

The examination of the knee joint complex should include a thorough and detailed history, a careful inspection and palpation of the knee for point tenderness, assessment of joint effusion, range-of-motion and strength testing, an evaluation of the ligaments for injury or laxity, an assessment of patella motion, and assessment of the integrity of the menisci. Accurate diagnosis requires knowledge of knee anatomy, common pain patterns in knee injuries, frequently encountered causes of knee pain, as well as specific physical examination skills.[3]

 Clinical Pearl

Broadly speaking, acute knee injuries fall into one of six categories: (1) contusions, (2) fractures or physeal injuries, (3) ligamentous injuries, (4) meniscal tears, (5) musculotendinous strains, and (6) extensor mechanism injuries, patellar subluxation or dislocation.[8]

History

The complete history should include information about how and when the injury occurred (onset), how the patient characterizes the symptoms, and whether the patient has had any previous knee disorders.[9]

 Clinical Pearl

Patients with knee problems often report pain, instability, stiffness, swelling, locking, or weakness.

In addition, the clinician should ask questions about:

- The location (anterior, medial, lateral, or posterior knee) (Table 9-1) (Figure 9-1 to 9-4), quality (e.g., dull, sharp, achy), severity, and duration of the patient's symptoms.
- The presence or absence of mechanical symptoms (locking, popping, giving way), and joint effusion (timing, amount, recurrence).
  - A history of locking episodes suggests a meniscal tear.
  - A sensation of popping at the time of injury suggests ligamentous injury, probably a complete rupture of a ligament (third-degree tear) (Table 9-2).
  - Episodes of giving way are consistent with some degree of knee instability and may indicate patellar subluxation or ligamentous rupture.
- The degree of dysfunction and disability.[10]
- Previous episodes and interventions for their knee pain, including the use of medications, supporting devices, and physical therapy.

 Clinical Pearl

The anterior cruciate ligament (ACL) and the medial collateral ligament (MCL) are the most commonly injured knee ligaments. The lateral collateral ligament (LCL) and the posterior cruciate ligament (PCL) are rarely injured.

Table 9-1 Differential Diagnosis of Knee Pain by Anatomic Site

Anterior Knee Pain	Medial Knee Pain	Lateral Knee Pain	Posterior Knee Pain
Patellar subluxation or dislocation	Medial collateral ligament sprain	Lateral collateral ligament sprain	Popliteal cyst (Baker's cyst)
Tibial apophysitis (Osgood–Schlatter lesion)	Medial meniscal tear	Lateral meniscal tear	Posterior cruciate ligament injury
Jumper's knee (patellar tendonitis)	Pes anserine bursitis	Iliotibial band tendonitis	Gastrocnemius muscle strain or rupture
Patellofemoral pain syndrome (chondromalacia patellae)	Medial plica syndrome	Popliteus tenosynovitis	Plantaris muscle strain or rupture
	Saphenous nerve neuritis (a burning quality)	Popliteus tendon rupture	Hamstring muscle/ tendon disorder
Tears of the menisci	Hoffa's disease.	Tibiofibular disorder	
Medial synovial plica syndrome	Semimembranosus tendonitis	Biceps femoris tendonitis	
Inflammatory or degenerative arthritis		Osteochondral fracture of the lateral femoral condyle	
Tumors of the joint			
Ligament injuries that mimic patellar instability			
Osteochondritis dissecans of the medial femoral condyle			
Prepatellar bursitis			
Inflammation of the patellar fat pad			
Sindig–Larsen– Johansson syndrome			

The patient's age and gender can provide some initial clues (Table 9-3).

 Clinical Pearl

Conditions that can cause chronic knee pain include arthritis, sepsis, overuse syndromes, and tumors.

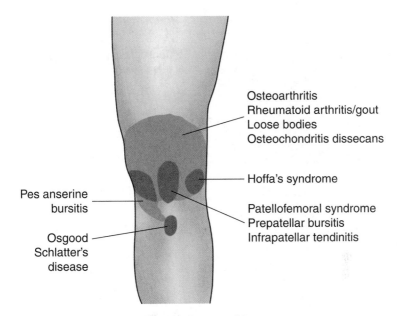

Osteoarthritis
Rheumatoid arthritis/gout
Loose bodies
Osteochondritis dissecans

Hoffa's syndrome

Pes anserine
bursitis

Patellofemoral syndrome
Prepatellar bursitis
Infrapatellar tendinitis

Osgood
Schlatter's
disease

Figure 9-1 Anterior knee pain and the possible causes.

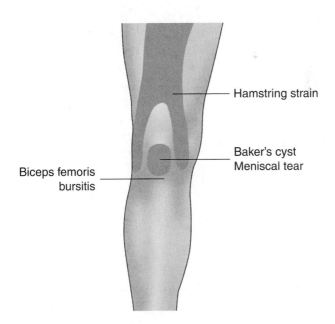

Hamstring strain

Baker's cyst
Meniscal tear

Biceps femoris
bursitis

Figure 9-2 Posterior knee pain and the possible causes.

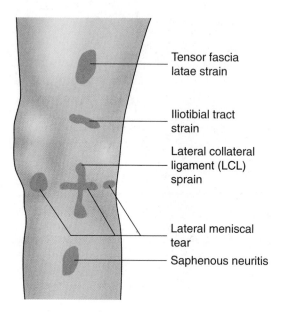

Figure 9-3 Lateral knee pain and the possible causes.

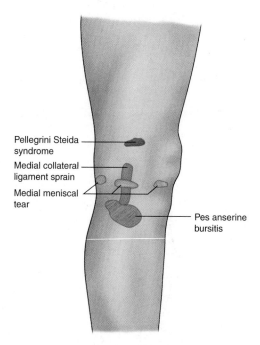

Figure 9-4 Medial knee pain and the possible causes.

Table 9-2 Common Ligamentous and Meniscal Injuries

Structure	Mechanism of Injury	Subjective Complaints
MCL	Most commonly involves external valgus or rotational force while leg is firmly planted. Often associated with ACL injury	Localized swelling and tenderness over injured area
ACL	Commonly involves noncontact pivoting/twisting mechanism while foot is planted; noncontact hyperextension; sudden deceleration; forced internal rotation; sudden valgus impact	Reports of being unable to continue activity; hearing "pop" in the knee; extreme pain at time of injury; acute knee swelling (within 1–2 hours of injury)
Meniscus	Usually caused by noncontact injury; rotational/torsional force applied to flexed knee with foot firmly planted	Reports of swelling developing within 12 hours of injury; localized swelling and tenderness over injured area. History of popping, clicking, or locking with knee motions

Information about the patient's activity level can provide the clinician with useful clues. For example, active patients are more likely to have acute ligamentous sprains and overuse injuries such as pes anserine bursitis and medial plica syndrome. Patients with overuse injuries often describe a precipitating event and gradual onset of symptoms.

Table 9-3 Common Causes of Knee Pain by Age Group and Gender

Children and Adolescents	Young Adults (20–45 years)	Older Adults (50+ years)
Females: patellar tracking problems such as patellar subluxation and patellofemoral pain syndrome Males: tibial apophysitis (Osgood–Schlatter lesion) and patellar tendonitis. Both: Jumper's knee (patellar tendonitis) Referred pain: slipped capital femoral epiphysis, others Osteochondritis dissecans	Patellofemoral pain syndrome (chondromalacia patellae) Medial plica syndrome Pes anserine bursitis Trauma: ligamentous sprains (anterior cruciate, medial collateral, lateral collateral), meniscal tear Inflammatory arthropathy: rheumatoid arthritis, Reiter's syndrome Septic arthritis	Osteoarthritis Crystal-induced inflammatory arthropathy: gout, pseudogout Popliteal cyst (Baker's cyst)

Clinical Pearl

Overuse injuries can be caused by both extrinsic factors such as poor training techniques or inadequate footwear, and intrinsic factors such as poor flexibility or structural abnormalities.[10]

Aggravating and alleviating factors, drugs or interventions used, and the injury's relationship to a specific activity also need to be identified.[11]

 Clinical Pearl

The timing and amount of joint effusion are important clues to the diagnosis:

• Rapid onset (within 2 hours) of a large, tense effusion suggests rupture of the anterior cruciate ligament or fracture of the tibial plateau with resultant hemarthrosis.

• Slower onset (24–36 hours) of a mild to moderate effusion is consistent with meniscal injury or ligamentous sprain.

• Recurrent knee effusion after activity is consistent with meniscal injury.

The position of the joint at the time of the traumatic force dictates which anatomic structures are at risk for injury; hence, an important aspect of obtaining the patient's history for acute injuries is to allow him/her to describe the position of the knee and direction of forces at the time it was injured.[12] Twisting injuries are somewhat less specific in terms of determining the injured structure as they can be associated with anterior cruciate ligament tears, meniscal tears, or patellar subluxation or dislocation.[8]

 Clinical Pearl

The primary stabilizers of the knee joint complex are the ACL, which is responsible for restricting anterior translation of the tibia; the PCL, which is responsible for restricting posterior translation of the tibia; the MCL, which restricts medial translation (valgus stress); and the LCL, which restricts lateral translation (varus stress).

Pain that is not alleviated with rest could indicate a nonmechanical source of pain, or a chemically induced source such as an inflammatory reaction. A hot and swollen joint without a history of trauma should provoke suspicions about hemophilia, rheumatoid arthritis, an infection, or gout.

 Clinical Pearl

Septic arthritis may develop in patients of any age, but crystal-induced inflammatory arthropathy is more likely in adults.

Systems Review

Knee pain can be referred to the knee from

- The lumbosacral region (L3 to S2 segments)
- The hip (hip joint pathology, such as slipped capital femoral epiphysis)
- The peripheral nerves of the lumbosacral plexus

 Clinical Pearl

Pain that is constant and burning in nature should alert the clinician to the possibility of reflex sympathetic dystrophy, gout, or radicular pain. Intermittent pain usually indicates a mechanical problem (meniscus).

Tests and Measures

Observation

The patient should be observed while he or she walks, stands, sits, and in nonweight bearing.[10] When possible the clinician should compare the involved knee with the asymptomatic knee. The clinician should observe the knees in standing in both the coronal (bowlegs, genu varum; knock knees, genu valgum) and sagittal planes (flexion or hyperextension, genu recurvatum). Normally, when a patient stands with their feet together, the medial aspects of both knees and ankles are also in contact.[8] With the patient standing, the clinician observes whether the pelvis is level, the knees symmetrical and the leg lengths equal.[13] The position of the patellar should be noted.

Clinical Pearl

When viewing the patellar, the clinician should note whether the patellar points straight ahead, tilts inward, outward, or is rotated in any way. Rotation and tilt may be caused by adaptively shortened structures in the lower extremities that alter the position of the patellar.

 Clinical Pearl

Knees with more than 15 degrees of misalignment in any plane (varus, valgus, recurvatum) do not do well if subject to ligamentous disruption.[14]

In addition, assessing the hip and ankle joints is important as problems in these joints can exacerbate knee injuries or cause referred knee pain:

- Increased anteversion (internal rotation) of the femur often occurs in combination with external torsion (external rotation) of the tibia.[8] This pattern of misalignment predisposes the patient to patellofemoral problems.
- Pronation of the foot or pes planus (flatfoot) can cause internal rotation of the femur, which also predisposes the patient to patellofemoral joint dysfunction.

The injured knee should be inspected for bruising, abrasions, surgical scars, erythema, discoloration, and swelling. The presence of bruising, swelling, or erythema is an important piece of information regarding the nature and severity of the injury.[3] Swelling in the knee may be suggested by the loss of the peri-patellar groove on either side of the patella.

The musculature above and below the knee should be symmetric bilaterally. In particular, the vastus medialis obliquus of the quadriceps should be evaluated to determine if it appears normal or shows signs of atrophy. Thigh atrophy can have significant detrimental effects on both patellar tracking and knee performance.[8] A well-defined gastrocnemius is usually indicative of an active lifestyle.[14]

During gait, the clinician should observe for antalgia, step length, pelvic tilt, and cadence.[3]

 Clinical Pearl

The major motion at the knee during the gait cycle occurs in the sagittal plane, including an arc of motion from full extension to approximately 60 degrees of flexion, and is characterized by two flexion waves.[2] The stance phase knee flexion wave peaks early in stance, which allows the quadriceps muscle to function as a shock absorber, whereas the swing phase knee flexion wave facilitates foot clearance and limb advancement.[2]

 Clinical Pearl

In the normal gait cycle, the knee comes to full extension only at heel strike. During stance phase, slight flexion occurs, and it is the contraction of the quadriceps at this point that prevents giving way. At toe-off, the knee flexes to about 40 degrees and continues to flex through mid-swing to approximately 65 degrees. At this point, the quadriceps contract to begin acceleration of the leg, with the knee returning to full extension once again at heel strike. At heel strike, the hamstrings must contract in order to decelerate the leg.

 Clinical Pearl

Swelling above the patella is most likely a joint effusion; below the patella, prepatellar bursitis; and behind the knee, a popliteal cyst.[2] Generalized swelling may be due to an effusion in the joint. With the patient supine, large knee effusions fill in the normal recesses on either side of the patella.[8] This can be confirmed using the *ballottement sign*.

Palpation

The knee is palpated and assessed for pain, warmth, and effusion employing a logical sequence and compared with the uninjured side (Table 9-4).

 Clinical Pearl

A detailed knowledge of the bony and soft tissue surface anatomy is of critical importance when trying to make a specific diagnosis in the knee.

Table 9-4 Palpation Points About the Knee

Area	Structure to Palpate
Medial knee	Medial tibial plateau
	Tibial tubercle
	Medial femoral condyle
	Medial femoral epicondyle
	Adductor tubercle
	Medial collateral ligament
	Tendons of the sartorius, gracilis, and the semitendinosus muscles
	Pes anserine bursa
Lateral knee	Lateral tibial plateau
	Lateral (Gerdy's) tubercle
	Lateral femoral condyle
	Lateral femoral epicondyle
	Head of the fibular
	Lateral meniscus
	Lateral collateral ligament
	Iliotibial band
	Common fibular nerve
Anterior knee	Patella
	Trochlear groove
	Prepatellar bursa
	Quadriceps
	Patella tendon/tibial tubercle
	Infrapatellar bursae (superficial and deep)
Posterior knee	Hamstring tendons
	Two heads of the gastrocnemius muscle
	Popliteal pulse
	Posterior tibial nerve

The results from the palpation exam should be correlated with other findings. The knee can be positioned in 30 degrees of flexion or 90 degrees of flexion. The former position allows the cruciate ligaments to be relaxed and allows for better palpation of the anterior half of the menisci.[14] The latter position brings the menisci more anteriorly, and the collateral ligaments more posteriorly and allows the femoral condyle to be more easily palpated.[14]

Clinical Pearl

The presence of an increase in temperature of the skin overlying the knee joint should be determined before the other tests are performed.

Point tenderness should be sought, particularly at the patella (all four poles), tibial tubercle, anterolateral (Figure 9-5), and anteromedial (Figure 9-6) joint line, medial joint line, and lateral joint line. Specific structures to be palpated include the quadriceps muscle, patella, patella tendon, iliotibial band, lateral collateral ligament, medial collateral ligament, medial hamstrings, lateral hamstrings, and the pes anserinus. Tenderness and/or differences in temperature between these structures when compared to the uninvolved knee suggest inflammation. The popliteal fossa, through which the principal neurovascular structures of the knee (popliteal artery and vein, tibial nerve, common fibular nerve) pass, should also be palpated.

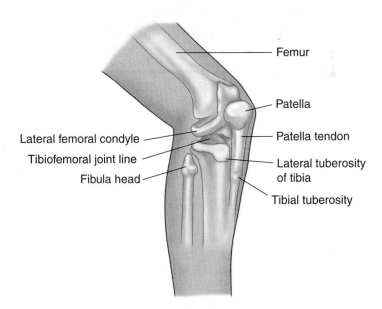

Figure 9-5 Palpable structures on the anterolateral aspect of the knee.

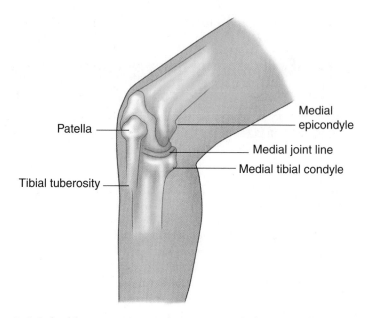

Figure 9-6 Palpable structures on the anteromedial aspect of the knee.

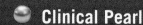

Clinical Pearl

Quadriceps tendonitis or rupture causes tenderness at the superior pole of the patella, whereas patellar tendonitis (jumper's knee) or rupture creates tenderness at the inferior pole.

Active Range of Motion With Passive Over Pressure

Range of motion testing for the tibiofemoral joint should include assessment of knee flexion and extension, tibial internal, and external rotation. Normal knee motion (Figure 9-7)(Table 9-5) has been described as 0 degree of extension to 140 degrees of flexion, although hyperextension (5 degrees –10 degrees) is frequently present to varying degrees.[15] The range of motion testing can often be diagnostic and provides the clinician with some clues as to the cause of the problem (Figure 9-8). It is important to examine the uninvolved knee first to allay any patient fears and to determine what the normal range of motion is. In addition, observation of the uninvolved knee can afford the clinician information about the patellofemoral joint and the tracking of the patella.[3]

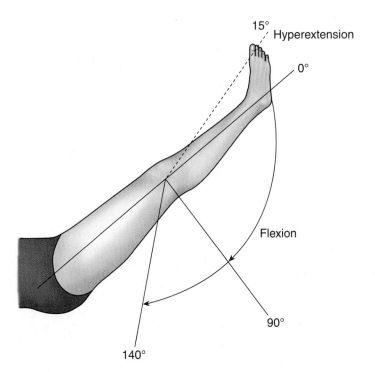

Figure 9-7 Normal knee motion.

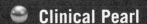

Clinical Pearl

Common causes for decrease in range of motion of the knee include:
- Effusion within the knee joint
- Meniscal tear
- Loose body within the joint
- Osteoarthritic changes

Patella Motion Tests

Probably the most important part of the patellofemoral examination is the observation of the dynamics of patellar tracking in weight bearing and non-weight bearing. The patella does not follow a straight path as the knee moves, but instead follows a curved path.

Table 9-5 Normal Ranges and End-feels at the Knee

Motion	Range of Motion (Degrees)	End-feel
Flexion	0–140	Tissue approximation or tissue stretch
Extension	0–15	Tissue stretch
External rotation of the tibia on the femur	30–40	Tissue stretch
Internal rotation of the tibia on the femur	20–30	Tissue stretch

 Clinical Pearl

Excessive lateral tracking of the patella as the patient nears full extension ('J' sign) is a common finding with patellofemoral dysfunction.[8] The clinician should also observe for signs of quadriceps lag, which results from weakness of the quadriceps muscle, causing the patient to have difficulty in completing the last 10 degrees to 15 degrees of knee extension.

The various contact areas of the patella are engaged at different parts of the range of motion (Table 9-6). Pain elicited in some but not all of the range provides the clinician with valuable information about the diagnosis and the ranges to avoid during the intervention.

Ankle Motions
Ankle motions are tested because a number of structures share a common relationship with the foot and ankle and the knee joint complex.

Hip Motions
A number of muscles cross both the hip and the knee. These include the rectus femoris, the gracilis, the sartorius, and the hamstrings. Adaptive shortening of any of these structures may cause alterations in postural mechanics and gait. The hip rotators can also influence other aspects of the lower kinetic chain.

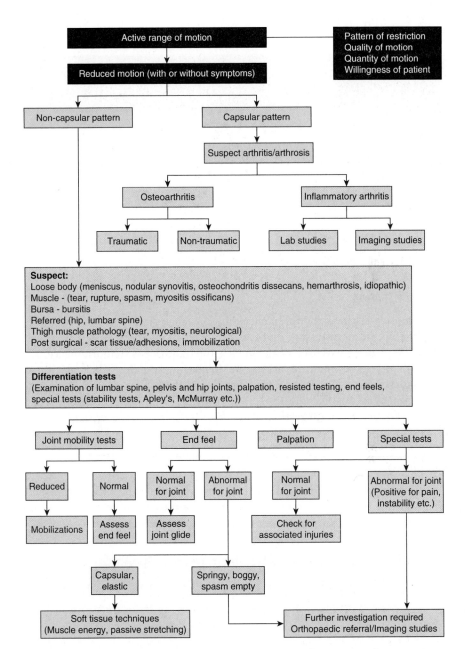

Figure 9-8 Examination sequence in the presence of symptom-free or incomplete active range of motion at the knee.

Table 9-6 Patella Contact During Ranges

Knee Range of Flexion (Degrees)	Facet Contact
0	No contact
15–20	Inferior pole
45	Middle pole
90	All facets
Full flexion (140)	Odd facet and lateral aspect

Strength Testing

Gross muscle testing is useful in checking for deficits in the lower extremities (Table 9-7). Strength testing involves the performance of resisted isometric tests. The primary extensor of the knee is the quadriceps (femoral nerve, L2, L3, L4), and the primary flexors are the hamstring muscles (tibial portion of the sciatic nerve, L5, S1). For each of the tests, the joint is placed as close to its open packed position (Table 9-8) as possible to minimize any joint compression forces. Strength testing of the hip, foot, and ankle muscles should also be included.

Functional Tests

Functional outcome following knee injury must consider the patient's perspective, and not just objective measurements of instability. Functional motion requirements of the knee vary according to the specific task.

 Clinical Pearl

In normal level ground walking, 60 degrees to 70 degrees of knee flexion is required. This requirement increases to 80 degrees to 85 degrees with stair climbing, and to 120 degrees to 140 degrees for running.[16] Approximately 120 degrees of knee flexion is necessary for activities such as squatting to tie a shoelace or to don a sock.[17]

Table 9-7 Muscles of the Knee: Their Actions, Nerve Supply, and Nerve Root Derivation

Action	Muscles Acting	Nerve Supply	Nerve Root Derivation
Flexion of knee	Biceps femoris	Sciatic	L5, S1–S2
	Semimembranosus	Sciatic	L5, S2–S2
	Semitendinosus	Sciatic	L5, S1–S2
	Gracilis	Obturator	L2–L3
	Sartorius	Femoral	L2–L3
	Popliteus	Tibial	L4–L5, S1
	Gastrocnemius	Tibial	S1–S2
	Tensor fascia latae	Superior gluteal	L4–L5
Extension of knee	Rectus femoris	Femoral	L2–L4
	Vastus medialis	Femoral	L2–L4
	Vastus intermedius	Femoral	L2–L4
	Vastus lateralis	Femoral	L2–L4
	Tensor fascia latae	Superior gluteal	L4–L5
Internal rotation of flexed leg (nonweight bearing)	Popliteus	Tibial	L4–L5
	Semimembranosus	Sciatic	L5, S1–S2
	Semitendinosus	Sciatic	L5, S1–S2
	Sartorius	Femoral	L2–L3
	Gracilis	Obturator	L2–L3
External rotation of flexed leg (nonweight bearing)	Biceps femoris	Sciatic	L5, S1–S2

Special Tests

Special tests for the knee joint complex are dependent on the clinician's needs, the structure of each joint and the subjective complaints (Table 9-9). These tests are only performed if there is some indication that they would be helpful in arriving at a diagnosis. The special tests help confirm or implicate a particular structure and may also provide information as to the degree of tissue damage (Table 9-10).

Stress Testing

The stress tests are used to determine the integrity of the joint, ligaments and the menisci. The goal of the stress tests is to identify the degree of separation

Table 9-8 Close and Open Packed Positions of the Knee Joints

Joint	Close Pack Position	Open Pack Position
Tibiofemoral	Full extension, lateral rotation of the tibia	25 degrees of flexion
Patellofemoral	Full flexion	<20 degrees of flexion

and the quality, or end-feel of the separation. Intact ligaments have an abrupt and firm end-feel, whereas sprained ligaments have a soft or indistinct end-feel depending on the degree of injury. A comparison should always be made with the uninvolved knee before a determination is made. It is important to remember that both pain and swelling can hamper the sensitivity of these tests.[10] Serious functional instability of the knee appears to occur unpredictably. The reasons for such discrepancies are unknown, but they may be due to[5]

• Varying definitions of instability
• Varying degrees of damage of the ACL[18,19]
• Different combinations of injuries[20]
• Different mechanisms of compensation for the loss of the ACL
• Differences in rehabilitation
• The diverse physical demands and expectations of different populations

Medial stability

Valgus Stress
The clinician applies a strong valgus force, with a counter force applied at the lateral femoral condyle (Figure 9-9). Normally, there is little or no valgus movement in the knee, and, if present, should be less than the amount of varus motion. Under normal conditions, the end-feel is firm. With degeneration of the medial or lateral compartments varus and valgus motions may be increased, while the end-feels will be normal.

With the knee tested in full extension, any demonstrable instability is usually very significant. Pain with this maneuver is caused by an increase in tension of the medial collateral structures, or the connection of these structures with the medial meniscus. If pain or an excessive amount of motion is detected compared with the other extremity, a hypermobility or instability should be suspected. The following structures may be implicated:

• Superficial and deep fibers of the MCL
• Posterior oblique ligament

Table 9-9 Subjective Complaint, Potential Diagnosis, and Confirmatory Test

Subjective Complaint	Potential Diagnosis	Confirmatory Test (s)
My knee hurts when I get up from a chair or go up steps	Patellofemoral dysfunction	Patellofemoral grind test
My knee gives out when I step down from the curb	Subluxation/dislocation of the patella	Patella apprehension test
My knee locks	Medial meniscus tear Loose body within the knee joint	McMurray test and Apley grinding and distraction tests
My knee feels swollen and tight	Fluid within the knee	Patellar effusion tests
My knee buckles; it gives out	Unstable knee joint (torn collateral or cruciate ligament) Medial meniscus tear Lumbar disc herniation	Valgus and varus stress tests, anterior drawer, Lachman, Posterior sag, meniscus tests, neurologic screen (DTR, strength, and sensation testing)
I cannot straighten my knee out	Fluid in the knee Torn meniscus	Meniscus tests, patellar ballottement test, bounce home test
I have pain on the inside of my leg	Torn medial collateral ligament Bursitis, pes anserinus bursa	Valgus stress test Palpation of the pes anserinus bursa
I made a quick turn wile playing sports while my foot was planted, and my leg suddenly collapsed and the knee became swollen	Medial meniscus tear	Apley test and McMurray test
I have swelling in the back of my knee	Popliteal cyst	Palpation of popliteal fossa
I landed heavily on the front of my knee and it hurts	Patellar fracture Chondromalacia Fat pad syndrome Prepatellar bursitis Infrapatellar bursitis	Radiograph Palpation
I cannot move my knee in any direction without pain	Infected knee joint	Joint aspiration

Table 9-10 Common Special Tests of the Tibiofemoral Join

Structure Assessed	Test	Reliability/Validity Studies	Comments
Medial collateral ligament (MCL)	Valgus stress	Study 1:[1] sensitivity—86%	Specificity not reported
		Study 2:[2] sensitivity—96%	Retrospective study. Nonstandardized clinical examination was used. Specificity not reported
		Study 3:[3] inter-rater reliability in extension—68%; inter-rater reliability in 30° flexion—56%	Varied physical therapist experience. Standardized examination techniques were not used. Sensitivity or specificity not reported
Lateral collateral ligament (LCL)	Varus stress	Study 1:[1] sensitivity—25%	Only four patients studied. Specificity not reported
Posterior cruciate ligament (PCL)	Posterior drawer	Study 1:[4] sensitivity—90%; specificity—99%	Double-blinded, randomized, controlled study
	Posterior sag sign	Study 1:[4] sensitivity—79%; specificity 100%	Double-blinded, randomized, controlled study
	Quadriceps active	Study 1:[5] sensitivity—98%; specificity—100%	Study was neither blinded nor randomized
		Study 2:[4] sensitivity—54%; specificity 97%	Double-blinded, randomized, controlled study
Anterior cruciate ligament (ACL)	Anterior drawer (A significant hemarthrosis, protective hamstring spasm, or a tear of the posterior horn of the medial meniscus may cause false negatives with this test.[6])	Study 1:[7] sensitivity (acute injuries)—22.2%; sensitivity (chronic injuries)—53.8%; specificity (acute plus chronic)—>97%	Retrospective study. Testing performed only under anesthesia
		Study 2:[1] sensitivity—41%; sensitivity (under anesthesia): 86%	Prospective study
		Study 3:[8] sensitivity (acute injuries)—33%; sensitivity (chronic injuries)—95%	Specificity not assessed
		Study 4:[9] sensitivity (acute injuries)—70%; sensitivity (under anesthesia)—91%	Retrospective study. Specificity not reported
		Study 5:[10] sensitivity (acute injuries)—40%; sensitivity (chronic injuries)—95.2%	Specificity not reported
		Study 6:[11] sensitivity (under anesthesia)—79.6%.	Retrospective study. Testing performed only under anesthesia. Specificity not reported

(continued on following page)

Structure Assessed	Test	Reliability/Validity Studies	Comments
	Lachman (A significant hemarthrosis, protective hamstring spasm, or a tear of the posterior horn of the medial meniscus may cause false negatives with this test.[6])	Study 1:[6] sensitivity—95%.	Specificity not reported
		Study 2:[9] sensitivity—99%	Retrospective study. Specificity not reported
		Study 3:[7] sensitivity (under anesthesia)—84.6%; specificity (under anesthesia)—95%	Retrospective study. Testing performed only under anesthesia
		Study 4:[11] sensitivity (under anesthesia)—98.6%	Retrospective review study. Testing performed only under anesthesia. Specificity not reported
		Study 5:[10] sensitivity (acute injuries)—80%; sensitivity (chronic injuries)—98.8%.	
		Study 6:[8] sensitivity (acute injuries)—87%; sensitivity (chronic injuries)—94%	Specificity not assessed
	Pivot shift	Study 1:[12] sensitivity—95%; specificity—100%	Sample size inadequate to determine specificity
		Study 2:[7] sensitivity—98.4%; specificity—>98%	Retrospective study. Testing performed only under anesthesia
		Study 3:[9] sensitivity—35%; sensitivity (under anesthesia)—98%	Retrospective study. Specificity not reported
Meniscus	McMurray	Study 1:[13] sensitivity—16%; specificity—98%	Prospective study. Interexaminer reliability was only fair
		Study 2:[14] sensitivity—29%; specificity—95%	Prospective study
		Study 3:[15] sensitivity—37%; specificity—77%	Prospective study
		Study 4:[16] sensitivity—58%	Prospective evaluation. Specificity not reported
	Apley grind	Study 1:[14] sensitivity—16%; specificity—80%	Prospective study
		Study 2:[15] sensitivity—13%; specificity—90%	Prospective blinded study

(continued on following page)

Table 9-10 *(continued from previous page)*

Structure Assessed	Test	Reliability/Validity Studies	Comments
	Bounce home	There are no studies in the literature that discuss the sensitivity, specificity, positive predictive value, or negative predictive value of this maneuver	

Data from

1. Harilainen A. Evaluation of knee instability in acute ligamentous injuries. *Ann Chir Gynaecol.* 1987;76:269–273.

2. Garvin GJ, Munk PL, Vellet AD. Tears of the medial collateral ligament: magnetic resonance imaging findings and associated injuries. *Can Assoc Radiol J.* 1993;44:199–204.

3. McClure PW, Rothstein JM, Riddle DL. Intertester reliability of clinical judgments of medial knee ligament integrity. *Phys Ther.* 1989;69:268–275.

4. Rubinstein RA, Jr., Shelbourne KD, McCarroll JR, et al. The accuracy of the clinical examination in the setting of posterior cruciate ligament injuries. *Am J Sports Med.* 1994;22:550–557.

5. Daniel DM, Stone ML, Barnett P, et al. Use of the quadriceps active test to diagnose posterior cruciate-ligament disruption and measure posterior laxity of the knee. *J Bone Joint Surg Am.* 1988;70:386–391.

6. Torg JS, Conrad W, Kalen V. Clinical diagnosis of anterior cruciate ligament instability in the athlete. *Am J Sports Med.* 1976;4:84–93.

7. Katz JW, Fingeroth RJ. The diagnostic accuracy of ruptures of the anterior cruciate ligament comparing the Lachman's test, the anterior drawer sign, and the pivot-shift test in acute and chronic knee injuries. *Am J Sports Med.* 1986;14:88–91.

8. Jonsson T, Althoff B, Peterson L, et al. Clinical diagnosis of ruptures of the anterior cruciate ligament. *Am J Sports Med.* 1982;10:100–102.

9. Donaldson WF, Warren RF, Wickiewicz TL. A comparison of acute anterior cruciate ligament examinations. *Am J Sports Med.* 1985;13:5–10.

10. Mitsou A, Vallianatos P. Clinical diagnosis of ruptures of the anterior cruciate ligament: a comparison between the Lachman test and the anterior drawer sign. *Injury.* 1988;19:427–428.

11. Kim SJ, Kim HK. Reliability of the anterior drawer test, the pivot shift test, and the Lachman test. *Clin Orthop Relat Res.* 1995;317:237–242.

12. Lucie RS, Wiedel JD, Messner DG. The acute pivot shift: clinical correlation. *Am J Sports Med.* 1984;12:189–191.

13. Evans PJ, Bell GD, Frank C. Prospective evaluation of the McMurray test. *Am J Sports Med.* 1993;21:604–608.

14. Fowler PJ, Lubliner JA. The predictive value of five clinical signs in the evaluation of meniscal pathology. *Arthroscopy.* 1989;5:184–186.

15. Kurosaka M, Yagi M, Yoshiya S, et al. Efficacy of the axially loaded pivot shift test for the diagnosis of a meniscal tear. *Int Orthop.* 1999;23:271–274.

16. Anderson AF, Lipscomb AB. Clinical diagnosis of meniscal tears. Description of a new manipulative test. *Am J Sports Med.* 1986;14:291–293.

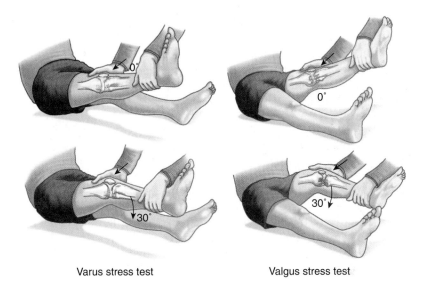

Varus stress test   Valgus stress test

Figure 9-9 Valgus test of the knee.

- Posterior–medial capsule
- Medial capsular ligament
- Anterior cruciate ligament
- Posterior cruciate ligament

The test is then repeated at 30 degrees of flexion (Figure 9-9) to further assess the MCL, the posterior oblique ligament, and the PCL. MCL injuries are classified into three grades. In grade I injuries, the MCL is tender and swollen but does not exhibit increased laxity with valgus testing. Increased laxity of the valgus test, but with a firm end-feel, while the knee is positioned in 30 degrees of flexion usually denotes a tearing, of at least a grade II tearing of the middle third of the capsular ligament and the parallel fibers of the MCL. An indefinite end-feel characterizes a grade III tear with either valgus test.

The posterior fibers of the MCL can be isolated, by placing the knee in 90 degrees of flexion with full external rotation of the tibia.[21] The femur is prevented from rotating by the clinician's shoulder. The clinician places one hand on the dorsum of the foot and the other on the heel, and an external rotation force is applied using the foot as a lever.

Lateral stability

Varus Stress
The clinician applies a strong varus force, with a counter force applied at the medial femoral condyle (Figure 9-9). To be able to assess the amount of varus

movement, the clinician should repeat the maneuver several times, applying slight overpressure at the end of the range of motion. Under normal conditions, the end-feel is firm, after slight movement.

If this test is positive for pain or excessive motion as a compared with the other extremity the following structures may be implicated:

- Lateral collateral ligament (LCL)
- Lateral capsular ligament
- Arcuate-popliteus complex
- Anterior cruciate ligament
- Posterior cruciate ligament

If the instability is gross, one or both cruciate ligaments may be involved, as well as, occasionally, the biceps femoris tendon and the iliotibial band, leading to a rotary instability, if not in the short term, certainly over a period of time.[22]

The test is then repeated at 30 degrees of flexion (Figure 9-9) and the tibia in full external rotation to further assess the LCL, the posterior–lateral capsule and the arcuate-popliteus complex.

Anterior stability

A number of tests have been advocated for testing the integrity of the ACL. Two of the more commonly used ones are the anterior drawer test and the Lachman. The Lachman test is a modification of the anterior drawer test.

Anterior Drawer Test

The patient is positioned in supine, hip flexed to 45 degrees and the knee flexed to 90 degrees. The clinician fixates the leg to be tested by sitting on the patient's foot (Figure 9-10). Using both hands, the clinician grasps the lower leg of the patient just distal to the joint space of the knee and place the thumbs, either in the joint space, or just distal to it, to assess mobility. It is important that all muscles around the knee be relaxed to allow any translatory movement to occur. With both hands, the clinician now abruptly pulls the lower leg forward. This test is positive when an increased anterior movement of the tibia occurs compared with the other extremity.

The Lachman Test

The Lachman test is one of the easiest and most accurate diagnostic measures used to assess ACL injuries.[23] A number of factors can influence the results of the Lachman test. These include

- an inability of the patient to relax,
- the degree of knee flexion,
- the size of the clinician's hand,
- the stabilization (and thus relaxation) of the patient's thigh.

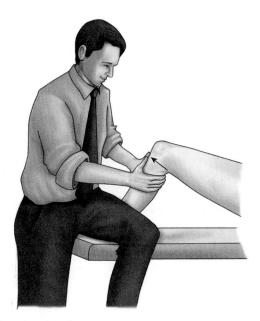

Figure 9-10 The anterior drawer.

According to Weiss et al.,[24] these factors can be minimized by the use of the modified Lachman test. In this test, the patient is positioned supine with their feet resting firmly on the end of the table and their knees flexed 10 degrees to 15 degrees. The clinician stabilizes the distal end of patient's femur using their thigh rather than their hand as in the Lachman test, and then attempts to displace patient's tibia anteriorly (Figure 9-11). If the tibia moves forward, and the concavity of the patellar tendon/ligament becomes convex, the test is considered positive.

The grading of knee instability is as follows:[25-27]

1+ (mild): 5 mm or less
2+ (moderate): 5 to 10 mm
3+ (serious): more than 10 mm
False negatives with this test can occur.

Posterior stability

The PCL is very strong and is rarely completely torn. It is typically injured in a dashboard injury, or in knee flexion activities (kneeling on the patella). A number of tests have been advocated to test the integrity of the PCL:[21]

Gravity (Godfrey) Sign

The patient is positioned in supine with the knee flexed to about 90 degrees. The clinician assesses the contour of the tibial tuberosity. If there is a rupture

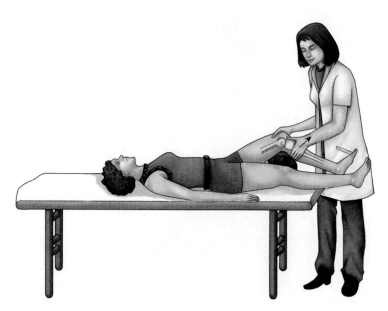

Figure 9-11 The Modified Lachman's.

(partial) of the PCL, the tibial tuberosity on the involved side will be less visible than on the noninvolved side.[28] This is caused by an abnormal posterior translation, resulting from a rupture of the PCL. In cases of doubt, the patient can be asked to contract the hamstrings slightly by pushing their heels into the clinician's hands. This will usually result in an increase in the posterior translation of the tibia. This maneuver is often performed as a quick test for integrity of the PCL.

Posterior Sag Sign

Patient positioned in supine with the hip flexed to 45 degrees and the knee flexed to 90 degrees. In this position, the tibia rocks back or sags back on the femur if the posterior cruciate ligament is torn. Normally, the medial tibial plateau extends 1 cm anteriorly beyond the femoral condyle when the knee is flexed 90 degrees. If this step off is lost, the step off test is considered positive.

Posterior Drawer

The patient is positioned in supine with the knee flexed to 90 degrees. The clinician attempts a posterior displacement of the tibia on the femur (Figure 9-12).

Quadriceps Active Test

The patient is positioned in supine with the knee flexed to 90 degrees in the posterior drawer test position. The foot is stabilized by the clinician, and the

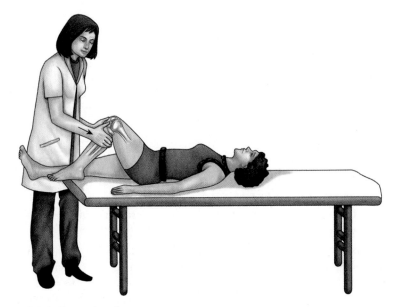

Figure 9-12 Posterior drawer test.

patient is asked to slide the foot gently down the table. Contraction of the quadriceps muscle in the PCL deficient knee results in an anterior shift of the tibia of 2 mm or more.

Multidirectional stability
Rotary or complex instabilities occur when abnormal or pathological movement is present in two or more planes. The ligamentous laxities, present at the knee joint in these situations, allow motion to take place around the sagittal, coronal, and the horizontal axis.

Posterior–Lateral Instability
This type of instability is relatively rare, as it requires complete posterior cruciate laxity. It occurs when the lateral tibial plateau subluxes posteriorly on the femur, with the axis shifting posteriorly and medially to the medial joint area. With a hyperextension test, this posterior displacement is obvious and has been labeled the external rotation recurvatum sign.

Active Posterolateral Drawer Test[29]
The patient sits with the foot on the floor in neutral rotation and the knee flexed to 80 degrees to 90 degrees. The patient is asked to isometrically contract the hamstrings, while the clinician stabilizes the foot. A positive result for the test is a posterior subluxation of the lateral tibial plateau.

Hughston's Posterior–Lateral Drawer Test[26,27]

The patient is positioned in supine with the involved leg flexed at the hip to 45 degrees, the knee flexed to 80 degrees to 90 degrees, and the lower leg in slight external rotation.[30] The clinician pushes the lower leg posteriorly. If the tibia rotates posteriorly during the test, the test is positive for posterior–lateral instability, and indicates that the following structures may have been injured:

- Posterior cruciate ligament
- Arcuate-popliteus complex
- Lateral collateral ligament
- Posterior–lateral capsule

The one-plane medial and lateral stability tests can be used to help differentiate further which lateral and posterior–lateral structures are affected.

Hughston's External Rotational Recurvatum Test[26,27]

This test is used to detect an abnormal relationship between the femur and tibia in knee extension. The patient is positioned in supine with their legs straight, and the clinician positioned at the foot of the table. The clinician gently grasps the great toes of both feet at the same time, and lifts the feet from the table, while focusing on the tibial tuberosity of both legs. The patient must be completely relaxed. In the presence of a posterior–lateral rotary instability, the knee moves into relative hyperextension at the lateral side of the knee, and the tibia externally rotates.[30]

Posterior–Medial Rotary Instability

Hughston's Posterior–Medial Drawer Test

The patient is positioned in supine with the involved leg flexed at the hip to 45 degrees, the knee flexed to 80 degrees to 90 degrees, and the lower leg in slight internal rotation.[30] The clinician pushes the lower leg posteriorly. If the tibia rotates posteriorly during the test, the test is positive for posterior–medial instability, and indicates that the following structures may have been injured:

- Posterior cruciate ligament
- Posterior oblique ligament
- Medial collateral ligament
- Posterior–medial capsule
- Anterior cruciate ligament

The one-plane medial and lateral stability tests can be used to help differentiate further which medial and posterior–medial structures are affected.

Anterior–Lateral Rotary Instability

The pathology for this condition almost certainly involves the PCL and, clinically, the instability allows the medial tibial condyle to sublux posteriorly, as the axis of motion has moved to the lateral joint compartment.[22]

The diagnosis of anterior–lateral instability is based on the demonstration of a forward subluxation of the lateral tibial plateau as the knee approaches extension and the spontaneous reduction of the subluxation during flexion, in the lateral pivot shift test.[22] This form of instability usually occurs when the individual is either decelerating or changing direction, and the sudden shift of the lateral compartment is experienced as a "giving way" phenomenon, often associated with pain.[22]

Pivot-Shift Test
Since the majority of patients with an ACL rupture complain of a "giving-way" sensation, the pivot shift test is regarded in current literature as capable of identifying rotational instability.[31–33]

There are two main types of clinical tests to determine the presence of the pivot shift, the reduction test and the subluxation test.

- In the reduction test, the knee is flexed from full extension under a valgus moment.[34] A sudden reduction of the anteriorly subluxed lateral tibial plateau is seen as the pivot shift.[35]

- The subluxation test is effectively the reverse of the reduction test.[27] However, only 35% to 75% of patients whose knees pivot while the patient is under anesthesia will experience such a pivot when awake.[36–39] The test begins with patient's knees extended. The clinician internally rotates the patient's tibias with one hand and applies a valgus stress to the patient's knee joint with the other (Figure 9-13). As the clinician gradually flexes the patient's ACL-deficient knee joint, the patient's subluxed anterior tibia snaps back into normal alignment at 20 degrees to 40 degrees of flexion.[31]

 Clinical Pearl

There is little agreement in the literature with regard to the sensitivity of the pivot shift test, which varies between 0% and 98%.[38,40,41]

The pivot shift can be positive with an isolated ACL injury,[38,42] or a tear or stretching of the lateral capsule,[43,44] although an injury to the MCL reduces the likelihood of a pivot shift even with ACL injury.[38,45]

MacIntosh (True Pivot-shift)
The MacIntosh test[46] is the most frequently used test to detect anterior–lateral instability, although Hughston,[27] Slocum, and Losee[44] have all described variations, with the latter author having received credit for describing the instability simultaneously, and independently, from MacIntosh.

The clinician picks up the relaxed leg by grasping the ankle, and flexes the leg by placing the heel of the other hand over the lateral head of the

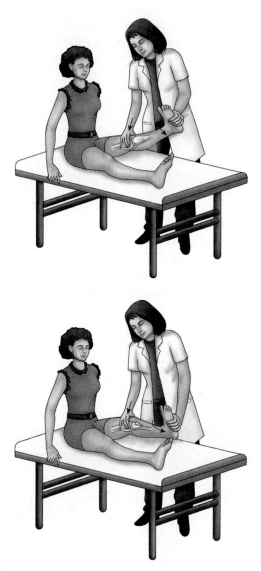

Figure 9-13 Pivot shift test.

gastrocnemius. The knee is then extended and a slight valgus stress is applied to its lateral aspect to support the tibia. Under the influence of gravity, the femur falls backwards and, as the knee approaches extension, the tibial plateau sub-luxes forward. This subluxation can be accentuated by gently internally rotating the tibia with the hand that is cradling the foot and ankle. At this point, a strong valgus force is placed on the knee by the upper hand, thereby impinging the subluxed tibial plateau against the lateral femoral condyle, by jamming the two joint surfaces together. This will prevent easy reduction as the tibia is then flexed on the femur. At approximately 30 degrees to 40 degrees of flexion, the displaced tibial plateau will suddenly reduce, often in a dramatic fashion.

Anterior–Medial Instability

Patients who demonstrate excessive anterior medial tibial condylar displacement during the anterior drawer test are exhibiting anterior–medial instability, as the axis of motion has moved to the lateral joint compartment.[22] The pathology involves the ACL, the MCL, and the posterior medial capsule.[22]

Slocum Test

The Slocum test is designed to assess for both rotary and anterior instabilities.[47] The patient is positioned in supine and their knee is flexed to 80 degrees to 90 degrees, with the hip flexed to 45 degrees. The foot of the involved leg is first placed in 30 degrees of internal rotation. Excessive internal rotation results in a tightening of the remaining structures and can lead to false negatives. The clinician sits on the foot to maintain its position, and pulls the tibia forward (Figure 9-14). A positive test results from movement occurring primarily on the lateral side of the knee, and indicates a lesion to one or more of the following structures:

- Anterior cruciate ligament
- Posterior–lateral capsule
- Arcuate popliteus complex
- Lateral collateral ligament
- Posterior cruciate ligament

If this test is positive, the second part of the test, which assesses anterior–medial rotary instability, is less reliable.[48]

The second half of the test is similar to the first, except that the patient's foot is placed in about 15 degrees of external rotation. Again, by placing the foot in too much external rotation, the clinician runs the risk of false negatives during testing. Movement occurring primarily on the medial side of the knee during testing is a positive result, and indicates a lesion to one or more of the following structures:

- Medial collateral ligament
- Posterior oblique ligament
- Posterior–medial capsule
- Anterior cruciate ligament

Patellar Stability Tests

Patellar stability is assessed by gently pushing the patella medially and laterally while the knee is relaxed in a position of 90 degrees of flexion. This position is used because this is the position when all of the retinacula are on stretch. If this test is positive for laxity, further testing is needed. The further testing involves application of medial, and lateral, patellar glides, tilts, and

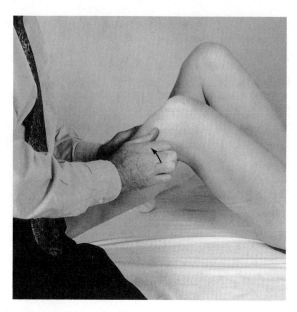

Figure 9-14 Slocum test.

rotations, with the knee in relaxed extension, and noting any limitations of motion, or excessive excursion.[49]

The apprehension test may also be used if patella instability is suspected. The patient lies supine and the knee is positioned in 30 degrees of flexion. In this position, the patella is at a point where, in most patients, it is about to engage in the femoral groove. The clinician slowly pushes the patella in a lateral direction. Patients who anticipate patellar dislocation will demonstrate visible apprehension or involuntary contraction of the quadriceps with this maneuver.

Meniscal Lesion Tests

McMurray's test[21]

The McMurray test was originally developed to diagnose posterior horn lesions of the medial meniscus.

The patient is positioned in supine and the clinician maximally flexes the hip and knee. This is performed by grasping the dorsum of the patient's foot in such a way that the thumb is lateral, the index and middle fingers are medial, and the ring and little fingers hold the medial edge of the foot (Figure 9-15). One hand is placed against the lateral aspect of the patient's knee (Figure 9-15). By rotating the patient's lower leg several times, the clinician can assess whether the patient is fully relaxed. While the lower leg is slightly externally rotated, the ipsilateral hand moves the patient's foot in a varus direction. The knee is flexed as far as comfortable, after which the foot is brought into a valgus direction with simultaneous internal rotation of the lower leg. The clinician then gently extends the knee to about 120 degrees, and at the same time exerts valgus pressure on the knee with the hand (Figure 9-15). This test is positive when a palpable click, or audible thump, is elicited that is also painful. It is thought that pain with passive external rotation implicates lesions of the posterior horn of the lateral meniscus, while pain with passive internal rotation implicates a lesion of the posterior horn of the medial meniscus, although false-positives are common.

Apley grind test[50]

The patient is positioned in the prone position with their knee flexed to 90 degrees. The patient's thigh rests on the table (Figure 9-16). The clinician applies internal and external rotation with compression to the lower leg, noting any pain, and the quality of motion. Pain with this maneuver may indicate a meniscal lesion.

Bounce home

The patient is positioned in supine with the patient's foot cupped in the clinician's hand. With the patient's knee completely flexed, the knee is passively allowed to extend. The knee should extend completely, or bounce home into extension with a sharp endpoint. If extension is not complete or has a rubbery end-feel, there is likely a torn meniscus or some other blockage present.

Steinmann's tenderness displacement test[21]

Steinmann's test is useful to distinguish meniscal pathology from injury to the ligament or osteophytes. The patient is positioned sitting on the edge of the table, with the knee hanging over at 90 degrees of flexion. Alternatively, the patient is positioned in supine lying with the clinician holding the knee at 90 degrees of flexion. The test consists of two parts:

1. The tibia is rotated laterally then medially. The test is positive if lateral pain is elicited on medial rotation and medial pain is elicited on lateral rotation. The test is repeated in various degrees of knee flexion.

2. Joint line tenderness is elicited. The knee is flexed and joint line is palpated. A positive test is indicated if the tenderness moves posteriorly with increasing flexion. The knee is extended and joint line palpated again. A positive test is indicated if the tenderness moves anteriorly when the knee is extended. The test is repeated in various degrees of flexion and extension.

Clinical Pearl

If, during the Steinmann's test, the most painful site is found in the joint space at the level of the MCL, the test is less reliable, because both the medial meniscus and the ligament move posteriorly during flexion.

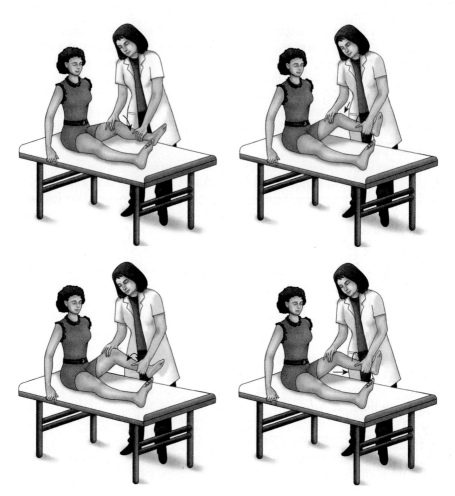

Figure 9-15 McMurray's test.

Special Tests for Specific Diagnoses

Plical Irritation

Plical irritation has a characteristic pattern of presentation. The anterior pain in the knee is episodic and associated with painful clicking, giving-way, and the feeling of something catching in the knee. Careful palpation of the patellar retinaculum and fat pad, with the knee extended and then flexed, can be used to detect tender plicae, and for the differentiation of tenderness within the fat pad, from tenderness over the anterior horn of the menisci.

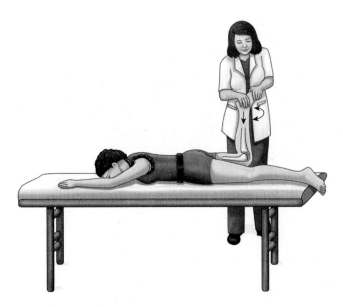

Figure 9-16 Apley's grind test.

Patellar Mobility and Retinaculum Tests

Patella glides can be used to examine for retinacular mobility. The patella should be able to translate at least 33% of its width both medially and laterally (Figure 9-17). Inability to do this indicates tightness of the retinacula. Hypermobility of the patella is demonstrated if the patella can be translated 100% of its width medially or laterally.

Hamstring Flexibility

The popliteal angle is the most popular method reported in the literature for assessing hamstring tightness especially in the presence of a knee flexion contracture.[51] Hamstring flexibility can also be assessed with a passive straight leg raise, while ensuring that the lumbar spine is flattened on the treatment table and the pelvis is stabilized. However, this method may be used only if there is full extension at the knee of the leg being examined. Normal hamstring length should allow 80 degrees to 85 degrees of hip flexion, when the knee is extended and the lumbar spine is flattened.[49]

ITB Flexibility

The cardinal sign for iliotibial contracture is that in the supine patient an abduction contracture is present when the hip and knee are extended, but is eliminated by flexion of the hip and knee.[52]

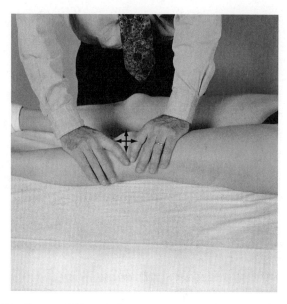

Figure 9-17 Patellar mobility testing.

Quadriceps Flexibility

Placing the patient prone and passively flexing the knee, bringing the heel toward the buttocks, examine quadriceps flexibility. The lumbar spine is monitored and stabilized if necessary to prevent motion. The heel should touch the buttocks.

Wilson Test

The Wilson test is used to assess the presence of osteochondritis dissecans. The test is performed with the patient supine. The clinician flexes the hip and knee 90 degrees and internally rotates the tibia. The knee is then slowly extended. The test is positive when the patient reports pain as the knee reaches approximately 20 degrees to 30 degrees of flexion and when pain is relieved with external rotation of the tibia while maintaining the same flexion angle.

Neurovascular Status

The neurovascular assessment should include pulse, sensation, and reflex testing. A working knowledge of the dermatomes and myotomes around the knee is essential. The L3 dermatome (femoral nerve) supplies the anterior thigh just above the knee, L4 the anteromedial portion of the knee and the leg (saphenous nerve), and L5 the anterolateral portion of the knee and leg (sural and peroneal nerves).[3] The skin over the posterior aspect of the knee is mostly innervated by the S2 dermatome.[3]

Imaging Studies

Plain Radiography

The Ottawa Knee Rules provide guidelines for when radiographs of the knee are necessary.[53] These rules aim to identify patients with clinically significant knee fractures, defined as a bone fragment at least 5 mm in breadth or an avulsion fracture associated with complete disruption of tendons or ligaments. The Ottawa guidelines recommend knee radiographs when one or more of the following are present: age 55 or older, tenderness at the head of the fibula, no bone tenderness of the knee other than the patella, inability to flex the knee to 90 degrees, and the inability to bear weight or walk more than four steps immediately after injury. Exclusion criteria include age younger than 18 years, isolated superficial skin injuries, injuries more than 7 days old (recent entries being reevaluated), patients with altered levels of consciousness, and paraplegia or multiple injuries. These rules were found to demonstrate near 100% sensitivity for knee fractures and reduce the need for radiographs by 28%.[54]

The Pittsburgh knee decision rules for radiography are based on the following indications:

1. The mechanism of injury is either blunt trauma or a fall.
2. The patient is younger than 12 years or older than 50 years of age.
3. The injury causes an inability to walk more than four weight-bearing steps in the emergency department.

Exclusion criteria:

1. Knee injuries sustained more than 6 days before presentation.
2. Patients with only superficial lacerations and abrasions.
3. History of previous surgeries or fractures on the affected knee.
4. Patients being reassessed the same injury.

According to one study,[55] utilization of these rules yield 99% sensitivity and 60% specificity for knee fractures.

When radiographs are indicated, anteroposterior and lateral views are usually supplemented with five additional views.

• The anteroposterior view is helpful for evaluating the distal femoral physis, the proximal tibial physis, the tibial intercondylar eminence, and the patella.
  • The tunnel or notch view is an anteroposterior radiograph with the knee flexed 20 degrees. This view shows the articular surfaces of the distal femoral condyles and is used when osteochondritis dissecans is suspected.

- The alignment view, a standing anteroposterior view of the entire lower extremity (including the hip, knee, and ankle joints), allows for assessment of anatomic, mechanical, and weight-bearing axes, and compartment space narrowing.
- The lateral view is useful for evaluating the position of the patella and the tibial tubercle.
- Two oblique views may be ordered secondarily to better appreciate minimally displaced fractures about the knee.
- Varus and valgus stress views may reveal physeal fractures and collateral ligament injury or laxity.
- The sunrise or sulcus view is used to assess the congruity of the patellofemoral articulation.

Magnetic Resonance Imaging

Magnetic resonance imaging (MRI), although rarely needed in the initial diagnostic workup, can highlight both soft tissue and bone, confirm or clarify a diagnosis, and can sometimes play an important role in surgical planning. The soft tissues include the menisci, cruciate and collateral ligaments, and synovial lining of the joint space. Osseous structures defined uniquely by MRI include articular cartilage, physeal cartilage, subchondral bone, periosteum, and marrow elements.

Plain tomograms or computed tomographic (CT) scans may be helpful in diagnosing tibial plateau fractures and osteochondral fractures.[8]

Examination Conclusions—The Evaluation

Following the examination, and once the clinical findings have been recorded, the clinician must determine a specific diagnosis or a working hypothesis, based on a summary of all of the findings. This diagnosis can be structure related (medical diagnosis) (Table 9-11), or a diagnosis based on the preferred practice patterns as described in the Guide to Physical Therapist Practice.[56]

INTERVENTION

The rehabilitation procedures chosen to progress the patient will depend on the type of tissue involved, the extent of the damage, and the stage of healing (See Chapter 3). The intervention must be related to the signs and symptoms present rather than the actual diagnosis.

Table 9-11 Differential Diagnosis of Common Causes of Knee Pain

Condition	Patient Age	Mechanism of Injury	Area of Symptoms	Symptoms Aggravated by	Observation	AROM	PROM	End-feel	Resisted	Tenderness with Palpation
Patellofemoral syndrome	20–50	Gradual Macrotrauma Microtrauma	Anterior knee	Prolonged sitting Stairs Kneeling	Possible soft tissue thickening/ swelling at anterior knee	Usually no limited ranges	Pain at end range knee flexion	Usually unremarkable	Usually no pain with resisted tests	Anterior knee especially with patella compression
Patellar tendonitis	15–50	Gradual (repeated eccentric overloading during deceleration activities)	Anterior knee	Squatting, jumping	Usually unremarkable	Usually unremarkable	Pain at end range knee flexion	Usually unremarkable	May have pain with resisted knee extension	Over the patellar tendon, inferior or superior to the patella
Quadriceps muscle tear	20–40	Sudden overload	Anterior thigh	Squatting	Possible bruising over anterior thigh/ knee Possible swelling over anterior thigh/ knee	Limited knee flexion	Pain with combined hip extension and knee flexion	Spasm/empty depending on extent of injury	Pain with resisted hip flexion Pain with resisted knee extension	Anterior thigh
Knee osteoarthritis	50+	Gradual due to microtrauma Macrotrauma	Generalized knee	Weight bearing	Possible soft tissue thickening/ swelling around knee	Loss of motion in a capsular pattern	Pain at end range knee flexion and extension	Unremarkable	Generalized weakness	Typically posterior knee if present at all

(continued on following page)

Table 9-11 *(continued from previous page)*

Condition	Patient Age	Mechanism of Injury	Area of Symptoms	Symptoms Aggravated by	Observation	AROM	PROM	End-feel	Resisted	Tenderness with Palpation
Anterior cruciate ligament sprain/tear	15–45	Trauma to knee (sudden deceleration, an abrupt change of direction, valgus force, rotary force) while foot is fixed	Varies according to number of associated structures involved Typically associated with immediate swelling of knee (acute hemarthrosis)	Weight bearing	Knee swelling	Loss of some knee flexion and extension (depending on extent of swelling)	Pain at end ranges	Loss of firm end feel with Lachman/ anterior drawer	Pain with resisted knee rotation	Depends on associated injuries
Collateral ligament injury	Varies	Trauma to contralateral aspect of knee (valgus or varus)	Distal femur on medial or lateral aspect depending on whether MCL or LCL is involved	Varus stress (LCL) Valgus stress (MCL)	Swelling may be present depending on extent of trauma	Depends on extent of trauma	Possible pain at end range of tibial rotation	Depends on extent of injury	Usually negative	Distal medial femur to medial joint line (MCL) Distal lateral femur to lateral joint line (LCL)

Prepatellar bursitis	15-50	Direct trauma to anterior aspect of knee. History of prolonged kneeling	Anterior knee	Kneeling	Local swelling, fluctuation	Unremarkable	Sometimes passive flexion is painful	Usually unremarkable	Usually unremarkable	Anterior aspect of knee
Patellar subluxation/ dislocation	Varies	Twisting injury with the femur internally rotating on a fixed foot, although there may be no history of trauma	Varies according to tissues involved	Weight bearing	Dependent on the degree of trauma	Dependent on extent of trauma	Dependent on extent of trauma, usually apprehension present	Spasm/empty	Usually unable to perform secondary to pain	Lateral femoral condyle, retinacular, patellar facet
Lumbar disc pathology	20-50	Gradual Sudden overload of lumbar spine	L3 dermatome	Trunk flexion Bearing down	May have associated trunk deviation	Usually pain with trunk flexion	Unremarkable	May have painful SLR	Fatiguable weakness in associated myotome	May have tenderness over involved spinal segment

COMMON ORTHOPEDIC CONDITIONS

ANTERIOR CRUCIATE LIGAMENT TEAR

Diagnosis

Anterior Cruciate Ligament (ACL) tear—ICD-9: 844.2.

 Clinical Pearl

The cruciate ligaments are intra-articular and extrasynovial because of the posterior invagination of the synovial membrane. These ligaments differ from those of other joints in that they restrict normal, rather than abnormal, motion. The tensile strength of the ACL is equal to that of the knee collaterals, but is half that of the PCL. ACL injuries occur most commonly in individuals aged 14–29 years.

Description

An injury to the ACL has terminated many a promising sports career. ACL injury factors have been divided into intrinsic and extrinsic factors.

- Intrinsic factors include a narrow intercondylar notch, larger Q-angles, weak ACL, generalized overall joint laxity, and lower extremity malalignment.
- Extrinsic factors include abnormal quadriceps and hamstring interactions, altered neuromuscular control, shoe-to-surface interface, playing surface, gender (ACL injury rates are two to eight times higher in women than in men participating in the same sports), and athlete's playing style.

 Clinical Pearl

The ACL is a unique structure and is one of the most important ligaments to knee stability, serving as a primary restraint to anterior translation of the tibia relative to the femur, and a secondary restraint to both internal and external rotation in the nonweight-bearing knee.

Subjective Findings

An accurate history includes the description of the onset of symptoms, duration, and progression of pain, history of a traumatic event, activities that worsen the pain, and previous treatments and outcomes.

- Twisting or hyperextension of the knee mechanism of injury
- Sensation of their knee "popping" or "giving out" as the tibia subluxes anteriorly
- Pain
- Immediate dysfunction
- Instability in the involved knee and the inability to walk without assistance
- Immediate swelling (acute hemarthrosis) of the involved knee

Objective Findings

- Large hemarthrosis
- Pain
- Positive special tests for anterior stability
- Involvement of other knee structures (medial meniscus, MCL, etc.)

Confirmatory/Special Tests

- Anterior drawer. Sensitivity: 0.41; specificity 0.95.
- Lachman (most sensitive for acute ACL rupture—sensitivity: 0.82; specificity 0.97).[1]
- Pivot-shift: The pivot shift is the anterior subluxation of the lateral tibial plateau that occurs when the lower leg is stabilized in (almost) full extension, whereby further flexion produces a palpable spring-like reduction. Sensitivity: 0.82; specificity 0.98.

The Lachman test has two advantages over the anterior drawer test in 90 degrees of knee flexion:

1. All parts of the ACL are more or less equally taut.
2. In acute lesions it is often impossible to position the knee in 90 degrees flexion because of a hemarthrosis.

 Clinical Pearl

In a study of patients with an ACL rupture, the Lachman test was positive in 80% of nonanesthetized patients and 100% of anesthetized patients. In comparison, the anterior drawer sign was positive in 9% of nonanesthetized patients and 52% of anesthetized patients.[2]

 Clinical Pearl

In a meta-analysis which looked at 28 studies to assess the accuracy of clinical tests for diagnosing ACL ruptures Benjaminse et al.[3] found the pivot shift test to be very specific both in acute as well as in chronic conditions, and recommended that both the Lachman and pivot shift test be performed in cases of suspected ACL injury.

 Clinical Pearl

The goal of the special tests is to identify the degree of separation and the quality, or end-feel of the separation. Intact ligaments have an abrupt and firm end-feel, whereas sprained ligaments have a soft or indistinct end-feel depending on the degree of injury.

 Clinical Pearl

During the examination, it is important for the clinician to examine the patient's contralateral knee for baseline comparisons. This especially is true in children who have inherent or congenital laxities, such as knock-knee (genu valgum) or saber legs (genu recurvatum).

Medical Studies

Radiographs (AP, lateral, and tunnel views) can identify arthritic changes that may be associated with chronic rotary instability from ACL deficiencies. They also can demonstrate avulsion fractures of the tibial spine, or hypoplastic intracondylar notches with diminished tibial spines, which indicate a congenital absence of the cruciate ligaments.

Magnetic resonance imaging (MRI) scans are useful for diagnosing ACL injuries, although their use in discriminating between complete and partial

ACL tears is limited. Diagnostic MRI scans, however, can detect associated meniscal tears that routine radiographs cannot show.

 Clinical Pearl

Both MRI scans and radiographs are necessary to assess whether young athletes' growth plates are closed or open, a factor that may affect treatment decisions.

Differential Diagnosis

- Osteochondral injury
- Meniscal injury
- Tibial plateau fracture
- Patellar dislocation/subluxation
- Patellar tendon/quadriceps rupture
- Posterior cruciate ligament tear

 Clinical Pearl

Isolated ACL injuries are rare because the ACL functions in conjunction with other structures of the knee.

Intervention

Clinicians must consider many factors when determining the best treatment options for patients with ACL injuries. Patients with either partial (grades I and II) ACL tears (negative pivot shifts), or "isolated" ACL tears, who lead a less active lifestyle, and participate in linear, nondeceleration activities are considered to be candidates for conservative intervention. For the middle-aged and older athlete, physical therapy often is the treatment of choice, unless the patient plans to participate in sports activities that expose the knees to vigorous twisting forces.

ROM exercises, which are initiated as early as possible, must be performed carefully, so as not to further aggravate soft tissue injury, and prolong pain and effusion.

Most authors stress the importance of strengthening the quadriceps, gastrocnemius-soleus, and hamstrings muscles to prevent, or minimize, atrophy and maintain or improve strength.

Clinical Pearl

Failure of the pain and effusion to resolve, and ROM to improve, should arouse suspicion of a displaced torn meniscus.

Prognosis

Symptomatic ACL deficiencies in young athletes' knee joints are subject to the same long-term detrimental effects that occur in adult athletes. Young athletes also may be more predisposed to more long-term degenerative knee conditions as the result of more years of chronic rotary knee instabilities from ACL deficiencies.

1. Katz JW, Fingeroth RJ. The diagnostic accuracy of ruptures of the anterior cruciate ligament comparing the Lachman's test, the anterior drawer sign, and the pivot-shift test in acute and chronic knee injuries. *Am J Sports Med.* 1986;14:88-91.
2. DeHaven KE. Diagnosis of acute knee injuries with hemarthrosis. *Am J Sports Med.* 1980;8:9-14.
3. Benjaminse A, Gokeler A, van der Schans CP. Clinical diagnosis of an anterior cruciate ligament rupture: a meta-analysis. *J Orthop Sports Phys Ther.* 2006;36:267-288.

BAKER'S (POPLITEAL) CYST

Diagnosis

Baker's (popliteal) cyst—ICD-9: 727.51.

Description

A Baker's cyst is an abnormal collection of synovial fluid in the fatty layers of the popliteal fossa. It is the most common synovial cyst in the knee. On occasion, the cyst can become so large that it protrudes through the soft tissues, just proximal to the popliteal fossa, between the heads of the gastrocnemius.

 Clinical Pearl

A Baker's cyst develops in the popliteal bursa located in the posteromedial aspect of the knee joint. This normally thin bursa (must be distinguished from the more common dilated semimembranosus bursa) communicates with the knee joint and becomes more prominent when synovitis or trauma creates excessive joint fluid that then enters into the popliteal bursa.

Subjective Findings

The subjective findings typically include the following:

- Complaints of tightness/swelling behind the knee or pain down the back of the leg (larger cyst or ruptured cyst).
- No history of trauma.

Objective Findings

The physical examination typically reveals the following findings:

- With the patient in the prone position and the leg fully extended, an oblong mass is palpable and visible in the medial popliteal fossa.
- Active knee flexion may be limited by 10 degrees to 15 degrees with a large cyst.

Confirmatory/Special Tests

A tentative diagnosis is based on the presence of a palpable, popliteal mass when all other causes have been ruled out.

Medical/Imaging Studies

Radiographs of the knee are usually negative but may show the outline of the cyst or show calcification present within the cyst.

Diagnostic ultrasound can be used to define the size and extent of the cyst.

Differential Diagnosis

- Deep venous thrombosis
- Medial gastrocnemius muscle strain
- Exertional compartment syndrome
- Inflammatory arthritis
- Superficial phlebitis
- Meniscal tear

Intervention

The intervention for large cysts that interfere with knee function is to aspirate the abnormal accumulation of fluid. However, this provides only transient relief, so treatment should be directed at the cause of increased synovial fluid (intra-articular lesion, severe arthritis).

Prognosis

The long-term prognosis depends on the underlying process affecting the knee and the success related to treating those processes.

COLLATERAL LIGAMENT SPRAIN

Diagnosis

Collateral ligament sprain—Medial (ICD-9: 844.1); Lateral (ICD-9: 844.0).

Description

The medial and lateral collateral ligaments are outside the joint and stabilize the knee against valgus and varus stresses, respectively.

 Clinical Pearl

The medial collateral ligament (MCL) is more commonly injured than the lateral collateral ligament (LCL). Injuries to the collateral ligaments can occur alone or in association with a meniscal tear or an anterior or posterior cruciate ligament tear.

Subjective Findings

An accurate history includes the description of the onset of symptoms, duration, and progression of pain, history of a traumatic event, activities that worsen the pain, and previous treatments and outcomes.

- Localized swelling or stiffness.
- Medial or lateral pain and tenderness, depending on which ligament is injured.

 Clinical Pearl

Most patients are able to ambulate after an acute collateral ligament injury.

Objective Findings

The physical examination typically reveals the following:

- The MCL may be tender along its entire course. Isolated tenderness at the most proximal or distal extent of the MCL may signify an avulsion type injury.
- The LCL may be tender anyway along its course.
- Positive varus (LCL) and valgus (MCL) stress tests applied first within the knee in full extension and then at 30 degrees of flexion (to relax the cruciate ligaments and posterior capsule). Laxity in full extension indicates a more extensive injury that likely includes the anterior and posterior cruciate ligaments plus the posterior capsule.

 Clinical Pearl

The MCL is best palpated with the knee in slight flexion, but the LCL is best examined with the leg in the figure-of-four position.

Confirmatory/Special Tests

- Abduction valgus stress test
- Adduction varus stress test

 Clinical Pearl

Unlike the valgus stress test, the varus test has been shown to be highly unreliable with many false negative findings.

Medical Studies

AP and lateral radiographs, although usually negative, may reveal an avulsion from the femoral origin of the MCL or the fibular insertion of the LCL.

Differential Diagnosis

- Anterior cruciate ligament tear
- Tibial plateau fracture
- Posterior cruciate ligament tear

- Patellar subluxation or dislocation with spontaneous reduction
- Osteochondral fracture
- Meniscal tear
- Epiphyseal fracture of the distal femur

Intervention

The intervention for isolated grade I–II collateral ligament tears usually is conservative. Even grade III MCL tears are also treated conservatively with the use of a hinge brace and a gradual return to full weight bearing over the course of 4 to 6 weeks. Grade III LCL tears that involve a tear of the posterolateral capsular complex are best treated surgically to avoid late instability, especially in varus knees.

Prognosis

Frank instability is very uncommon after an isolated collateral ligament injury.

MEDIAL GASTROCNEMIUS STRAIN

Diagnosis

Medial gastrocnemius strain—ICD-9: 844.9. Also referred to as tennis leg.

Description

A medial gastrocnemius strain typically results from an acute, forceful push-off with the foot joint in activities such as hill running, jumping, or tennis. Acute strains of the medial head of the gastrocnemius are most common in athletes over 30 years of age.

Subjective Findings

The subjective findings typically include the following:

- Complaints of a pulling or tearing sensation in the calf.
- The patient may hold the ankle in plantar flexion to avoid placing tension on the injured muscle.

Objective Findings

The physical examination typically reveals the following findings:

- Tenderness and swelling over the medial gastrocnemius. Most of the tenderness occurs over the medial gastrocnemius musculotendinous junction.

- Pain aggravated with passive dorsiflexion.
- Inability to perform a single-leg toe raise.
- Negative Thomson test.
- Peripheral pulses are intact.

Confirmatory/Special Tests

No specific confirmatory/special tests are necessary to diagnose this condition.

Medical/Imaging Studies

No specific medical/imaging tests are necessary to diagnose this condition. Plain radiographs may be appropriate if an avulsion fracture is suspected.

Differential Diagnosis

- Achilles tendonitis.
- Achilles tendon rupture.
- Popliteal (Baker's) cyst rupture.
- Plantaris tendon rupture.
- Posterior tibial tendon tendonitis/rupture.
- Chronic exertional compartment syndrome (posterior).
- Deep vein thrombosis.

Intervention

The intervention depends on the stage of healing. In the acute stage the goal is to control the pain and inflammation using rest, ice, compression, and elevation. Gentle active and passive range of motion exercises are then initiated before progressing to strengthening exercises for the plantar flexors (stationary cycling, leg presses, and heel raises). Once the athlete is pain free with full and symmetric ROM and full strength is regained, sports-specific activities can be resumed. Strengthening and stretching of the injured area should continue for several months to overcome the increased risk for reinjury due to the deposition of scar tissue that is involved in the healing process.

Prognosis

A strain of the medial gastrocnemius typically responds very well to conservative management. Persistent symptoms indicate the need for further examination.

MENISCAL TEAR

Diagnosis

Meniscal tear—ICD-9: 836.0 (Medial); 836.1 (Lateral). Also referred to as a cartilage injury.

Description

Because of the interrelationship of the menisci with other structures of the knee, a torn meniscus is the most common cause of mechanical symptoms in the knee. With aging, the meniscal tissue degenerates and can delaminate, thus making it more susceptible to splitting from shear stress, resulting in horizontal cleavage tears.[629] Without the menisci, the loads on the articular surfaces are increased significantly, leading to a greater potential for articular cartilage injuries and degenerative arthritis.

 Clinical Pearl

Meniscal lesions usually occur when the patient attempts to turn, twist, or change direction when weight bearing, but they also can occur from contact to the lateral or medial aspect of the knee while the lower extremity is planted. Because the menisci are without pain fibers, it is the tearing and bleeding into the peripheral attachments as well as traction on the capsule that most likely produce the patient's symptoms.

Subjective Findings

The typical subjective findings include:

- Reports of a significant twisting injury to the knee, although older patients with degenerative tears may have a history of minimal or no trauma.
- History of swelling, popping, or clicking. In some cases, large unstable fragments of meniscal tissue can lead to a "locked" knee.
- Pain along the joint line, particularly with twisting or squatting activities.

 Clinical Pearl

The shape and location of the meniscal tear determines the symptoms and clinical findings.

Objective Findings

The physical examination typically reveals:

- Tenderness over the medial or lateral joint line.
- Some degree of effusion.
- Forced flexion and circumduction (internal and external rotation of the foot) frequently elicit pain on the side of the knee with the meniscal tear—see confirmatory/special tests.

Confirmatory/Special Tests

- McMurray
- Apley's Test
- Steinmann's Tenderness Displacement Test

Medical Studies

AP, lateral, and axial patellofemoral views are indicated for patients with a history of trauma or an effusion. For patients with chronic conditions, the AP and lateral views should be weight bearing.

MRI is highly specific and sensitive for meniscal pathology.

 Clinical Pearl

A weight bearing AP view with the knee flexed to 45° is sensitive for early osteoarthritis and is recommended in older patients.

Differential Diagnosis

- Anterior cruciate ligament tear
- Loose body
- Medial collateral ligament tear
- Crystal disease
- Osteoarthritis
- Osteochondritis dissecans
- Patellar subluxation or dislocation
- Pes anserine bursitis
- Tibial plateau fracture
- Saphenous neuritis

Intervention

At the time of writing, four conservative approaches exist for the intervention of meniscal injuries: rehabilitation, meniscectomy, meniscus repair, and allograft transplantation. The choice of intervention depends on the several factors, including age, activity demands, size and location of the tear, and collateral tissue damage.

The conservative intervention for meniscal tears focuses on the resolution of impairments such as swelling, restricted range of motion, and strength, using exercises, bracing, and oral medications.

Prognosis

Unless a tear is acute, peripheral, and stable, the relative avascularity of the middle third and inner third of both menisci indicates a poor healing potential in these areas. If the knee is locked or cannot be fully extended, the torn meniscal fragment is displaced and must be treated surgically.

OSGOOD SCHLATTER'S DISEASE

Diagnosis

Osgood Schlatter's disease—ICD-9: 732.4. Also known as osteochondritis of inferior patella, osteochondritis of the tibial tuberosity, or tibial tubercle traction apophysitis.

Description

Osgood Schlatter's disease is a form of periostitis of the tibial apophysitis type that manifests as a partial avulsion of the tibial tuberosity with subsequent osteonecrosis of the fragmented bone.

 Clinical Pearl

Although traditionally associated with pubescent males, it is now typical of females involved in athletic activity, particularly soccer and gymnastics.

Subjective Findings

An accurate history includes the description of the onset of symptoms, duration, and progression of pain, history of a traumatic event, activities that worsen the pain, and previous treatments and outcomes. Subjective reports include the following:

- Gradually increasing pain and swelling below the involved knee.
- Involvement in sporting activities that involve running, jumping, and landing.

Objective Findings

The physical examination typically reveals the following:

- Prominence over the tibial tubercle. Mild swelling may also be evident.
- Pinpoint tenderness over the tibial tuberosity.
- Passive range of motion reveals limitation of knee flexion.
- Active range of motion of knee flexion is painful at end ranges.
- Resisted knee extension typically reproduces the pain.
- Flexibility testing may reveal adaptive shortening of the hamstrings, quadriceps, and calf muscles.

Confirmatory/Special Tests

The diagnosis for this condition is based on the patient age, history, and physical findings.

Medical Studies

AP and lateral radiographs of the knee may be normal or show soft tissue swelling. Small spicules of heterotopic ossification may be seen.

 Clinical Pearl

When a patient has bilateral symptoms, radiographs are rarely needed.

Differential Diagnosis

- Neoplasm
- Pes anserinus bursitis
- Avulsion of the tibial tubercle
- Sindig–Larsen–Johansson apophysitis

Intervention

The ultimate treatment decision is based upon a variety of factors, including the patient's overall medical condition, severity, and duration of symptoms, expectations, associated knee pathology, and surgeon preference. The typical intervention for this condition involves activity modification to limit the pain, quadriceps stretching, and knee pads to be used for kneeling activities.

Prognosis

This condition is self-limiting and spontaneously remitting over a period of 6 to 24 months as the tibial tubercle ossifies.

OSTEOARTHRITIS OF THE KNEE

Diagnosis

Osteoarthritis of the knee—ICD-9: 721.6. Also referred to as degenerative joint disease.

Description

Osteoarthritis of the knee can involve each of the three compartments (medial, lateral, and the patellofemoral joint) individually or in combination. The medial compartment is the area most frequently involved.

 Clinical Pearl

Secondary osteoarthritis of the knee usually occurs in individuals with a significant history of trauma to the knee.

 Clinical Pearl

Established risk factors for osteoarthritis of the knee include physically demanding occupations, particularly in jobs that involve kneeling or squatting, older age, female sex, evidence of osteoarthritis in other joints, obesity, and previous injury or surgery of the knee.

Subjective Findings

An accurate history includes the description of the onset of symptoms, duration, and progression of pain, history of a traumatic event, activities that worsen the pain, and previous treatments and outcomes. Typical subjective complaints include:

- Insidious onset of pain/stiffness
- Pain with weight bearing
- May have complaints of buckling, locking, or giving way
- Difficulty climbing or descending stairs

Objective Findings

The physical examination usually reveals:

- Angular deformity through the knee (varus or valgus).
- Effusion (mild to severe).
- Diffuse tenderness along the joint lines.
- Loss of active range of motion in a capsular pattern.
- Reflexive dysfunction of the quadriceps muscle.

Confirmatory/Special Tests

The diagnosis of osteoarthritis of the knee is made based on a combination of patient history, physical examination, and radiographic views.

Medical Studies

Weight-bearing AP radiographs of both knees in full extension will show narrowing of the joint space. The overall condition of the patellofemoral and tibiofemoral joints may be further assessed with lateral and axial patellofemoral views. In addition, weight-bearing AP radiographs with the knee in approximately 40 degrees of flexion can help identify narrowing of the articular surface because they profile different weight-bearing areas of the tibia and femur. The intercondylar notch (tunnel) view often will reveal osteophytes as well as demonstrate osteochondral loose bodies.

 Clinical Pearl

Radiographic findings of degenerative arthritis include asymmetric joint narrowing, bone sclerosis, periarticular cysts, and osteophytes.

Differential Diagnosis

- Disc herniation (L3–L4)
- Meniscal tear
- Osteonecrosis of the femur or tibia
- Pigmented villonodular synovitis

- Septic arthritis
- Tendonitis/bursitis
- Primary hip pathology

Intervention

The ultimate treatment decision is based upon a variety of factors, including the patient's overall medical condition, severity, and duration of symptoms, expectations, associated pathology, and surgeon preference. Exercises to strengthen the quadriceps, such as quad-setting exercises and isometric exercises, are becoming accepted as useful conservative treatment for osteoarthritis of the knee. In addition to exercises that improve lower extremity strength, range of motion, and cardiovascular endurance, it is now being recommended that exercise therapy programs also include techniques to improve balance and coordination, and provide patients with an opportunity to practice various skills that they will likely encounter during normal day activities. The conservative intervention for osteoarthritis of the knee also includes NSAIDs, cortisone injections, patient education, weight loss, thermal modalities, and shoe inserts. Finally, the patient is instructed in principles of joint protection, and advised to seek alternatives to prolonged standing, kneeling, and squatting.

 Clinical Pearl

Isokinetic and concentric exercises must be prescribed carefully to avoid excessive compressive forces or shear forces at the knee.

Prognosis

Osteoarthritis is a progressive condition, although the symptoms can be somewhat controlled using medication, mechanical aids, shoe inserts, non-impact exercises, and strengthening. Severe functional limitations and pain at rest or at night indicate a failure of conservative management and the need for surgical treatment.

PATELLAR TENDONITIS (JUMPER'S KNEE)

Diagnosis

Patellar tendonitis (Jumper's knee)—ICD-9: 726.64.

Clinical Pearl

Some authors feel that the term *patellar tendonitis* is a misnomer because the patellar "tendon," which connects two bones, is in fact a ligament.

Description

Patellar tendonitis (jumper's knee) is an overuse condition that is frequently associated with eccentric overloading during deceleration activities (e.g., repeated jumping and landing, downhill running).

 Clinical Pearl

Patellar tendonitis occurs at the inferior pole of the patella or at its insertion at tibial tubercle, whereas quadriceps tendonitis occurs at the superior pole of the patella.

Subjective Findings

An accurate history includes the description of the onset of symptoms, duration, and progression of pain, history of a traumatic event, activities that worsen the pain, and previous treatments and outcomes. The typical subjective findings include:

- History of jumping or kicking sports.
- Anterior knee pain.
- Pain that is noted immediately at the end of exercise or following sitting that has been preceded by exercise.
- Pain with sitting, squatting, or kneeling.
- Pain with climbing or descending stairs, jumping, or running.

Objective Findings

The physical examination typically reveals the following:

- Localized tenderness at either the inferior pole of the patella, at tibial tubercle, or both.
- Active range of motion of the knee is typically normal.
- Pain with passive hyperflexion of the knee.
- Pain with resisted knee extension.

Confirmatory/Special Tests

The diagnosis of tendonitis is based on a detailed history, and careful palpation of the tendon in both flexion and extension.

Medical Studies

AP and lateral radiographs of the knee typically are negative, but lateral views may show small osteophytes or heterotopic ossification at the inferior pole of the patella.

Differential Diagnosis

- Anterior or posterior cruciate ligament injury.
- Septic arthritis of the knee.
- Partial rupture of the knee extensor mechanism.
- Patellofemoral syndrome.
- Inflammatory condition.

Intervention

The intervention for this condition occurs in three stages:

1. Relative rest from aggravating activities.
2. Regaining pain-free active motion, flexibility of the quadriceps and hamstrings, and exercises focusing on pain-free quadriceps strengthening.
3. Gradual resumption of the activities that caused the symptoms.

Prognosis

Patellar tendonitis is usually a self-limiting condition that responds to rest, stretching, eccentric strengthening, bracing, and other conservative techniques. Surgical intervention is usually required only if significant tendonosis develops.

PATELLOFEMORAL PAIN SYNDROME

Diagnosis

Patellofemoral pain syndrome (PFPS)—ICD-9: 717.7. Also referred to as patellofemoral dysfunction or patellofemoral arthralgia.

Description

A relatively common disorder that is diagnosed based on the presence of anterior or retropatella knee pain associated with prolonged sitting or with weight-bearing activities that load the patellofemoral joint, such as squatting, kneeling, running, and ascending and descending steps.

Subjective Findings

- Reports of anterior knee pain with going up or down stairs or hills; instability of patella with activities.
- There is usually no history of trauma and swelling is uncommon.
- More common in female than male patients.

Objective Findings

- Observation may reveal valgus alignment of the knees, femoral anteversion (increased internal rotation compared with external rotation), and abnormal tracking.
- Quadriceps weakness.
- Generalized laxity of the patellofemoral ligaments.

Confirmatory/Special Tests

- Retinacula Test: The patient is placed in the side-lying position, and the knee is fully flexed. This position tightens the iliotibial band. The clinician applies a medial and oblique force to the patella with the thumbs. Approximately 0.5 to 1 cm of patella motion should be available.
- Ober's Test: The Ober test is designed to assess iliotibial band length.
- Fairbank's Apprehension Test for Patellar Instability: Best performed with the patient supine and the patient's leg supported at approximately 30 degrees of knee flexion. The clinician applies a laterally directed force to the medial aspect of the patella, attempting to sublux it laterally while applying a small amount of passive flexion to the knee.
- The McConnell Test: This test involves manual compression to the patella with the palm of the hand at various angles of knee flexion to compress the articulating facets. Although the findings have little bearing on the overall intervention, they can guide the clinician as to which knee flexion angles to avoid during exercise.

Medical Studies

Radiographs of the knee (sunrise/Merchant view is essential).

Differential Diagnosis

- Patellofemoral arthritis, subluxation, or instability
- Plica syndrome
- Osgood Schlatter disease
- Chondromalacia patella
- Jumper's knee
- Osteochondritis dissecans
- Hip disorders

 Clinical Pearl

Hip disorders should be considered as a cause of knee pain complaints in children.

Intervention

Current evidence-based treatment approaches include taping, strengthening of the hip musculature and quadriceps, manual therapy to the lower quarter, and the fitting of foot orthoses. The goals of treatment are to improve patellofemoral tracking and alignment, to reduce pain and swelling, and to retard the development of patellofemoral arthritis.

Prognosis

The prognosis for this condition is uniformly good. Preventive exercises cannot be over emphasized.

PLICA SYNDROME

Diagnosis

Plica syndrome—ICD-9: 717.9 (unspecified internal derangement of the knee); 727.00 (synovitis and tenosynovitis, unspecified).

Description

A plica is a normal fold in the synovium. The most common plica in the knee is called the anterior or inferior plica, or mucous ligament. The plicae to the medial and lateral sides of the patella, which run in a horizontal plane from the fat pad to the side of the patellar retinaculum, are referred to as the superomedial or superolateral plicae or the suprapatellar membrane, or the medial or lateral synovial shelf.

A plica that becomes inflamed and thickened from trauma or overuse may interfere with normal joint motion. The plica syndrome has been associated with anterior pain as well as clicking, catching, locking, or pseudolocking of the knee, and it may even mimic acute internal derangement of the knee.

 Clinical Pearl

The severity of symptoms is not proportional to the size or breadth of the synovial plica. There also appears to be no correlation between the duration of symptoms and the presence of pathologic changes in the plica.

Subjective Findings

The subjective findings typically include the following:

- Reports of an insidious onset of knee pain, although the onset may be related to a fall or injury.
- Activity-related aching in the anterior or anteromedial aspects of the knee.
- There may be a painful snapping or popping in the knee.

Objective Findings

The physical examination typically reveals the following findings:

- Tenderness according to the location of the symptomatic plica. Careful palpation of the patellar retinaculum and fat pad, with the knee extended and then flexed, can be used to detect tender plicae, and for the differentiation of tenderness within the fat pad, from tenderness over the anterior horn of the menisci.
- May be able to reproduce the snapping or popping at approximately 60 degrees of knee flexion with passive extension.

Confirmatory/Special Tests

The diagnosis of plica syndrome is based on patient history and the findings from the physical examination.

Medical/Imaging Studies

Plicae are not visualized well on plain radiographs, but a double-contrast arthrogram may demonstrate a suprapatellar plica or an anterior plica. A skyline radiograph may demonstrate a synovial shelf.

Differential Diagnosis

- Meniscal tear
- Septic arthritis
- Quadriceps or patellar tendonitis
- Osteochondritis dissecans
- Prepatellar bursitis
- Patellofemoral instability

Intervention

The conservative intervention for plica syndrome involves stretching of the quadriceps, hamstrings, and gastrocnemius as well as isometric strengthening, cryotherapy, ultrasound, patellar bracing, anti-inflammatory medication, and an altered sports-training schedule.

Prognosis

When patients are truly symptomatic, or when conservative measures have failed, surgical excision is usually curative.

PREPATELLAR BURSITIS

Diagnosis

Prepatellar bursitis—ICD-9: 726.65.

Description

The prepatellar bursa can become inflamed or infected (septic bursitis) as a result of trauma to the anterior knee, such as a direct blow, or from chronic irritation from activities that require extensive kneeling.

 Clinical Pearl

The prepatellar bursa on the anterior aspect of the knee is superficial and lies between the skin and the bony patella. It is one of two bursae in the body that can become infected.

Subjective Findings

The subjective findings typically include the following:

- Complaints of knee swelling and knee pain just over the front of the knee.

Objective Findings

The physical examination typically reveals the following findings:

- Observation of swelling directly over the inferior portion of patella.
- Palpation reveals bursal sac tenderness (acute) or bursal sac thickening (chronic).
- Normal active range of motion of the knee.

Confirmatory/Special Tests

Fluid analysis is the only special test indicated.

Medical/Imaging Studies

AP and lateral radiographs should be obtained in patients with chronic pain to rule out bony conditions. Otherwise, radiographs are unnecessary to make the diagnosis.

Differential Diagnosis

- Inflammatory arthritis
- Medial meniscal tear
- Osteoarthritis of the knee
- Patellar tendonitis
- Patellar fracture
- Saphenous nerve entrapment
- Septic knee/bursitis/arthritis
- Tumor

Intervention

The goals of the intervention are to decrease inflammation using cryotherapy and patient education on activity modification. Those patients with identifiable adaptive shortening of the quadriceps, hamstrings or iliotibial band are instructed on proper stretching techniques.

Prognosis

Approximately half of traumatic bursitis resolves spontaneously. Approximately 10% progress to chronic bursitis and may require bursectomy.

REHABILITATION LADDER

KNEE

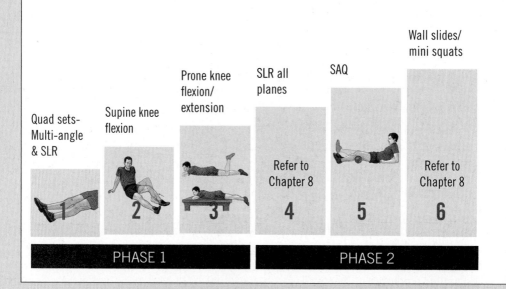

The purpose of these training ladders is to provide the clinician with a safe and progressive framework of exercises that are designed to allow the patient to improve in an efficient manner. The patient begins at the appropriate step, which is based on the stage of healing and the goal of the intervention.

- Phase 1: Acute—pain management, restoration of full passive range of motion, and restoration of normal accessory motion.
- Phase 2: Subacute—active range of motion exercises and early strengthening.
- Phase 3: Chronic—specific strengthening with a strong emphasis on enhancing dynamic stability.

The degree of movement and the speed of progression are both guided by the signs and symptoms. Once the patient is able to perform an exercise

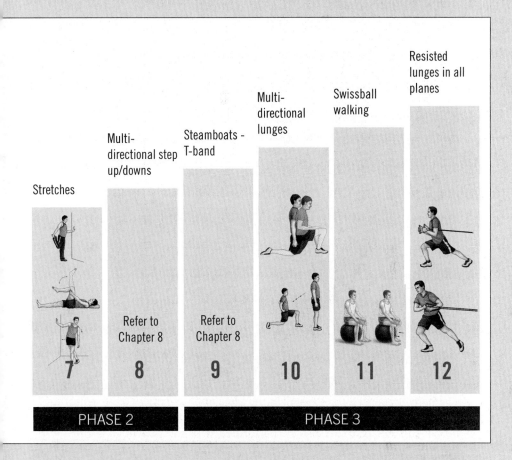

for 8–12 reps without pain, he/she progresses up to the next exercise step. This continues until the patient attempts an exercise that reproduces the pain. At this point, the patient returns to the last exercise that he/she was able to perform without pain and performs that exercise 5 times/day for 1 to 2 days before attempting to progress again. The patient is advanced through the training ladders to the appropriate point, with particular attention paid to patient response to treatment in terms of changes in symptoms, swelling, degree of irritability, or motion. In addition, muscle imbalances are addressed with appropriate flexibility exercises.

Once the patient is able to perform the last exercise of Phase 3 (Step 12 of the ladder), he or she can move on to functional and sport-specific training (Phase 4) as appropriate, which focus on power and higher-speed exercises similar to sport specific demands.

1. Quad sets and SLR

The patient is position in supine, or sitting in a chair (with the heel on the floor), or long sitting with the knee of the involved leg extended, and the uninvolved leg is flexed. The patient is asked to contract the quadriceps isometrically (1), which causes the patella to glide proximally. The contraction is held for 10 seconds. During the contraction, the patient is asked to dorsiflex the ankle. Once the quadriceps set is completed without pain, the patient is then asked to perform a straight leg raise by lifting the leg approximately 15 degrees off the bed.

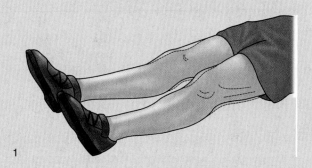

1

2. Supine knee flexion

The patient is positioned in supine, either on a bed (2a) or against a wall (2b). The patient is asked to slowly flex the knee until a gentle stretch sensation is felt. This position is held 10 seconds and the exercise is repeated a further 10 times. This exercise can also be performed with the patient in sitting. With the foot firmly planted on the floor, the patient is asked to move forward in the chair.

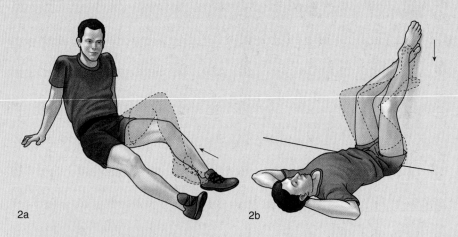

2a   2b

3. Prone knee range of motion

To increase knee extension, the patient is positioned in prone with the thigh supported so that the hip and knee are extended as much as possible (3a). Gravity is used to slowly extend the knee (4). To increase knee flexion, the patient is positioned in prone and is asked to flex the knee as far as tolerated (3b).

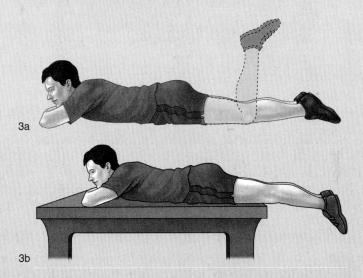

3a

3b

4. SLR in all planes

Refer to Chapter 8 for full description.

5. Short arc quads

The patient is positioned in supine or long sitting with a rolled towel under the knee to support it in flexion (5). The patient is asked to extend the knee against gravity.

🔵 Clinical Pearl

Modifications to the short arc quad exercise include:

Patient positioned in the short sitting position at the edge of the table with the seat of a wheeled stool placed under the heel to stop knee flexion at the desired angle. The patient is then asked to extend the knee by pushing the stool away.

The short arc terminal extension can be combined with a straight leg raise.

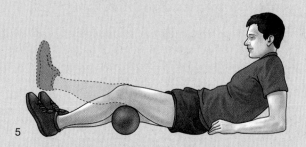

5

6. Wall slides/partial squats
Refer to Chapter 8 for full description.

7. Stretches
The quadriceps (7a), hamstrings (7b), and iliotibial band (ITB) (7c) are stretched. To stretch the ITB, the patient is positioned in standing with the involved leg closest to the wall (7). The patient is asked to cross the involved leg behind the uninvolved leg and then to lean the pelvis toward the wall while dropping the shoulder (7) furthest away from the wall, thereby imparting a stretch to the ITB.

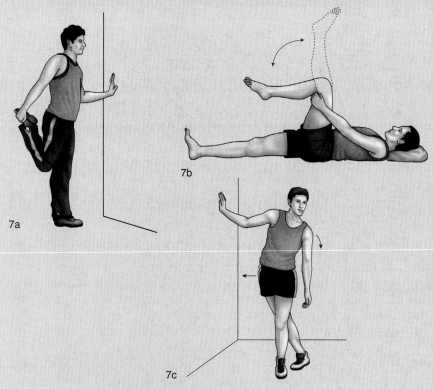

7a

7b

7c

8. Multidirectional step ups
Refer to Chapter 8 for full description.

9. Steamboats
Refer to Chapter 8 for full description.

10. Multidirectional lunges
The patient is positioned in standing. Starting with a forward lunge (10a), the patient is then progressed into lunging in a variety of directions including backwards (10b), and to both sides.

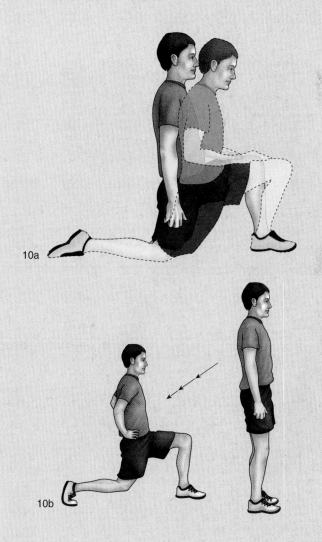

11. Swissball walking

The patient is positioned sitting on a Swissball so that the feet are flat on the ground (11). The patient is asked to start walking around the clinic while staying on the Swissball.

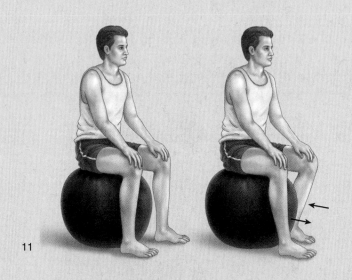

12. Resisted lunging.

A length of sports cord is attached to a stable structure. While holding on to the unattached end of the cord the patient performs a series of lunges in a variety of directions including forwards (12a) and sideways (12b).

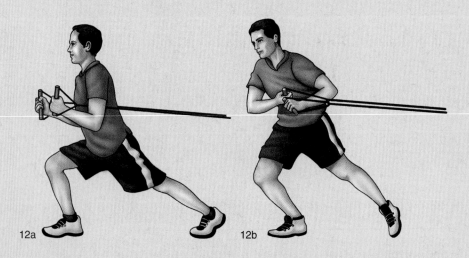

REFERENCES

1. Dye SF. An evolutionary perspective of the knee. *J Bone and Joint Surg.* 1987;69A:976–983.
2. Davids JR. Pediatric knee. Clinical assessment and common disorders. *Pediatr Clin North Am.* 1996;43:1067–1090.
3. Mendelsohn CL, Paiement GD. Physical examination of the knee. *Prim Care.* 1996;23:321–328.
4. Wojtys EM, Huston LJ. Neuromuscular performance in normal and anterior cruciate ligament-deficient lower extremities. *Am J Sports Med.* 1994;22:89–104.
5. Frank CB, Jackson DW. The science of reconstruction of the anterior cruciate ligament. *J Bone Joint Surg.* 1997;79:1556–1576.
6. Gray H. The joints: articulation of the lower limb. In: Clemente CD, ed. *Anatomy of the Human Body.* 13th ed.. Philadelphia: Lea & Febiger; 1985: 309–310, 397, 401.
7. Pick TP, Howden R. *Gray's Anatomy.* 15th ed. New York: Barnes & Noble Books; 1995.
8. Rothenberg MH, Graf BK. Evaluation of acute knee injuries. *Postgrad Med.* 1993;93:75–82, 85–86.
9. Clancy WG. Evaluation of acute knee injuries. In: Finerman G, ed. *American Association of Orthopaedic Surgeons, Symposium on Sports Medicine: The Knee.* St Louis: CV Mosby; 1985: 185–193.
10. Austermuehle PD. Common. knee injuries in primary care. *Nurse Pract.* 2001;26:32–45; quiz 46–47.
11. Bergfeld JA, Ireland ML, Wojtys EM. Pinpointing the cause of acute knee pain. *Patient Care Arch.* 1997;31:100–117.
12. Solomon DH, Simel DL, Bates DW, et al. The rational clinical examination. Does this patient have a torn meniscus or ligament of the knee? Value of the physical examination. *JAMA* 2001;286:1610–1620.
13. Brinker MR, Miller MD. *Fundamentals of Orthopedics.* Philadelphia, PA: WB Saunders; 1999.
14. Feagin JA, Jr. The office diagnosis and documentation of common knee problems. *Clin Sports Med.* 1989;8:453–459.
15. Barber-Westin SD, Noyes FR, Andrews M. A rigorous comparison between the sexes of results and complications after anterior cruciate ligament reconstruction. *Am J Sports Med.* 1997;25:514–526.
16. Reinking MF. Knee anatomy and biomechanics. In: Wadsworth C, ed. *Disorders of the Knee—Home Study Course.* La Crosse, WI: Orthopaedic Section, APTA, Inc.; 2001.
17. Laubenthal KN, Smidt GL, Kettelkamp DB. A quantitative analysis of knee motion for activities of daily living. *Phys Ther.* 1972;52:34–42.
18. Rauch G, Wirth T, Dorner P, et al. Is conservative treatment of partial or complete anterior cruciate ligament rupture still justified? An analysis of the recent literature and a recommendation for arriving at a decision. *Zeitschr Orthop.* 1991;129: 438–446.
19. Sommerlath K, Odensten M, Lysholm J. The late course of acute partial anterior cruciate ligament tears. A nine to 15-year follow-up evaluation. *Clin Orthop Rel Res.* 1992;281:152–158.

20. Terry GC, Norwood LA, Hughston JC, et al. How iliotibial tract injuries of the knee combine with acute anterior cruciate ligament tears to influence abnormal anterior tibial displacement. *Am J Sports Med.* 1993;21:55–60.
21. Winkel D, Matthijs O, Phelps V. *Examination of the Knee.* Maryland, MD: Aspen; 1997.
22. Reid DC. Knee ligament injuries, anatomy, classification, and examination. In: Reid DC, ed. *Sports Injury Assessment and Rehabilitation.* New York: Churchill Livingstone; 1992: 437–493.
23. Liu SH, et al. The diagnosis of acute complete tears of the anterior cruciate ligament. *J Bone Joint Surg.* 1995;77:586.
24. Weiss JR, Irrgang JJ, Sawhney R, et al. A functional assessment of anterior cruciate ligament deficiency in an acute and clinical setting. *J Orthop Sports Phys Ther.* 1990;11:372–373.
25. Hanten WP, Pace MB. Reliability of measuring anterior laxity of the knee joint using a knee ligament arthrometer. *Phys Ther.* 1987;67:357–359.
26. Hughston JC, Andrews JR, Cross MJ, et al. Classification of knee ligament instabilities. Part 2. *J Bone Joint Surg.* 1976;58A:173–179.
27. Hughston JC, Andrews JR, Cross MJ, et al. Classification of knee ligament instabilities. Part 1. *J Bone Joint Surg.* 1976;58A:159–172.
28. Strobel M, Stedtfeld HW. *Diagnostic Evaluation of the Knee.* Berlin: Springer-Verlag; 1990.
29. Shino K, Horibe S, Ono K. The voluntary evoked posterolateral drawer sign in the knee with posterolateral instability. *Clin Orthop.* 1987;215:179–186.
30. Hughston JC, Norwood LA. The posterolateral drawer test and external rotation recurvatum test for posterolateral rotary instability of the knee. *Clin Orthop.* 1980;147:82–87.
31. Jensen K. Manual laxity tests for anterior cruciate ligament injuries. *J Orthop Sports Phys Ther.* 1990;11:474–481.
32. Jakob RP, Stäubli HU, Deland JT. Grading the pivot shift. *J Bone Joint Surg.* 1987;69B:294–299.
33. Noyes FR, Grood ES, Cummings JF, et al. An analysis of the pivot shift phenomenon. *Am J Sports Med.* 1991;19:148–155.
34. Bull AM, Andersen HN, Basso O, et al. Incidence and mechanism of the pivot shift. An in vitro study. *Clin Orthop Rel Res.* 1999;363:219–231.
35. Galway HR, Beaupre A, MacIntosh DL. Pivot shift: a clinical sign of symptomatic anterior cruciate deficiency. *J Bone Joint Surg.* 1972;54B:763–764.
36. Bach BR, Jr., Jones GT, Sweet FA, et al. Arthroscopy-assisted anterior cruciate ligament reconstruction using patellar tendon substitution. Two- to four-year follow-up results. *Am J Sports Med.* 1994;22:758–767.
37. Daniel DM, Stone ML, Riehl B. Ligament surgery: the evaluation of results. In: Daniel DM, Akeson WH, O'Connor JJ, eds. *Knee Ligaments, Structure, Function and Repair.* New York: Raven Press; 1990: 521–534.
38. Donaldson WF, Warren RF, Wickiewicz TL. A comparison of acute anterior cruciate ligament examinations. *Am J Sports Med.* 1985;13:5–10.
39. Norwood LA, Andrews JR, Meisterling RC, et al. Acute anterolateral rotatory instability of the knee. *J Bone Joint Surg.* 1979;61A:704–709.

40. DeHaven KE. Diagnosis of acute knee injuries with hemarthrosis. *Am J Sports Med*. 1980;8:9–14.
41. Otter C, Aufdemkampe G, Lezeman H. Diagnostiek van knieletsel en relatie tussen de aanwezigheid van knieklachten en de resultaten van functionele testen en Biodex-test, In Jaarboek 1994 Fysiotherapie Kinesitherapie. Houten: Bohn, Stafleu, van Loghum; 1994: 195–228.
42. Harilainen A, Sandelin J, Osterman K, et al. Prospective preoperative evaluation of anterior cruciate ligament instability of the knee joint and results of reconstruction with patellar ligament. *Clin Orthop*. 1993;297:17–22.
43. Losee RE. Concepts of the pivot shift. *Clin Orthop*. 1983;172:45–51.
44. Losee RE, Johnson TR, Southwick WO. Anterior subluxation of the lateral tibial plateau. A diagnostic test and operative repair. *J Bone Joint Surg*. 1978;60A:1015–1030.
45. Gerber C, Matter P. Biomechanical analysis of the knee after rupture of the anterior cruciate ligament and its primary repair: an instant-centre analysis of function. *J Bone Joint Surg*. 1983;65B:391–399.
46. MacIntosh DL, Galway RD. The lateral pivot shift: a symptomatic and clinical sign of anterior cruciate insufficiency. *85th Annual Meeting of American Orthopaedic Association*, Tucker's Town, Bermuda; 1972.
47. Slocum DB, Larson RL. Rotatory instability of the knee. *J Bone and Joint Surg*. 1968;50A:211–225.
48. Slocum DB, James SL, Larson RL, et al. Clinical test for anterolateral rotary instability of the knee. *Clin Orthop Relat Res*. 1976;118:63–69.
49. Grelsamer RP, McConnell J. Examination of the patellofemoral joint, *The Patella: A Team Approach*. Maryland: Aspen; 1998: 109–118.
50. Apley AG. The diagnosis of meniscus injuries: Some new clinical methods. *J Bone and Joint Surg*. 1947;29B:78–84.
51. Kuo L, Chung W, Bates E, et al. The hamstring index. *J Pediatr Orthop*. 1997;17:78–88.
52. Gautam VK, Anand S. A new test for estimating iliotibial band contracture. *J Bone Joint Surg*. 1998;80B:474–475.
53. Steill IG, Wells HA, Hoag RH, et al. Implementation of the Ottawa Knee Rule for the use of radiography in acute knee injuries. *JAMA*. 1997;278:2075–2079.
54. Stiell IG, Greenberg GH, Wells GA, et al. Prospective validation of a decision rule for the use of radiography in acute knee injuries. *JAMA*. 1996;275:611–615.
55. Seaberg DC, Yealy DM, Lukens T, et al. Multicenter comparison of two clinical decision rules for the use of radiography in acute, high-risk knee injuries. *Ann Emerg Med*. 1998;32:8–13.
56. Guide to physical therapist practice. *Phys Ther*. 2001;81:S13–S95.

QUESTIONS

1. Which of the two knee menisci is the larger and thicker?
2. Classify each of the following joints: superior tibiofibular, inferior tibiofibular, tibiofemoral, patellofemoral.

3. Which knee ligaments are intra-articular but extrasynovial?
4. Which portion of the meniscus is vascular?
5. What is the function of the posterior oblique ligament (POL)?
6. What is the major function of the posterior cruciate ligament?
7. Describe the symptoms of an irritated plica.
8. What is the normal amount of tibial torsion?
9. Which of the two knee meniscus is most commonly injured?
10. what is the Q-angle?
11. What is bipartite patella?
12. What is Hoffa's disease?
13. What is the weight-bearing status of most patients following a total knee arthroplasty?
14. What diagnosis should you suspect in a patient you are treating following knee arthroplasty who has developed increased calf swelling and localized tenderness?
15. List the four sites of potential fibular nerve entrapment.
16. What is the capsular pattern of the tibiofemoral joint?
17. Which aspect of the medial meniscus produces locking with flexion if damaged?
18. Which of the menisci is oval and which is round?
19. How should you position the patient's knee in order to manual muscle test the popliteus muscle?
20. Does the popliteus produce external rotation of the femur in weight bearing or nonweight bearing?
21. Which of the knee ligaments, the collaterals or the cruciates prevent external rotation of the tibia?
22. In the valgus stress test, which of the MCL fibers are tested with the knee positioned in 90 degrees° of flexion?
23. What is the correct term for "sabre legs"?
24. During what part in the range is superior articulating facet of the patella in contact with the femur?
25. What peripheral nerve is labile around the neck of the fibula?
26. Which thigh muscle has some fibers that participate in the oblique popliteal ligament?

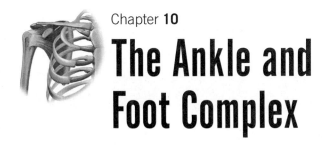

Chapter **10**

The Ankle and Foot Complex

OVERVIEW

Despite the fact that the ankle complex is endowed with multiple structural supports, it is the most commonly injured part in the body.[1] As elsewhere, injuries to this area can be either microtraumatic or macrotraumatic. Due to the many articulations, ligament and muscular attachments, and a complex biomechanical arrangement, obtaining an accurate diagnosis necessitates a thorough knowledge of surface anatomy and biomechanics combined with the findings of a detailed history and physical examination.

● Clinical Pearl

Foot problems may result from trauma, congenital abnormalities, overuse, systemic illness, or poorly fitting shoes. Epidemiologically, lateral ankle sprains are the most common sports injuries.

Anatomy

The majority of the support provided to the ankle and foot joints (Table 10-1) comes by way of the arrangement of the ankle mortise and by the numerous ligaments found here (Table 10-2). Further stabilization is afforded by an abundant number of tendons that cross this joint complex (Table 10-3) (Table 10-4) (Figures 10-1 through 10-3). These tendons are also involved in producing foot and ankle movements and are held in place by retinaculi.

Examination

The exact form of the examination of the foot and ankle complex is very dependent on the acuteness of the condition.

Table 10-1 The Joints of the Foot and Ankle: Their Open-packed, Close-packed Positions, and Capsular Patterns

Joints of the Hindfoot	Open-pack Position	Close-pack Position	Capsular Pattern
Tibiofibular joint	Plantar flexion	Maximum dorsiflexion	Pain on stress
Talocrural joint	10 degrees plantar flexion and midway between inversion and eversion	Maximum dorsiflexion	Plantar flexion, dorsiflexion
Subtalar joint	Midway between extremes of range of motion	Supination	Varus, valgus
Joints of the Midfoot			
Midtarsal joints	Midway between extremes of ROM	Supination	Dorsiflexion, plantar flexion, adduction, medial rotation
Joints of the Forefoot			
Tarsometatarsal joints	Midway between extremes of range of motion	Supination	None
Metatarsophalangeal joints	10 degrees extension	Full extension	Great toe: Extension, flexion 2nd-5th toes: Variable
Interphalangeal joints	Slight flexion	Full extension	Flexion, extension

◉ Clinical Pearl

An inability to bear weight, severe pain, and rapid swelling indicate a serious injury such as a capsular tear, fracture, or grade III ligament sprain.[2-5] In such cases the patient should be referred for further medical examination.

History

The clinician must determine whether the onset was the result of an injury or whether the symptoms occurred gradually. Information about the mechanism

Table 10-2 Ankle and Foot Joints and Associated Ligaments

Joint	Associated Ligament	Fiber Direction	Motions Limited
Distal tibiofibular	Anterior tibiofibular	Distolateral	Distal glide of fibula
			Plantar flexion
	Posterior tibiofibular	Distolateral	Distal glide of fibular
			Plantar flexion
	Interosseous		Separation of tibia and fibula
Talocrural	Deltoid (medial collateral) Superficial		
	Tibionavicular	Plantar–anterior	Plantar flexion, abduction
	Tibiocalcaneal	Plantar, plantar-	Eversion, abduction
	Posterior tibiotalar	post	Dorsiflexion, abduction
	Deep	Plantar–posterior	
	Anterior tibiotalar	Anterior	Eversion, abduction, plantar flexion
	Lateral or fibular collateral		
	Anterior talofibular		Plantar flexion
		Anterior–medial	Inversion
			Anterior displacement of foot
	Calcaneofibular		Inversion
		Posterior–medial	Dorsiflexion
	Posterior talofibular		Dorsiflexion
		Horizontal (lateral)	Posterior displacement of foot
	Lateral talocalcaneal		Inversion
			Dorsiflexion
	Anterior capsule	Posterior–medial	Plantar flexion
	Posterior capsule		Dorsiflexion
Subtalar	Interosseous talocalcaneal		
	Anterior band	Proximal-anterior-lateral	Inversion
			Joint separation
	Posterior band		Inversion
		Proximal-posterior-lateral	Joint separation
	Lateral talocalcaneal		
	Deltoid		
	Lateral collateral	(See talocrural)	Dorsiflexion
	Posterior talocalcaneal	(See talocrural)	Eversion
	Medial talocalcaneal	(See talocrural)	Inversion
	Anterior talocalcaneal (cervical ligaments)	Vertical Plantar–anterior Plantar-posterior-lateral	

(continued on following page)

Table 10-2 *(continued from previous page)*

Joint	Associated Ligament	Fiber Direction	Motions Limited
Main ligamentous support of longitudinal arches	Long plantar	Anterior, slightly medial	Eversion
	Short plantar		Eversion
	Plantar calcaneonavicular	Anterior	Eversion
	Plantar aponeurosis	Dorsal-anterior medial	Eversion
		Anterior	
Midtarsal or transverse	Bifurcated		Joint separation
	Medial band	Longitudinal	Plantar flexion
	Lateral band	Horizontal	Inversion
	Dorsal talonavicular	Longitudinal	Plantar flexion of talus on navicular
	Dorsal calcaneocuboid	Longitudinal	Inversion, plantar flexion
	Ligaments supporting the arches		
Intertarsal	Numerous ligaments named by two interconnected bones (dorsal and plantar ligaments)		Joint motion in direction causing lig tightness
			Flattening of transverse arch
	Interosseous ligaments connecting cuneiforms, cuboid, and navicular		
	Ligaments supporting arches		
Tarsometatarsal	Dorsal, plantar, and interosseous		Joint separation
Intermetatarsal	Dorsal, plantar, and interosseous		Joint separation
			Joint separation
	Deep transverse metatarsal		Flattening of transverse arch
Metatarsophalangeal	Fibrous capsule		
	Dorsally, thin-separated from extensor tendons by bursae		Flexion
			Extension
	Inseparable from deep surface of plantar and collateral ligaments	Plantar-anterior	Flexion, abduction, or adduction in flexion
			Extension
	Collateral		
	Plantar, grooved for flexor tendons		

Joint	Associated Ligament	Fiber Direction	Motions Limited
Interphalangeal	Collateral		Flexion, abduction, or adduction in flexion
	Plantar		Extension
	Extensor hood replaces dorsal ligaments		Flexion

Table 10-3 Intrinsic Muscles of the Foot

Muscle	Proximal	Distal	Innervation
Extensor digitorum brevis	Distal superior surface of calcaneus	Dorsal surface of second through fourth toes, base of proximal phalanx	Deep peroneal S1 and S2
Abductor hallucis	Tuberosity of calcaneus and plantar aponeurosis	Base of proximal phalanx, medial side	Medial plantar L5 and S1 (L4)
Adductor hallucis	Base of second, third, and fourth metatarsals and deep plantar ligaments	Proximal phalanx of first digit lateral side	Medial and lateral plantar S1 and S2
Lumbricals	Medial and adjacent sides of flexor digitorum longus tendon to each lateral digit	Medial side of proximal phalanx and extensor hood	Medial and lateral plantarL5, S1, and S2 (L4)
Plantar interossei			
First	Base and medial side of third metatarsal	Base of proximal phalanx and extensor hood of third digit	Medial and lateral plantar S1 and S2
Second	Base and medial side of fourth metatarsal	Base of proximal phalanx and extensor hood of fourth digit	
Third	Base and medial side of fifth metatarsal	Base of proximal phalanx and extensor hood of fifth digit	
Dorsal interossei			
First	First and second metatarsal bones	Proximal phalanx and extensor hood of second digit medially	Medial and lateral plantar S1 and S2
Second	Second and third metatarsal bones	Proximal phalanx and extensor hood ofsecond digit laterally	
Third	Third and fourth metatarsal bones	Proximal phalanx and extensor hood of third digit laterally	
Fourth	Fourth and fifth metatarsal bones	Proximal phalanx and extensor hood of fourth digit laterally	
Abductor digiti minimi	Lateral side of fifth metatarsal bone	Proximal phalanx of fifth digit	Lateral plantar S1 and S2

Table 10-4 Extrinsic Muscle Attachments and Innervation

Muscle	Proximal	Distal	Innervation
Gastrocnemius	Medial and lateral condyle of femur	Posterior surface of calcaneusthrough Achilles tendon	Tibial S2 (S1)
Plantaris	Lateral supracondylar line of femur	Posterior surface of calcaneus through Achilles tendon	Tibial S2 (S1)
Soleus	Head of fibula, proximal third of shaft, soleal line and midshaft of posterior tibia	Posterior surface of calcaneus through Achilles tendon	Tibial S2 (S1)
Tibialis anterior	Distal to lateral tibial condyle, proximal half of lateral tibial shaft, and interosseous membrane	First cuneiform bone, medial and plantar surfaces and base of first metatarsal	Deep fibular (peroneal) L4 (L5)
Tibialis posterior	Posterior surface of tibia, proximal two thirds posterior of fibula, and interosseous membrane	Tuberosity of navicular bone, tendinous expansion to other tarsals and metatarsals	Tibial L4 and L5
Fibularis longus	Lateral condyle of tibia, head and proximal two thirds of fibula	Base of first metatarsal and first cuneiform, lateral side	Superficial fibular (peroneal) L5 and S1 (S2)
Fibularis brevis	Distal two thirds of lateral fibular shaft	Tuberosity of fifth metatarsal	Superficial fibular (peroneal) L5 and S1 (S2)
Fibularis tertius	Lateral slip from extensor digitorum longus	Tuberosity of fifth metatarsal	Deep fibular (peroneal) L5 and S1
Flexor hallucis brevis	Plantar surface of cuboid and third cuneiform bones	Base of proximal phalanx of great toe	Medial plantar S3 (S2)
Flexor hallucis longus	Posterior distal two thirds fibula	Base of distal phalanx of great toe	Tibial S2 (S3)
Flexor digitorum brevis	Tuberosity of calcaneus	One tendon slip into base of middle phalanx of each of the lateral four toes	Medial and lateral plantar S3 (S2)
Flexor digitorum longus	Middle three fifths of posterior tibia	Base of distal phalanx of lateral four toes	Tibial S2 (S3)
Extensor hallucis longus	Middle half of anterior shaft of fibula	Base of distal phalanx of great toe	Deep fibular (peroneal) L5 and S1

(continued on following page)

Muscle	Proximal	Distal	Innervation
Extensor hallucis brevis	Distal superior and lateral surfaces of calcaneus	Dorsal surface of proximal phalanx	Deep fibular (peroneal) S1 and S2
Extensor digitorum longus	Lateral condyle of tibia proximal anterior surface of shaft of fibula	One tendon to each lateral four toes, to middle phalanx and extending to distal phalanges	Deep fibular (peroneal) L5 and S1

should include, when, where, and how the injury occurred. Details about the mechanism of injury allow the clinician to infer the pathological status and structures involved, although it must be remembered that the patient's recollection of the mechanism frequently does not correspond to the structures damaged.[6,7] Where possible, the position of the foot and ankle at the time of the injury should also be determined.

⬤ Clinical Pearl

Most ankle injuries occur when the foot is plantar flexed, inverted, and adducted (Table 10-5)[8]. This same mechanism can also lead to

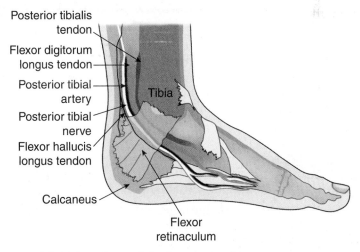

Posterior tibialis tendon
Flexor digitorum longus tendon
Posterior tibial artery
Posterior tibial nerve
Flexor hallucis longus tendon
Calcaneus
Tibia
Flexor retinaculum

Figure 10-1 Medial tendons of the foot and ankle.

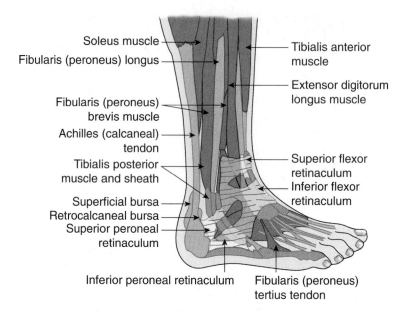

Soleus muscle

Fibularis (peroneus) longus

Fibularis (peroneus) brevis muscle

Achilles (calcaneal) tendon

Tibialis posterior muscle and sheath

Superficial bursa

Retrocalcaneal bursa

Superior peroneal retinaculum

Inferior peroneal retinaculum

Tibialis anterior muscle

Extensor digitorum longus muscle

Superior flexor retinaculum

Inferior flexor retinaculum

Fibularis (peroneus) tertius tendon

Figure 10-2 Lateral aspect of the foot and ankle.

more serious conditions such as a malleolar or talar dome fracture. A dorsiflexion injury with associated snapping and pain on the lateral aspect of the ankle that rapidly diminishes may indicate a tear of the fibular (peroneal) retinaculum.[9]

Information about the time of injury, the time of the onset of swelling, and its location are important. Most often the patients can point to the location of the initial pain. The patient may note hearing a "snap," "crack," or "pop" at the time of injury, which could indicate a ligamentous injury or a fracture.

 Clinical Pearl

It is worth remembering that the clinical presentation of subtle fractures can be similar to that of ankle sprains, and these fractures are frequently missed on the initial examination.

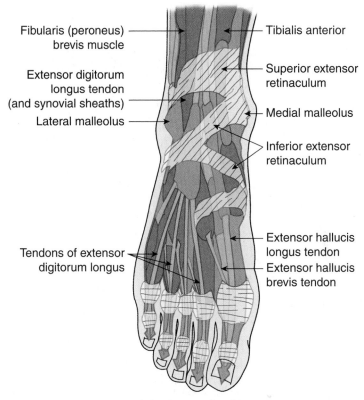

Fibularis (peroneus) brevis muscle

Extensor digitorum longus tendon (and synovial sheaths)

Lateral malleolus

Tibialis anterior

Superior extensor retinaculum

Medial malleolus

Inferior extensor retinaculum

Extensor hallucis longus tendon

Extensor hallucis brevis tendon

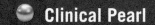

Tendons of extensor digitorum longus

Figure 10-3 Anterior aspect of the foot and ankle.

Determining the location of the pain can provide some clues as to the cause (Figure 10-4). The site and severity of the pain can be measured using a body diagram and visual analogue scale, respectively.

Clinical Pearl

A stress fracture, or tendonitis, typically has a localized site of pain, whereas diffuse pain is associated with compartment syndromes.

The distribution of pain is important, and the clinician should rule out whether the pattern is dermatomal, from a peripheral nerve, or referred from a distal structure (refer to Systems Review).[10]

Table 10-5 Summary and Comparison of Common Foot and Ankle Fractures

Fracture Type	Mechanism of Injury	Examination Findings*
Talar dome (lateral)	Inversion with dorsiflexion	Tenderness anterior to the lateral malleolus, along the anterior border of the talus
Talar dome (medial)	Inversion with plantar flexion or atraumatic	Tenderness posterior to the medial malleolus, along the posterior border of the talus
Lateral talar process	Rapid inversion with dorsiflexion	Point tenderness over the lateral process (anterior and inferior to the lateral malleolus)
Posterior talar process (lateral tubercle)	Hyperplantar flexion or forced inversion	Tenderness to deep palpation anterior to the Achilles tendon over posterolateral talus Plantar flexion may reproduce pain.
Posterior talar process (medial tubercle)	Dorsiflexion with pronation	Tenderness to deep palpation between the medial malleolus and the Achilles tendon
Anterior process of the calcaneus	Inversion with plantar flexion can lead to an avulsion fracture. Forced dorsiflexion can cause a compression fracture.	Point tenderness over the calcanealcuboid joint (approximately 1 cm inferior and 3 to 4 cm anterior to the lateral malleolus)

AP = anteroposterior; NWBSLC = nonweight-bearing, short leg cast.
*Data from reference 8.

Information should be gleaned about activities that aggravate the symptoms. For example, pain with forced dorsiflexion and eversion, and with squatting activities, may suggest ankle instability. Pain after activity suggests an overuse, or chronic injury. Pain during an activity suggests stress on the injured structure.

If there is no traumatic event, the clinician must determine if there has been a change in exercise or activity intensity (increased mileage with runners), training surface, or changes in body weight, or shoe wear (causal agents).[6,7]

• Increased symptoms associated with an increase in exercise or activity intensity likely indicate an overuse injury.

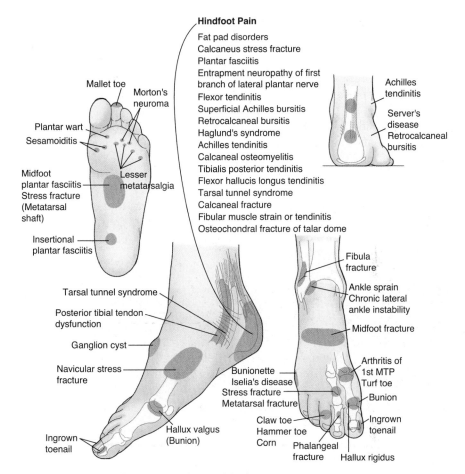

Hindfoot Pain

Fat pad disorders
Calcaneus stress fracture
Plantar fasciitis
Entrapment neuropathy of first branch of lateral plantar nerve
Flexor tendinitis
Superficial Achilles bursitis
Retrocalcaneal bursitis
Haglund's syndrome
Achilles tendinitis
Calcaneal osteomyelitis
Tibialis posterior tendinitis
Flexor hallucis longus tendinitis
Tarsal tunnel syndrome
Calcaneal fracture
Fibular muscle strain or tendinitis
Osteochondral fracture of talar dome

Mallet toe
Morton's neuroma
Plantar wart
Sesamoiditis
Midfoot plantar fasciitis
Stress fracture (Metatarsal shaft)
Lesser metatarsalgia
Insertional plantar fasciitis

Achilles tendinitis
Server's disease
Retrocalcaneal bursitis

Tarsal tunnel syndrome
Posterior tibial tendon dysfunction
Ganglion cyst
Navicular stress fracture
Ingrown toenail
Hallux valgus (Bunion)

Fibula fracture
Ankle sprain
Chronic lateral ankle instability
Midfoot fracture
Arthritis of 1st MTP
Turf toe
Bunion
Ingrown toenail

Bunionette
Iselia's disease
Stress fracture
Metatarsal fracture
Claw toe
Hammer toe
Corn
Phalangeal fracture
Hallux rigidus

Figure 10-4 Pain location and possible diagnoses.

- Complaints of cramping may accompany muscular fatigue or intermittent claudication from arterial insufficiency.
- Increased symptoms when walking or running on uneven terrain as compared with an even terrain may suggest ankle instability.
- Increased symptoms when walking or running on hard surfaces as compared to a stiffer surface may suggest a lack of shock absorbency of the foot or shoe.

Additionally, questions regarding past medical history, previous ankle injury, goals of the patient regarding functional results, and level and intensity of sports involvement are important to individualize the intervention.

Systems Review

As symptoms can be referred distally to the foot and ankle from a host of other joints and conditions, the clinician must be able to differentially diagnose from the presenting signs and symptoms. The cause of the referred symptoms may be neurological or systemic in origin. If a disorder involving a specific nerve root (L4, L5, S1, or S2) is suspected, the necessary sensory, motor, and reflex testing should be performed. Peripheral nerve entrapments, although not common, may also occur in this region, and often go unrecognized. These include Morton neuroma and entrapment of the tibial nerve or its branches, the deep fibular (peroneal) nerve, superficial fibular (peroneal) nerve, sural and saphenous nerves.[11]

Systemic problems that may involve the leg, foot, and ankle include diabetes mellitus (peripheral neuropathy), osteomyelitis, gout and pseudogout, sickle cell disease, complex regional pain syndrome, peripheral vascular disease, and rheumatoid arthritis.

 Clinical Pearl

A systemic problem, such as rheumatoid arthritis, may be associated with other signs and symptoms, including other joint pain, although the other joint pain may also be the result of overcompensation in the rest of the kinetic chain.

Warning signs at the ankle and foot, which should alert the clinician to a more insidious condition, include the following:

- Immediate and continuous inability to bear weight, which may indicate a fracture.
- Nocturnal pain, which may indicate a malignancy, hemarthrosis, fracture, or infection.
- Gross pain during valgus motions, which may indicate compression of a fractured lateral malleolus.
- Pain and weakness during resisted eversion, which may indicate fracture of the fifth metatarsal bases.
- Calf pain and/or tenderness, swelling with pitting edema, increased skin temperature, superficial venous dilatation, or cyanosis may indicate the presence of a deep vein thrombosis (DVT), which requires immediate medical attention.

- Gross tenderness during pressure on the distal fibula, which may indicate a fibular fracture.
- Feelings of warmth or coldness in the foot. An abnormally warm foot can indicate local inflammation, but can also originate from a tumor in the pelvis or lumbar region.[12] An abnormally cold foot usually indicates a vascular problem.[12]

Tests and Measures

Observation

Assessment of the foot and ankle begins as the patient enters the examination room with observation of the patient's gait pattern, and static standing posture. The observation of the foot and ankle complex can provide the clinician with a wealth of information, including clues about static and dynamic, and structural or mechanical foot abnormalities.

 Clinical Pearl

It is extremely important to observe the entire kinetic chain when assessing the foot, and ankle. Weight-bearing and nonweight-bearing alignment and postures of the lower extremity are compared where possible.

 Clinical Pearl

A patient with an acquired flatfoot from posterior tibial tendon dysfunction will have increased valgus at the calcaneus and more than two visible toes ("too many toes" sign) when viewed from behind.

 Clinical Pearl

An important part of the examination of the foot and ankle is the gait assessment. Gait is best observed with the patient barefoot. If an antalgic gait is present the clinician must determine why to help rule out weight-bearing pain from other structures within the kinetic chain. Gait abnormalities may result from neuromuscular weakness, soft-tissue contractures, lower extremity malignment, or pain (see Chapter 3).

The leg, foot, and ankle are observed for the presence of bruising, cyanosis, erythema, pallor, skin breakdown, swelling, or unusual angulation. Cyanosis and pallor indicate problems with vascular supply.[13] The appearance of bluish–black plaques on the posterior and posterior–lateral aspect of one or both heels in a young distance runner is found in a condition called *black-dot heel*, which results from a shearing stress or a pinching of the heel between the counter and the sole of the shoe at heel strike during running.

 Clinical Pearl

Retromalleolar swelling could suggest a tear of the fibularis (peroneus) brevis tendon.

Swelling and pain on the posterior aspect of the distal fibula may indicate a traumatic fibularis (peroneal) tendon subluxation.[14]

Swelling only on the anterolateral aspect of the ankle joint can indicate an anterolateral ankle impingement. This can be confirmed if pain is elicited with passive forced ankle dorsiflexion, and extreme ankle eversion and inversion.[15]

Callus formation on the sole of the foot is an indicator of dysfunction. Calluses provide the clinician with an index to the degree of shear stresses applied to the foot, and clearly outline abnormal weight-bearing areas.[16] In adequate amounts, calluses provide protection, but in excess, may cause pain.

 Clinical Pearl

Callus formation under the second and third metatarsal heads could indicate excessive pronation in a flexible foot, or Morton neuroma if just under the former. A callus under the fifth, and sometimes the fourth, metatarsal head may indicate an abnormally rigid foot.

The weight bearing and wear patterns of the shoes should be noted. The greatest amount of wear on the sole of the shoe should occur beneath the ball of the foot, in the area corresponding to the first, second, and third metatarsophalangeal (MTP) joints and slight wear to the lateral side of the heel.

⊜ Clinical Pearl

Old running shoes belonging to patients who excessively pronate tend to display overcompression of the medial arch of the midsole and extensive wear of the lateral regions of the heel counter and medial forefoot. The upper portion of the shoe should demonstrate a transverse crease at the level of the MTP joints. A stiff first MTP joint can produce a crease line that runs obliquely, from forward and medial to backward and lateral.[17]

The cup, at the rear of the shoe, which is formed by the heel counter, should be vertical and symmetrical with respect to the shoe.[18] A medial inclination of the cup, with bulging of the lateral lip of the counter, indicates a pronated foot.[17] A lateral bulge of the heel counter indicates a supinated foot. Scuffing of the top of the shoe might indicate tibialis anterior weakness.[19]

With the patient standing, the transverse and longitudinal arches should be grossly evaluated for accentuation or collapse.

The nonweight-bearing component of the examination is initiated by having the patient seated on the edge of the bed, feet dangling. In this position, the feet should adopt an inverted and plantar-flexed pose. A mobile or nonstructural flat foot will take on a more normal configuration in nonweight bearing, whereas a fixed or structural flat foot will maintain its planus state. By placing one hand on the patella, and the other hand on the tips of the malleoli, the clinician should note approximately 20 degrees to 30 degrees of external rotation of the ankle in relation to the knee.[20]

Palpation

Careful palpation, which can provide vital information in identifying the source of symptoms, should be performed with the involved and uninvolved leg, foot, and ankle to differentiate tenderness of specific structures (Figures 10-1 through 10-3 and Figure 10-5). Areas of localized swelling and ecchymosis over the ligaments on the medial or lateral aspects of the foot and ankle should be noted. In addition, the clinician should note the borders of ecchymosis, the temperature and tautness of the shin, as well as the suppleness of the soft tissues.[13]

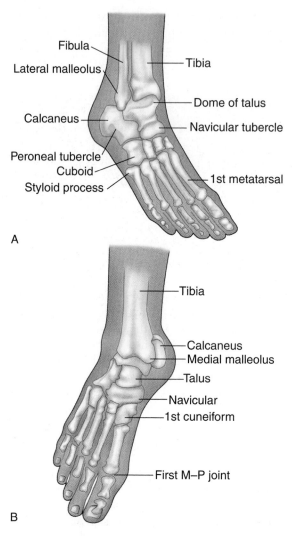

Figure 10-5 Palpation points.

Clinical Pearl

Inflamed tendons are often characterized by swollen tendon sheaths, pain with direct palpation, and pain with both active movement and passive stretching of the tendon.[13] Partial rupture of tendons may present with an enlarged, bulbous thickening of the tendon at the rupture site.[13]

Posterior Aspect of Foot and Ankle

Achilles tendon
The Achilles tendon is inspected for contour changes such as swelling, erythema, and thickening. Any gaps or nodules in the tendon and specific sites of pain should be carefully examined. Palpable gaps in the tendon, accompanied by an inability to rise up on the toes could indicate a rupture of the tendon. The most common site of Achilles tendon rupture is 2 to 6 cm proximal to the insertion of the Achilles tendon into the calcaneus.[13]

Calcaneus
At the distal end of the Achilles tendon is the calcaneal tuberosity. The posterior aspect of the calcaneus and surrounding soft tissue is palpated for evidence of exostosis ("pump bump" or Haglund deformity), and associated swelling (retrocalcaneal bursitis). The inferior medial process of the calcaneus, just distal to the weight-bearing portion serves as the attachment of the plantar fascia and is often tender with plantar fasciitis.

Anterior and Anterior–Medial Aspect of Foot and Ankle
While reading the next section, the reader may find it helpful to remove a shoe and sock and self-palpate.

Great toe and the phalanges
Beginning medially, the clinician locates and palpates the great toe and its two phalanges. The first metatarsal bone is more proximal, the head of which should be palpated for tenderness on the lateral aspect (bunion), and inferior aspect (sesamoiditis).

Moving laterally from the phalanges of the great toe, the clinician palpates the phalanges and metatarsal heads of the other four toes.

Tenderness of the 2nd metatarsal head could indicate the presence of Freiberg disease, an osteochondritis of the 2nd metatarsal head.

🌑 Clinical Pearl

A callus under the 2nd and 3rd metatarsal head may indicate a fallen metatarsal arch.

Palpable tenderness in the region of the third and fourth metatarsal heads could indicate a Morton neuroma, especially if walking barefoot relieves the characteristic sharp pain between the toes of this condition. Tenderness on the lateral aspect of the fifth metatarsal head could indicate the presence of a *tailor* bunion.

Cuneiform
The first cuneiform is located at the proximal end of the first metatarsal, and is palpated for tenderness.

Navicular
The navicular is the most prominent bone on the medial aspect of the foot. The navicular tuberosity can be located by moving proximally from the medial aspect of the first cuneiform. The talonavicular joint line lies directly proximal to the navicular tuberosity. In addition, the posterior tibialis, which can be made more prominent with resisted plantar flexion, adduction, and supination, can be used as a reference because it inserts on the plantar surface of the navicular (see later). Tenderness of the navicular could indicate the presence of a fracture, or osteochondritis of the navicular (Köhler disease).

2nd and 3rd cuneiforms
These two bones can be palpated by moving laterally from the first cuneiform. Tenderness of these bones may indicate a cuneiform fracture.

Dorsal pedis pulse
The pulse of the dorsal pedis artery, a branch of the anterior tibial artery, can be palpated over the cuneiform bones, between the first and second cuneiform, or between the first and second metatarsal bones.

Medial malleolus
The medial malleolus is palpated for swelling or tenderness. Moving proximally from the anterior aspect of the medial malleolus, the distal aspect of the tibia is palpated. Distal to that is the talus bone. Moving distal from the tibia, the clinician palpates the long extensor tendons, the tibialis anterior, and the extensor retinaculum. The tendon of the tibialis anterior is visible at the level of the medial cuneiform and the base of the 1st metatarsal bone, especially if the foot is positioned in dorsiflexion and supination.

 Clinical Pearl

Tenderness along the posterior and inferior aspect of the medial malleolus, which can radiate distally to the medial arch, could indicate the presence of flexor hallucis longus tendonitis.[13]

Tarsal tunnel

The tarsal tunnel is a fibroosseous tunnel located just posterior to the medial malleolus on the inside of the ankle. The roof of the tarsal tunnel is formed by the deep fascia of the leg and the deep transverse fascia. The proximal and inferior borders of the tunnel are formed by inferior and superior margins of the flexor retinaculum. The superior aspect of the calcaneus, the medial wall of the talus, and the distal–medial aspect of the tibia form the floor of the tunnel. The tendons of the flexor hallucis longus muscle, flexor digitorum longus muscle, tibialis posterior muscle, the posterior tibial nerve, and the posterior tibial artery pass through the tarsal tunnel.

 Clinical Pearl

> Irritation of the posterior tibial nerve can be detected by applying gentle localized percussion over the area of the nerve entrapment (Tinel sign). A positive test is the reproduction of a tingling sensation in the distribution of the posterior tibial nerve (see Special Tests).

Talus

The talus can be located by moving from the distal aspect of the medial malleolus along a line joining the navicular tuberosity. Its location can be made easier by everting and inverting the foot. Eversion causes the talar head to become more prominent, whereas inversion causes the head to be less visible.

Sustentaculum tali

Distal and inferior to the medial malleolus, a shelf-like bony prominence of the calcaneus (the sustentaculum tali) can be palpated. At the dorsal aspect of the sustentaculum tali, the talocalcaneal joint line can be palpated.

Posterior tibialis tendon

This tendon is palpable at the level of the medial malleolus especially with the foot held in plantar flexion and supination. Distal and medial to this tendon, the crossing of the flexor digitorum longus and flexor hallucis tendons can be felt. Palpation of the posterior tibialis tendon along its course will often identify specific areas of pain in the region of synovitis or partial tendon rupture.[13]

Posterior tibial artery

The posterior tibial artery can be located posterior to the medial malleolus, and anterior to the Achilles tendon.

Medial (deltoid) ligaments

These ligaments are usually palpated as a group on the medial aspect of the ankle. The medial (deltoid) ligaments are divided into superficial and deep ligaments. The palpable, although difficult to differentiate, superficial ligaments include the tibionavicular, calcaneotibial, and the superficial posterior talotibial ligament. It is worth remembering that isolated injury to these ligaments is rare. It is difficult to diagnose these injuries by physical examination alone—often stress radiographs in external rotation[21] and valgus talar tilt[22] are needed to confirm suspicion.[13]

Anterior and Anterior–Lateral Aspect of the Foot and Ankle

Tibial crest

The tibial crest is palpated for tenderness, which may indicate the presence of shin splints. Swelling in this area may indicate the presence of anterior compartment syndrome. The muscles of the lateral compartment (fibularis [peronei]) and anterior compartment (tibialis anterior, and the long extensors) are palpated here for swelling or tenderness. Swelling or tenderness of these structures usually indicates inflammation.

Lateral malleolus

The lateral malleolus is located at the distal aspect of the fibula. Distal to the lateral malleolus is the calcaneus.

Fibularis (peroneus) longus

The tendon of the fibularis (peroneus) longus runs superficially behind the lateral malleolus. Resisted pronation and plantar flexion of the foot makes the tendon more prominent. Tenderness along the lateral calcaneal wall to the cuboid may indicate tendonitis of the fibularis (peroneus) longus.[13]

● Clinical Pearl

Pain with resisted plantar flexion and pronation over the tendon will help implicate the fibularis (peroneus) longus tendon.[14]

Fibularis (peroneus) brevis

The origin for the fibularis (peroneus) brevis is more distal to the fibularis (peroneus) longus and lies deeper. It becomes superficial on the lateral aspect of the foot at its insertion at the tuberosity of the 5th metatarsal.

Clinical Pearl

Tenderness over the posterior and distal aspect of the lateral malleolus may indicate tendonitis of the fibularis (peroneus) brevis.[13] Pain with resisted plantar flexion and abduction over the tendon will help implicate the fibularis (peroneus) brevis tendon.[14]

Anterior talofibular ligament (ATFL)
The ATFL can be palpated two to three fingerbreadths anterior–inferior to the lateral malleolus.[2] This is usually the area of most extreme tenderness following an inversion sprain. The anterior aspect of the distal tibiofibular syndesmosis may also be tender following this type of sprain.

Calcaneofibular ligament (CFL)
The CFL can be palpated one to two fingerbreadths inferior to the lateral malleolus.[2]

Posterior talofibular ligament (PTFL)
The PTFL can be palpated posterior–inferior to the posterior edge of the lateral malleolus.[2]

Sinus tarsi
The sinus tarsi is visible as a concave space between the lateral tendon of the extensor digitorum longus muscle and the anterior aspect of the lateral malleolus. The origin of the extensor digitorum brevis is at the level of this tunnel.

Cuboid
The cuboid bone can be palpated by moving distally about one finger width from the sinus tarsi.

Active and Passive Range of Motion

Range of motion (ROM) testing is divided into active range of motion (AROM) (Figure 10-6), and passive range of motion (PROM) with overpressure to assess the end feel. AROM tests are used to assess the patient's willingness to move and the presence of movement restriction patterns such as a capsular or noncapsular pattern. The end feel may provide the clinician with information as to the cause of a motion restriction. The normal ROMs, and end-feels, for the lower leg, ankle, and foot are outlined in Table 10-6. The open- and close-packed positions, and capsular patterns are outlined in Table 10-1.

General AROM of the foot and ankle in the nonweight-bearing position is assessed first, with painful movements being performed last. Weight-bearing tests are then performed. In addition to the foot and ankle tests, the clinician should also assess hip and knee ROM.

If the symptoms are experienced in the hindfoot during the general tests, then passive, active, and resisted inversion and eversion of the heel must be tested. If these and the weight-bearing tests are negative, there is probably no immediate need to proceed with a more detailed examination, although this may have to be done if no other region can be inculpated. However, a more detailed articular scanning examination is required if the symptoms increase and/or the ROM decreases, or an abnormal end feel is detected.

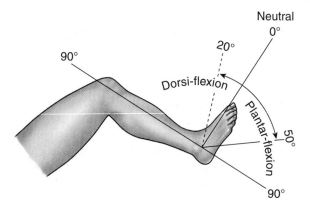

Figure 10-6 ROM of the foot and ankle. (Reproduced with permission from reference 23).

Table 10-6 Normal Ranges of Motion, and End Feels, for the Lower Leg, Ankle, and Foot

Motion	Normal Range (Degrees)	End Feel
Plantar flexion	30 degrees –to 50 degrees	Tissue stretch
Dorsiflexion	20 degrees	Tissue stretch
Hindfoot inversion (supination)	20 degrees	Tissue stretch
Hindfoot eversion (pronation)	10 degrees	Tissue stretch
Toe flexion	Great toe: MTP, 45 degrees ; IP, 90 degrees	Tissue stretch
	Lateral fo degrees r toes: MTP, 40 degrees; PIP, 35 degrees DIP, 60°	
Toe extension	Great toe: MTP, 70 degrees; IP, 0 degree	Tissue stretch
	Lateral four toes: MTP, 40 degrees; PIP, 0 degree; DIP, 30 degrees	

DIP = distal interphalangeal; IP = interphalangeal; MTP = metatarsophalangeal; PIP = proximal interphalangeal.

Distal Tibiofibular Joint

Specific motion at this joint cannot be produced voluntarily. However, the function of this joint can be assessed indirectly by asking the patient to twist around both feet in each direction while weight bearing, or with weight-bearing dorsiflexion.

Dorsiflexion

The patient is positioned in supine, with the knee slightly flexed and supported by a pillow, while the clinician stands at the foot at the table, facing the patient.

Active dorsiflexion is initially performed with the knee flexed. Care must be taken to prevent pronation at the subtalar and oblique midtarsal joint during dorsiflexion. This can be achieved by slightly inverting the foot to lock the longitudinal arch.[20] Passive overpressure is applied. With the knee flexed to 90 degrees, the length of the soleus muscle is examined. Passive overpressure into dorsiflexion when the knee is flexed assesses the joint motion, as well as the soleus length. The soleus is implicated if pain is produced in this test, especially if resisted plantar flexion is painful or more painful with the knee flexed than with the knee extended.

To assess the length of the gastrocnemius, the patient is positioned in supine with the knee extended, and the ankle is positioned in subtalar neutral. The patient is then asked to dorsiflex the ankle. Passive overpressure into dorsiflexion is applied. The normal range is 20 degrees.[24] If the gastrocnemius is shortened, dorsiflexion of the ankle will be reduced as the knee is extended and increased as the knee is flexed. A muscular end feel should be felt with the knee extended, and a capsular end feel should be felt with the knee flexed.

Plantar Flexion

The patient is positioned in supine, with the leg supported by a pillow, while the clinician stands at the foot at the table, facing the patient. The patient is asked to plantar flex the ankle. Plantar flexion of the ankle is approximately 30 degrees to −50 degrees.[25] When tested in weight bearing with the unilateral heel raise, heel inversion should be seen to occur. Failure of the foot to invert may indicate instability of the foot/ankle, or posterior tibialis dysfunction, or adaptive shortening.[26]

 Clinical Pearl

Ankle plantar flexion and dorsiflexion are sagittal plane motions that occur primarily of the talocrural joint.

Hindfoot Inversion and Hindfoot Eversion

Subtalar joint motion is extremely important to normal foot function. A loss of eversion causes weight bearing to occur along the lateral side of the ankle joint. The patient is positioned in prone. Both hindfoot inversion and hindfoot eversion are tested by lining up the longitudinal axis of the leg and vertical axis of the calcaneus. Passive motion of hindfoot inversion is normally 20 degrees.[25] The amount of hindfoot eversion is normally 10 degrees.[25]

 Clinical Pearl

Hindfoot inversion and eversion occur primarily at the subtalar or talocalcaneal articulation. There is usually twice as much inversion as eversion, but the calcaneus should move at least to vertical passively and functionally.

Great Toe Motion

The patient is positioned in supine, with the leg supported by a pillow, while the clinician stands at the foot at the table, facing the patient. Active extension of the great toe is performed and assisted passively without dorsiflexing the first ray. Extension of the great toe occurs primarily at the MTP joint. Passive extension of the great toe at the MTP joint should demonstrate elevation of the medial longitudinal arch (windlass effect), and external rotation of the tibia.[27] MTP joint extension of between 55 degrees and 90 degrees is necessary at terminal stance,[28-30] depending on length of stride, shoe flexibility, and toe-in/toe-out foot placement angle.[31] Forty-five degrees of first MTP flexion, and 90 degrees of interphalangeal (IP) joint flexion are considered normal.[20]

 Clinical Pearl

An inability to spread or fan the toes may indicate loss of intrinsic muscle function.

Strength Testing

Isometric tests are carried out in the extreme range, and if positive, in the neutral range. The straight plane motions of ankle dorsiflexion, plantar flexion, inversion, and eversion are tested initially. Pain with any of these tests requires a more thorough examination of the individual muscles. The individual isometric muscle tests can give the clinician information about patterns of weakness other than from spinal nerve root or peripheral nerve palsies and can also help to isolate the pain generators.

 Clinical Pearl

Weakness on isometric testing needs to be analyzed for the type (increasing weakness with repeated contractions of the same resistance indicating a palsy versus consistent weakness with repeated contractions, which could suggest a deconditioned muscle, or a significant muscle tear), and the pattern of weakness (spinal nerve root, nerve trunk, or peripheral nerve). A painful weakness is invariably a sign of serious pathology, and depending on the pattern, could indicate a fracture or a tumor. However, if a single motion is painfully weak this could indicate muscle inhibition due to pain.

Ankle

Gastrocnemius and plantaris muscles

If no weakness is apparent, a test is performed in the functional position, standing with the knee extended and the opposite foot off the floor. Technically, one heel raise through full ROM while standing with support on one leg scores a 3/5

(Fair) with manual muscle testing with five single-limb heel raises scoring a 4/5 (Good), and 10 single-limb heel raises scoring a 5/5 (Normal). From a functional viewpoint, a wider range of scoring can sometimes prove more useful.

Soleus muscle

The soleus muscle produces plantar flexion of the ankle joint, regardless of the position of the knee. To determine the individual functioning of the soleus as a plantar flexor, the knee is flexed to minimize the effect of the gastrocnemius muscle. To test the soleus, the patient stands with some degree of knee flexion, and then rises up on toes. Ten to 15 raises performed in this fashion are considered normal, 5 to 9 raises are graded as Fair, 1 to 4 raises are graded as Poor, and 0 repetitions is graded as nonfunctional.

Tibialis anterior muscle

The tibialis anterior muscle produces the motion of dorsiflexion and inversion. The knee must remain flexed during the test to allow complete dorsiflexion. The patient's foot is positioned in dorsiflexion and inversion. The leg is stabilized, and resistance is applied to the medial–dorsal aspect of the forefoot into plantar flexion and eversion. Weakness indicates a lesion involving the L4 nerve root or the deep fibular (peroneal) nerve.

Tibialis posterior muscle

The tibialis posterior muscle produces the motion of inversion in a plantar-flexed position. The leg is stabilized in the anatomical position, with the ankle in slight plantar flexion. Resistance is applied to the medial border of the forefoot into eversion and dorsiflexion.

Fibularis (peroneus) longus, fibularis (peroneus) brevis, and fibularis (peroneus) tertius muscles

The lateral compartment muscles and the fibularis (peroneus) tertius muscle produce the motion of eversion. The patient is positioned in supine with the foot over the edge of the table and the ankle in the anatomical position. Resistance is applied to the lateral border of the forefoot. Weakness of the fibularis (peroneus) longus and brevis indicates injury or dysfunction of the fibularis (peroneus) tendons or a lesion involving the superficial fibular (peroneus) nerve.

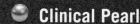

Clinical Pearl

Pain elicited on the lateral aspect of the midfoot with resisted eversion of the foot and plantar flexion of the first ray could indicate a complete rupture of the fibularis (peroneus) longus tendon.[14]

Digits
Grades for the toes differ from the standard format because gravity is not considered a factor.

0: No contraction.
Trace or 1: Muscle contraction is palpated, but no movement occurs.
Poor or 2: Subject can partially complete the ROM.
Fair or 3: Subject can complete the test range.
Good or 4: Subject can complete the test range, but is able to take less resistance on the test side than on the opposite side.
Normal or 5: Subject can complete the test range and take maximal resistance on the test side as compared with the normal side.

Flexor hallucis brevis and longus muscles
The flexor hallucis brevis and flexor hallucis longus muscles produce MTP joint flexion, and IP joint flexion. The foot is maintained in midposition. The first metatarsal is stabilized, and resistance is applied beneath the proximal and distal phalanx of the great toe into toe extension.

 Clinical Pearl

The flexor hallucis muscle is the easiest and most specific muscle to assess for S1 nerve root dysfunction.

Flexor digitorum brevis and longus muscles
The flexor digitorum longus and brevis muscles produce IP joint flexion. The motion is tested with the foot in the anatomical position. If the gastrocnemius muscle is shortened preventing the ankle from assuming the anatomical position, the knee is flexed. The toes may be tested simultaneously.

The foot is held in the midposition and the metatarsals are stabilized. Resistance is applied beneath the distal and proximal phalanges.

Extensor hallucis longus and brevis muscles
The extensor hallucis longus and the extensor hallucis brevis muscles produce the motion of extension of the IP and MTP joints. The foot is maintained in midposition. Resistance is applied to the dorsum of both phalanges of the first digit into toe flexion.

Clinical Pearl

The extensor hallucis muscle is the easiest and most specific muscle to assess for L5 nerve root dysfunction.

Extensor digitorum longus and brevis muscles
The extensor digitorum longus and the extensor digitorum brevis muscles produce the motion of extension at the MTP and IP joints of the lateral four digits from a flexed position. Resistance is applied to the dorsal surface of the proximal and distal phalanges into toe flexion.

Intrinsic Muscles of the Foot
The intrinsic muscles of the foot are tested with the patient in either the supine or sitting position. Most subjects are unable to voluntarily contract the intrinsic muscles of the foot individually.

Abductor hallucis muscle
The metatarsals are stabilized and resistance is applied medially to the distal end of the first phalanx.

Adductor hallucis muscle
The metatarsals are stabilized and resistance is applied to the lateral side of the proximal phalanx of the first digit.

Lumbrical muscles
The lateral four metatarsals are stabilized and resistance is applied to the middle and distal phalanges of the lateral four digits.

Plantar interossei muscles
The lateral three metatarsals are stabilized and resistance is applied to the middle and distal phalanges.

Dorsal interossei and abductor digiti minimi muscles
The metatarsals are stabilized and resistance is applied:

- Dorsal interossei: Applied to the middle and distal phalanges.

- Abductor digiti minimi: Applied to the lateral side of the proximal phalanx of the fifth digit.

Functional Examination

Abnormal biomechanics have been implicated in overuse injuries of the foot and ankle. These abnormalities can occur in the spine, hip, knee, ankle, or foot. Many of the abnormalities that occur in the ankle or foot can be addressed using orthotics or a trial of arch support taping. The functional assessment should include evaluating individuals standing, walking, and when necessary, running with a focus on calcaneal position, arch height, and great toe extension.

Passive Articular Mobility

Passive articular mobility tests assess the accessory motions available between the joint surfaces. These include tests of the accessory glides of the joint, and tests involving joint compression and joint distraction. As with any other joint complex, the quality and quantity of joint motion must be compared with the results from the uninvolved side to determine the level of joint involvement and so that comparisons can be made. For these tests, the patient is positioned in supine or side lying.

Long-Axis Distraction

The clinician stabilizes the proximal segment and applies traction to the distal segment. This test is performed at the talocrural joint (Figure 10-7), the subtalar joint (Figure 10-8), the MTP joints, and the IP joints.

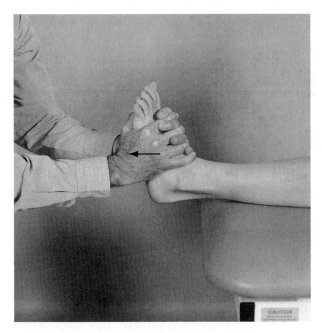

Figure 10-7 Long axis distraction of the talocrural joint.

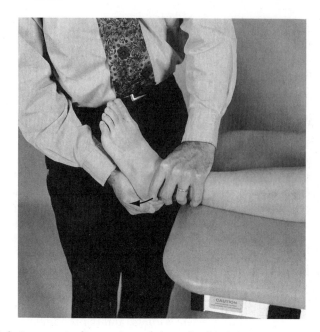

Figure 10-8 Long axis distraction of the subtalar joint.

Anterior-Posterior Glide

To test the anterior movement, the clinician stabilizes the tibia and fibula and draws the talus and foot forward (Figure 10-9). Pulling the tibia forward on the talus and foot (Figure 10-10) tests the posterior movement.

The anterior–posterior glides can also be applied to the midtarsal, tarsometatarsal, MTP, and IP joints.

Tibial Excursion

Tibial excursion in an anterior and posterior direction occurs during dorsiflexion and plantar flexion respectively. This motion may be assessed in the nonweight-bearing position. The calcaneus and talus are fixed, and the tibia and fibula are glided in an anterior and posterior direction (Figure 10-11).[32]

Abduction–Adduction (Subtalar)

The patient is positioned in supine, with the knee slightly flexed and supported by a pillow. The clinician faces the patient. The clinician grasps the forefoot and places it into adduction and abduction. The amount and quality of the motions, as compared with the other foot, are compared. The range of adduction is generally twice that of abduction, approximately 30 degrees and 15 degrees, respectively.[3]

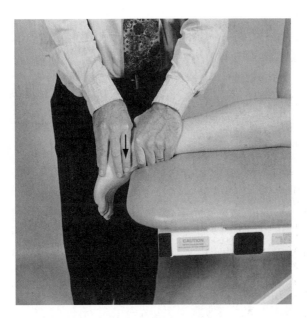

Figure 10-9 Anterior glide of the talus.

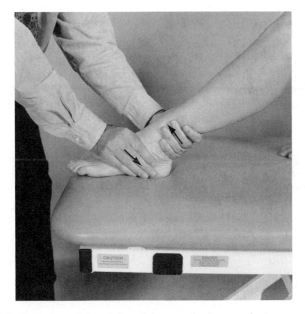

Figure 10-10 Anterior glide of the tibia, producing a relative posterior glide of the talus.

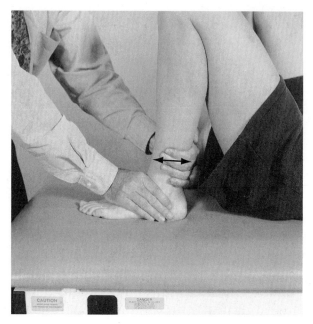

Figure 10-11 Tibial excursion.

Calcaneal Inversion-Eversion

The patient is positioned in supine, with the knee slightly flexed and supported by a pillow, while the clinician faces the patient. The clinician grasps the calcaneus in one hand, while the other hand is placed on the forefoot, to lock the talus. The calcaneus is passively inverted (varus) and everted (valgus) on the talus. The amount and quality of the motions, as compared with the other foot, are compared.

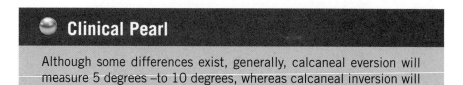

⬤ Clinical Pearl

Although some differences exist, generally, calcaneal eversion will measure 5 degrees –to 10 degrees, whereas calcaneal inversion will measure 20 degrees to 30 degrees.[20,25,33]

Transverse Tarsal Joints (Talonavicular and Calcaneocuboid)

The patient is positioned in supine with the knee flexed approximately 60 degrees and the heel resting on the table. Using one hand, the clinician grasps

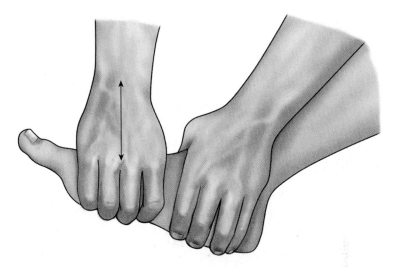

Figure 10-12 Mobility testing the transverse tarsal joints.

and fixes the talus and calcaneus at the level of the talar neck. The other hand grasps the navicular using the navicular tubercle as a landmark (Figure 10-12) and then glides the cuboid dorsally or plantarly on the calcaneus.

Midtarsal Joint Motion
The rotational movements of the midtarsal joint, which allow the forefoot to twist on the rearfoot can be observed in the nonweight-bearing position. The clinician stabilizes the calcaneus with one hand, while inverting and everting the foot with the other hand.[32]

Cuboid Motion
The patient is positioned in prone and the patient's knee is flexed. Using one hand, the clinician grasps the calcaneus, locking it, while with the thumb and index of the other hand, the clinician grasps the cuboid and moves it dorsally and ventrally. The clinician notes the quality and quantity of motion.

Navicular Motion
The patient is positioned in supine with the knee flexed approximately 60 degrees and the heel resting on the table. Using one hand, the clinician grasps and fixes the navicular. With the other hand, the clinician grasps the cuneiforms and moves them dorsally and ventrally (Figure 10-13). The quality and quantity of motion is noted and compared with the other side.

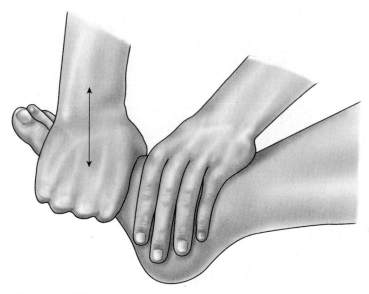

Figure 10-13 Mobility testing the naviculocuneiform joints.

Cuneiform Motion

The patient is positioned in supine with the knee flexed approximately 60 degrees and the heel resting on the table. The clinician grasps and locks the cuneiforms, and then moves the metatarsal joints on the navicular.

First MTP Joint (1st Ray) Motion

The patient is positioned in supine, with the clinician seated at the foot of the table facing away from the patient. The foot to be examined is positioned on a pillow in the clinician's lap. The clinician grasps and locks the first MTP joint, before grasping the great toe first metatarsal joint and moving it into extension and flexion (posteriorly and anteriorly, respectively) (Figure 10-14).

Limited range may result from a combination of biomechanical factors such as excessive pronation or joint glide restriction.[34] To examine the conjunct rotation of the metatarsals, the clinician locks the second metatarsal to evaluate the first, and locks the third to evaluate the second. The quantity and quality of motion is noted and compared with the other side.

Fifth Metatarsal Motion

The patient is positioned in prone. Using one hand, the clinician grasps the cuboid and stabilizes it. With the other hand, the clinician grasps the fifth metatarsal and moves it dorsally and ventrally. To examine the rotatory motion of the

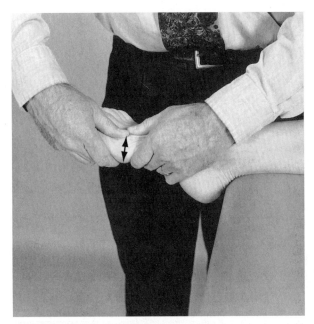

Figure 10-14 Testing the first MTP joint motion.

metatarsal, the clinician locks the fourth metatarsal and examines motion of the fifth. To examine motion of the fourth metatarsal, the third metatarsal is locked. The quality and quantity of motion is noted and compared with the other side.

Phalangeal Motion
The patient is positioned in supine, with the clinician seated at the foot of the table facing away from the patient. The foot to be examined is positioned on a pillow in the clinician's lap. The clinician grasps the metatarsal and locks it with one hand. With the other hand the first phalanx articulating with that metatarsal is grasped. After applying slight traction, the clinician examines the posterior, anterior, abduction, adduction, and rotatory motions. The quantity and quality of motion is noted and compared with the other side.

Special Tests

Special tests are merely confirmatory tests and should not be used alone to form a diagnosis. Selection for their use is at the discretion of the clinician and is based on a complete patient history. The results from these tests are used in conjunction with the other clinical findings. To assure accuracy with these tests, both sides should be tested for comparison.

Ligamentous Stress Tests

The examination of the ligamentous structures in the ankle and foot is essential, not only because of their vast array, but also because of the amount of stability that they provide. Positive results for the ligamentous stability tests include excessive movement as compared with the same test on the uninvolved extremity, pain, depending on the severity, or apprehension.

Mortise/syndesmosis

There are no studies in the literature that discuss the sensitivity, specificity, positive predictive value, or negative predictive value of the tests for syndesmotic injury.

Squeeze (Distal Tibiofibular Compression) Test

To perform the squeeze test, the clinician squeezes the tibia and fibula together at a point about 6 to 8 inches below the knee in the midshaft of the lower leg.[35] Pain felt in the anterolateral aspect of the distal third of the leg may indicate a compromised syndesmosis, if the presence of a tibia and/or fibula fracture, calf contusion, or compartment syndrome has been ruled out.[9,36]

 Clinical Pearl

In a study using fresh human cadavers, the squeeze test produced motion at the distal tibiofibular joint, causing the tibia and fibula to separate.[37]

Clunk (Cotton) Test

The patient is positioned in supine with their foot over the end of the bed. One hand is used to stabilize the distal leg, while the clinician uses the other hand to grasp the heel and move the calcaneus medially and laterally.[38] A clunk can be felt as the talus hits the tibia and fibula if there has been significant mortise widening.[2]

Alternatively, the patient can be positioned in supine with their knee flexed to the point where the ankle is in the position of full dorsiflexion. The clinician applies overpressure into further dorsiflexion by grasping the femoral condyles with one hand and leaning down into the table. The clinician uses the other hand to pull the tibia (crura) anteriorly. Because the ankle is in its close-packed position, no movement should be felt.

Posterior Drawer Test

The posterior drawer test can also be used to test for the presence of instability at the inferior tibiofibular joint. The patient is supine. The hip and knee are fully flexed to provide as much dorsiflexion of the ankle as possible. This drives the wide anterior part of the talus back into the mortise. An anterior stabilizing force is then applied to the cruris, and the foot and talus are translated posteriorly. If the inferior tibiofibular joint is stable, there will be no drawer available, but if there is instability, there will be a drawer.

Lateral collaterals
The lateral collaterals resist inversion and consist of the anterior talofibular, calcaneofibular, and posterior talofibular. An additional function of the lateral ligaments of the ankle is to prevent excessive varus movement, especially during plantar flexion. In extreme plantar flexion, the mortise no longer stabilizes the broader anterior part of the talus, and varus movement of the ankle is then possible. The degree of displacement with these tests can be graded from 1+ to 3+ in excessive movement as compared with the uninvolved ankle.

The Anterior Drawer Test
The anterior drawer stress test is performed to estimate the stability of the ATFL.[39–41] The test is performed with the patient sitting at the end of the bed or lying supine with their knee flexed to relax the gastrocnemius–soleus muscles and the foot supported perpendicular to the leg.[42,43] The clinician uses one hand to stabilize the distal aspect of the leg, while the other hand grasps the patient's heel and positions the ankle in 10 degrees to 15 degrees of plantar flexion. The heel is very gently pulled forward, and, if the test is positive, the talus, and with it the foot, rotates anteriorly out of the ankle mortise, around the intact medial (deltoid) ligament, which serves as the center of rotation. Comparisons are made with the contralateral ankle to avoid any false positives.

 Clinical Pearl

> Opinions vary as to how much difference in displacement is normal with the anterior drawer test, with standards ranging from greater than 2 mm[44] to greater than 4 mm.[1,39,45,46]

This test has limited reliability, particularly if it is negative, or if it is performed without anesthesia in the presence of muscle guarding.[47]

The Dimple Sign
If pain and spasm are minimal, the presence of "a dimple" located just in front of the tip of the lateral malleolus, during the anterior drawer test is a

positive indication for a rupture of the ATFL.[48] This results from a negative pressure created by the forward movement of the talus, which draws the skin inward at the side of ligament rupture.[49] This dimple sign is also seen with a combined rupture of the ATFL and calcaneofibular ligaments.[48]

 Clinical Pearl

The dimple sign is only present within the first 48 hours of injury, and cannot be elicited in ankles examined at 7 days or more after injury, due to organized hematoma and repair tissue blocking the communication between the joint and the subcutaneous tissues.[48]

Gungor Test[50]

The Gungor test can be used to evaluate the anterior displacement of the talus from the ankle mortise. This test is preferable to the anterior drawer test if the ankle is swollen and the patient is guarding.[13] The patient is positioned in prone with the ankle hanging past the end of the examination table and the toes facing downward. The heel is then pressed downward to force the talus anteriorly within the ankle mortise. A positive sign is noted when the skin becomes taut and the Achilles tendon becomes increasingly defined.[50]

Talar Tilt

To perform this test, the clinician medially supports the tibia with one hand, and forcibly inverts the lateral aspect of the heel with the other hand. If comparison of the medial and lateral aspects of the ankle while the foot is everted and inverted demonstrates a difference of greater than 25% between the medial and lateral openings, a positive talar tilt test is noted.[1] Other findings may include a soft end feel, or lateral dimpling.[51] Overall, the literature does not support the use of the talar tilt test as a diagnostic tool.

 Clinical Pearl

With an inverted ankle, strain on the CFL is highest in dorsiflexion; thus, when the ankle is dorsiflexed or in a neutral position, the CFL is the lateral ligament most often injured in inversion sprains.[52] Although isolated CFL tears are uncommon, CFL tears in combination with ATFL tears are the second most common injury pattern (20% of injuries).[52,53] Midsubstance rupture of the CFL remains the most common injury pattern, although a number of fibula or calcaneus avulsion-type injury patterns exist.[53]

ATFL Test

The patient is positioned in supine. The cruris is gripped with the stabilizing hand, using a lumbrical grip, while the other hand grasps over the mortise and onto the neck of talus, so that the index fingers are together at the point between fibula and talus. The clinician moves the patient's foot into plantar flexion and full inversion, and a force is applied in an attempt to adduct (distract) the calcaneus, thereby gapping the lateral side of the ankle. Pain on the lateral aspect of the ankle with this test, and/or displacement depending on severity, may indicate a sprain of the ligament.

Inversion Stress Maneuver

The inversion stress maneuver is a test that attempts to assess CFL integrity.[40] The patient is positioned supine. The cruris is gripped with the stabilizing hand, while the moving hand cups the heel. The ankle is dorsiflexed via the calcaneus to a right angle (total dorsiflexion is impractical) and inverted. An adduction, and anterior–medial translation of the calcaneus is then applied tending to gap the lateral side of the joint. Pain on the lateral aspect of the ankle with this test, and/or displacement depending on severity, may indicate a sprain of the ligament.

Posterior Talofibular

The patient is either prone or supine, and the cruris is gripped or the fibula stabilized. The patient's leg is stabilized in internal rotation, and the foot is placed in full dorsiflexion. The clinician externally rotates the heel/calcaneus, thereby moving the talar attachment of the ligament away from the malleolus. Pain on the lateral aspect of the ankle with this test, and/or displacement depending on severity, may indicate a sprain of the ligament.

Medial (deltoid) ligament complex

The medial (deltoid) ligaments function to resist eversion. Given their strength, these ligaments are only usually injured as the result of major trauma.

Kleiger (External Rotation) Test

The Kleiger (external rotation) test[35,54,55] is a general test to assess the integrity of the medial (deltoid) ligament complex, but can also implicate the syndesmosis if pain is produced over the anterior or posterior tibiofibular ligaments and the interosseous membrane.[36,56,57] If this test is positive, further testing is necessary to determine the source of the symptoms. Information about the mechanism of injury can afford the clinician some clues. Trauma involving external rotation tends to disrupt the deep medial (deltoid) ligaments before disruption of the superficial medial (deltoid) ligaments.[13] In contrast, trauma involving abduction disrupts the superficial medial (deltoid) ligaments, while the deep ligaments remain intact.[58]

The patient sits with their legs dangling over the end of the bed, with the knee flexed to 90 degrees, and foot relaxed. The clinician stabilizes the lower leg with one hand and, using the other hand, grasps the foot and rotates it laterally (Figure 10-15). Pain on the medial and lateral aspect of the ankle, and/or displacement of the talus from the medial malleolus, depending on severity, with this test may indicate a tear of the medial (deltoid) ligament.

Clinical Pearl

The Kleiger test has also been used to identify syndesmotic injury. However, there are no studies in the literature that discuss the sensitivity, specificity, positive predictive value, or negative predictive value of this maneuver in detecting syndesmotic lesions.

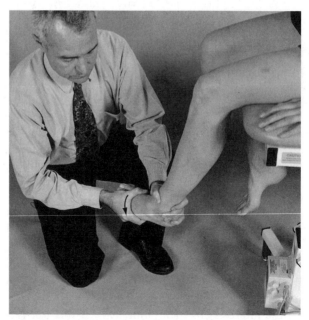

Figure 10-15 Kleiger test.

Patla Test for Tibialis Posterior Length[26]

The patient is positioned in prone, with the knee flexed to 90 degrees. The clinician stabilizes the calcaneus in eversion and the ankle in dorsiflexion with one hand. With the other hand, the clinician contacts the plantar surface of the bases of the second, third, and fourth metatarsals with the thumb, while the index and middle fingers contact the plantar surface of the navicular. The clinician then pushes the navicular and metatarsal heads dorsally and compares the end feel and patient response with the uninvolved side. A positive test is indicated with reproduction of the patient's symptoms.

Tendon Tests

Peroneal longus (fibularis) tendon subluxation[59]

To test for fibularis (peroneal) tendon subluxation, the patient is positioned in prone with the knee of the involved leg flexed to approximately 90 degrees. After inspection of the posterior lateral fibula for any obvious dislocation, the ankle is actively dorsiflexed and everted against resistance. This test dramatically recreates the fibularis longus tendon dislocation if positive.[13]

Thompson test for acute achilles tendon rupture

In this test, the patient is positioned in prone, or in kneeling with the feet over the edge of the bed. With the patient relaxed, the clinician gently squeezes the calf muscle (Figure 10-16) and observes for the production of plantar flexion. An absence of plantar flexion indicates a complete rupture of the Achilles tendon.[60] Although this test may be good for detecting acute Achilles tendon ruptures, it does not accurately detect chronic ruptures.[13,61]

Matles test for chronic achilles tendon rupture

The Matles test is the preferred test for detecting a chronic rupture of the Achilles tendon.[61] The patient is positioned in prone. The patient is asked to bend the knee to approximately 90 degrees. As the patient flexes the knee, the clinician observes the position of the foot and ankle. Normally the foot is slightly plantar flexed as the knee is flexed to 90 degrees. However, if there is an Achilles tendon rupture, the involved foot will either be in a neutral or a dorsiflexed position.[13,61]

Too many toes' sign for posterior tibialis tendon dysfunction

This is more an observation than a test. The patient is asked to stand in a normal relaxed position, while the clinician views the patient from behind. If the heel is in valgus, the forefoot abducted, or the tibia externally rotated more than normal, the clinician will observe more toes on the involved side than on the normal side.[62]

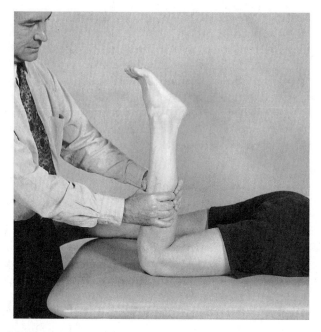

Figure 10-16 Thompson test.

Anterior tibialis tendon rupture test

Although not a specific test in the true sense, a combination of clinical findings can strongly suggest the presence of an anterior tibialis tendon rupture. These include the following:[13,63-65]

- A palpable defect between the extensor retinaculum and the insertion site of the tendon.

- A retracted bulbous proximal stump of the tendon on the anteromedial aspect of the ankle.

- Inability to perform active dorsiflexion beyond ankle and subtalar joint neutral position.

- Diminished ankle dorsiflexion by 10 degrees to 15 degrees from normal, especially with flexion of the hallux.

- Some degree of foot-drop or a steppage-type gait, unless there is substitution of the extensor hallucis longus or other toe extensors.

- Evidence of foot slap with gait.

- Difficulty with heel walking.

Articular Stability Tests

Navicular drop test

The navicular drop test is a method by which to assess the degree to which the talus plantar flexes in space on a calcaneus that has been stabilized by the ground, during subtalar joint pronation.[66,67]

The clinician palpates the position of the navicular tubercle as the patient's foot is nonweight bearing but resting on the floor surface with the subtalar joint maintained in neutral. The clinician then attempts to quantify inferior displacement of the navicular tubercle as the patient assumes 50% weight bearing on the tested foot.[31] A navicular drop, which is greater than 10 mm from the neutral position to the relaxed standing position, suggests excessive medial longitudinal arch collapse of abnormal pronation.[67,68]

Feiss Line[69]

The Feiss line test is another test used to assess the height of the medial arch using the navicular position. With the patient nonweight bearing, the clinician marks the apex of the medial malleolus and the plantar aspect of the first MTP joint, and a line is drawn between the two points. The navicular is palpated on the medial aspect of the foot, and an assessment is made as to the position of the navicular relative to the imaginary line. The patient is then asked to stand with his or her feet about 3 to 6 inches apart. In weight bearing, the navicular normally lies on or very close to the line. If the navicular falls one third of the distance to the floor, it represents a first-degree flatfoot; if it falls two thirds of the distance, it represents a second-degree flatfoot, and if it rests on the floor, it represents a third-degree flatfoot.

Talar rock

The talar rock[70] is an articular stability test for the subtalar joint. The test is performed with the patient positioned in side lying, their hip and knee flexed. The clinician sits on the table with their back to the patient, and places both hands around the ankle just distal to the malleoli. The clinician applies a slight distraction force to the ankle, before applying a rocking movement to the foot in an upward or downward direction. A "clunk" is felt at the end of each of the movements if the test is positive.

Passive foot rotation

This test assesses the integrity of the midtarsal and tarsometatarsal joints. A rotational movement is applied to the midtarsal and tarsometatarsal joints. At the midtarsal joint, the proximal row of the tarsal bones (navicular, calcaneus, and talus) is stabilized, and the distal row (cuneiforms and cuboid) is rotated in both directions. At the tarsometatarsal joints, the distal row of the tarsals is stabilized and the metatarsals are rotated in both directions.

Neurovascular Status

Homan sign

The patient is positioned in supine with their knee extended. The clinician stabilizes the thigh with one hand, and passively dorsiflexes the patient's ankle with the other. Pain in the calf with this maneuver may indicate a positive Homan sign for deep vein thrombosis (DVT), especially if there are associated signs including pallor and swelling in the leg and a loss of the dorsal pedis pulse.

 Clinical Pearl

A positive Homan sign has been found to be insensitive, nonspecific, and is present in fewer than 30% of documented cases of DVT,[71,72] and the performance of the test may increase the risk of producing a pulmonary embolism.

Buerger test

The patient is positioned in supine with the knee extended. The clinician elevates the patient's leg to about 45 degrees and maintains it there for at least 3 minutes. Blanching of the foot is positive for poor arterial circulation, especially if, when the patient sits with the legs over the end of the bed, it takes 1 to 2 minutes for the limb color to be restored.

Morton test[73]

The patient is positioned in supine. The clinician grasps the foot around the metatarsal heads and squeezes the heads together. The reproduction of pain with this maneuver indicates the presence of a neuroma, or a stress fracture.

Duchenne test[73]

The patient is positioned in supine with their legs straight. The clinician pushes through the sole on the first metatarsal head, and pushes the foot into dorsiflexion. The patient is asked to plantar flex the foot. If the medial border dorsiflexes and offers no resistance while the lateral border plantar flexes, a lesion of the superficial fibular (peroneal) nerve, or a lesion of the L4, L5, and S1 nerve root is indicated.

Tinel sign

There are two locations around the ankle from where the Tinel sign can be elicited. The anterior tibial branch of the deep fibular (peroneal) nerve can be tapped on the anterior aspect of the ankle. The posterior tibial nerve may be tapped behind the medial malleolus at the entrance to the tarsal tunnel.

Tingling or paresthesias with these tests is considered a positive finding for peripheral nerve entrapment.

Dorsal pedis pulse
The dorsal pedis pulse can be palpated just lateral to the tendon of the extensor hallucis longus over the dorsum of the foot.

Neurological Tests

Symptoms are commonly referred to the leg, foot and ankle from the lumbar spine, pelvis, hip, or knee.

> ### ● Clinical Pearl
>
> Important neurological structures that pass through the ankle and terminate in the foot are the saphenous, superficial fibular (peroneal), deep fibular (peroneal), posterior and anterior tibial nerves, and the sural nerve.

Symptoms can also be referred to the foot and ankle from the L4–S2 nerve roots (sciatic) but also from a host of other conditions. The applicable sensory, motor, and reflex testing should be performed if a disorder related to a spinal nerve root (L4–S2) or peripheral nerve is suspected. A neurogenic cause of foot pain must be considered in a patient, especially if the pain is refractory. The patient usually complains of pain that is poorly localized, which is aggravated by activity, but may also occur at rest. Any difference in sensation between extremities should be noted and can be mapped out in more detail using a pinwheel. The segmental and peripheral nerve innervations are listed in Chapter 3. Common reflexes tested in this area are the Achilles reflex (S1–2), and the posterior tibial reflex (L4–5).

The pathological reflexes (Babinski, and Oppenheim) are tested if an upper motor neuron lesion is suspected.

Imaging Studies

Various imaging studies can be used to assist in the diagnosis of foot and ankle injuries.

Radiography
Standard radiographs are usually the first imaging test to be performed (Table 10-7). The standard radiographic views of the foot are the AP, lateral,

Table 10-7 Ottawa Ankle Rules for Foot and Ankle Radiographic Series in Patients With Acute Ankle Injury

An ankle radiographic series is required only if patient has pain in malleolar zone and any one of the following findings:	A foot radiographic series is required only if patient has pain in midfoot zone and any one of the following findings:
Bone tenderness at the posterior edge or tip of the lateral malleolus	Bone tenderness at the base of the fifth metatarsal
Bone tenderness at the posterior edge or tip of the medial malleolus	Bone tenderness at the navicular
Inability to bear weight both immediately and in emergency department	Inability to bear weight both immediately and in emergency department

Data from references 74 and 75.

and 45 degrees oblique views. These tests are performed if osseous pathology is suspected. Bone tenderness in the posterior half of the lower 6 cm of the fibula or tibia, and an inability to bear weight immediately after injury are indications to obtain radiographs to rule out fracture of the ankle.[74-76]

If there is bone tenderness over the navicular and/or fifth metatarsal, and an inability to bear weight immediately after injury then radiographs of the foot are indicated.[74,75]

Other roentgenographic techniques include arthrography, fibularis (peroneal) tenography, and magnetic resonance imaging (MRI). These tests are primarily used to highlight soft-tissue injuries.

Examination Conclusions: The Evaluation

Following the examination, and once the clinical findings have been recorded, the clinician must determine a specific diagnosis or a working hypothesis, based on a summary of all of the findings. This diagnosis can be structure-related (medical diagnosis) (Table 10-8), or a diagnosis based on the preferred practice patterns as described in the *Guide to Physical Therapist Practice*.[77]

INTERVENTION

The rehabilitation procedures chosen to progress the patient will depend on the type of tissue involved, the extent of the damage, and the stage of healing (see Chapter 3). The intervention must be related to the signs and symptoms present rather than the actual diagnosis.

Table 10-8 Differential Diagnosis of Common Causes of Leg, Foot, and Ankle Pain

Condition	Patient Age	Mechanism of Injury	Area of Symptoms	Symptoms Aggravated By	Observation	AROM	PROM	Resisted	Special Tests	Tenderness With Palpation
Gastrocnemius strain	20 to 40	Sudden overload	Upper calf	Heel raise	Antalgic gait	Painful and limited DF	Pain with overpressure into DF Restricted range of DF with knee extended	Pain on PF		Mid to upper calf
Plantar fasciitis	20 to 60	Gradual with no known cause	Sole of foot (under heel)	Weight bearing especially first thing in the morning	Unremarkable Flattened arches Pronated foot	Full and pain free	Pain with overpressure into great toe extension	Weak foot intrinsics	Pressure applied over plantar fascial insertion site on the calcaneus	Plantar aspect of heel
Achilles tendonitis	20 to 40	Overuse	Posterior ankle	Jumping, running	Minor swelling of posterior ankle	Painful and limited DF	Pain with overpressure into DF Restricted range of DF with knee extended	Pain on PF		Posterior ankle
Posterior tibialis tendonitis	20 to 40	Overuse with a flat pronated foot	Medial ankle, along the course of the tendon	Activities involving weight bearing plantar flexion	Possible peritendinous swelling over medial ankle	Pain on eversion Pain on PF	Pain with overpressure into eversion Pain with overpressure into PF	Pain on resisted inversion with the foot plantarflexed	Rule out tear with heel raise symmetry	Medial ankle

(continued on following page)

Table 10-8 *(continued from previous page)*

Condition	Patient Age	Mechanism of Injury	Area of Symptoms	Symptoms Aggravated By	Observation	AROM	PROM	Resisted	Special Tests	Tenderness With Palpation
Morton's neuroma	40 to 60	Gradual with no known cause	Sole of foot	Weight bearing	Pronated foot Flattened arches	Full and pain free	Pain with overpressure into toe extension	Strong and painless		Web spaces of toes
Retrocalcaneal bursitis	Varies	Direct irritation of bursa, usually from shoe	Hindfoot	Friction	Possible swelling, erythema of hindfoot	Usually unremarkable	Usually unremarkable	Usually unremarkable	Palpation	Just above the insertion site of the Achilles tendon on the calcaneus
Anterior tibialis tendonitis	15 to 45	Overuse	Anterior lower leg	Activities involving repetitive dorsiflexion	Unremarkable	Pain combined PF and inversion	Pain with overpressure into PF	Pain on DF		Anterolateral lower leg
Tarsal tunnel syndrome	25 to 50	Posttraumatic, neoplastic, inflammatory, rapid weight gain, fluid retention, abnormal foot/ ankle mechanics, or a valgus foot deformity	Medial malleolus, distribution of posterior tibial nerve up the leg, or down into the medial arch, plantar surface of the foot and toes	Excessive dynamic pronation in walking or running	Pronated foot, pes planus, possible swelling	Full and pain free	Pain with extreme plantar flexion and eversion	Weak toe flexion (late)	Positive Tinel over tarsal tunnel	No tenderness usually

Midfoot Sprain	15 to 40	High impact landing sports Foot twisted when in fixed position	Midfoot	Walking on toes	Usually unremarkable	Usually unremarkable	Usually unremarkable	Usually unremarkable	Weight-bearing lateral and anterior-posterior radiographs	Generalized tenderness of midfoot
Medial tibial stress syndrome	15 to 30	Overuse	Anterior lower leg Posterior-medial lower leg	Exercise involving involved lower extremity		Pain combined PF and inversion	Full and pain free	Pain on PF Pain on eversion		Posteromedial calf
Metatarsal stress fracture	15 to 45	Overuse	Forefoot	Weight bearing activities	Possible edema over fracture site	Usually unremarkable	Usually unremarkable	Usually unremarkable	Palpation, ultrasound, tuning fork, bone scan, MRI, CT scan	Maximal point tenderness over the bone at the fracture site
Referred	Varies	Symptoms can be referred from the lumbar spine, hip, knee, or from systemic diseases such as diabetes mellitus (DM), spondyloarthropathy (Reiter syndrome)	May be dermatomal if spinal nerve involved; stocking-like if DM, bilateral heels if Reiter's	Activities unrelated to foot and ankle; unrelated to activity	Varies, but may be unremarkable	Usually unremarkable	Usually unremarkable	Usually unremarkable, but weakness may be present if spinal nerve root involved	Sensation, DTR, lab tests	Tenderness of joint if spondyloarthropathy

AROM = active range of motion; PROM = passive range of motion

COMMON ORTHOPEDIC CONDITIONS

ACHILLES TENDONITIS

Diagnosis

Achilles tendonitis—ICD-9: 726.71.

Description

Achilles tendonitis is the most common form of tendonitis in runners and track athletes. Considered the thickest and strongest tendon in the body, the calcaneal tendon is about 15 cm long, begins at the midleg, and receives muscular fibers almost to its termination. The Achilles tendon has a relatively poor blood supply, particularly in an area known as the critical zone that exists at 4.5 cm above the tendon insertion.

 Clinical Pearl

The Achilles tendon is placed under extreme and rapid eccentric loading forces during such activities as running, standing up while cycling, ballet, gymnastics, soccer, and basketball.

Subjective Findings

- Gradual onset of pain and swelling in the Achilles tendon 2 to 3 cm proximal to the insertion of the tendon, which is exacerbated by activity.
- Some patients will present with pain and stiffness along the Achilles tendon when rising in the morning or pain at the start of activity that improves as the activity progresses.

Objective Findings

- Tenderness and warmth to palpation along the tendon.
- Decreased active and passive dorsiflexion.
- Gait analysis of the involved side may reveal antalgia, premature heel-off, excessive pronation, and the involved lower extremity held in external rotation.
- Involved lower extremity held in external rotation during gait.
- There is often pain with resisted testing of the gastrocnemius–soleus complex.

Clinical Pearl

Tenderness that is located 2 to 6 cm proximal to the insertion is indicative of noninsertional tendonitis, whereas pain at the bone–tendon junction is more indicative of insertional tendonitis.

Confirmatory/Special Tests

The diagnosis is based on the history and physical findings.

Medical Studies

Lateral radiographs may show a calcaneal spur or calcific deposit at the insertion of the tendon, but it is not an acute finding.

Differential Diagnosis

- Retrocalcaneal bursitis.
- Metabolic diseases.
- Arthritis and chondropathic diseases of the ankle joint.
- Tibia vara.
- Os trigonum.
- A calcaneal contusion.
- Plantar heel pain.
- Calcaneal stress fracture.
- Stress fractures of the fibula or tibia.

Intervention

The conservative intervention, which almost always involves modification of extrinsic factors (training errors including a sudden increase in mileage, excessive hill running, and improper shoes), includes Achilles stretching, eccentric strengthening of the calf muscles, the correction of any lower chain asymmetries (low back, pelvic, and hip flexor asymmetries; knee flexion contracture; femoral anteversion; and foot pronation), electrotherapeutic modalities as appropriate, the use of a heel lift, and correct shoe wear, and orthotics—appropriately designed orthoses made from a mold of the foot held in subtalar neutral and nonweight bearing can be of significant benefit.

Prognosis

Surgery to debride a degenerative tendon and remove calcific deposits is indicated if the patient is unresponsive to nonsurgical measures for 9 months.

ANKLE SPRAIN

Diagnosis

Ankle sprain—ICD-9: 845.0.

Description

A sprain of a ligament is defined as an injury that stretches the fibers of the ligament.

 Clinical Pearl

The ankle joint complex is the most frequently injured region in athletics.

 Clinical Pearl

In the neutral position or dorsiflexion, the ankle is stable because the widest part of the talus is in the mortise. However, in plantar flexion, ankle stability is decreased as the narrow posterior portion of the talus is in the mortise.

Subjective Findings

An accurate history includes the description of the onset of symptoms, duration and progression of pain, history of a traumatic event, activities that worsen the pain, and previous treatments and outcomes.

Objective Findings

Although a physical examination is reliable for the diagnosis of an ankle fracture, the reliability for detecting lateral ankle sprains may not be as definitive, especially if the examination is performed immediately after the injury.

Clinical Pearl

Dynamic stability is provided to the lateral ankle by the strength of the fibularis (peroneus) longus and brevis tendons.

Confirmatory/Special Tests

- Anterior drawer test (anterior talofibular ligament): ankle positioned in 30 degree plantar flexion and slight internal rotation.
- Inversion stress test: ankle positioned in full dorsiflexion. Clinician applies inversion stress to the heel to test the calcaneofibular ligament.

Sign/Symptom	Grade I	Grade II	Grade III
Loss of functional ability	Minimal	Some	Great
Pain	Minimal	Moderate	Severe
Swelling	Minimal	Moderate	Severe
Ecchymosis	Usually not	Frequently	Yes
Difficulty bearing weight	No	Usually	Almost always

 Clinical Pearl

The ATFL, which is the least elastic of the lateral ligaments, is involved in 60% to 70% of all ankle sprains, whereas 20% involve both the ATFL and CFL.

Medical Studies

Due to the difficulty of assessing the magnitude of injury during the acute stage, ancillary studies such as stress radiography and arthrography may be used to supplement the physical examination. MRI may be of some benefit in patients with equivocal examinations.

Differential Diagnosis

- Talotibial impingement syndrome.
- Osteochondritis dissecans.

- Acute rupture of the peroneal retinaculum.
- Fracture.

 Clinical Pearl

A clinician examining the foot and ankle needs to be aware of other potential pathologies that should be considered when an adolescent patient is referred to physical therapy with the diagnosis of ankle sprain. These pathologies include osteochondrosis, osteochondritis dissecans, accessory ossicle, anterior impingement syndrome, sinus tarsi syndrome, tarsal coalition, and epiphyseal fractures.

Intervention

The ultimate treatment decision is based on a variety of factors, including the patient's overall medical condition, severity and duration of symptoms, expectations, associated foot and ankle pathology, and surgeon preference.

Prognosis

The prognosis for ankle sprains is inversely proportional to the severity and grade of the injury. If left untreated, ankle sprains can lead to chronic instability and impairment.

 Clinical Pearl

Approximately one third of the population, that sustains injury to the lateral ligaments of the ankle, complains of residual dysfunction as long as 9 months after the injury.

HALLUX RIGIDUS

Diagnosis

Hallux rigidus—ICD-9: 735.2. Also known as a great toe arthritis or hallux limitus.

Description

Hallux rigidus is characterized by decreased dorsiflexion of the first MTP joint, and pain and swelling in the dorsal aspect of the joint. Two types of hallux rigidus have been described:

- Adolescent: the adolescent type is consistent with an osteochondritis dissecans or localized articular disorder.
- Adult: the adult type is a more generalized degenerative arthritis.

 Clinical Pearl

The MTP joint of the great toe is the most common site of arthritis in the foot.

Subjective Findings

The subjective findings typically include the following:

- Pain and stiffness of the great toe, especially as the toe moves into dorsiflexion (walking or running up hills, climbing stairs, or during the toe-off phase of gait).
- The patient may also experience tingling and numbness on the dorsum of the toe due to compression of the cutaneous nerves.

Objective Findings

The physical examination typically reveals the following findings:

- Tenderness is usually present on palpation of the dorsal, and especially lateral, aspects of the joint.

Confirmatory/Special Tests

The diagnosis of hallux rigidus is made on the basis of stiffness of the great toe with loss of extension at the MTP joint.

Medical/Imaging Studies

Anteroposterior (AP) and lateral radiographs demonstrate loss of first MTP joint space, the formation of dorsal and lateral osteophytes on the metatarsal head, and occasionally loose fragments about the joint.

Differential Diagnosis

- Gout.
- Hallux valgus.
- Turf toe.

Intervention

The initial intervention involves shoe modifications, rest, and nonsteroidal anti-inflammatory drugs. A shoe with an extra-depth toe box can be helpful to decrease dorsal pressure on the first MTP joint, whereas a stiff-soled shoe or a rigid custom orthotic with a Morton extension can be helpful in limiting toe dorsiflexion. A rocker-bottom sole can also help to decrease the extension of the hallux during normal gait. An intra-articular corticosteroid injection may be considered as a temporizing measure.

Prognosis

If symptoms increase, or when conservative measures fail, surgical intervention (cheilectomy) may provide the solution.

HALLUX VALGUS

Diagnosis

Hallux valgus—ICD-9: 735.0. Also referred to as bunion, or metatarsus primus varus.

Description

Hallux valgus is the term used to describe a deformity of the first MTP joint in which the proximal phalanx is deviated laterally with respect to the first metatarsal. The term has been expanded to include varying degrees of metatarsus primus varus/valgus deviation of the proximal phalanx, medial deviation of the first metatarsal head, and bunion formation.

 Clinical Pearl

Hallux valgus has been observed to occur almost exclusively in populations that wear shoes, although some predisposing anatomic factors make some feet more vulnerable than others to the effects of extrinsic factors. Women have been observed to have hallux valgus at a rate of 9:1 compared with men. Hallux valgus has also been reported to affect 22% to 36% of adolescents.

Subjective Findings

The subjective finding typically includes the following:

• Complaints of pain and swelling, aggravated by shoe wear.

Objective Findings

The physical examination typically reveals the following findings:

• Observation may reveal a hypertrophic bursa over the medial eminence of the first metatarsal.

• There may be pronation (inward rotation) of the great toe with resultant callus on the medial aspect.

🌑 Clinical Pearl

The deformity results from a lateral subluxation of the FHL muscle, which transforms the FHL and brevis from flexors to adductors, which pull the proximal interphalangeal joint medially and the distal interphalangeal joint laterally.

Confirmatory/Special Tests

The diagnosis of hallux valgus is made based on subjective history, physical findings, and the results of imaging studies.

Medical/Imaging Studies

The severity of the bunion deformity is graded by measuring forefoot angles on weight-bearing AP radiographs of the foot.

Differential Diagnosis

• Hallux varus.
• Hallux rigidus.
• Gout.

Intervention

The intervention for hallux valgus is conservative in mild to moderate cases. The intervention for the bunion includes wider shoes and orthotics. Achilles stretching should be used in cases of Achilles contracture. A simple toe spacer can be used between the first and second toes, and a silicone bunion pad placed over the bunion may be helpful in alleviating direct pressure on the prominence. In cases of pes planus associated with hallux valgus, a medial longitudinal arch support with Morton extension under the first MTP joint may also alleviate symptoms.

Prognosis

If pain persists, structural realignment of the first metatarsal is usually necessary because the bunion deformity becomes more severe and decompensated.

HEEL PAD SYNDROME (PLANTAR FASCIITIS)

Diagnosis

Heel pad syndrome (Plantar fasciitis) —ICD-9: 728.71.

Description

Heel pad syndrome, often referred to as plantar fasciitis, is an inflammatory process resulting from a number of factors including prolonged standing, repetitive stress, and abnormal foot alignment (pronated or a cavus type foot).

 Clinical Pearl

> Plantar fasciitis is common among dancers, tennis players, basketball players, and other athletes whose sport involves running.

Subjective Findings

- History of pain and tenderness on the plantar medial aspect of the heel, especially during initial weight bearing in the morning or after a prolonged period of nonweight bearing.
  - The heel pain often decreases during the day but worsens with increased activity (such as jogging, climbing stairs, or going up on the toes) or after a period of sitting.

Objective Findings

- Localized pain on palpation along the medial edge of the fascia or at its origin on the anterior edge of the calcaneus, although firm finger pressure is often necessary to localize the point of maximum tenderness.

Confirmatory/Special Tests

To test for plantar heel pain, the fascia needs to be put on stretch with a bowstring type test. The patient's heel is manually fixed in eversion. The clinician takes hold of the first metatarsal and places it in dorsiflexion before extending the big toe as far as possible. Pain should be elicited at the medial tubercle.

Medical Studies

Radiographs may show a bone spur at the origin of the fascia, but it is not an acute finding.

Differential Diagnosis

The differential diagnosis for plantar fasciitis is extensive and includes:

- Inflammatory spondyloarthropathies. These disorders should be considered when multiple joints or areas are involved.
- Tarsal tunnel syndrome (entrapment of the tibial nerve).
- Calcaneal stress fracture. The history for calcaneal stress fractures usually involves a sudden increase in a running activity, such as that seen in a military recruit at boot camp or a reservist.
- Nerve entrapment. Positive percussion (Tinel sign) on the medial aspect of the heel should lead to a suspicion of entrapment of the nerve to abductor digiti quinti or a tarsal tunnel syndrome.
- Tumors. Tumors in this area are quite rare, presenting as palpable masses or bony erosions of the calcaneus.
- Atrophy of the heel pad.
- Infections. As with infections in other parts of the body, there will usually be some swelling and/or erythema, and a history of malaise or fever.
- Neuropathy (diabetic, alcoholic). A history of burning pain, numbness, or paresthesias can often be elicited in patients with neuropathic pain. A thorough neurological examination will confirm the diagnosis.
- The fatpad syndrome. Pain while hopping on the toes may help distinguish this entity from the fatpad syndrome.
- Sever disease.

Intervention

The lack of a universal intervention for plantar heel pain, and the poor level of long-term success, likely stems from its many causes. The intervention for plantar heel pain should include the following:

- Rest or at least elimination of any activity that continually provides axial loading of the heel and tensile stresses on the fascia.
- Shoes that provide good shock absorption at the heel and support to the medial longitudinal arch and plantar fascia band should be recommended to the patient.

- Orthotics, but only after careful examination of the footwear, to ensure a firm, well-fitting heel counter, good heel cushioning, and an adequate longitudinal arch support.
- Strengthening exercises for the foot intrinsics.
- A regimen of stretching of the gastrocnemius and the medial fascial band performed before arising in the morning and after sedentary periods during the day, as well as before and after exercise.

Prognosis

Almost 90% of patients with plantar heel pain who undergo a conservative intervention improve significantly within 12 months, although approximately 10% can develop persistent and often disabling symptoms.

METATARSAL STRESS FRACTURE

Diagnosis

Metatarsal Stress fracture—ICD-9: 825.25. The second and third metatarsals are the most frequently injured.

Description

A stress or fatigue fracture is a break that develops in bone after cyclical, submaximal loading. Extrinsic factor that may result in stress fractures of the leg and foot are running on hard surfaces, improper running shoes, or sudden increases in jogging or running distance.

 Clinical Pearl

Patients who abruptly increase their training, whether it be training mileage, time spent in high-impact activities, or training intensity, are susceptible to metatarsal stress fractures.

Subjective Findings

The typical subjective findings include the following:
- Pain and swelling on weight bearing.

- History of a sudden increase in activity, change in running surface, or even prolonged walking.

Objective Findings

Intrinsic factors to consider when evaluating stress fractures include malalignment of the lower extremity, particularly excessive pronation. The physical examination typically reveals swelling, ecchymosis, and tenderness over the fractured metatarsal.

Confirmatory/Special Tests

The diagnosis for a metatarsal stress fracture is based on the history and physical examination, with confirmation from imaging studies.

Medical Studies

AP, lateral, and oblique radiographs of the foot may demonstrate a fracture.

 Clinical Pearl

A stress fracture of a metatarsal may not show up on radiographs for 2 to 3 weeks, although a technetium bone scan is positive as early as 48 to 72 hours after onset of symptoms.

Differential Diagnosis

- Metatarsalgia.
- Lisfranc fracture.
- Lisfranc dislocation or sprain.
- Morton (interdigital) neuroma.

Intervention

The intervention for nondisplaced metatarsal neck and shaft fractures includes the use of a short leg cast, fracture brace, or wooden sole shoe. Weight bearing is permitted as tolerated.

Prognosis

Fractures of the metatarsal bones usually heal with nonsurgical treatment; however, a zone 2 fracture of the proximal diaphysis of the fifth metatarsal requires more extensive immobilization, and a zone 3 fracture of this bone may result in nonunion or delayed union.

MORTON NEUROMA

Diagnosis

Interdigital (Morton) neuroma—ICD-9: 355.6 (mononeuritis of lower limb; lesion of plantar nerve). Also known as intermetatarsal neuroma or plantar neuroma.

 Clinical Pearl

A Morton neuroma is not a true neuroma but rather a perineural fibrosis of the common digital nerve as it passes between the metatarsal heads.

Description

An interdigital neuroma, or Morton neuroma, is a mechanical entrapment neuropathy of the interdigital nerve. The entrapment may occur as the nerve courses on the plantar side of the distal aspect of the transverse intermetatarsal ligament, where it is vulnerable to traction injury and compression during the toe-off phase of running or during repetitive positions of toe rise.

 Clinical Pearl

The most commonly involved nerve is the third interdigital nerve, between the third and fourth metatarsal heads, followed in incidence by the second interdigital nerve and, rarely, the first and fourth interdigital nerves.

Subjective Findings

The subjective findings typically include the following:

• Complaints of forefoot burning, cramping, tingling, and numbness in the toes of the involved interspace, with occasional proximal radiation in the foot.

- Symptoms are aggravated by wearing high heels or tight, restrictive shoes.
- Night pain is rare.

Objective Findings

The physical examination typically reveals the following findings:

- Palpable isolated tenderness in the region of the third and fourth metatarsal heads.
- Pain is relieved by walking barefoot.

 Clinical Pearl

Careful palpation of the MTP joint, metatarsal head, and proximal phalanx should be performed to rule out localized joint or bone pathology, such as MTP joint synovitis, stress fracture, or Freiberg's disease, which can also cause symptoms of forefoot pain.

Confirmatory/Special Tests

Morton Test. The patient is positioned in supine. The clinician grasps the foot around the metatarsal heads and squeezes the heads together. The reproduction of pain with this maneuver indicates the presence of a neuroma, or a stress fracture.

Medical/Imaging Studies

Medical/imaging studies are not typically required for this condition.

Differential Diagnosis

- Stress fracture.
- Metatarsophalangeal synovitis.
- Hammer toe.
- Metatarsalgia.

Intervention

The intervention initially entails avoiding the offending activity, cross-training in lower-impact sports, and modification of footwear. A switch to wider, more accommodating shoes with soft soles and better shock absorption will often improve symptoms. A metatarsal pad, such as an adhesive-backed felt pad, placed proximal to the symptomatic interspace is helpful. The metatarsal pad can also be incorporated into a custom-made full-length semirigid orthotic. A trial of nonsteroidal anti-inflammatory drugs is indicated in an attempt to decrease inflammation around the interdigital nerve. A trial of vitamin B_6 has been used successfully in the treatment of carpal tunnel syndrome and may also be useful in the treatment of interdigital neuritis.

Prognosis

If symptoms persist or recur, surgical excision of the neuroma or division of the transverse metatarsal ligament is indicated.

POSTERIOR TIBIAL TENDON DYSFUNCTION

Diagnosis

Posterior tibial tendon dysfunction—ICD-9: 726.72. Also referred to as acquired flatfoot, and posterior tibial tendon insufficiency.

Description

Posterior tibial dysfunction is a complex disorder of the hindfoot. Controversy exists as to whether persisting rotational instability after ankle sprain may cause posterior tibial dysfunction or vice versa. Demographically, the classic presentation is an overweight woman over 55 years of age.

 Clinical Pearl

The primary function of the tibialis posterior muscle is to invert and plantar flex the foot. It also provides support to the medial longitudinal arch. The tendon is lined with a tenosynovial sheath that can become inflamed, producing a tenosynovitis.

Subjective Findings

Subjectively, the patient complains of the following:

• Insidious onset of pain. The pain is usually felt in one of three locations:

- Distal to the medial malleoli in the area of the navicular.
- Proximal to the medial malleoli.
- At the musculotendinous origin (medial shin splints), or insertion.
- Swelling on the medial aspect of the ankle.

 Clinical Pearl

Posterior tibialis tendonitis is seen relatively frequently in dancers, joggers, and ice skaters, especially in those participants with a pronated foot and flattened longitudinal arch.

Objective Findings

The physical examination typically reveals the following:

- Swelling and tenderness posterior and inferior to the medial malleolus, along the course of the posterior tibial tendon, and to its insertion into the navicular.
- The medial arch is decreased or completely flattened.
- The heel shows increased valgus, and with advanced changes, the forefoot is in abduction.
  - When viewed from behind, more than two toes will be visible on the affected foot (the "too many toes" sign) because of the forefoot abduction and hindfoot valgus.
- Pain on resisted ankle plantar flexion and inversion.
- With a complete rupture, the navicular subluxes inferiorly, and the patient ambulates in a flat-footed position as they are unable to produce any toe-off.

 Clinical Pearl

Patients with dysfunction or rupture of the posterior tibial tendon cannot perform a complete heel rise on the affected leg, and when this test is performed while standing on both legs, normal inversion of the heel does not occur.

Confirmatory/Special Tests

- Patla Test for tibialis posterior.
- Feiss line.
- Too many toes sign.

Medical Studies

Plain radiographs are rarely helpful, although weight-bearing AP and lateral radiographs reveal a flat foot, with alignment changes at the talonavicular and other joints.

MRI or bone scan may also aid in the diagnosis.

Differential Diagnosis

- Congenital pes planus.
- Tarsal coalition.
- Medial malleolus stress fracture.
- Medial ankle laxity.
- Lisfranc fracture-dislocation.

Intervention

The intervention for posterior tibialis dysfunction depends on the cause, but the overall approach includes tibialis posterior stretching, strengthening, orthotics, occasional casting, and icing.

Prognosis

A progressive, painful flatfoot with gait disturbance is common. When conservative management fails, surgical debridement of the tendon may be indicated.

RETROCALCANEAL BURSITIS

Diagnosis

Retrocalcaneal bursitis—ICD-9.

Description

Retrocalcaneal bursitis involves the irritation of a small bursa located between the Achilles tendon and the posterior aspect of the ankle.

Clinical Pearl

The retrocalcaneal bursa functions to lubricate the tendon and the talus bone when the foot is in extreme plantar flexion.

Subjective Findings

The subjective findings typically include the following:

- Posterior ankle pain.
- Pain with walking.

Objective Findings

The physical examination typically reveals the following findings:

- Local tenderness and swelling in the soft tissues behind the ankle, especially just posterior to the talus.
- An increase in symptoms when the ankle is passively moved into extreme plantar flexion.
- Resistive testing is pain-free.
- Active ROM of the foot and ankle is normal.

Confirmatory/Special Tests

No special testing is indicated.

Medical Studies

Imaging studies are not normally necessary unless a stress fracture of the calcaneus is suspected.

Differential Diagnosis

- Calcaneal stress fracture.
- Arthritis of the ankle.
- Tarsal tunnel syndrome.

Intervention

The aim of the intervention is to reduce the swelling and inflammation in the bursa and to prevent a recurrence. The treatment of choice is Achilles tendon stretching exercises.

Prognosis

Retrocalcaneal bursitis usually responds well to conservative management. Local corticosteroid injections can be used in recalcitrant cases.

TARSAL TUNNEL SYNDROME

Diagnosis

Tarsal tunnel syndrome—ICD-9: 355.5.

Description

Tarsal tunnel syndrome (TTS) is an entrapment neuropathy of the tibial nerve as it passes through the anatomic tunnel between the flexor retinaculum and the medial malleolus. In addition, the terminal branches of the tibial nerve, the medial and lateral plantar (posterior tibial) nerves may be involved. Etiological factors for TTS can be classified as internal or external. Internal factors include anatomical variations such as an accessory flexor digitorum longus muscle. External factors include excessive pronation, which can tighten the flexor retinaculum and the calcaneonavicular ligament.

 Clinical Pearl

Anterior tarsal tunnel syndrome involves entrapment of the deep fibular (peroneal) nerve.

Subjective Findings

The subjective findings typically include the following:

• Gradual or sudden onset of diffuse, poorly localized pain along the medial ankle.

• There may be complaints of paresthesias along the medial ankle and into the arch.

• The pain is often worse after walking or other exercise and also may occur at night.

Objective Findings

The physical examination typically reveals the following findings:

- Tenderness over the tarsal tunnel just posterior to the medial malleolus.
- Percussion over the tibial nerve (Tinel sign) should reproduce the symptoms.

Confirmatory/Special Tests

- Tinel sign.

Medical/Imaging Studies

Radiographs of the foot and ankle unnecessary to rule out bony pathology, but the radiographs are usually normal. Electrodiagnostic testing may identify tibial nerve entrapment but the results can be unreliable.

Differential Diagnosis

- Plantar heel pain.
- Chronic heel pain syndrome.
- Complex regional pain syndrome.
- Diabetic/peripheral neuropathy.
- Flexor hallucis longus tenosynovitis.
- Posterior tibial tendon dysfunction.

Intervention

Conservative intervention for TTS includes the use of orthotics to correct biomechanical gait abnormalities. Specifically a foot orthosis with a rearfoot varus post can limit excessive pronation. In cases of early excessive rearfoot pronation and subtalar joint pronation at heel strike, an orthosis with a deepened heel cup can help to control rearfoot motion. In cases of severe hyperpronation, a rearfoot wedge may be helpful.

Prognosis

Surgical intervention (nerve decompression) is used as a last resort.

TURF TOE

Diagnosis

Turf toe—ICD-9: 845.12 (sprains and strains of ankle and foot; metatarsophalangeal joint).

Description

The term "turf toe" refers to a sprain of the first MTP joint of the great toe, which most commonly occurs with hyperextension but may occur with hyperflexion, and varus and valgus stresses of the first MTP joint.

 Clinical Pearl

Hypermobility of the first ray has been implicated in numerous conditions frequently accompanied by excessive or prolonged sspronation, including lesser metatarsalgia, acquired flatfoot, posterior tibialis tendonitis, plantar fasciitis, and shin splints.

 Clinical Pearl

With forced hyperflexion of the hallux, tearing of the plantar plate and collateral ligaments can occur. In the more severe injury, the capsule can actually tear off of the metatarsal head. A fracture of the sesamoids can also occur, and dorsal dislocation of the first MTP joint is possible.

Subjective Findings

The subjective findings typically include the following:

- Complaints of a red, swollen, stiff first MTP joint. The joint may be tender both plantarly and dorsally. Players may have a limp and be unable to run or jump because of pain.
- A history of a single dorsiflexion injury or multiple injuries to the great toe.

Objective Findings

Clanton and Ford[1] have classified the severity of turf toe injuries from grades I to III:

- A grade I sprain is a minor stretch injury to the soft tissue restraints with little pain, swelling, or disability.

[1]Adapted from reference 78.

- A grade II sprain is a partial tear of the capsuloligamentous structures with moderate pain, swelling, ecchymosis, and disability.
- A grade III sprain is a complete tear of the plantar plate with severe swelling, pain, ecchymosis, and inability to bear weight normally.

Confirmatory/Special Tests

No specific confirmatory/special test exists.

Medical/Imaging Studies

Radiographs of the foot should be obtained to rule out fracture of the sesamoids or metatarsal head articular surface and to check joint congruity.

Differential Diagnosis

- Hallux rigidus.
- Sesamoid stress fracture.
- Gout.

Intervention

The initial intervention for turf toe is rest, ice, a compressive dressing, and elevation. A nonsteroidal anti-inflammatory medication is often recommended. The toe should be taped to limit dorsiflexion with multiple loops of tape placed over the dorsal aspect of the hallucal proximal phalanx and criss-crossed under the ball of the foot plantarly, or a forefoot steel plate can be used. PROM and progressive resistance exercises are begun as soon as symptoms allow. Patients with grade I sprains are usually allowed to return to sports as soon as symptoms allow, sometimes immediately. Patients with grade II sprains usually require 3 to 14 days rest from athletic training. Grade III sprains usually require crutches for a few days and up to 6 weeks rest from sports participation. A return to sports training too early after injury could result in prolonged disability. Return to play is indicated when the toe can be dorsiflexed 90 degrees.

Prognosis

Turf toe typically develops into a chronic injury, and long-term results include decreased first MTP joint motion, impaired push-off, and hallux rigidus. Fifty percent of athletes will have persistent symptoms 5 years later.

REHABILITATION LADDER

ANKLE AND FOOT

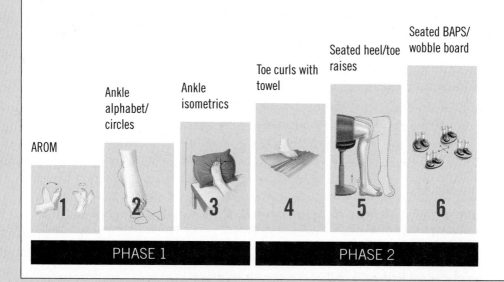

The purpose of these training ladders is to provide the clinician with a safe and progressive framework of exercises that are designed to allow the patient to improve in an efficient manner. The patient begins at the appropriate step, which is based on the stage of healing and the goal of the intervention.

- Phase 1: Acute—pain management, restoration of full passive range of motion, and restoration of normal accessory motion.
- Phase 2: Subacute—active range of motion exercises and early strengthening.
- Phase 3: Chronic—specific strengthening with a strong emphasis on enhancing dynamic stability.

The degree of movement and the speed of progression are both guided by the signs and symptoms. Once the patient is able to perform an exercise for

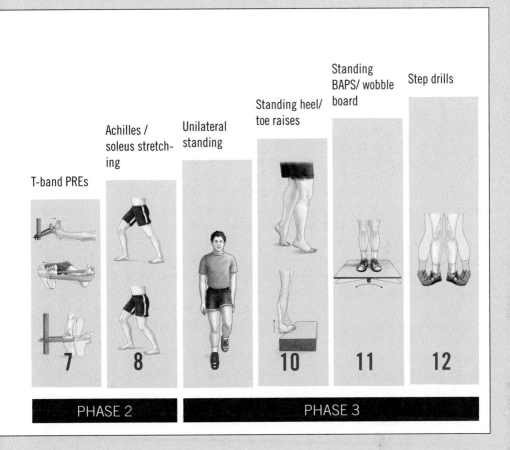

Standing BAPS/ wobble board

Step drills

Standing heel/ toe raises

Achilles / soleus stretch-ing

Unilateral standing

T-band PREs

7   8   10   11   12

PHASE 2   PHASE 3

8–12 reps without pain, he or she progresses up to the next exercise step. This continues until the patient attempts an exercise that reproduces the pain. At this point, the patient returns to the last exercise that he or she was able to perform without pain and performs that exercise five times per day for 1 to 2 days before attempting to progress again. The patient is advanced through the training ladders to the appropriate point, with particular attention paid to patient response to treatment in terms of changes in symptoms, swelling, degree of irritability, or motion. In addition, muscle imbalances are addressed with appropriate flexibility exercises.

Once the patient is able to perform the last exercise of Phase 3 (Step 12 of the ladder), he or she can move on to functional and sport-specific training (Phase 4) as appropriate, which focus on power and higher-speed exercises similar to sport specific demands.

1. AROM of the ankle

The patient is positioned in supine or long sitting. The patient is asked to move the ankle actively into inversion (1a), eversion, dorsiflexion (1b), and plantarflexion.

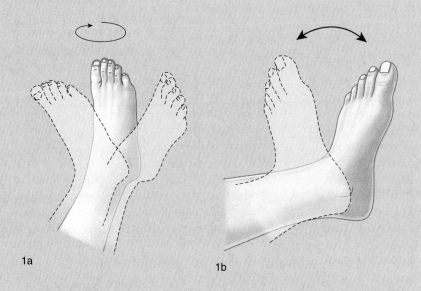

1a   1b

2. Ankle alphabet

The patient is positioned in supine or long sitting. The patient is asked to move the ankle actively as though tracing the letters of the alphabet (2).

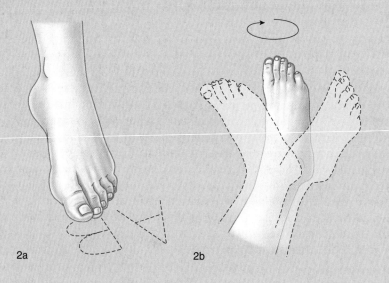

2a   2b

3. Ankle isometrics
The patient is positioned in supine a long sitting. The patient is asked to perform an isometric contraction into plantarflexion (3a), eversion (3b), inversion (3c), and dorsiflexion (3d).

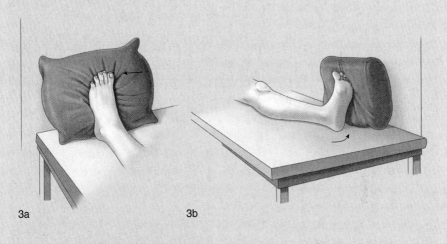

3a   3b

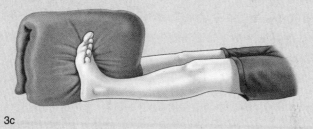

3c

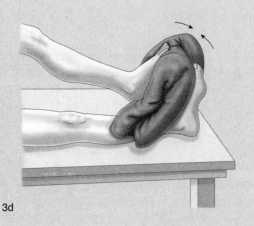

3d

4. Towel toe curl

The patient is positioned in sitting with their foot resting on a towel. The patient is asked to pull the towel along the floor using the foot into eversion and inversion, or by scrunching the toes (4). Resistance can be added to this exercise by placing a weight at the end of the towel.

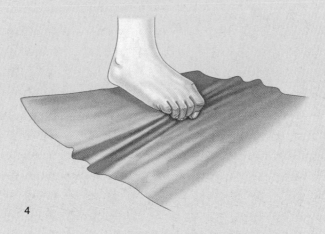

4

5. Seated toe-heel raise

The patient is positioned in sitting so that the foot rest flat on the floor. The patient is asked to alternately raise the heel and then the toes off the floor (5).

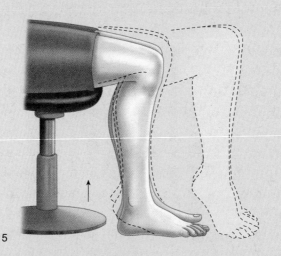

5

6. Seated wobble board

The patient is positioned in sitting with the feet resting on a wobble board (6). The patient is asked to move the wobble board initially in straight planes and then in multiple directions.

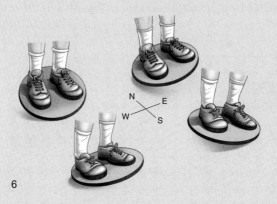

6

7. Resistive exercises

Exercise tubing is placed around the patient's foot and the patient is asked to move the foot into dorsiflexion (7a), eversion (7b), inversion (7c), and plantarflexion.

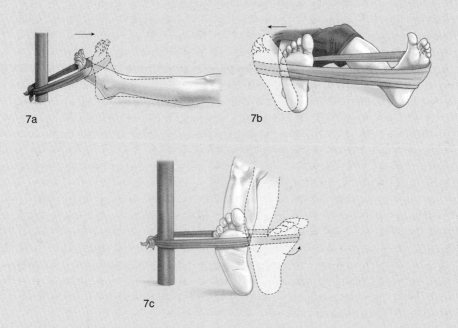

7a

7b

7c

8. Achilles tendon and soleus stretch

The patient is positioned in standing facing a wall. The patient is asked to stride forward with one foot, keeping the heel of the back foot flat on the floor (8a). The patient is then asked to shift the bodyweight forward onto the front foot while maintaining the knee of the back leg in extension. The procedure is the same for the soleus stretch, except that the knee of the back leg is flexed (8b).

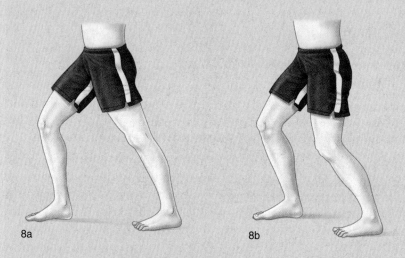

8a   8b

9. Unilateral standing

Refer to Chapter 8 for full description.

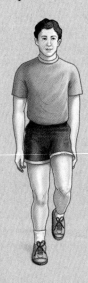

9

10. Standing heel raises
The patient is positioned in standing. The patient is asked to raise both heels from the floor. The exercise is progressed so that the patient is standing on the involved leg only and is asked to perform a heel raise on a flat surface (10a). Once this can be accomplished, the patient performs the exercise on a step (10b).

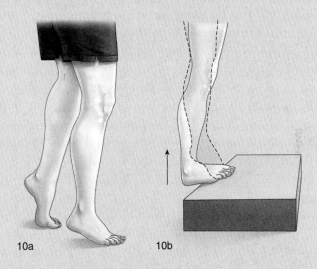

10a   10b

11. Standing exercises on a wobble board
The patient is positioned in standing and then performs a series of exercises using the wobble board (11).

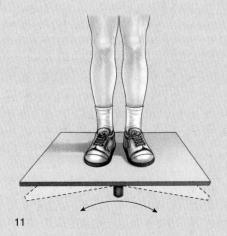

11

12. Step exercises

The patient is positioned in standing and performs a series of stepping exercises (12) in multiple directions.

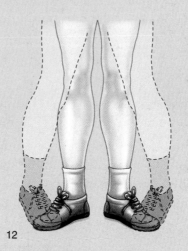

12

REFERENCES

1. Childs S. Acute ankle injury. *Lippincott's Primary Care Practice*. 1999;3: 428–440.

2. Adamson C, Cymet T. Ankle sprains: evaluation, treatment, rehabilitation. *Maryland Med J*. 1997;46:530–537.

3. Bordelon RL. Clinical assessment of the foot. In: Donatelli RA, ed. *Biomechanics of the Foot and Ankle*. Philadelphia, PA: WB Saunders; 1990:85–98.

4. Brostrom L. Sprained ankles: III. Clinical observations in recent ligament ruptures. *Acta Chir Scand*. 1965:130:560–569.

5. Cox JS. The diagnosis and management of ankle ligament injuries in the athlete. Athl *Training*. 1982;18:192–196.

6. Safran MR, Zachazewski JE, Benedetti RS, et al. Lateral ankle sprains: a comprehensive review part 2: treatment and rehabilitation with an emphasis on the athlete. *Med Sci Sports Exerc*. 1999;31:S438–S447.

7. Safran MR, Benedetti RS, Bartolozzi AR, III., et al. Lateral ankle sprains: a comprehensive review: part 1: etiology, pathoanatomy, histopathogenesis, and diagnosis. *Med SciSports Exerc*. 1999;31:S429–S437.

8. Judd, D.B. and D.H. Kim. Foot fractures frequently misdiagnosed as ankle sprains. *Am Fam Phys*. 2002;66:785–794.

9. Marder RA. Current methods for the evaluation of ankle ligament injuries. *J Bone and Joint Surg*. 1994;76A:1103–1111.

10. Magee DJ. Lower leg, ankle, and foot.In: Magee DJ, ed. *Orthopedic Physical Assessment*. Philadelphia, PA: W.B. Saunders; 2002:765–845.

11. Kelikian H, Kelikian AS. *Disorders of the Ankle*. Philadelphia, PA: W. B. Saunders; 1985.

12. Winkel D, Matthijs O, Phelps V. Examination of the ankle and foot. In: Winkel D, Matthijs O, Phelps V, eds. *Diagnosis and Treatment of the Lower Extremities*. Maryland, MD: Aspen; 1997:375–401.

13. Lee TK, Maleski R. Physical examination of the ankle for ankle pathology. *Clin Podiatr Med Surg*. 2002;19:251–269.

14. Sammarco GJ, Mangone PG. Diagnosis and treatment of peroneal tendon injuries. *Foot Ankle Surg*. 1986;6:197–205.

15. Guhl JF. *Soft Tissue (Synovial) Pathology, Ankle Arthroscopy: Pathology and Surgical Technique*. 2nd ed. Thorofare, NJ: Slack Publishing; 1993:93–135.

16. Reid DC. *Sports Injury Assessment and Rehabilitation*. New York, NY: Churchill Livingstone; 1992.

17. Hertling D, Kessler RM. *Management of Common Musculoskeletal Disorders: Physical Therapy Principles and Methods*. 3rd ed. Philadelphia, PA: Lippincott Williams & Wilkins; 1996.

18. Baxter DE. The heel in sport. *Clin Sports Med*. 1994;13:683–693.

19. Appling SA, Kasser RJ. Foot and ankle. In: Wadsworth C, ed. *Current Concepts of Orthopedic Physical Therapy - Home Study Course*. La Crosse, WI: Orthopaedic Section, APTA; 2001.

20. Mann RA. Biomechanical approach to the treatment of foot problems. *Foot Ankle*. 1982;2:205–212.

21. Brand RL, Collins MDF. Operative management of ligamentous injuries to the ankle. *Clin Sports Med*. 1982;1:117–130.

22. Leith JM, McConkey JP, Li D, et al. Valgus stress radiography in normal ankles. *Foot Ankle Int*. 1997;18:654–657.

23. Luttgens K, Hamilton N. *Kinesiology: Scientific Basis of Human Motion*. 10th ed. New York, NY: McGraw-Hill; 2002:567.

24. Leach RE, Dizorio E, Harvey RA. Pathologic hindfoot conditions in the athlete. *Clin Orthop*. 1983;177:116–121.

25. Root M, Orien W, Weed J. *Clinical Biomechanics: Normal and Abnormal Function of the Foot*. Los Angeles, LA: Clinical Biomechanics Corp.; 1977.

26. Patla CE, Abbott JH. Tibialis posterior myofascial tightness as a source of heel pain. diagnosis and treatment. *J Orthop Sports Phys Ther*. 2000;30:624–632.

27. Rose GK, Welton GA, Marshall T. The diagnosis of flat foot in the child. *J Bone Joint Surg*. 1985;67B:71–78.

28. Bojsen-Möller F, Lamoreux L. Significance of dorsiflexion of the toes in walking. *Acta Orthop Scand*. 1975;50:471–479.

29. Buell T, Green DR, Risser J. Measurement of the first metatarsophalangeal joint range of motion. *J Am Podiat Med Assn*. 1988; 78:439–448.

30. Joseph J. Range of movement of the great toe in men. *J Bone Joint Surg*. 1954; 36B:450–457.

31. Gross MT. Lower quarter screening for skeletal malalignment - suggestions for orthotics and shoewear. *J Orthop Sports Phys Ther*. 1995;21:389–405.

32. Donatelli R. Normal anatomy and pathophysiology of the foot and ankle. In: Wadsworth C, eds. *Contemporary Topics on the Foot and Ankle*. La Crosse, WI: Orthopedic Section, APTA Inc.; 2000.
33. Inman VT. *The Joints of the Ankle*. Baltimore: Williams & Wilkins; 1991.
34. Katcherian DA. Pathology of the first ray. In: Mizel MS, Miller RA, Scioli MW, eds. *Orthopaedic Knowledge Update, Foot and Ankle*. Rosemont, IL: American Academy of Orthopaedic Surgeons; 1998:157–159.
35. Brosky T, Nyland A, Nitz A, et al. The ankle ligaments: consideration of syndesmotic injury and implications for rehabilitation. *J Orthop Sports Phys Ther*. 1995;21:197–205.
36. Hopkinson WJ, St Pierre P, Ryan JB, et al. Syndesmosis sprains of the ankle. *Foot Ankle Int*. 1990;10:325–330.
37. Teitz CC, Harrington RM. A biomechanical analysis of the squeeze test for sprains of the syndesmotic ligaments of the ankle. *Foot Ankle Int*. 1998;19: 489–492.
38. Peng JR. Solving the dilemna of the high ankle sprain in the athlete. *Sports Med Arthrosc Rev*. 2000;8:316–325.
39. Anderson KJ, Lecocq JF. Operative treatment of injury to the fibular collateral ligaments of the ankle. *J Bone Joint Surg*. 1954;36A:825–832.
40. Hollis JM, Blaiser RD, Flahiff CM. Simulated lateral ankle ligamentous injury: change in ankle stability. *Am J Sports Med*. 1993;23:672–677.
41. Johnson EE, Markolf K. The contribution of the anterior talofibular ligament to ankle laxity. *J Bone Joint Surg*. 1983;65A:81–88.
42. Landeros O, Frost HM, Higgins CC. Anteriorly unstable ankle due to trauma: a report of 29 cases. *J Bone Joint Surg*. 1996;48A:1028.
43. Landeros O, Frost HM, Higgins CC. Post traumatic anterior ankle instability. *Clin Orthop*. 1968;56:169–178.
44. Wedmore IS, Charette J. Emergency department evaluation and treatment of ankle and foot injuries. *Emerg Med Clin North Am*. 2000;18:86–114.
45. Gould N, Selingson D, Gassman J. Early and late repair of lateral ligaments of the ankle. Foot Ankle. 1980;1:84–89.
46. Staples OS. Rupture of the fibular collateral ligaments of the ankle. *J Bone Joint Surg*. 1975;57A:101–107.
47. Frost HM, Hanson CA. Technique for testing the drawer sign in the ankle. *Clin Orthop*. 1977;123:49–51.
48. Aradi AJ, Wong J, Walsh M. The dimple sign of a ruptured lateral ligament of the ankle: brief report. *J Bone Joint Surg [Br]*. 1988;70B:327–328.
49. van Dijk CN, Lim LSL, Bossuyt PMM, et al. Physical examination is sufficient for the diagnosis of sprained ankles. *J Bone Joint Surg [Br]*. 1996;78B: 958–962.
50. Birrer RB, Fani-Salek MH, Totten VY, et al. Managing ankle injuries in the emergency department. *J Emerg Med*. 1999;17:651–660.
51. Beynnon BD, Renstrom PA, Alosa DM, et al. Ankle ligament injury risk factors: a prospective study of college athletes. *J Orthop Res*. 2001;19:213–220.
52. Martin LP, Wayne JS, Monahan TJ, et al. Elongation behavior of calcaneofibular and cervical ligaments during inversion loads applied in an open kinetic chain. *Foot Ankle Int*. 1998;19:232–239.

53. Sugimoto K, Takakura Y, Samoto N, et al. Subtalar arthrography in recurrent instability of the ankle. *Clin Orthop Relat Res.* 2002;394:169–176.
54. Kleiger B. Mechanisms of ankle injury. *Orthop Clin North Am.* 1974;5:127–146.
55. Hockenbury RT, Sammarco GJ. Evaluation and treatment of ankle sprains - clinical recommendations for a positive outcome. *Phys Sports Med.* 2001;24:57–64.
56. Alonso A, Khoury L, Adams R. Clinical tests for ankle syndesmosis injury: reliability and prediction of return to function. *J Orthop Sports Phys Ther.* 1998;27:276–284.
57. Katznel A, Lin M. Ruptures of the ligaments about the tibiofibular syndesmosis. *Injury.* 1984;25:170–172.
58. Rasmussen O, Kroman-Andersen C. Experimental ankle injuries: analysis of the traumatology of the ankle ligaments. *Acta Orthop Scand.* 1983;54:356–362.
59. Safran MR, O'Malley D, Jr., Fu FH. Peroneal tendon subluxation in athletes: new exam techniques, case reports, and review. *Med Sci Sports Exerc.* 1999;31:S487–S492.
60. Thompson TC, Doherty JH. Spontaneous rupture of tendon of Achilles: a new clinical diagnostic test. *J Trauma.* 1962;2:126–129.
61. Maffulli N. The clinical diagnosis of subcutaneous tear of the Achilles tendon. A prospective study in 174 patients. *Am J Sports Med.* 1998;26:266–270.
62. Johnson KA. Posterior tibial tendon. In: Baxter DE, ed. *The Foot and Ankle in Sport.* St Louis, MO: C.V. Mosby; 1995.
63. Kausch T, Rutt J. Subcutaneous rupture of the the tibialis anterior tendon: review of the literature and a case report. *Arch Orthop Trauma Surg.* 1998;117:290–293.
64. Miller RR, Mahan KT. Closed rupture of the anterior tibial tendon: a case report. *J Am Pod Med Assn.* 1998;88:394–399.
65. Omari AM, Lee AS, Parsons SW. The clinical presentation of chronic tibialis anterior tendon insufficiency. *Foot Ankle Surg.* 1999;5:251–256.
66. Picciano AM, Rowlands MS, Worrell T. Reliability of open and closed kinetic chain subtalar joint neutral positions and navicular drop test. *J Orthop Sports Phys Ther.* 1993;18:553–558.
67. Mueller MJ, Host JV, Norton BJ. Navicular drop as a composite measure of excessive pronation. *J Am Podiat Med Assn.* 1993;83:198–202.
68. Brody DM. Techniques in the evaluation and treatment of the injured runner. *Orthop Clin North Am.* 1982;13:541–558.
69. Palmer ML, Epler M. *Clinical Assessment Procedures in Physical Therapy.* Philadelphia, PA: J.B. Lippincott; 1990.
70. Mennell JM. *Foot Pain.* Boston, MA: Little, Brown and Co.; 1969.
71. McRae SJ, Ginsberg JS. Update in the diagnosis of deep-vein thrombosis and pulmonary embolism. *Curr Opin Anaesthesiol.* 2006;19:44–51.
72. Aschwanden M, Labs KH, Engel H, et al. Acute deep vein thrombosis: early mobilization does not increase the frequency of pulmonary embolism. *Thromb Haemost.* 2001;85:42–46.
73. Evans RC. Illustrated Essentials in Orthopedic Physical Assessment. St. Louis, MO: Mosby-Year book Inc.; 1994.
74. Stiell IG, Greenberg GH, McKnight RD, et al. Decision rules for the use of radiography in acute ankle injuries: refinement and prospective validation. *JAMA.* 1994;269:1127–1132.

75. Stiell IG, McKnight RD, Greenberg GH, et al. Implementation of the Ottawa Ankle Rules. *JAMA*. 1994;271:827–832.
76. Leddy JJ, Smolinski RJ, Lawrence J, et al. Prospective evaluation of the Ottawa Ankle Rules in a University Sports Medicine Center. With a modification to increase specificity for identifying malleolar fractures. *Am J Sports Med*. 1998;26:158–165.
77. Guide to physical therapist practice. *Phys Ther*. 2001;81:S13–S95.
78. Clanton TO, Ford JJ. Turf toe injury. *Clin Sports Med*. 1984;13:731–41.

QUESTIONS

1. What are the major anatomic divisions of the bones of the foot?
2. Of the four muscular layers on the plantar aspect of the foot, moving from superficial to deep, which three muscles make up the first layer?
3. What is another name for the "spring" ligament?
4. Where is the sinus tarsi located?
5. What bones make up the midfoot?
6. Moving from medial to lateral, name the distal tarsal bones.
7. What is the only tendon to attach to the talus?
8. Which is the largest tarsal bone?
9. Which tarsal bone is the most prone to avascular necrosis?
10. What are the two major ligaments associated with the calcaneocuboid joint?
11. Which structures form the Lisfranc joint?
12. What is primary function of the tibialis posterior muscle?
13. What is the main function of the fibular (peroneal) muscles?
14. Which nerve provides cutaneous distribution to the medial aspect of the foot?
15. Pronation and supination are considered triplanar motions. Which three body plane motions are involved in pronation?
16. What is the close-packed position of the talocrural joint?
17. What is the close-packed position for the subtalar joint?
18. What is tarsal tunnel syndrome?
19. Where in the foot is the most common site of a neuroma?
20. What is a pilon ankle fracture?
21. What is a Jones fracture?
22. How is an adaptive shortened gastrocnemius differentiated from an adaptive shortened soleus muscle?
23. Which special test is used to detect an Achilles tendon rupture?

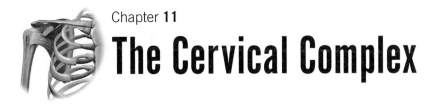

Chapter **11**

The Cervical Complex

OVERVIEW

With stability being sacrificed for mobility, the cervical complex is rendered more vulnerable to both direct and indirect trauma.

> ### ⬤ Clinical Pearl
>
> The cervical complex can be the source of many pain syndromes, including neck, upper thoracic and periscapular syndromes, cervical radiculopathy, and shoulder and elbow syndromes.[1] These syndromes may result from a vast array of causes, ranging from acute minor sprains to chronic degenerative changes.[2]

Neck pain usually resolves in days or weeks, but can recur and become chronic. Due to the proximity of the temporomandibular joint (TMJ) to both the craniovertebral joints and the cervical spine proper, dysfunction of this joint must always be given consideration when examining this complex.

ANATOMY

The cervical complex consists of the craniovertebral joints, the cervical spine proper, and the TMJ. The craniovertebral joints connect the cervical spine proper to the head.

> ### ⬤ Clinical Pearl
>
> The two major ligaments of the craniovertebral joints are as follows:
>
> • Transverse: retains the odontoid process in contact with the anterior arch during cervical flexion and extension.

• Alar functions to limit rotation of the craniovertebral region at C1–2.

The cervical spine proper, consisting of seven vertebrae, is one of the key links in the upper kinetic chain as, together with the craniovertebral joints, it is responsible for the control of head, and thus eye motion. For the most part, the muscles of the cervical complex (Table 11-1) function to support and move the head (Tables 11-2 and 11-3). Given the number of degrees of freedom available at the neck, it is likely that the muscles are organized as functional synergies. Synergies are conceptualized as units of control, incorporating the muscles around the joint that will act together in a functional

Table 11-1 Attachments and Innervation of Cervical Muscles

Muscle	Proximal	Distal	Innervation
Upper trapezius	Superior nuchal line Ligamentum nuchae	Lateral third of clavicle and the acromion process	Spinal accessory
Levator scapulae	Transverse processes of upper four cervical vertebrae	Medial border of scapula at level of scapular superior angle	Dorsal scapular C5 (C3 and C4)
Splenius capitis	Inferior ligamentum nuchae, spinous process of C7 and T1–4 vertebrae	Mastoid process, occipital bone, and lateral third of superior nuchal line	Cervical spinal nerve and ventral primary rami of cervical spinal nerves
Splenius cervicis	Spinous processes of T3–6 vertebrae	Posterior tubercles of C1–3	
Scalenus			
Anterior	Anterior tubercles of C3–6	Superior crest of first rib	Ventral primary rami of cervical spinal nerves
Middle	Posterior tubercles of C2–7	Superior crest of first rib	
Posterior	Posterior tubercles of C5–7	Outer surface of second rib	
Longus colli	Anterior tubercles of C3–5	Tubercle of the atlas, anterior	Ventral primary rami of cervical
	Anterior surface of C5–7, T1–3	Tubercles of C5 and C6, anterior surface of C2–4	spinal nerves
Longus capitis	Anterior tubercles of C3–6	Inferior occipital bone, basilar portion	Ventral primary rami of cervical spine nerves

Table 11-2 Prime Movers of the Cervical Spine: Extensors and Flexors

	Extensor Muscles	Flexor Muscles
Prime Movers	Accessory Muscles	Prime Movers
Trapezius	Multifidus	Sternocleidomastoid—anterior fibers
Sternocleidomastoid—posterior fibers	Suboccipitals	Accessory muscles
Iliocostalis cervices	Rectus capitis posterior major and minor	Prevertebral muscles
Longissimus cervices	Obliquus capitis superior	Longus coli
Splenius cervices	Obliquus capitis inferior	Longus capitis
Splenius capitis		Rectus capitis anterior
Interspinales cervices		Scalene group
Spinalis cervices		Scalenus anterior
Spinalis capitis		Infrahyoid group
Semispinalis cervices		Sternohyoid
Semispinalis capitis		Omohyoid
Levator scapulae		Sternothyroid
		Thyrohyoid

fashion.[3] Under this concept, the central nervous system needs only trigger a synergic unit to produce a specific movement, instead of communicating with each individual muscle.[3] Synergistic movement incorporates both agonist and antagonist muscle groups, which results in a greater level of control.

 Clinical Pearl

The atlanto-occipital joint primarily allows flexion and extension, whereas the atlanto-axial (A-A) articulation primarily provides rotation (approximately 50% of all cervical rotation). Unlike the

Table 11-3 Prime Movers of the Cervical Spine: Rotation and Side Bending

Muscles of Rotation and Side Bending	
Ipsilateral Side Bending	**Ipsilateral Rotation**
Longissimus capitis	Splenius capitis
Intertransversarii posteriores	Splenius cervices
Cervices	Rotatores breves cervices
Multifidus	Rotatores longi cervices
Rectus capitis lateralis	Rectus capitis posterior major
Intertransversarii anteriores cervices	Obliquus capitis inferior
Scaleni	
Iliocostalis cervicis	
Contralateral Rotation	**Ipsilateral Side Bending and Contralateral Rotation**
Obliquus capitis superior	Sternocleidomastoid Scalenus anterior Multifidus Longus colli
Ipsilateral Side Bending and Ipsilateral Rotation	
Longus coli	
Scalenus posterior	

segments of the cervical spine proper, the craniovertebral region lacks the articular stability of those segments below. Indeed, injuries to the A-A complex account for approximately 25% of all cervical spine injuries.[4]

Vertebrae C3 through C7 allow for varying degrees of flexion, extension, side bending, and rotation as an interdependent group. Movements of flexion center on C5 and C6 and extension movements center on C6 and C7.[5]

Intervertebral discs (IVDs) are found from C2–3 and below, and are subjected to significant deformation during flexion and extension. Eight pairs of cervical spinal nerves exit bilaterally through the intervertebral foramina.

Clinical Pearl

Each spinal nerve is named for the vertebra above which it exits; for example, the C6 nerve exits above the C6 vertebra.

The TMJ is a synovial, compound modified ovoid bicondylar joint, formed between the articular eminence of the temporal bone, the intra-articular disc and the head of the mandible. The mandible works like a class-three lever, with its joint as the fulcrum. There is agreement among the experts that postural impairments of the cervical, and upper thoracic spine, can produce both pain and impairment of the TMJ.[6] Located between the articulating surface of the temporal bone, and the mandibular condyle, is a fibrocartilaginous disc (sometimes inappropriately referred to as a "meniscus"). The TMJ is primarily supplied from three nerves that are part of the mandibular division of the fifth cranial (trigeminal) nerve.

EXAMINATION

The cervical complex is an area of the body that needs to be examined with caution, especially when there is a history of acute and recent trauma of the neck because of the potential for the examination itself to be harmful.[7] The initial examination should focus on general appearance (including skin lesions such as rashes), vital signs (pulse, blood pressure, and temperature), mental status and speech, gait, balance and coordination, cranial nerve and long tract examination, visual fields, acuity, and skull palpation.[8]

Clinical Pearl

The examination of the cervical complex must be graduated and progressive so that the testing can be discontinued at the first signs of serious pathology.[7]

An examination algorithm for the cervical spine proper is outlined in Figure 11-1. Based on the findings from this examination, an examination

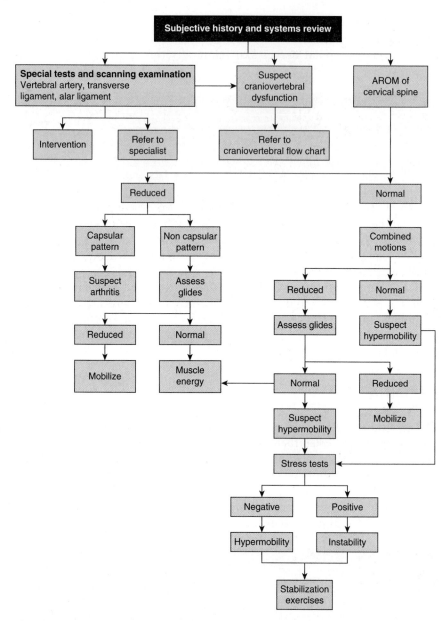

Figure 11-1 Algorithm for examination of the cervical spine proper.

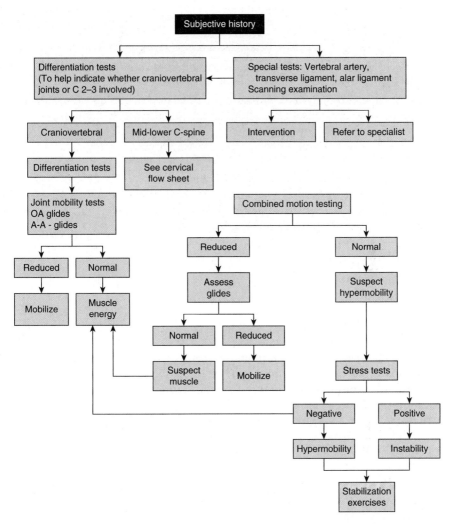

Figure 11-2 Algorithm for examination of the craniovertebral joints.

of the TMJ and craniovertebral joints may be warranted (Figure 11-2). In general, the occipito-atlantal (O-A) joint is examined and treated before the A-A joint to avoid confusion between findings from the combined tests of both joints.

Although most conditions involving neck and upper limb symptoms can be diagnosed after a careful history and physical examination, in cases of significant trauma, imaging studies may be required to exclude a fracture or instability.

Clinical Pearl

Due to the proximity of the cranial structures, the clinician should develop the habit of quickly screening patients with neck and head pain for their ability to orient to time, place and name, concentrate, reason and process information, make judgments, communicate effectively, and recall information.

Clearing tests for the cervical complex include
- Vertebral artery tests
- Sharp–Purser test
- Articular stability tests
- Transverse ligament test
- Alar ligament test
- TMJ tests

History

The history often gives the clinician clues as to the patient's chief complaint (pain, paresthesia, numbness, weakness, or stiffness), the source of the patient's symptoms, the nature (constant, intermittent, or variable) and location (head, neck, shoulder, arm, and hand) (Figure 11-3) of the involved structure (Table 11-4), the severity of the condition, and the activities or positions that appear to aggravate or improve the patient's condition (Table 11-5). In addition, asking the patient to describe his or her symptoms over a 24-hour period can provide the clinician with valuable information about positions and activities that aggravate or relieve the symptoms and about the duration of the symptoms. Questions about head and facial pain should also be asked (Table 11-6).

 Clinical Pearl

Pain that increases with activity or within a few hours after activity, but settles down with rest or a change in position is commonly referred to as mechanical pain. Conditions that have a mechanical origin are usually improved with rest, although they may worsen initially on retiring.[9]

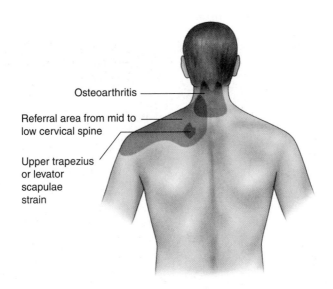

Osteoarthritis

Referral area from mid to
low cervical spine

Upper trapezius
or levator
scapulae
strain

Figure 11-3 Pain location and possible diagnoses.

The patient's sleeping position and habits should be investigated. Pain caused by sustained positions may awaken the patient at night, but is usually relieved with a change of position. Patients who report difficulty sleeping due to pain may have an inflammatory condition.

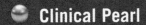 **Clinical Pearl**

Pain that persists or worsens despite rest and intervention, pain that persists around the clock, or pain that worsens at night raises suspicion for a metabolic or neoplastic condition, or for psychosocial factors that prolong recovery.[10]

It is important to determine:

• If the presenting symptoms were caused by trauma or surgery, or if the onset of pain occurred gradually. Questions should focus on any history of trauma during birth or childhood, as well as more recently.

Table 11-4 Pain Location and Possible Causes

Pain Location	Possible Cause
Head	Upper cervical spine
Localized pain	Muscle strain Ligament sprain Facet degeneration Disc degeneration
Upper trapezius region	Spinal nerve root irritation (C3)
Shoulder and lateral upper arm	Shoulder impingement
Radial forearm and thumb, and occasionally the index finger	Spinal nerve root irritation (C4)
Posterior arm, dorsal (occasionally ventral) forearm, and the index and middle fingers	Spinal nerve root irritation (C5) Spinal nerve root irritation (C5–6) Spinal nerve root irritation (C7)
Medial arm, ulnar forearm, and the ring and little fingers	Spinal nerve root irritation (C 8) Thoracic outlet syndrome Ulnar nerve neuropathy
Scapular region	Lower cervical nerve roots, discs, spinal longitudinal ligaments, and facet joints
Upper extremity in nondermatomal distribution	Thoracic outlet syndrome Cervical myelopathy

- If there are any emotional factors in the patient's background that may provoke habitual head protrusion or muscular tension.
- If the patient is aware of any parafunctional habits (cheek biting, nail biting, pencil chewing, teeth clenching, or bruxism).
- The behavior of symptoms over a 24-hour period. This information assists the clinician in formulating causal relationships.
- Whether the symptoms are improving or worsening.
- The relationship of eating to the symptoms. Alcohol, chocolate, and other foods can cause head pain in some individuals, suggesting a vasomotor-related pain.

Table 11-5 Differential Diagnosis of Cervical Spondylosis, Cervical Myelopathy, Spinal Stenosis, Thoracic Outlet Syndrome, and Posterolateral Disc Herniation

	Cervical Spondylosis (Osteoarthritis)	Cervical Myelopathy	Spinal Stenosis	Thoracic Outlet Syndrome	Posterolateral Cervical Disc Herniation
Pain	Unilateral	Not usually painful unless there is an associated radiculopathy	Unilateral or bilateral	May or may not be pain	Unilateral (commonly) or bilateral
Distribution of pain	Into affected dermatomes	Upper extremity (nondermatomal)	Usually several dermatomes affected	Upper extremity (nondermatomal)	Into affected dermatomes
Pain worsened by	Cervical extension	Cervical extension	Cervical extension	Shoulder retraction and depression	Cervical flexion
Pain relieved by	Positioning Cervical flexion	Positioning	Rest Cervical flexion	Positioning depending on type	Positioning
Age group affected	>45 years >60 years	40–60 years 50–70 years	11–70 years Most common: 30–60 years	Diverse	17–60 years
Instability	Possible	Possible	No	No	No
Levels commonly affected	C5-6, C6-7	C4–5, 5–6	Varies	C8–T1	C5–6
Onset	Slow	Slow	Slow	Slow	Sudden
Deep tendon reflexes	Hyporeflexive	Hyporeflexive in UE Hyporeflexive in LE	Hyporeflexive	Unremarkable or hyporeflexive	Hyporeflexive
Diagnostic imaging	Radiographs diagnostic	MRI and/or CT myelography	MRI	Radiograph	Diagnostic when clinical signs support

Table 11-6 Normal Active Range of Motion of the Cervical Complex

Movement	Range (degrees)
Flexion	80–90
Extension	70
Side bending	20–45
Axial rotation	70–90

- The patient's past dental and orthodontic history.
- Whether the patient has experienced any "locking" of the jaw. The patient may report the jaw suddenly "catching" or "getting stuck," which usually is related to an internal derangement.[11] Locking implies an inability to fully open or close the jaw. Locking usually is preceded by reciprocal clicking (see the discussion of range of motion testing, later).

 Clinical Pearl

Locking of the jaw in the closed position is often caused by the condyle assuming a position that is posterior or anteromedial to the disc.

Chronic head, neck, and back pain often are associated with psychogenic causes. Psychiatric disorders, usually, are manifested in patients whose afflictions seem to be excessive or persist beyond what would be normal for that condition.

The chronicity of the symptoms can afford the clinician with some clues[10]:

- Muscle strains usually resolve within a few days to a couple of weeks
- Ligament sprains may take up to a couple of months
- Disc injuries or herniations with radiculopathy can take 3 to 6 months for full recovery.

There are three cardinal features of temporomandibular disorders, which can be local or remote:

1. *Restricted jaw function.* A history of limited mouth opening, which may be intermittent or progressive, is a key feature of TMD. Patients may describe a generalized tight feeling, which may indicate a muscular disorder, or capsulitis, or the sensation that the jaw suddenly "catches" or "locks," which usually is related to mechanical interferences in the joint (internal derangement).[12] Associated signs of an internal derangement include pain and deviation of mandibular movements during opening and closing.

2. *Joint noises.* The presence of joint noises (crepitus) of the TMJ may or may not be significant, because joint sounds occur in approximately 50% of healthy populations.[13] Some joint sounds, such as "soft" crepitus, are not audible to the clinician, so a stethoscope may be required. "Hard" crepitus, often described as gravelly or grating, is a diffuse sustained noise that occurs during a considerable portion of the opening or closing cycle, or both, and is an evidence of a change in osseous contour.[14] Clicking is a brief noise that occurs at some point during opening, closing, or both.

 Clinical Pearl

Jaw clicking during mouth opening or closing may be suggestive of an internal derangement consisting of an anterior disc displacement with reduction.[15,16]

 Clinical Pearl

TMJ sounds should be described and related to symptoms. Joint noise is, of itself, of little clinical importance in the absence of pain.[17,18]

---

3. *Orofacial pain.* Approximately half of all cases of TMD are masticatory myalgias.[19] Pain should be evaluated carefully in terms of its onset, nature, intensity, site, duration, aggravating and relieving factors, and, especially, how it relates to the other features such as joint noise and restricted mandibular movements.[12] Orofacial pain associated with mouth opening or closing, and jaw crepitus is suggestive of osteoarthrosis, capsulitis, or

internal derangement consisting of an anterior disc displacement with reduction.[15,16,20–23]

Clinical Pearl

In a study by Magnusson and colleagues,[24] five different scales of self-assessment of pain were tested in patients with TMJ disorders. The precision and sensitivity and the capacity to register memory of pain and discomfort were compared for each of the five scales. From these results, the behavior rating scale can be recommended when measuring pain and discomfort in patients with TMJ disorders.

Clinical Pearl

Clinicians often see patients with a TMD who present with nonspecific symptoms such as neck pain, headaches, earaches, and tinnitus. However, because these symptoms are not considered specific for TMDs, other possible causes should be sought and ruled out during the systems review.[25–27]

Localized pain generally points to muscle strains, ligament sprains, and facet or disc (degenerative) processes, although these structures commonly radiate pain to the thoracic spine, the periscapular, the upper chest or upper trapezius (Table 11-4).

Clinical Pearl

Cervical facet dysfunction can be either primary (following a direct injury to the facet) or secondary (the result of a degenerative process to the facet, or dysfunction of the IVD and associated structures). The patient with a cervical facet dysfunction typically reports diffuse nonspecific neck pain in the posterior neck and/or scapular area, which is exacerbated by specific neck motions—closing pattern (decreased extension, and side bending/rotation to the involved side) of the spine. Physiologically, degenerative changes to the cervical spine produces a thickening and sclerosis of the subchondral bone, and development of osteophytes or bone spurs, resulting in a narrowing of the joint space, and a loss of shock absorption capabilities.

Symptoms that radiate into the upper limbs frequently stem from cervical radiculitis, although myofascial radiation patterns occur occasionally.[10] Radicular or referred pain may be accompanied by sensorimotor symptoms.[28]

 Clinical Pearl

Cervical disc lesions can be grouped as follows:

- Disc bulge: involves bulging of the disc margin beyond the endplates of the adjacent vertebral levels.

- Disc protrusion: involves tearing of the nucleus pulposus through a small portion of the annulus fibrosis.

- Disc extrusion: involves expansion of the nucleus pulposus through the outer lamina of the annulus fibrosis.

- Disc sequestration: the nucleus pulposus becomes detached from the annulus and typically resides within the spinal cord canal.

The neurological examination attempts to differentiate between nerve root and spinal cord compression (Table 11-5). Other differential diagnostic considerations for upper limb symptoms include thoracic outlet syndrome (see Special Tests) and peripheral nerve entrapments.[29]

 Clinical Pearl

Cervical zygapophyseal joint pain is typically unilateral, and described by the patient as a dull ache. Occasionally, the pain can be referred into the craniovertebral or interscapular regions.

Pain may also be referred to the tip of the acromion or scapular region via the cutaneous branches of the upper thoracic dorsal rami.[30]

The rib articulations of cervicothoracic region may produce local pain, or refer pain to the suprascapular fossa or shoulder.[31]

 Clinical Pearl

Neck pain accompanied by widespread musculoskeletal pain raises the strong possibility of fibromyalgia, whereas neck pain with synovitis of peripheral joints suggests an inflammatory arthropathy such as rheumatoid arthritis.[32] Generalized aching and the presence of trigger points characterize myofascial pain syndromes. In the cervical complex, myofascial pain can occur as a secondary tissue response to an IVD or zygapophyseal joint injury.[33]

A report of vertigo, although potentially problematic, is not in of itself a contraindication to the continuation of the examination. Differential diagnosis for complaints of dizziness includes primary central nervous system diseases, vestibular and ocular involvement, and, more rarely, metabolic disorders.[34] Careful questioning can help in the differentiation of central and peripheral causes of vertigo.

• Central vertigo is usually due to a disturbance of the vestibular system, which can produce sensations of head and body rotations, to and fro movements, or up and down movements.

• Peripheral vertigo is manifested with general complaints such as unsteadiness, and feeling lightheaded .

Cervical vertigo may be produced by localized muscle changes and receptor irritation.[35] Dizziness provoked by head movements or head positions could indicate an inner ear dysfunction. Dizziness provoked by specific cervical motions, particularly extension or rotation, may also indicate a vertebral artery compromise.

 Clinical Pearl

The vertebral artery is a branch of the subclavian artery. The basilar artery and vertebral artery form the vertebrobasilar system, which directly supplies the pons, medulla, thalamus, cerebellum, midbrain, and occipital region of the cortex. Occlusion of the vertebral or basilar arteries can occur as a result of cervical rotation or cervical rotation coupled with cervical extension. Common signs and symptoms of such occlusion include dizziness and gait disturbances.

Finally, it is important for the clinician to determine whether the patient has had successive onsets of similar symptoms in the past, as recurrent injury tends to have a detrimental affect on the potential for recovery. If it is a recurrent injury, the clinician should note how often, and how easily, the injury has recurred, and the success, or failure of previous interventions.

 Clinical Pearl

For the purposes of the examination, it is important to establish a baseline of symptoms so that the clinician is able to determine whether a particular examination movement aggravates or lessens the patient's symptoms. All symptoms presented should be recorded on a body diagram, even those that may initially appear unrelated. If pain is the major symptom, the clinician should attempt to quantify the pain using a pain rating scale. It is also appropriate at this time to establish the patient's goals.

Mechanism

The clinician must determine whether trauma occurred and the exact mechanism.

- In acute sprains and strains, patients typically relate an activity that precipitated the onset of their symptoms. This may have involved lifting or pulling a heavy object, an awkward sleeping position, a hyperextension injury, or a prolonged static posture.
- In whiplash-associated disorders, patients generally describe an accident in which they were unexpectedly struck from the rear, front, or side. Rotational injuries can also occur.

If there were neurological symptoms following the trauma (paresthesias, dizziness, ringing in the ears (tinnitus), visual disturbances, or loss of consciousness), more severe damage should be suspected.[36] If the patient reports electric shock-like symptoms when looking downward (neck flexion), the clinician should consider the possibility of inflammation or irritation of the meninges (Lhermitte sign).[37–39]

Clinical Pearl

Lhermitte symptom or "phenomenon" is not so much a test as it is a symptom. The test is currently described as being performed in a variety of ways, although it is most commonly described as passive cervical flexion to end range with the patient seated. A positive test is indicated by the presence of an electric shock-like sensation that radiates down the spinal column into the upper or lower limbs when flexing the neck. It also may be precipitated by extending the head, coughing, sneezing, bending forward, or moving the limbs. A positive test is described to occur with cervical spinal cord pathology from a variety of conditions, including multiple sclerosis, spinal cord tumor, cervical spondylosis, and radiation myelitis. However, there are currently no reports in the literature investigating the interexaminer reliability of the test.

 Clinical Pearl

An insidious onset of symptoms could suggest postural, degenerative, or myofascial origins, a disease process, such as ankylosing spondylitis, cervical spondylosis, thoracic outlet syndrome, or facet syndrome. An insidious onset may also indicate the presence of a serious pathology such as a tumor.

Systems Review

The cervical complex houses many vital structures. These include the spinal cord, the vertebral artery, and the brain stem. Given the high density of neurological structures in this region, dysfunction of this region can refer symptoms to areas quite distal. It is extremely important for the clinician to approach this area with caution and to rule out the presence of serious pathology.

 Clinical Pearl

Nonorganic findings consistent with abnormal illness behavior include[40]:

• Complaints of pain with light touch or pinching of the skin over the cervical region.

- Complaints of widespread tenderness with local palpation in the cervical or upper thoracic region.

- Neck pain with rotation of the head, trunk, and pelvis in unison while standing, and limited neck rotation—less than 50% of normal in each direction.

- Diminished sensation in a pattern not corresponding to a specific dermatome of the nerve root or peripheral nerve.

- Giveaway weakness on motor testing.

- Signs of overreaction.

General health questions provide information about the status of the cardiopulmonary system, the presence or absence of systemic disease, and information about medications the patient may be taking which might impact the examination or intervention. Where applicable, the patient should be examined for central and peripheral neurological deficit, neurovascular compromise, and serious skeletal injury such as fractures or craniovertebral ligamentous instability. Warning signs in the cervical region include the following:

- An unexplained weight loss, which could suggest cancer
- Evidence of compromise to two or three spinal nerve roots
- A gradual increasing of pain. Normally pain subsides over time
- An expansion of symptoms in terms of the regions involved. The area of symptoms should decrease with time as healing occurs
- Spasm with passive range of motion of the neck
- Visual disturbances. The cranial nerves should be assessed if there are complaints about vision, or the patient appears to have problems with speech and/or swallowing. Such disturbances could indicate a cranial bleed or an upper motor neuron lesion
- Painful and weak resistive testing
- Hoarseness. Hoarseness may be the result of cranial nerve involvement or pharyngeal damage. In cases of a motor vehicle accident, hoarseness may occur as a reaction to the inhalation of the chemicals released by the deployment of the airbag
- Horner syndrome
- T1 palsy (weakness and atrophy of the intrinsic muscles of the hand)
- Side bending away from the painful side causes pain (if this is the only motion that causes pain).

Clinical Pearl

It must be remembered that every cervical patient, especially the ones with a history of a hyperextension mechanism, is at potential risk for serious head and neck injuries, including compromise of the vertebral artery.

The following signs and symptoms demand a cautious approach or an appropriate referral:

- Recent trauma of 6 weeks or less
- An acute capsular pattern of the neck. According to Cyriax,[41] the capsular pattern of the cervical spine proper is full flexion in the presence of limited extension, and symmetrical limitation of rotation and side bending. The presence of a capsular pattern may indicate arthritis
- Severe movement loss of head and neck motion, whether capsular or non-capsular
- Strong spasm
- Segmental paresis
- Segmental or multi segmental hypo/hyper or areflexia (see next section)
- Other neurological signs and/or symptoms
- Constant or continuous pain
- Moderate-to-severe radiating pain
- Moderate-to-severe headaches
- Tinnitus (ringing in the ear)
- Facial pain. Patients with referred pain in the region of the trigeminal nerve (CN V) commonly have an underlying disorder of the upper cervical spine, such as A-A instability caused by rheumatoid arthritis.[42,43] In addition, trigeminal neuralgia can refer pain along the course of the trigeminal nerve. The trigeminal nerve has three major branches: the ophthalmic, the maxillary, and the mandibular. All three of these branches carry sensory information, but the mandibular nerve has both sensory and motor functions. Tumors, viral infections of the trigeminal nerve, or swelling in the brain, have all been hypothesized as potential sources of nerve dysfunction[44–46]
- History of loss of consciousness.
- Psychological changes (memory loss or forgetfulness, difficulties with problem solving, reduced motivation, irritability, anxiety and/or depression, insomnia).

Clinical Pearl

Symptoms that respond to mechanical stimuli in a predictable manner are usually considered to have a mechanical source. Symptoms
that show no predictable response to mechanical stimuli are unlikely
to be mechanical in origin, and their presence should alert the clinician to the possibility of a more sinister disorder or one of central
initiation, autonomic, or affective nature.[47]

Vascular Compromise

The existence of dizziness or seizures always warrants further investigation. It
is not always an easy task for the clinician to determine whether the presenting
dizziness is due to a disturbed afferent input from the cervical complex, which
can be extremely rewarding to treat, or whether the cause is more serious.[7]
For example, dizziness provoked by head movements may indicate an inner
ear or vertebral artery problem. A history of falling without loss of consciousness (drop attack) is strongly suggestive of vertebral artery compromise.[48]
Testing of the vertebral artery should be considered if the observation and
history reveal any of the signs and symptoms that have been linked, directly or
indirectly to vertebral artery insufficiency, which include the following:

- Wallenberg, Horner, and similar syndromes
- Bilateral or quadrilateral paresthesia
- Hemiparesthesia
- Ataxia
- Nystagmus
- Drop attacks
- Periodic loss of consciousness
- Lip anesthesia
- Hemifacial para/anesthesia
- Dysphasia
- Dysarthria

Headache or Facial Pain

A history of headaches may or may not be benign, depending on the frequency and
severity. Differential diagnosis is important, especially in light of the fact that there
is considerable overlap between tension headaches, cervicogenic headaches, cervical, trigeminal and glossopharyngeal neuralgia, Lyme disease, migraines without

aura, and TMJ dysfunction.[49] A determination must be made as to the location frequency and intensity of the headaches, and whether a certain position alters the headache. If the patient reports relief of pain and referred symptoms with the placement of the hand or arm of the affected side on top of the head, this is the Bakody sign and is usually indicative of a disc lesion of the C4 or C5 level.[50]

 Clinical Pearl

In general, the TMJ and the upper three cervical joints all refer symptoms to the head, whereas the mid-to-low cervical spine typically refers symptoms to the shoulder and arm.[51-53]

Cervicogenic headaches, which can be mild, moderate, or severe, tend to be unilateral, and located in the suboccipital region with referral to the frontal, retro-orbital, and temporal areas.[54,55]

 Clinical Pearl

The more serious causes of headache without a history of trauma include spontaneous subarachnoid hemorrhage, meningitis, pituitary tumor, brain tumor, and encephalitis.

Facial pain can be the consequence of temporomandibular dysfunction, temporal arteritis, acute sinusitis, orbital disease, glaucoma, trigeminal neuralgia, referred pain, and herpes zoster.

 Clinical Pearl

Pain that is centered immediately in front of the tragus of the ear and that projects to the ear, temple, cheek, and along the mandible is highly diagnostic for TMD.[56]

Balance Disturbance

Early indications of a balance disturbance can occur during the history or systems review with correct questioning. A simple question such as "Do you have difficulty with walking or with balance?" can provide the clinician with valuable information. Positive responses may indicate a cervical myelopathy or a systemic neurological impairment.[57]

Clinical Pearl

Myelopathy may occur with compression of the spinal cord, and is more likely to occur at the C5–6 level, because in this region the spinal cord is at its widest and the spinal canal is at its narrowest.[58] Depending on the cause, the onset of myelopathy can be sudden or gradual. The patient typically complains of symptoms in multiple extremities, and clumsiness when performing fine motor skills. Objectively, the patient may demonstrate gait ataxia, positive pathological reflexes below the level of spinal pathology, and lower motor neuron signs at the level of spinal pathology.

Once the possibility of cervical, systemic, psychogenic, or ear or sinus problems has been ruled out, the next step is to consider the possibility of TMJ pain and impairment, particularly if the pain is accompanied by jaw clicking and limited mouth opening.[59]

Tests and Measures

Observation

Static observation of general posture, as well as the relationship of the head on the neck and the neck on the trunk, is observed while the patient is standing and sitting, both in the waiting area and in the examination room. The patient is observed in the sagittal, coronal, and transverse planes.

Clinical Pearl

A major contributor to cervicogenic pain is a lack of postural control due to poor neuromuscular function.[49,60–62]

The patient should have a smooth cervical lordosis with gentle transition into thoracic kyphosis. A "forward" head (ear forward of the acromion) or accentuated cervicothoracic hump creates a constant flexion moment of the head over the spine.[10] Similarly, flexed posturing at the hips from tight hip flexors results in a compensatory increase in the lumbar and cervical lordoses. Sustained postures, or fatigue overloading of the deep spinal and postural muscles, can result in increased joint compressive forces, and inefficient movement strategies.[63–66]

 Clinical Pearl

Torticollis is a rotational dysfunction of the upper neck musclulature. Although torticollis can be congenital, it may also be a physical manifestation or protective mechanism produced by an underlying pathology (trauma to the cervical spine, inflammation, neurological, or disease process). The adopted head posture of ipsilateral neck side bending and contralateral head rotation has been attributed to a sustained contraction of the sternocleidomastoid (SCM) muscle.

Thoracic outlet syndrome or other chronic strain patterns can be associated with obesity, or those patients with rounded shoulders, a hunched posture, or overdeveloped anterior chest wall muscles.

Palpation

Palpation is a key component of the evaluation for cervical myofascial pain. Examination of the skin overlying the spine has been found to be very helpful toward making a diagnosis as certain skin changes in a particular location may point in the direction of a dysfunctional spinal area.[67] The following muscle groups of the cervical complex should be palpated routinely:

- Trapezius: a large muscle group with upper, middle, and lower fibers. This muscle is susceptible to the effects of whiplash injury. The upper trapezius is greatly affected by postural insufficiency.
- Sternocleidomastoid: should be palpated along both sternal and clavicular heads.
- Posterior muscle groups: splenius, semispinalis, multifidi, and suboccipital muscles. All of these muscle groups can cause radiation of pain in or about the head.
- Scalenes: if tender, these can be assessed as a group by asking the patient to turn the head toward the painful side and pull the chin down into the supraclavicular fossa. The individual scalene muscles can be evaluated by stretching the head to the opposite side, looking straight forward (middle scalene), looking away (anterior scalene), and look toward the elbow (posterior scalene).[68]

The spinous processes and the interspinous ligaments from C2 through T1 are usually palpable during the assessment of flexion and extension. C7 is usually the longest spinous process, being referred to as the vertebra prominens, although, the spinous process of either C6 or T1 might be quite long as well.

Clinical Pearl

Exquisite bony tenderness may indicate a fracture; interspinous pain may be consistent with a ligament sprain, which is confirmed by pain in the same area during neck flexion.

The facet articulations are approximately a thumb's breadth to either side of the spinous process. Point tenderness here, especially with extension and rotation to the same side, suggests that the patient has facet joint pain. Finally, the surrounding soft tissues of the neck and shoulder girdle should be palpated. Trigger points of the paraspinal and shoulder girdle regions will refer pain to a more distal area.

Clinical Pearl

Tender points may indicate a localized muscle strain, in which case contraction of the muscle containing the tender point should cause pain.

An area that is tender to palpation but not painful during muscle contraction may represent pain referred from some other area. These patterns can also be identified during range-of-motion testing.

Active Range of Motion

The clinical examination of the mobility of the cervical complex should consist of a comparison between active and passive ranges, both in straight planes and with combined motions of the cervical complex. Normal ranges for the cervical spine are outlined in Table 11-6. Knowledge of cervical anatomy and kinematics should assist the clinician in determining the structure responsible based on the pattern of movement restriction (Table 11-7) noted in the physical examination.

Table 11-7 Positions and Movement Restriction Patterns of the Cervical Spine

Pattern/Position	Description
Capsular pattern	Side bending and rotation equally limited extension
Close-packed Position	Full extension
Open-packed Position	Slight extension
Closing restriction	Decreased extension and side bending and rotation toward the side of the restriction
Opening restriction	Decreased flexion and side bending and rotation away from the side of the restriction

Clinical Pearl

An acute or chronic closed-lock of the TMJ can result from a nonreducing deformed disc acting as an obstacle to the sliding condylar head. This condition can result from trauma, parafunctional habits (cheek biting, nail biting, pencil chewing, teeth clenching, or bruxism), malocclusion, disc adhesion, or inflammation. The signs and symptoms associated with this condition include the following:

• Deviation in mouth opening toward the involved side.

• Pain on palpation during mouth opening.

• Restrictions of joint mobility.

• Decreased protrusion with the mandible shifting toward the involved side.

To help determine whether the TMJ is contributing to the patient's symptoms, a quick TMJ screen is recommended. An accurate diagnosis of TMD involves a careful evaluation of the information gleaned from the history, systems review, and tests and measures. In most chronic cases, a behavioral or psychological examination is required.[18,53,69–74] Because postural dysfunctions are closely related to TMJ symptoms, the clinician should always perform a postural examination as part of a comprehensive examination of this joint. The TMJ screen involves having the patient open and close the mouth, while the clinician notes both the range and quality of movement. To help improve the accuracy of the range of motion testing, the clinician can palpate over the mandible heads during opening and closing to determine whether they move together. The clinician also notes any crepitus or clicking on opening and closing, and where they occur in the range.

 Clinical Pearl

The capsular pattern of the TMJ is limitation of mouth opening. If one joint is more involved than the other, the jaw laterally deviates to the involved side during opening.

The range of motion available at the cervical complex is the result of such factors as the shape and orientation of the zygapophyseal joint surfaces, the inherent flexibility of the restraining ligaments and joint capsules, and the height and pliability of the IVD.[75] In addition the range of motion is influenced by the range available in the craniovertebral joints and upper thoracic joints. Neck and head rotation could be considered as the functional motion of the craniovertebral joints, particularly the A-A joints.

 Clinical Pearl

Biomechanical studies have identified flexion and extension motion of the OA joint to be approximately 13 degrees. Side bending motion at the OA joint averages 8 degrees with negligible rotation.

Rotation is the key movement of the AA joint, which averages 47 degrees and is limited by the lateral atlantoaxial facet joint capsule and the opposite alar ligament.[68] There is 10 degrees of total flexion and extension at the AA joint with a negligible amount of side bending.

Range of motion ideally should be assessed actively using a goniometer placed at the external auditory meatus for flexion and extension, at the top of the head for rotation, and at the nares for side bending.[68]

 Clinical Pearl

During visual observation, the patient should be able to touch chin to chest with mouth closed (flexion between 90 degrees and 80

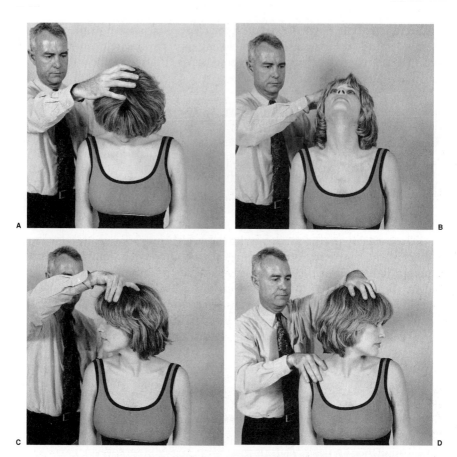

Figure 11-4 Cervical active range of motion with passive overpressure.

degrees), look almost straight up to the ceiling (extension of between 70 degrees and 90 degrees), rotate the chin to approach the shoulder (rotation of between 70 degrees and 90 degrees), and bend the ear toward the shoulder (side bending of between 20 degrees and 45 degrees) (Figure 11-4).[10]

The wide variations in ranges can result from the age of the patient being assessed. As with other joints in the body, the available range of motion typically decreases with age, the only exception being the rotation available at

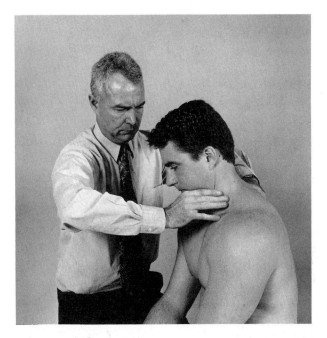

Figure 11-5 Short neck flexion.

C1–2, which may increase.[76] To better assess the craniovertebral joints, short neck flexion (Figure 11-5) and short neck extension (Figure 11-6) should be assessed. McKenzie[9] advocates the addition of neck protrusion and neck retraction to the range of motion examination, or to specific motions, to determine whether these additions affect the symptoms (see Combined Motion Testing).

Clinical Pearl

Using a goniometer, intraclass correlation coefficients have been found to range from 0.84 to 0.95 for intratester reliability, and between 0.73 and 0.92 for intertester reliability.[40]

Each of the motions is tested with a gentle overpressure (Figure 11-4), applied at the end of range if the active range appears to full and pain free. With the exception of rotation, the weight of the head usually provides sufficient overpressure.

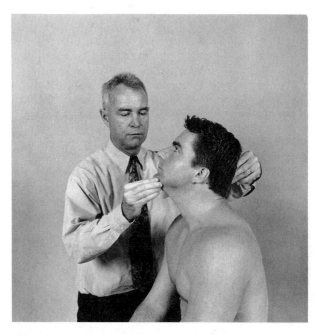

Figure 11-6 Short neck extension.

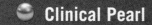

Clinical Pearl

It is necessary to apply overpressure even in the presence of pain, to get an end-feel. If the application of overpressure produces pain, the presence of an acute muscle spasm is possible. Caution must be taken when using overpressure in the direction of rotation, especially if the rotation is combined with ipsilateral side bending and extension, as this can compromise the vertebral artery.[77]

The clinician should evaluate the following:

• The quality and quantity of the motion. Quantity and quality of movement refers to the ability to achieve end range with curve reversal and without deviation from the intended movement plane.[78] Considerable emphasis should be placed on the amount and quality of flexion available, and the symptoms it provokes, as flexion is the only motion normally tolerated well by the cervical complex.

• The end-feel

- The symptoms provoked
- The willingness of the patient to move
- The presence of specific patterns of restriction.

Combined Motion Testing

As normal function involves complex and combined motions of the cervical complex, combined motion testing can also be used.

Using a biomechanical model, a restriction of cervical extension, side bending and rotation to the same side as the pain is termed a *closing* restriction. A restriction of the opposite motions (cervical flexion, side bending, and rotation to the opposite side of the pain) is termed an *opening* restriction. Opening restrictions are slightly more difficult to identify in the cervical spine proper because, frequently, there is no actual restriction of cervical flexion, but rather a restriction of rotation and side bending, along with reproduction of pain on the contralateral side.[79]

The results from these motions can be combined with the findings from the history and the single plane motions to categorize the symptomatic responses into one of three syndromes: postural, dysfunction, or derangement. This information can guide the clinician as to which motions to use in the intervention.

Key Muscle Testing

A focused examination of the myotome or "key muscles" is essential in any active patient complaining of neck pain, because a patient can have a pure motor radiculopathy with few or no extremity symptoms. In an athlete, maximal force must be applied when testing the major muscle groups to detect early weakness. There are numerous smaller muscles throughout this area, so resistance needs to be applied gradually.

Clinical Pearl

By repetitively loading the patient's resisting muscle with rapid, consecutive impulses, more subtle weakness can be detected. Even if the pressure overpowers the patient, the key is detecting asymmetries in strength or differences from one key muscle to the next.

During the resisted tests, the clinician looks for relative strength and fatigability. The muscles tested below are also used during the Cyriax upper quarter scanning examination. Alternates are given for each "myotome" or key muscle.

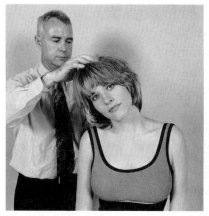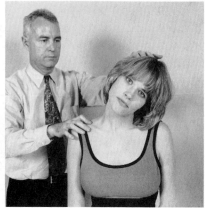

Figure 11-7 Resisted cervical side bending.

Resisted Cervical Rotation
Resisted cervical rotation tests the C2 "myotome".

Resisted Cervical Side Bending
Resisted side bending (Figure 11-7) tests the C3 "myotome".

Scapular Elevators (C2–4)
The clinician asks the patient to elevate their shoulders about one half of full elevation. The clinician applies a downward force on both shoulders while the patient resists (Figure 11-8).

Diaphragm (C4)
The clinician measures the amount of rib expansion that occurs with a deep breath using a tape measure. A comparison is made to a similar measurement at rest. Four measurement positions are used:

- Fourth lateral intercostal space
- Axilla
- Nipple line
- Tenth rib

Shoulder Abduction (C5)
The clinician asks the patient to abduct the arms to about 80 degrees to 90 degrees with the forearms in neutral. The clinician applies a downward force on the humerus while the patient resists (Figure 11-9).

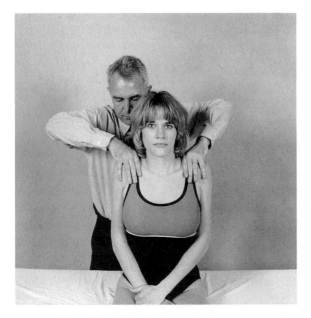

Figure 11-8 Resisted shoulder elevation.

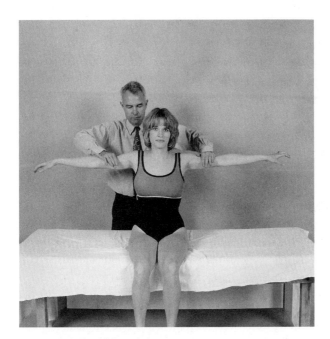

Figure 11- 9 Resisted shoulder abduction.

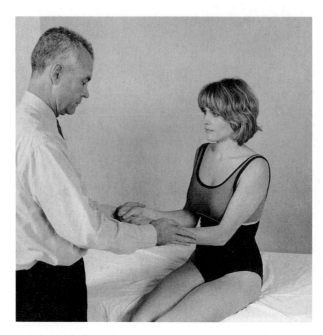

Figure 11-10 Resisted shoulder external rotation.

Shoulder External Rotation (C5)
The clinician asks the patient to put the arms by the sides, with the elbows flexed to 90 degrees and forearms in neutral. The clinician applies an inward force to the forearms (Figure 11-10).

Elbow Flexion (C6)
The clinician asks the patient to put the arms by the sides, with the elbows flexed to approximately 90 degrees and the forearms supinated. The clinician applies a downward force to the forearms (Figure 11-11).

Wrist Extension (C6)
The clinician asks the patient to place the arms by the sides, with the elbows flexed to 90 degrees and the forearms, wrists, and fingers in neutral. The clinician applies a downward force to the back of the patient's hands (Figure 11-12).

Shoulder Internal Rotation (C6)
The clinician asks the patient to put the arms by the sides, with the elbows flexed to 90 degrees and forearms in neutral. The clinician applies an outward force to the forearms (Figure 11-13).

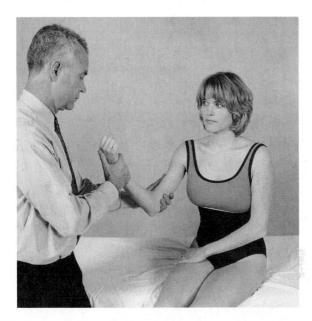

Figure 11-11 Resisted elbow flexion.

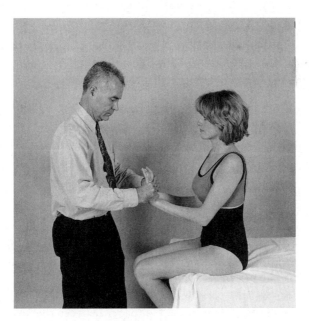

Figure 11-12 Resisted wrist extension.

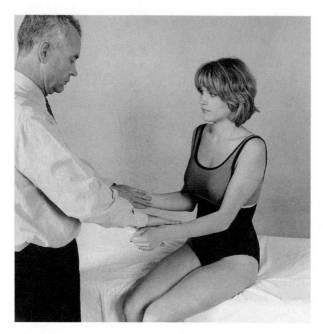

Figure 11-13 Resisted shoulder internal rotation.

Elbow Extension (C7)
The patient is seated with their elbow slightly flexed. The clinician stands to the side of the patient and tests the triceps by grasping the patient's forearms and attempting to flex their elbows (Figure 11-14).

Wrist Flexion (C7)
The clinician asks the patient to place the arms by the sides, with the elbows flexed to approximately 90 degrees and the forearms, wrists, and fingers in neutral. The clinician applies an upward force to the palm of the patient's hands (Figure 11-15).

Thumb Extension (C8)
The patient extends their thumb just short of full range of motion. The clinician stabilizes the proximal interphalangeal joint of the thumb with one hand and applies an isometric force into thumb flexion with the other (Figure 11-16).

Hand Intrinsics (T1)
The patient is asked to squeeze a piece of paper between the fingers while the clinician tries to pull it away (Figure 11-17).

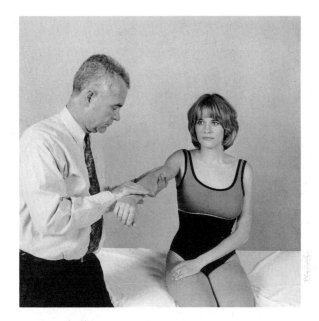

Figure 11-14 Resisted elbow extension.

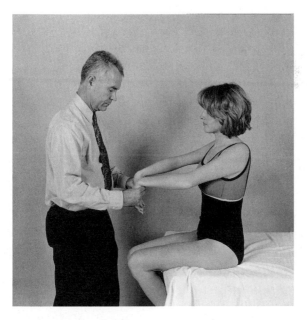

Figure 11-15 Resisted wrist flexion.

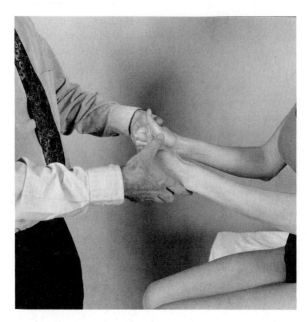

Figure 11-16 Resisted thumb extension.

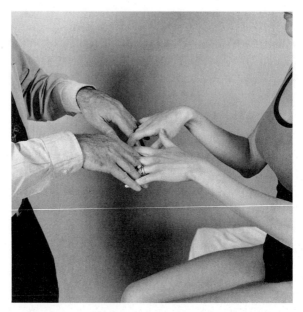

Figure 11-17 Strength test for finger adductors (hand intrinsics).

Temporalis
The patient is positioned sitting. The clinician palpates the side of the head in the temporal fossa region. The patient is asked to elevate and retract the mandible. Resistance can be applied using a tongue depressor placed between the teeth. Both sides are tested.

Masseter
The patient is positioned sitting. The clinician palpates the cheek, just above the angle of the mandible. The patient is asked to elevate the mandible, as in closing the jaw. Resistance can be applied using a tongue depressor placed between the teeth.

Lateral Pterygoid
The patient is positioned sitting. The clinician palpates the pterygoid at the neck of the mandible and joint capsule. The patient is asked to protrude and depress the mandible against manual resistance.

Medial Pterygoid
The patient is positioned sitting. The patient is asked to elevate and protrude the mandible. Resistance can be applied using a tongue depressor placed between the teeth.

Suprahyoid Muscles
The patient is positioned sitting. The clinician palpates the floor of the mouth. The patient is asked to press the tip of the tongue against the front teeth. Resistance can be applied to the surface of the hyoid bone in an attempt to protrude the tongue.

Infrahyoid Muscles
The patient is positioned sitting. The clinician palpates below the hyoid bone, immediately lateral to the midline. The patient is asked to swallow, while the clinician palpates for the movement of the hyoid and larynx.

Muscles of Facial Expression
This group of muscles, most of which are innervated by the facial nerve, can be assessed by having the patient attempt to make the specific facial expression attributed to each muscle (Table 11-8).

Muscle Length Testing

Upper Trapezius
The patient is positioned in supine. The patient's head is maximally flexed, inclined to the contralateral side, and ipsilaterally rotated (Figure 11-18).

Table 11-8 Muscles of Facial Expression

Muscle	Action	Innervation
Occipitofrontalis	Wrinkles forehead by raising eyebrows	Facial nerve
Corrugator	Draws eyebrows together, as in frowning	Facial nerve
Procerus	Draws skin on lateral nose upward, forming transverse wrinkles over bridge of the nose	Facial nerve
Nasalis	Dilates and compresses aperture of the nostrils	Facial nerve
Orbicularis oculi	Closes eyes tightly	Facial nerve
Superior levator palpebrae	Lifts upper eyelid	Oculomotor nerve
Orbicularis oris	Closes and protrudes lips	Facial nerve
Major and minor zygomatic	Raises corners of mouth upward and laterally, as in smiling	Facial nerve
Levator anguli oris	Raises upper border of lip straight up, as in sneering	Facial nerve
Risorius	Draws corners of mouth laterally	Facial nerve
Buccinator	Presses cheeks firmly against teeth	Facial nerve
Levator labii superioris	Protrudes and elevates upper lip	Facial nerve
Depressor anguli oris and platysma	Draws corner of mouth downward and tenses skin over neck	Facial nerve
Depressor labii inferioris	Protrudes lower lip, as in pouting	Facial nerve
Mentalis	Raises skin on chin	Facial nerve

While stabilizing the head, the clinician depresses the shoulder distally. A normal finding is free movement of about 45 degrees of rotation, with a soft motion barrier. Tightness of this muscle results in a restriction in the range of motion, and a hard barrier.

Levator Scapulae
The patient is positioned in supine. Starting from the neutral position, the clinician introduces a combination of full cervical spine flexion, contralateral rota-

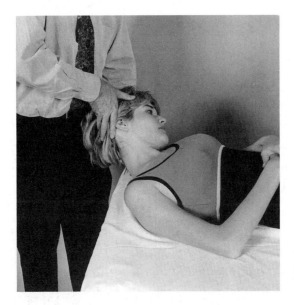

Figure 11-18 Muscle length test of upper trapezius.

tion, and then inclines the head toward the contralateral side (Figure 11-19). An evaluation is made as to the amount of restriction and tension, and whether pain is reproduced. The test is repeated on the other side for comparison.

Sternocleidomastoid
The patient is positioned in sitting with the clinician standing behind. From this position, the clinician palpates the clavicular and sternal origins of the sternocleidomastoid with the thumb and index finger. Starting from the neutral position, the clinician induces side-flexion of the neck to the contralateral side, and extension of the neck (Figure 11-20). The clinician stabilizes the scapula and rotates the patient's head and neck toward ipsilateral side.

Scalenes
The patient is positioned in sitting, with the clinician behind. The clinician fixates the shoulder girdle with one hand and with the other hand side bends the head to the contralateral side (Figure 11-21). The normal range of motion should be about 45 degrees.

Neurological Examination

The neurological examination is performed to assess the normal conduction of the central and peripheral nervous systems, and to help rule out such

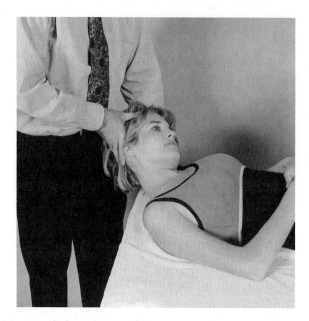

Figure 11-19 Muscle length test of levator scapulae.

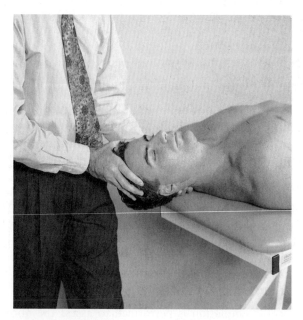

Figure 11-20 Muscle length test of sternocleidomastoid.

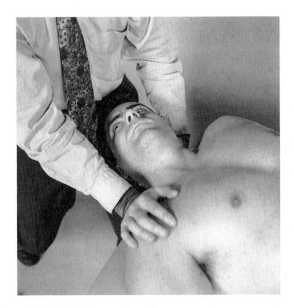

Figure 11-21 Muscle length test of scalenes.

conditions as brachial neuritis and thoracic outlet syndrome. The tests for the thoracic outlet syndrome are described under Special Tests.

Sensory (Afferent System)
The sensory examination can usually be eliminated from an otherwise straightforward presentation of neck pain. The wide variation of dermatomal innervation and the subjectivity of the test make the sensory examination less useful than motor or reflex testing. However, if the differential diagnosis of upper-limb dysesthesias includes a peripheral nerve entrapment, then checking for a sensory loss in a peripheral nerve distribution is useful.

The clinician instructs the patient to say "yes" each time they feel something touching their skin. The clinician notes any hypo- or hyperesthesia within the distributions. Light touch of hair follicles is used throughout the whole dermatome followed by pinprick in the area of hypoesthesia. Remember that there is normally no C1 dermatome!

Deep Tendon Reflexes
Absent or decreased reflexes are not necessarily pathological, especially in athletes who have well-developed muscles. The following reflexes should be checked for differences between the two sides:

- C5–6—Brachioradialis (Figure 11-22).

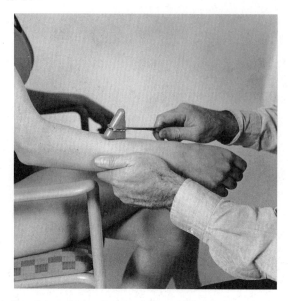

Figure 11-22 Brachioradialis deep tendon reflex (DTR).

- C6—Biceps (Figure 11-23).
- C7—Triceps (Figure 11-24).

Spinal Cord Reflexes
- Hoffman sign (Figure 11-25).
- Babinski (Figure 11-26).
- Lower limb tendon reflexes (Achilles, patellar).

Differing Philosophies
The next stage in the examination process depends on the clinician's background. For those clinicians heavily influenced by the muscle energy techniques of the osteopaths,[80] position testing is used to determine which segment to focus on. Other clinicians omit the position tests and proceed to the combined motion and passive physiological tests.

Position Testing
The patient is positioned in sitting and the clinician stands behind the patient. Using the thumbs, the clinician palpates the articular pillars of the cranial vertebra of the segment to be tested. The patient is asked to flex the neck, and the clinician assesses the position of the cranial vertebra relative to its caudal neighbor and notes which articular pillar of the cranial vertebra is

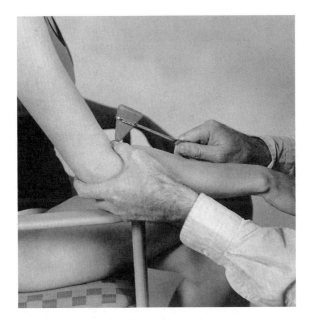

Figure 11-23 Biceps DTR.

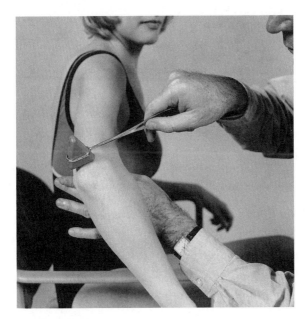

Figure 11-24 Triceps DTR.

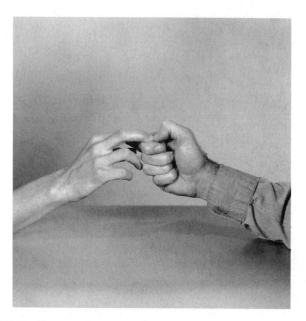

Figure 11-25 Hoffman reflex.

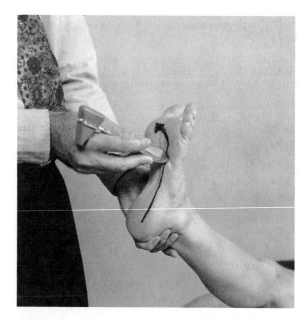

Figure 11-26 Babinski.

the most dorsal. A dorsal left articular pillar of the cranial vertebra relative to the caudal vertebra is indicative of a left rotated position of the segment in flexion.[80]

For example, a dorsal left articular pillar of C4 relative to C5 is indicative of a left rotated position of the C4–5 joint complex in extension.[80]

This test may also be performed with the patient supine. However, in sitting one can better observe the effect of the weight of the head on the joint mechanics.

Passive Physiological Intervertebral Mobility Testing

To test the intersegmental mobility of the midcervical region, the patient's neck is placed in the neutral position of the head on the neck, and the neck on the trunk. Once in this position, lateral glides are performed, beginning at C2 and progressing inferiorly. The lateral glides are usually tested in one direction before repeating the process on the other side. These lateral glides result in a relative side bending of the cervical spine proper in the opposite direction to the glide. Each spinal level is glided laterally to the left and right, while the clinician palpates for muscle guarding, range of motion, end-feel, and the provocation of symptoms. Lateral glides are performed as far inferiorly as possible.

Following this procedure, the areas where a restricted glide was found are targeted, and repetition of the lateral glides is performed in the extended and then flexed positions.

Cervical Stress Tests

Depending on the irritability of the segment, a variety of tests can be used to assess for instability. It is worthwhile starting gently with segmental palpation and gentle posterior–anterior pressures before progressing to the other techniques. The patient is positioned in supine and the following tests are performed to examine segmental stability.

Posterior–Anterior Spring Test

For anterior stability testing, the clinician places their thumbs over the posterior aspects of the transverse processes of the inferior vertebra of the segment being tested. The vertebra is then pushed anteriorly, and the clinician feels for the quality and quantity of movement. A rotational component can be added to the test by applying force on only one of the transverse processes.

For posterior stability testing, the thumbs are placed on the anterior aspect of the superior vertebra, and the index fingers are on the posterior aspect (neural arch) of the inferior.[81] The inferior vertebra is then pushed anteriorly on the superior one, producing a relative posterior shear of the superior segment.

To keep this test comfortable, the thumbs must be placed under (posterior) to the sternocleidomastoid, rather than over it, and merely function to stabilize the maneuver, exerting no pushing force.

Transverse Shear

The transverse shear test should not be confused with the lateral glide tests previously mentioned. The lateral glide tests are used to assess joint motion, whereas the transverse shear test assesses the stability of the segment. Although motion is expected to occur in the lateral glide test, no motion should be felt to occur with the transverse shear test.[82]

The inferior segment is stabilized and the clinician attempts to translate the superior segment transversely using the soft part of the MCP joint of the index finger.[81] The end-feel should be a combination of capsular, and slightly springy. The test is then reversed so that the superior segment is stabilized and the inferior segment is translated under it.

The test is repeated at each segmental level and for each side.

Anterior Shear—Transverse Ligament

The patient is positioned in supine with their head cradled in the clinician's hands. The clinician locates the anterior arches of C2 by moving around the vertebra from the back to the front using the thumbs. Once located, the clinician pushes down on the anterior arches of C2 with the thumbs toward the table, while the patient's occiput, and C1, cupped in the clinician's hands, is lifted, keeping the head parallel to the ceiling, but in slight flexion (Figure 11-27). The patient is instructed to keep their eyes open and to count backward aloud. The position is held for approximately 15 seconds or until an end-feel is perceived.

Coronal Stability—Alar Ligament

Rotation and side bending tighten the contralateral alar (rotation or side bending to the right tightens the left alar), whereas flexion typically tightens both alar ligaments.

The transverse process of C2 is palpated with one hand, while the patient's head is side bent or rotated (Figure 11-28). This is a test of immediacy. If the C2 spinous process does not move as soon as the head begins to rotate, laxity of the alar ligament should be suspected.

Sharp—Purser Test

This test was designed originally to test the sagittal stability of the A-A segment in patients with rheumatoid arthritis, because a number of pathological

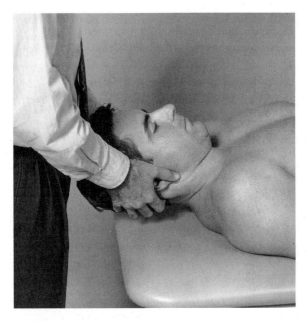

Figure 11-27 Anterior shear-transverse ligament test.

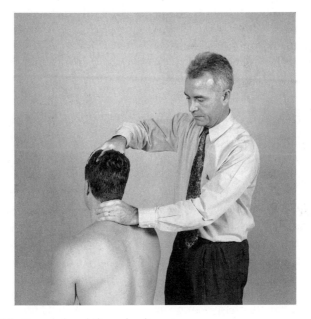

Figure 11-28 Coronal stability-alar ligament test.

conditions can affect the stability of the osseoligamentous ring of the median joints of this segment in this patient population. These changes result in degeneration and thinning of the articular cartilage between the odontoid process and the anterior arch of the atlas, or, occasionally, in softening of the dens. The aim of the test was to determine whether the instability was significant enough to provoke central nervous system's signs or symptoms.

 Clinical Pearl

The odontoid process is a vertical extension of the C2 vertebra that projects superiorly to articulate with the C1 vertebra. The process functions to provide stability while allowing for mobility between C1 and C2. Fractures of the odontoid process can result in entrapment or damage to either the brainstem or the spinal cord.

The patient is positioned in sitting. The patient is asked to segmentally flex the head and relate any signs or symptoms that this might evoke to the clinician. In addition, a positive test may be indicated by the patient hearing or feeling a clunk. Local symptoms, such as soreness, are ignored for the purposes of evaluating the test. If no serious signs or symptoms are provoked, the clinician stabilizes C2 with one hand and applies a posteriorly oriented force to the head. In the presence of a positive test, a provisional assumption is made that the symptoms are caused by excessive translation of the atlas, compromising one or more of the sensitive structures listed previously, and the physical examination is terminated.

 Clinical Pearl

Uitvlugt and Indenbaum[83] assessed the validity of the Sharp–Purser test in 123 outpatients with rheumatoid arthritis. The study findings indicated a predictive value of 85% and a specificity of 96%. The sensitivity was 88% when subluxation was greater than 4 mm.[83] The authors concluded that the Sharp–Purser test is a useful clinical examination to diagnose A-A instability.[83]

Confirmation is made with radiographic studies—an atlantoaxial displacement of greater than 3 mm on flexion–extension film is considered abnormal.

Clinical Pearl

Rheumatoid arthritis in the cervical spine is common in those patients with rheumatoid arthritis, occurring in approximately 50% of all cases.[84]

Distraction and Compression

The patient is supine and the clinician stands at the patient's head. The clinician cups the patient's occiput in one hand and rests the anterior aspect of the ipsilateral shoulder on the patient's forehead. The other hand stabilizes at a level close to the base of the neck.[81] An axial traction force is applied (neck distraction or axial manual traction test). The clinician notes the quality and quantity of motion. The test is then repeated except that an axial compression force is applied.

Pain reproduced with compression suggests the possibility of one or more of the following:

- IVD herniation
- A vertebral end plate fracture
- A vertebral body fracture
- Acute arthritis or joint inflammation of a zygapophysial joint
- Nerve root irritation, if radicular pain is produced

A reproduction of pain with cervical distraction suggests the presence of the following:

- A spinal ligament tear
- A tear or inflammation of the annulus fibrosis
- Muscle spasm
- Large disc herniation
- Dural irritability (if nonradicular arm or leg pain is produced).

Clinical Pearl

The interexaminer reliability of the neck distraction test has been found to be good.[85]

The neck distraction test has been found to have a specificity of 100% and a sensitivity of 40% to 43%.[86]

Functional Assessment Tests

The Neck Disability Index (NDI) is a patient survey instrument. Overall, no instrument is known to be significantly more advantageous than the NDI for the neck. The NDI is a revision of the Oswestry Index and is designed to measure the level of activity of daily living reduction in patients with neck pain.

 Clinical Pearl

The NDI has been widely researched and validated,[87] and the test/ retest reliability has been found to be 0.89.[87]

Special Tests

Temporomandibular Joint Screen

As the TMJ can refer pain to this region, the clinician is well advised to rule out this joint as the cause for the patient's symptoms.

The patient is asked to open and close the mouth, and to laterally deviate the jaw as the clinician observes the quality and quantity of motion, and notes any reproduction of symptoms.

Vertebral Artery Tests

Barre test

Barre test can be used to assess for vertebral artery insufficiency, especially if the patient is unable to lie supine. The patient is seated with the arms outstretched, forearms supinated. The patient is asked to close his or her eyes and move the head and neck into maximum extension and rotation. A positive test is one in which one of the outstretched arms sinks toward the floor and pronates, indicating the side of the compromise.

Hautard (Hautant, Hautart, or Hautarth) test[48,88]

As with Barre test, proprioceptive loss rather than dizziness is sought in Hautard test. The test has two parts. The patient is seated. Both arms are actively flexed to 90 degrees at the shoulders. The eyes are then closed for a few seconds while the clinician observes for any loss of position of one or both arms. If the arms move, the proprioception loss has a nonvascular cause. If the first part of the test is negative, the patient is asked to extend and rotate the neck. Because the second part of the test is performed to elicit a vascular cause for the dizziness, the eyes can be open or closed. Having the eyes open allows the clinician to observe for nystagmus and changes in pupil size. Each position is held for 10 to 30 seconds. If wavering of the arms occurs with the second part of the test, a vascular cause for the symptoms is suspected.

Cervical quadrant test[89]

The patient is positioned supine. The supine position is reported to result in an increase in passive motion at the cervical spine compared with sitting and may, therefore, better test the ability of the VA to sustain a stretch. The clinician passively moves the patient's head into extension and side bending. Maintaining this position, the clinician rotates the patient's head to the same side as the side bending and holds it there for 30 seconds. A positive test is one in which referring symptoms are produced if the opposite artery is involved.

DeKleyn–Nieuwenhuyse test[90]

The patient is positioned supine. The clinician passively moves the patient's head into extension and rotation. A positive test is one in which referring symptoms are produced if the opposite artery is involved. Despite its widespread appearance in a number of texts, this test is not recommended as an introductory test for the VA because of the severe traction stresses it places on the VA.[48]

Spurling Neck Compression Test

Spurling neck compression test (also referred to as foraminal compression test, neck compression test, or quadrant test) is useful to evaluate nerve root irritability. The patient's cervical complex is placed in extension and the head rotated toward the affected shoulder. An axial load is then placed on the spine by applying downward pressure through the patient's head. Reproduction of radicular symptoms (pain or paresthesias occurring distant from the neck, in the distribution of a cervical spinal nerve root) to the ipsilateral side to which the head is rotated is a positive test and indicates an irritation of the nerve root. If this maneuver causes only local pain, the discomfort is probably related to irritation of the facet or other posterior element, making a nerve-root process less likely.

 Clinical Pearl

There are few methodologically sound studies that assess the inter-examiner reliability, sensitivity, and specificity of Spurling neck compression test. The literature appears to indicate high specificity and low sensitivity.[68]

Shoulder Abduction Test

The shoulder abduction test is performed by asking the patient to actively abduct (or the clinician can passively abduct) the ipsilateral shoulder so that the hand rests on top of the head, with the patient either sitting or supine. Relief or reduction of ipsilateral cervical radicular symptoms is indicative of a positive test.

Finger Escape Sign

The finger escape sign is performed by asking the patient to hold his or her fingers in extension. The test is positive if the ring and small fingers gradually flex and abduct. A positive test is indicative of cervical myelopathy. The patient should further be observed for the ability to rapidly open and close his or her hands.

 Clinical Pearl

> The literature seems to indicate high specificity with low sensitivity for the shoulder abduction test.[68] Interestingly, incorporation of the abduction maneuver into a nonsurgical treatment program is reported as beneficial for patients with a positive test.[91]

Brachial Plexus Tests

Stretch test

This test is similar to the straight leg raise for the lower extremity as it stretches the brachial plexus. The patient is positioned in sitting. The patient is asked to side bend the head to the uninvolved side and to extend the shoulder and elbow on the involved side. Pain and paresthesia along the involved arm is indicative of a brachial plexus irritation.

Compression test

The patient is positioned in sitting. The patient is asked to side bend the head to the uninvolved side. The clinician applies firm pressure to the brachial plexus by squeezing the plexus between the thumb and fingers. Reproduction of shoulder or upper arm pain is positive for mechanical cervical lesions.[92]

Tinel sign

The patient is positioned in sitting. The patient is asked to side bend the head to the uninvolved side. The clinician taps along the trunks of the brachial plexus using the fingertips. Local pain indicates a cervical plexus lesion. A tingling sensation in the distribution of one of the trunks may indicate a compression or neuroma of one or more trunks of the brachial plexus.[93]

Upper Limb Tension Tests

The upper limb tension tests are equivalent to the straight leg raise test in the lumbar spine, and are designed to put stress on the neuromeningeal structures of the upper limb. Each test begins by testing the normal side first. Normal responses include the following:

- Deep stretch or ache in the cubital fossa
- Deep stretch or ache into the anterior or radial aspect of forearm and radial aspect of hand
- Deep stretch in the anterior shoulder area
- Sensation felt down the radial aspect of the forearm
- Sensation felt in the median distribution of the hand

Positive findings include:

- Production of patient's symptoms
- A sensitizing test in the ipsilateral quadrant alters the symptoms

Thoracic Outlet Tests

When performing thoracic outlet syndrome tests, evaluation for either the diminution or disappearance of pulse or reproduction of neurological symptoms indicates a positive test. However, the aim of the tests should be to reproduce the patient's symptoms rather than to obliterate the radial pulse, as more than 50% of normal, asymptomatic individuals will exhibit obliteration of the radial pulse during classic provocative testing.[94]

A baseline pulse should be established first, before performing the respective test maneuvers.

Adson vascular test

The patient extends their neck, turns their head toward the side being examined, and takes a deep breath. This test, if positive, tends to implicate the scalenes because this test increases the tension of the anterior and middle scalenes, and compromises the interscalene triangle.[95] the efficacy of this test remains controversial—one would expect that the scalene angle should increase not decrease with this maneuver thereby allowing more room for the brachial plexus, not less.

 Clinical Pearl

To date, no studies have been performed to document the reliability of the Adson test, although the specificity has been noted to range from 18% to 87%, but the sensitivity has been documented to approach 94%.[68,96]

Allen pectoralis minor test
The Allen test increases the tone of the pectoralis minor muscle. The shoulder of the seated patient is positioned in 90 degrees of glenohumeral abduction, 90 degrees of glenohumeral external rotation, and 90 degrees of elbow flexion on the tested side. Although the radial pulse is monitored, the patient is asked to turn their head away from the tested side. This test, if positive, tends to implicate pectoralis tightness as the cause for the symptoms.

Costoclavicular
During this test, the shoulders are drawn back and downward in an exaggerated military position to reduce the volume of the costoclavicular space. No studies are available that identify the sensitivity or specificity of this maneuver.

Hyperextension maneuver
The patient is positioned in sitting on the edge of a table. The clinician grasps the arm on the symptomatic side, passively depresses its shoulder girdle and then pulls the arm down toward the floor, while palpating the radial pulse. The patient is asked to extend the head and to turn away from the tested side. A positive test for TOS is indicated if there is an absence or diminishing of the pulse.

Roos test[97]
The patient is positioned in sitting. The arm is positioned in 90 degrees of shoulder abduction, and 90 degrees of elbow flexion. The patient is asked to perform slow finger clenching for 3 minutes. The radial pulse may be reduced or obliterated during this maneuver, and an infraclavicular bruit may be heard. If the patient is unable to maintain the arms in the start position for 3 minutes or reports pain heaviness or numbness and tingling, the test is considered positive for TOS on the involved side. This test is also referred to as the *Hands-up* test or the *elevated arm stress test* (EAST). Compared to the other tests for thoracic outlet syndrome, this test has a high false-positive rate.[68]

Overhead test
The overhead exercise test is useful to detect thoracic outlet arterial compression. The patient elevates both arms overhead, and then rapidly flexes and extends the fingers. A positive test is achieved if the patient experiences

heaviness, fatigue, numbness, tingling, blanching, or discoloration of a limb within 20 seconds.[95]

Hyperabduction maneuver (Wright test)[98]
This test is considered by many to be the best provocative test for thoracic outlet compression caused by compression in the costoclavicular space. The patient is asked to take a deep breath while the clinician passively abducts and externally rotates the patient's arm. There are no studies to date that have described the reliability, sensitivity, or specificity of this test.

Passive shoulder shrug
This simple, but effective test is used with patients who present with TOS symptoms to help rule out thoracic outlet syndrome. The patient is seated with their arms folded and the clinician stands behind. The clinician grasps the patient's elbows and passively elevates the shoulders up and forward. This position is maintained for 30 seconds. Any changes in the patient's symptoms are noted. The maneuver has the affect of slackening the soft tissues and the plexus.

Diagnostic Imaging

Diagnostic testing is most useful when it affects the intervention. However, if a patient does not progress as expected, diagnostic testing is indicated because the intervention strategy may need to change.

Radiographs

Plain radiographs of the cervical complex should be done with a history of significant trauma involving a direct blow to the neck or head. The basic evaluation includes anteroposterior (AP), lateral, right and left oblique, and AP odontoid views. Lateral flexion and extension views can help evaluate ligament stability.

An equivocal bony abnormality or persistent pain out of proportion to the clinical scenario may warrant a computed tomography scan. In most other painful conditions, including mild radiculopathy (motor strength 4/5 or greater), radiographs can be delayed until after a trial of conservative treatment. However, if at 4 to 6 weeks no significant improvement is apparent, the basic plain radiographic evaluation should be done to evaluate for anatomic structures or abnormalities that may be delaying healing.

Magnetic Resonance Imaging

Magnetic resonance imaging (MRI) is useful to evaluate for a mechanical compression that may be causing radiculopathy. MRI, however, shows only anatomy and gives no information about the physiological process that may be the cause. Correlating the images with the history and physical examination, therefore, establishes whether MRI pathology is clinically relevant. In mild cases of radiculopathy, MRI is not usually needed initially because most patients improve with conservative care. If, however, the patient's weakness progresses, pain is intractable, or 6 to 8 weeks of conservative intervention bring no improvement, an MRI is useful to identify the anatomic lesion.

Electromyography and Nerve Conduction

Needle electromyography (EMG) is useful in evaluating the physiological state of nerves and muscles in a patient who has upper-limb weakness and is not improving with therapy. EMG can help indicate whether an injured nerve is stable or actively denervating or whether reinnervation has occurred. It can also help distinguish between nerve root lesions and brachial plexopathy. EMG abnormalities, though, may not be seen for up to 21 days after onset of injury or symptoms, making it less useful in early stages.

Examination Conclusions—The Evaluation

Following the examination, and once the clinical findings have been recorded, the clinician must determine a specific diagnosis or a working hypothesis, based on a summary of all of the findings. This diagnosis can be structure related (medical diagnosis), or a diagnosis based on the preferred practice patterns as described in the Guide to Physical Therapist Practice.[99]

INTERVENTION

The success rates of physical therapy interventions depends on the type of tissue involved, the extent of the damage, and the stage of healing. The intervention approach is usually determined by the examination philosophy. Whatever the philosophy, the intervention must be related to the signs and symptoms present rather than the actual diagnosis.

 Clinical Pearl

Manipulation and patient education, which include stretching, have shown more success in treating nontraumatic neck pain groups than control groups.[100] There is also some evidence that supports the use of strengthening exercises combined with manual therapy,[101,102] and TENS with exercise[103] for chronic neck pain.

No present evidence-based reviews have been conducted on physical therapy interventions specifically for TMD. Feine and Lund concluded that there was no good evidence that any intervention reviewed (heat, cold, ultrasound, low intensity laser, TENS, mobilization/manipulation, and exercise) significantly reduced the symptoms associated with TMD.[104] Complicating matters is the fact that the majority of the symptoms associated with TMD are self-limiting and resolve without active intervention.[11] The chronic pain associated with TMD most likely occurs because of secondary factors. These factors include a fixed head forward posture, abnormal stress levels, depression, or oral parafunctional habits (such as bruxism). Based on a systematic review of 30 studies examining the effectiveness of exercise, manual therapy, electrotherapy, relaxation training, and biofeedback in the management of TMD, Medlicott and Harris[105] made the following recommendations:

- Active exercises and manual mobilizations may be effective.
- Postural training may be used in combination with other interventions, as independent effects of postural training are unknown.
- Low/midlaser therapy may be more effective than other electrotherapy modalities.[106]
- Programs involving relaxation techniques and biofeedback, electromyography training, and proprioceptive reeducation may be more effective than placebo treatment or occlusal splints.
- Combinations of active exercises, manual therapy, postural correction, and relaxation techniques may be effective.

COMMON ORTHOPEDIC CONDITIONS

CERVICAL HEADACHE

Diagnosis

Cervical headache—ICD-9: 784.0 (headache), 307.81 (tension headache). Also known as cervicogenic headache, occipital neuralgia, tension headache, and cephalalgia.

Description

From the upper cervical segments, neck pain may be referred to the head and manifested as headache. Cervical headaches (CHs) are loosely defined as "any headache beginning in the neck." With CHs, pain is precipitated or aggravated by specific neck movements or sustained neck posture. Generally speaking, a CH is a symptom of an underlying pathology.

 Clinical Pearl

CHs tend to be unilateral and accompanied by tenderness of the C2–3 articular pillars on the affected side.[107] The patient with a CH usually reports a dull aching pain of moderate intensity, which begins in the neck or occipital region and then spreads to include a greater part of the cranium.[108]

CHs can emerge from a number of sources, including[109]

- irritation of the posterior (dorsal) root ganglia and nerve root components caused by compression of the C2 posterior (dorsal) root ganglia between the C1 posterior arch and the superior C2 articular process[110];
- compression of the C2 anterior (ventral) ramus at the articular process of C1 to C2[111];
- entrapment of the C2 posterior (dorsal) root ganglia by the C1–2 epistrophic ligament.[112]

Subjective Findings

The subjective findings depend on the type of headache. The typical findings with a CH include the following:

- Reports of headache, described as a dull ache of moderate-to-severe intensity, occurring daily or at least two to three times per week.
- Headache upon awakening with slow increase in symptoms throughout day.
- Location of symptoms may be unilateral or bilateral, but the pain generally starts in the suboccipital region with subsequent radiation into the temporal, frontal, or retro-orbital regions.

 Clinical Pearl

The following associated symptoms could indicate a more serious cause of headache:

- Dizziness
- Bilateral or quadrilateral paresthesias/weakness

- Nausea and vomiting
- Blurred vision
- Difficulty swallowing
- Phonophobia or photophobia (suggestive of migraine)

Objective Findings

To help in the determination when examining a patient complaining of headache, the clinician is advised to follow the simple diagnostic clinical algorithm set out below[8]:

- Exclude possible intracranial causes on history and physical examination. If intracranial pathology is suspected, then an urgent workup is required, which may include neuroimaging studies and laboratory investigations.
- Exclude headaches associated with viral or other infective illness.
- Exclude a drug-induced headache or headache related to alcohol or substance abuse.
- Consider an exercise-related (or sex-related) headache syndrome.
- Differentiate between vascular, tension, cervicogenic, and other causes of headache. CHs are typically associated with limited mobility in the suboccipital region, tenderness of the suboccipital muscles, poor posture, and weakness of the scapulothoracic muscles and deep neck flexors.

Confirmatory/Special Tests

The diagnosis of CH is generally a diagnosis of exclusion.

Medical/Imaging Studies

Unless serious pathology is suspected, medical/imaging studies are not typically warranted for this diagnosis.

Differential Diagnosis

The differential diagnosis for CH is extensive and includes, but is not limited to, the following:

- Cerebrovascular accident
- Cervical strain or sprain
- Cervical myelopathy
- Meningitis
- Encephalitis

- Cervical spondylosis
- Cervical stenosis
- Concussion
- Upper cervical instability
- Brain tumor.

Intervention

Several interventions have been recommended for CHs, including posture training, manual therapy, exercise, rest, and minor analgesics.[113] Manual therapy studies have demonstrated positive effects at both the impairment (pain and muscle function) and the disability level, with most studies focusing on short-term outcomes.[114,115] Specifically, intervention should include

- increasing the strength and control of the abdominals;
- increasing the length of the anterior thorax muscles;
- increasing the length of the posterior cervical extensor muscles;
- improving the strength and decreasing the length of the posterior scapulothoracic muscles;
- increasing shoulder joint and cervical motion.
- Joint mobilization to the upper cervical spine where appropriate.[116]

 Clinical Pearl

McKenzie[9] recommends a home program of cervical retraction exercises to decrease CH symptoms and maintain correct cervical alignment. These exercises, which are performed throughout the day, are progressed based on changes in symptom location and intensity. If an exercise fails to reduce CH pain, a new component is added and the prior exercise is discontinued.[117]

For the prevention of chronic tension-type headaches, behavioral approaches commonly involve regular sleep and meals, stress coping, meditation, or relaxation strategies, and avoidance of initiating or trigger factors, including work-related or family stress and emotional problems.[113]

Prognosis

The prognosis varies greatly and depends on the cause of the headache.

Source: References 7, 9, 107–117.

CERVICAL RADICULOPATHY

Diagnosis

Cervical radiculopathy—ICD-9: Spondylosis (721.1); arthralgia of cervical spine (719.48), degeneration of cervical IVD (722.4), displacement of intravertebral disc (IVD) without myelopathy (722.0), and herniated disc (722.71). The diagnosis of cervical radiculopathy is based on the history of radicular pain and paresthesia, neurological impairment, and correlating abnormalities on x-rays.

Description

In addition to degenerative processes (osteophyte formation, foraminal narrowing, space occupying lesions), cervical radiculopathy can be caused by structural changes (bulge, protrusion, extrusion, or sequestration) in the cervical IVD. The two most common causes are cervical arthritis with foraminal encroachment, and a herniated nucleus pulposus. Whatever the cause, cervical radiculopathy typically includes

- an insidious onset, or history of repressive cervical spine loading or stress
- an impairment of upper extremity neurological function
- compression of spinal nerve, spinal cord, or both.

 Clinical Pearl

Patients with a cervical disc herniation are often younger, whereas patients with radicular symptoms due to cervical disc degeneration are often middle-aged, except at C7–T1, which is more common in the seventh and eighth decades.

Subjective Findings

- Onset of symptoms is usually insidious.
- Complaints of pain can vary, and can include headaches, neck pain, arm pain, scapular pain, and/or anterior chest pain with a dull ache to severe burning quality.
- Complaints of numbness or tingling in particular fingers. Neurological deficits should correspond with the offending cervical level:
  - C2 to C3 disc herniations are rare in either traumatic or spontaneous etiology. These herniations are difficult to identify on clinical examination because these patients usually have no specific motor weakness and reflex abnormality.

- Radiculopathy of the fourth cervical nerve root may be an unexplained cause of neck and shoulder pain. Difficulty with breathing during exercise may be reported in diaphragmatic involvement (C3–5).

- Radiculopathy of the fifth cervical nerve root can present with numbness in an "epaulet" distribution, beginning at the superior aspect of the shoulder and extending laterally to the midpart of the arm. The absence of pain with a range of motion of the shoulder and the absence of impingement signs at the shoulder help to differentiate radiculopathy of the fifth cervical nerve root from a pathological shoulder condition.

- Radiculopathy of the sixth cervical nerve root presents with symptoms radiating from the neck to the lateral aspect of the biceps, down the lateral aspect of the forearm, to the dorsal aspect of the web space between the thumb and index finger, and into the tips of those digits. Numbness occurs in the same distribution.

- The seventh cervical nerve root (C6–7 level) is the most frequently involved by cervical radiculopathy. The symptoms typically radiate along the back of the shoulder, often extending into the scapular region, down along the triceps, and then along the dorsum of the forearm and into the dorsum of the long finger.

- Radiculopathy of the eighth cervical nerve root usually presents with symptoms extending down the medial aspect of the arm and forearm and into the medial border of the hand and the ulnar two digits. Numbness usually involves the dorsal and volar aspects of the ulnar two digits and hand and may extend up the medial aspect of the forearm.

- Weakness may occur in advanced cases, especially with the grip strength and/or lifting strength.

- Clumsiness with activities involving finger dexterity tends to highlight involvement of the eighth cervical nerve root.

  - The function of the flexor digitorum profundus in the index and long fingers and of the flexor pollicis longus in the thumb can be affected by eighth cervical radiculopathy, but they are not affected by ulnar nerve entrapment.

  - With the exception of the adductor pollicis, the short thenar muscles are spared with ulnar nerve involvement but involved with eighth cervical or first thoracic radiculopathy.

  - Entrapment of the anterior interosseus nerve may masquerade as eighth cervical or first thoracic radiculopathy, but it does not cause the sensory changes or have thenar muscle involvement.

- Prior episodes of similar symptoms or localized neck pain are important for diagnosis and ultimate intervention.

- The symptoms are usually aggravated by sitting for prolonged periods, specific neck motions (extension or rotation of the head to the side of the pain), sleeping prone, and coughing or sneezing.
- The symptoms are usually eased by lying down, cervical spine support, sleeping with the head supported in either sidelying or supine, or the use of pain medications and thermal modalities.

 Clinical Pearl

Aggravation of the symptoms by neck extension often helps to differentiate a radicular etiology from muscular neck pain or a pathological condition of the shoulder with secondary muscle pain in the neck.

 Clinical Pearl

Leg symptoms associated with neck dysfunction, especially in the elderly, should arouse the suspicion of cervical spondylotic myelopathy.

Objective Findings

Numerous clinical examination findings are purported to be diagnostic of cervical radiculopathy including patient history, cervical range of motion limitations, neurological examination, and specific maneuvers (e.g., Spurling). Because the clinical presentation of cervical radiculopathy is so variable, it is advisable to use a combination of test results before making a diagnosis. Findings may include some or all of the following:

- Typically, the patient has a head list away from the side of injury and holds the neck stiffly.
- Active range of motion is usually reduced in the direction of pain, which is usually extension, rotation, and side bending, either toward or away from the affected nerve root. Same-side bending induces pain by an impingement of a nerve root at the site of the neural foramen.
- On palpation, a nonspecific finding is tenderness noted along the cervical paraspinals, along the ipsilateral side of the affected nerve root, and over the upper trapezius. There may also be muscle tenderness along muscles where the symptoms are referred (e.g., medial scapula, proximal arm, and

lateral epicondyle), as well as associated hypertonicity or spasm in these painful muscles.

- Manual muscle testing determines a nerve root level on physical examination and can detect subtle weakness in a myotomal, or key muscle, distribution.
  - Weakness of shoulder abduction suggests C5 pathology.
  - Elbow flexion and wrist extension weakness suggests a C6 radiculopathy.
  - Weakness of elbow extension and wrist flexion can occur with a C7 radiculopathy.
  - Weakness of thumb extension and ulnar deviation of the wrist is seen in C8 radiculopathies.
  - The sensory examination, quite subjective in as much as it requires patient response, may reveal a dermatomal pattern of diminished, or loss of, sensation. In addition, patients with radiculitis may have hyperesthesia to light touch and pinprick examination.
- Deep tendon reflexes. Any grade of reflex can be normal, so the asymmetry of the reflexes is most helpful:
  - The biceps brachii reflex occurs at the level of C5 to C6. The brachioradialis is another C5 to C6 reflex.
  - The triceps reflex tests the C7 to C8 nerve roots.
  - The pronator reflex can be helpful in differentiating C6 and C7 nerve root problems. If it is abnormal in conjunction with an abnormal triceps reflex, then the level of involvement is more likely to be C7. This reflex is performed by tapping the anterior aspect of the forearm, with the forearm in a neutral position and the elbow flexed.

Confirmatory/Special Tests

- Spurling. This test is performed by asking the patient to rotate the head to the uninvolved side and then the involved side. The clinician then carefully applies a downward pressure on the head with the head in neutral. The test is considered positive if pain radiates into the limb ipsilateral to the side at which the head is rotated. Neck pain with no radiation into the shoulder or arm does not constitute a positive test. Conditions such as stenosis, cervical spondylosis, osteophytes, or disc herniation are implicated with a positive test.
- Manual distraction of the head on the neck. Gentle manual cervical distraction can also be used with the patient supine as a physical examination test. A positive response is indicated by a reduction of neck or limb symptoms.
- Vertebral artery test. Studies would suggest that the traditional vertebral artery tests have very little, if any, diagnostic value, although testing persists. The clinician should use a combination of the patient's description of their

symptoms and medical history, and the more specific tests of blood flow before reaching a conclusion.

- Thoracic outlet tests (Adson, Halstead, Roos [EAST], and Wright).

Medical Studies

Radiographical studies may be recommended based on severity. A cervical spine series (including posteroanterior, lateral, and odontoid, and oblique views) are usually recommended. Plain films may show a loss of the normal cervical lordosis or foraminal encroachment as well as the formation of bone spurs. Patients with reflex loss or dramatic motor weakness are typically prescribed electrodiagnostic studies and MRI to help establish the diagnosis. MRI imaging is the most common method of diagnosing cervical disc pathology.

Differential Diagnosis

- Cervical strain or sprain
- Spinal stenosis
- Cervical spondylosis
- Cardiac pain
- Epidural abscess—polyradicular involvement may be seen
- Schwannomas, meningiomas, and benign or malignant vertebral body tumors
- Spinal cord/epidural tumor
- Peripheral nerve entrapment within the upper limb, including entrapment or compression of suprascapular, median, and ulnar nerves
  - Thoracic outlet syndrome
  - Brachial neuritis. Upper trunk brachial plexus disorders can be confused with a C5 or C6 radiculopathy.

 Clinical Pearl

A Pancoast tumor of the apical lung can involve the caudad cervical nerve roots and, additionally, the sympathetic chain.

Intervention

Little is known about the natural history of cervical radiculopathy, and there are few controlled randomized studies comparing operative with conservative intervention. Conservative intervention currently consists of

- Acute stage
  - Modified rest
  - Local icing and electrotherapeutic modalities such as electrical stimulation, and pulsed ultrasound to help reduce pain and inflammation
  - Manual or mechanical traction. Traction can be tried in an attempt to remove the compression from the nerve. The choice of patient position is determined by patient comfort and the ability of the clinician. Supine manual traction is easier to perform and is often more comfortable for the patient because the spine is unloaded.
  - Protection. A cervical collar may be used in severe cases to assist with activities of daily living.
  - Oral corticosteroid "dose-packs" and NSAIDs
- Subacute/chronic stages. Cervical and cervicothoracic stabilization exercises form the cornerstone of the therapeutic exercise progression. Based on tolerance, the patient is prescribed a progressive program of range of motion and then strengthening exercises as outlined at the end of the chapter. The strengthening exercise must include strengthening of the entire upper quadrant.

Prognosis

No research exists at present that addresses prognosis for a patient with cervical disc pathology—the majority of studies have used generic self-report measures, or measures of pain. Long–term results require attention to psychological stress, posture, and exercise. Surgical intervention is reserved for patients with persistent radicular pain who do not respond to conservative measures.

CERVICAL SPONDYLOSIS

Diagnosis

Cervical spondylosis—ICD-9: 721.0 (without myelopathy); 721.1 (with myelopathy); 723.0 (spinal stenosis in cervical region). This condition is also referred to as cervical arthritis or degenerative disc disease of the cervical spine.

Description

A chronic degenerative condition of the cervical spine that affects the vertebral bodies and IVDs of the neck as well as the contents of the spinal canal (nerve roots and/or spinal cord). Abnormalities in the osseous (bony spurs) and the fibroelastic boundaries (buckling of the ligamentum flavum, disc pathology) of the bony cervical spinal canal affect the availability of space for spinal cord and nerve roots, resulting in a stenosis. Myelopathy, radiculopathy, or both may occur.

 Clinical Pearl

Cervical myelopathy is the most prevalent spinal cord compression pathology in individuals over the age of 55. Narrowing of the spinal canal and resultant myelopathy are more common in older men. Typical symptoms of early cervical myelopathy may include palmar paresthesias in the upper extremities; difficulty with upper extremity dexterity, loss of balance, subtle gait changes, lower extremity weakness, and reports of incontinence.

Subjective Findings

Subjective complaints vary according to the anatomic level involved, but may include the following:

- Limited mobility of the cervical spine.
- Morning stiffness of the neck, which gradually improves throughout the day.
- A gradual onset of neck, shoulder, elbow, wrist, or hand pain (multiple nerve roots may be involved) of increased frequency and severity. Headaches may also be reported.
- Pain tends to worsen with upright positioning or activity.

 Clinical Pearl

No specific aggravating factors associated with cervical myelopathy have been found in the literature.

Objective Findings

It is important to assess the sensory and motor function of the upper and lower nerve roots, as well as gait (ataxia):

- The presence of upper motor neuron lesion (long tract) signs (Hoffmann, clonus, Babinski, and hyperreflexia) with myelopathy. Abnormal reflexes and motor and sensory dysfunction in patients with radiculopathy.

- Tenderness along the lateral neck or along the spinous processes posteriorly.
- Reduced motion in the sagittal plane, with a decrease in side bending. As the degeneration progresses, a capsular pattern develops. Cervical flexion may produce electric shock-like symptoms that travel down the spine, arms, or legs (*Lhermitte symptom*).

Confirmatory/Special Tests

As many of the clinical tests for cervical myelopathy have been shown to have relative poor sensitivity, it is recommended that the clinician use a cluster of tests (see chapter content) before reaching a diagnosis:

- Lhermitte symptom or "Phenomenon."
- Vertebral artery test.
- Craniovertebral ligament stress tests.
- Finger escape sign.
- Spurling.

Medical Studies

In the absence of pain, the finding of degenerative changes on radiographs should not be misconstrued as pathological. Anteroposterior and lateral views can be useful, but myelography, with CT, is usually the imaging test of choice to assess spinal and foraminal stenosis.

 Clinical Pearl

Degenerative findings occur most commonly at the C5–6 and C6–7 disc spaces.

Differential Diagnosis

- Cervical radiculopathy.
- Cerebrovascular accident.
- Spinal cord tumor.
- Metastatic tumor (night pain, sweats, fever, etc.)
- Rheumatoid arthritis.
- Peripheral neuropathy.
- Multiple sclerosis.
- Syringomyelia (loss of superficial abdominal reflexes, insensitivity to pain)

Intervention

In those cases where the clinician suspects the presence of serious pathology such as cervical myelopathy, the referring physician should be alerted. In all other cases, in addition to NSAIDs/epidural steroids, the intervention depends on the symptoms and level of involvement:

- Cervical spondylosis without radiculopathy or myelopathy
  - The use of electrotherapeutic modalities to control pain and increase the extensibility of the connective tissue. These modalities usually include moist heat, electrical stimulation, and ultrasound.
- Nerve irritation
  - Immobilization of the cervical spine may be considered to limit the motion of the neck and prevent further irritation. With the use of any of the braces, the patient's tolerance and compliance are considerations.
    - Soft cervical collars are recommended initially.
    - More rigid orthoses (e.g., Philadelphia collar, Minerva body jacket) can significantly immobilize the cervical spine.
- Molded cervical pillows to align the spine during sleep and provide symptomatic relief.
- Manual techniques to stretch the adaptively shortened tissues.
- Range-of-motion exercises as tolerated. These exercises initially are performed in the pain-free direction, and then in the direction of pain.
- As the patient regains motion, isometric exercises and cervical stabilization exercises are prescribed.

Prognosis

Surgical decompression and fusion may be necessary for patients with intractable pain, progressive neurological findings, or symptoms of cervical myelopathy and spinal cord compression.

CERVICAL STRAIN

Diagnosis

Cervical strain/sprain—ICD-9: 847.0. The term cervical strain includes ligamentous injuries, whereas a cervical strain involves a muscle injury in the neck. Several terms are used to describe this condition and include whiplash, wry neck (an acute form of torticollis), mechanical neck pain, and trapezius strain.

Description

Cervical strain/sprain can occur from a variety of traumatic or atraumatic mechanisms that result in irritation and compression of the cervical and upper back muscles.

Subjective Findings

- Onset may follow an incident of trauma or may be spontaneous. Conditions that are aggravated by flexion-based activities could implicate a transverse and/or alar ligament sprain, supraspinous and interspinous ligament sprain, fracture, disc protrusion, and muscle strain. Conditions are aggravated by extension-based activities could indicate central canal stenosis, facet joint dysfunction, spondylolisthesis, and muscle strain. Conditions aggravated by side bending could indicate an alar ligament sprain, fracture, lateral stenosis, facet joint dysfunction, uncovertebral joint dysfunction, and muscle strain. Chronic symptoms may require more investigation as symptoms may not be associated with a single tissue source.

 Clinical Pearl

Symptoms that fluctuate and that are accompanied with complaints of catching sensations, cracking/popping, and a history of neck injuries are indicative of a patient with degenerative disc disease.

- Complaints of pain, stiffness, and tightness in the upper back or shoulder. Pain is the chief complaint. Occipital headaches may also occur.
  - Pain and stiffness worse in the morning can be due to inflammation that worsens during the night due to decreased circulation and decreased muscle activation.
  - Pain and fatigue that is worse in the afternoon or evening implicates postural influences.
  - Pain at night during sleeping can be due to sleep position (sleeping prone requires cervical extension and rotation), or from moving the head and neck. However, symptoms that occur which are unrelated to movement can implicate cancer.
- The location of pain can vary[118,119]:
  - Pain from C3–4 disc can be felt in the C7 spinous process and the posterior border to the trapezius muscle. Symptoms from the zygapophyseal

joints at the same level can be felt in the posterior of the cervical region and head.

- Pain from C4–5 disc can be felt in the scapular spine and superior angle. Symptoms from the zygapophyseal joints at the same level can be felt in the posterolateral middle and lower cervical region to the top of the shoulder.

- Pain from C5–6 disc can be felt in the medial scapular border. Symptoms from the zygapophyseal joints at the same level can be felt in the posterolateral middle and primarily lower cervical spine and the top and lateral parts of the shoulder and caudally to the spine of the scapula.

- Pain from C6–7 disc can be felt in the inferior angle of the scapula. Symptoms from the zygapophyseal joints at the same level can be felt in the top and lateral parts of the shoulder extending caudally to the inferior border of the scapula.

- May complain of dysphagia, headaches, and/or visual disturbance.

- Symptoms are typically aggravated by cervical positions that stretch or elongate the involved tissue, or sustained postural positions.

- Symptoms are typically eased by lying down or supporting the cervical region.

Clinical Pearl

Questions about present and previous medications should be asked.

- Chronic use of analgesics can result in a rebound effect (an increase in frequency and severity of neck and head pain).

- Previous corticosteroid use may increase the risk of developing osteoporosis and therefore increase the likelihood of a fracture with a low-velocity mechanism of injury.

Objective Findings

- Tenderness over the transverse and spinous processes, or over the anterior vertebral body, depending on the structures involved.

- Depending on the severity of the strain, motion can be markedly restricted as a result of muscle guarding.

- Symptoms relieved by alleviating pressure or load of the specific tissue.

Clinical Pearl

Signs and symptoms to alert the clinician (red flags) include
- Central nervous system signs.
- Periodic loss of consciousness.
- Patient does not move the neck, even slightly (fractured dens).
- Painful weakness of the neck muscles (fracture).
- Gentle traction and compression are painful (fracture).
- Severe muscle spasm (fracture).
- Complaints of dizziness.

Confirmatory/Special Tests

Diagnosis is made based on subjective complaints, objective findings, and imaging studies as necessary.

- Manual distraction/compression of the head on the neck with the patient supine.
    1. Pain with distraction would tend to implicate muscle or ligament
    2. Pain with compression would tend to implicate articular surfaces and IVD.
- Vertebral artery test.
- Alar and transverse ligament stress tests.
- Sharp–Purser test, especially in those patients with a history of rheumatoid arthritis.

Medical Studies

Findings on plain films are typically normal, although there may be a loss of the cervical lordosis in moderate to severe cases. Anteroposterior, lateral, and open mouth radiographs are necessary if the patient has a history of trauma, associated neurological deficit, or if the patient is elderly. Cervical spine stability must first be verified before the diagnosis of cervical sprain can be made. The Canadian C-spine Rules recommend that radiographs should be performed in patients who present with trauma combined with the presence of a high risk factor including age greater than 65 years, dangerous mechanism, or paresthesias in the extremities.[120]

Differential Diagnosis

- Fracture (abnormal radiographs or history of osteoporosis)
- Dislocation and subluxation, especially with a history of trauma (whiplash)

- IVD injury (herniation, degeneration)

- Neurovascular compromise

- Rheumatoid disease (rheumatoid arthritis, ankylosing spondylitis). Rheumatoid disease can be associated with an atlantoaxial subluxation. The classic subjective history with this type of patient is a report of neck pain, the inability to keep the head from falling forward, with associated paresthesias in the hands when looking down.

- A history of Down syndrome or Klippel–Feil syndrome could indicate cervical instability

- Cervical spine tumor/infection (night pain, weight loss, history, fever, chills, sweats)

- Myofascial pain syndrome

- Symptom magnification/secondary gain (inconsistent or exaggerated findings).

Intervention

- Ice and electrical stimulation are applied to the neck during the first 48 to 72 hours to help control pain and inflammation. If necessary, a soft or hard collar can be used to help the neck rest while weight-bearing (standing or sitting).

- Aerobic activities, such as walking, are initiated as early as possible.

- Range-of-motion exercises in the pain-free ranges of flexion and rotation are initiated as early as possible to reduce the likelihood of hypomobility.

- Joint mobilizations. Hypermobility is common in the cervical spine (hypomobility is more common in the upper cervical spine). If the symptomatic segment is hypermobile, any reduction in symptoms depends on improving mobility of the adjacent segments. Improving joint mobility can take between one treatment and several treatments.

- A trial of cervical traction. Improvement with the application of traction suggests that the pathology involves a structure(s) that is sensitive to compression. A worsening of symptoms with cervical traction could implicate an error in application (direction, amount/duration of pull) a cervical hypomobility, or a cervical instability.

- Gentle cervical isometrics. Aggressive strengthening of the cervical musculature should not begin until full range of motion is restored. Strengthening of the trapezius muscle and other scapular stabilizers can be performed using upper extremity exercises, taking care to avoid an increase in symptoms. Increasing neuromuscular control may occur within 2 weeks, but improving muscle strength and endurance may take 6 weeks at minimum, and 8 to 12 weeks in the presence of pain or other pathology.

Clinical Pearl

If significant neck pain persists last 6 to 8 weeks, flexion and extension radiographs may be useful to exclude, or confirm, instability.

Prognosis

The condition is usually self-limiting and many patients improve within a few days to a few weeks. Factors associated with poor prognosis include the presence of occipital headaches, interscapular pain, and involvement in litigation or workers compensation claims. If pain persists for more than 3 months, more severe ligamentous, disc, associated zygapophysial joint injuries, or other factors should be suspected.

Source: References 118–120.

CRANIOVERTEBRAL LIGAMENT INJURY

Diagnosis

Craniovertebral ligament injury. ICD-9: 848.9 (unspecified site of sprain and strain). Also known as an upper cervical sprain/ligament tear.

Description

Sprain of either the alar or the transverse ligament of the upper cervical spine/ craniovertebral region. This type of injury can result in instability and subsequent compromise of the spinal cord, vertebral artery, and/or the brainstem.

Subjective Findings

The subjective findings typically include some or all of the following:
- History of trauma (whiplash), chronic rheumatoid arthritis, Down syndrome.
- Extreme hesitancy when asked to move the head or neck in any direction.
- Bilateral paresthesias in the hands and feet.
- Bowel and bladder disturbances.
- Dizziness.
- Tinnitus (ringing in the ears).
- Blurred vision.
- Nausea.

- Diplopia (double vision).
- Dysarthria.
- Dysphagia (difficulty with swallowing).
- Drop attacks.

Objective Findings

The physical examination, undertaken with great care, typically reveals the following findings:

- Limitation of both active and passive range of motion.
- Neurological signs may or may not be present.
- Cranial nerve signs may or may not be present (depends on the extent of the injury).
- Ataxic gait.
- Pathologic reflexes.

Confirmatory/Special Tests

- Positive ligament testing for the injured structure (alar or transverse ligament) in combination with both subjective complaints and objective findings.

Medical/Imaging Studies

- Anterior widening of the atlantodens interval of more than 5 mm on the flexion view suggests incompetence of the transverse ligament.
- MRI testing is used to confirm the diagnosis.

Differential Diagnosis

- Odontoid fracture
- Cervical pathology
- Cerebrovascular accident
- Chiari malformation

Intervention

This condition warrants immediate medical referral while ensuring stabilization of the cervical spine (collar).

Prognosis

Surgical outcomes for these patients is usually good and without severe complications. Depending on the surgical procedure (internal fixation, arthrodesis) the patient may lose some cervical mobility.

REHABILITATION LADDER

CERVICAL SPINE

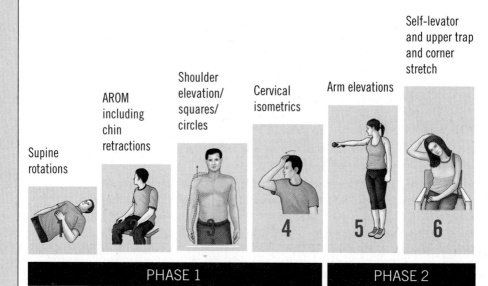

Self-levator and upper trap and corner stretch

Arm elevations

Cervical isometrics

Shoulder elevation/ squares/ circles

AROM including chin retractions

Supine rotations

PHASE 1 | PHASE 2

The purpose of these training ladders is to provide the clinician with a safe and progressive framework of exercises that are designed to allow the patient to improve in an efficient manner. The patient begins at the appropriate step, which is based on the stage of healing and the goal of the intervention.

- Phase 1: Acute—pain management, restoration of full passive range of motion, and restoration of normal accessory motion.
- Phase 2: Subacute—active range of motion exercises and early strengthening.
- Phase 3: Chronic—specific strengthening with a strong emphasis on enhancing dynamic stability.

The degree of movement and the speed of progression are both guided by the signs and symptoms. Once the patient is able to perform an exercise for

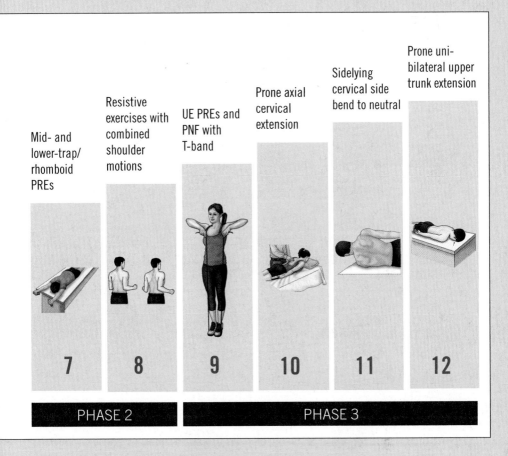

Mid- and lower-trap/rhomboid PREs

Resistive exercises with combined shoulder motions

UE PREs and PNF with T-band

Prone axial cervical extension

Sidelying cervical side bend to neutral

Prone uni-bilateral upper trunk extension

7   8   9   10   11   12

PHASE 2   PHASE 3

8–12 reps without pain, he or she progresses up to the next exercise step. This continues until the patient attempts an exercise that reproduces the pain. At this point, the patient returns to the last exercise that he or she was able to perform without pain and performs that exercise five times per day for 1 to 2 days before attempting to progress again. The patient is advanced through the training ladders to the appropriate point, with particular attention paid to patient response to treatment in terms of changes in symptoms, swelling, degree of irritability or motion. In addition, muscle imbalances are addressed with appropriate flexibility exercises.

Once the patient is able to perform the last exercise of Phase 3 (Step 12 of the ladder), he or she can move on to functional and sport-specific training (Phase 4) as appropriate, which focus on power and higher-speed exercises similar to sport-specific demands.

1. Supine rotations

The patient is positioned in supine with the head resting comfortably on a pillow. The patient is asked to slowly turn the head to one side and then to the other.

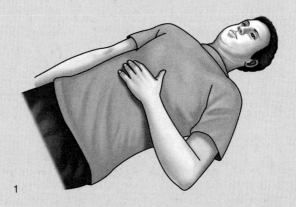

2. Active range of motion

The patient is positioned in sitting or standing. The patient is asked to actively move the head and neck into rotation (2a), flexion/extension (2b), side bending (2c), and to perform a chin tuck (2d).

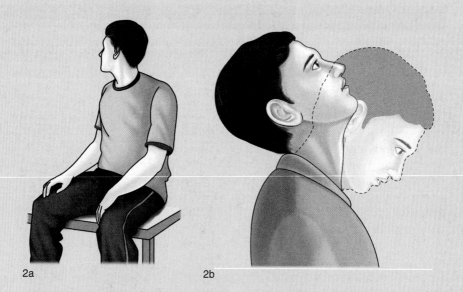

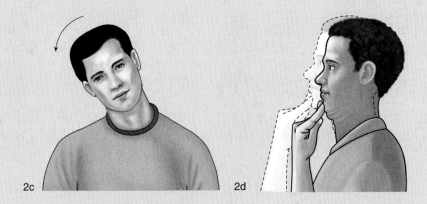

2c   2d

3. Shoulder elevation/circles/squares

The patient is positioned in sitting or standing. The patient is asked to raise the shoulders (3a), perform shoulder circles (3b), or perform shoulder squares (3c).

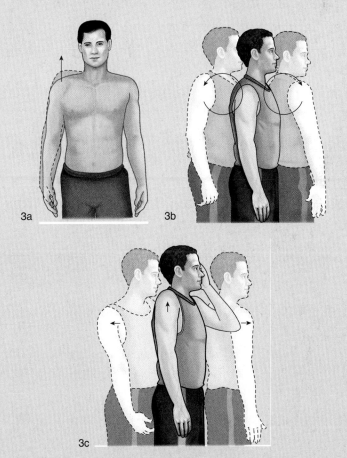

3a   3b

3c

4. Cervical isometrics

The patient is positioned in sitting or standing. The patient is asked to perform an isometric contraction into flexion (4a), rotation (4b), side bending
(4c), and extension (4d).

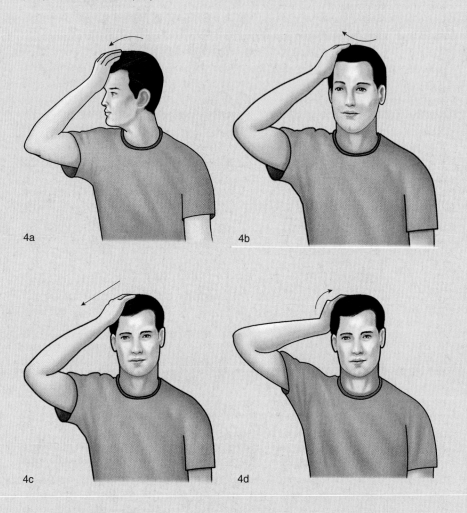

5. Arm elevation

The patient is positioned in sitting or standing. The patient is asked to raise
the arm in a variety of directions first without a weight and then with a weight
in the hand as tolerated (5).

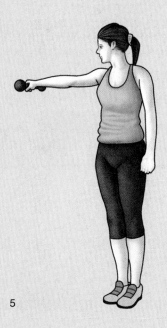

5

6. Cervical stretches

The patient is positioned in sitting. Instructions are given to the patient as to how to self-stretch the levator scapula (6a), and the upper trapezius (6b). The patient is then asked to perform a corner stretch (6c).

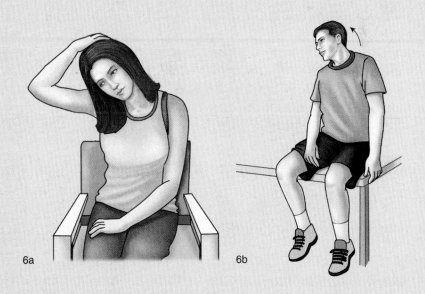

6a   6b

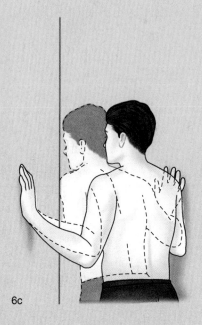

6c

7. Scapulothoracic PREs
The patient is positioned in prone. The patient performs exercises for the
lower trapezius (7a), middle trapezius (7b), and the rhomboids (7c).

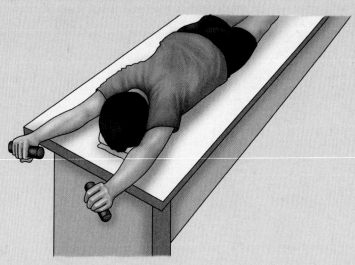

7a

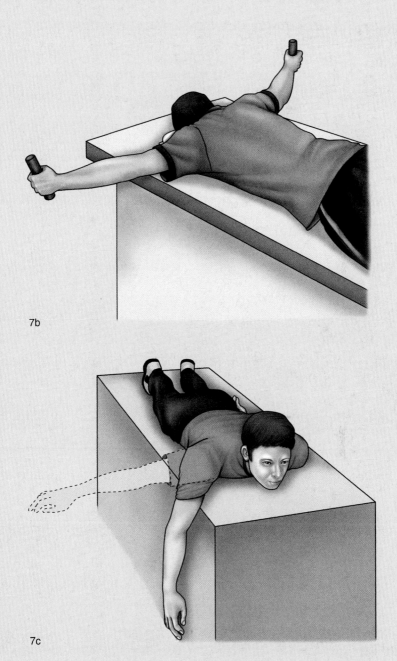

7b

7c

8. Resistive exercises with combined shoulder motions

See Chapter 5 for full description. Exercises should include scaption and rowing sets.

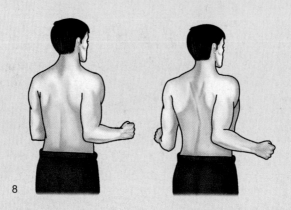

8

9. UE PREs including PNF

The patient is asked to perform a series of upper extremity PREs including PNF patterns (9a–9c).

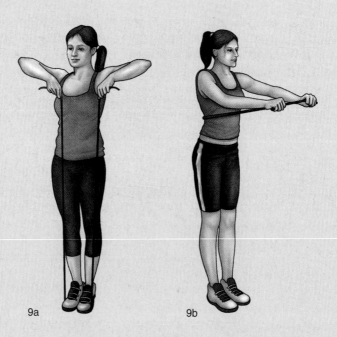

9a   9b

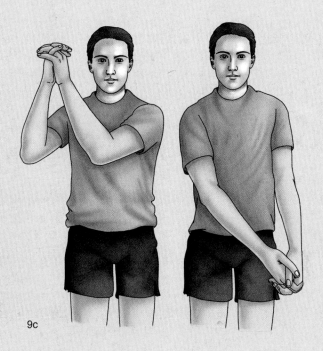

9c

10. Prone axial cervical extension

The patient is positioned in prone lying with their forehead resting on a small towel. The patient is asked to lift the forehead off the towel, keeping the chin tucked in a neutral cervical spine position. The position is held for 10 seconds.

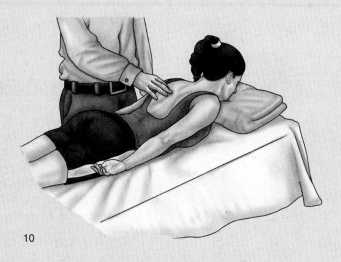

10

11. Sidelying side bends

The patient is positioned in sidelying. The patient is asked to side bend the cervical spine toward the ceiling against gravity. The position is held for 10 seconds.

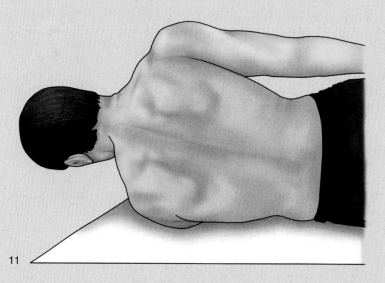

11

12. Prone uni-bilateral upper trunk extension

The patient is positioned in prone lying. The patient is asked to raise the head and one arm off the table and to hold the position for 10 seconds. The exercise can be made more difficult by asking the patient to lift the head and both arms together off the table.

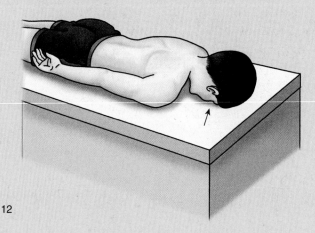

12

REFERENCES

1. Maigne J-Y. Cervicothoracic and thoracolumbar spinal pain syndromes. In: Giles LGF, Singer KP, eds. *Clinical Anatomy and Management of the Thoracic Spine*. Oxford, UK: Butterworth-Heinemann; 2000:157–168.

2. Jull GA. Physiotherapy management of neck pain of mechanical origin. In: Giles LGF, Singer KP, eds. *Clinical Anatomy and Management of Cervical Spine Pain. The Clinical Anatomy of Back Pain*. London, UK: Butterworth-Heinemann; 1998:168–191.

3. Keshner EA. Motor control of the cervical spine. In: Boyling JD, Jull GA, eds. *Grieve's Modern Manual Therapy: The Vertebral Column*. Philadelphia, PA: Churchill Livingstone; 2004:105–117.

4. Vieweg U, Meyer B, Schramm J. Differential treatment in acute upper cervical spine injuries: a critical review of a single-institution series. *Surg Neurol*. 2000;54:203–210; discussion 210–211.

5. Bland JH. Diagnosis of thoracic pain syndromes. In: Giles LGF, Singer KP, eds. *Clinical Anatomy and Management of the Thoracic Spine*. Oxford, UK: Butterworth-Heinemann; 2000:145–156.

6. Bell WE. *Orofacial Pains: Classification, Diagnosis, Management*. 3rd ed. Chicago, IL: New Year Medical Publishers; 1985.

7. Meadows J. *A Rationale and Complete Approach to the Sub-acute Post-MVA Cervical Patient*. Calgary, AB: Swodeam Consulting; 1995.

8. McCrory P. Headaches and exercise. *Sports Med*. 2000;30:221–229.

9. McKenzie RA. *The Cervical and Thoracic Spine: Mechanical Diagnosis and Therapy*. Waikanae, NZ: Spinal Publications; 1990.

10. Aptaker RL. Neck pain: Part 1: narrowing the differential. *Phys Sports Med*. 1996;24:26–38.

11. Carlsson GE, LeResche L. Epidemiology of temporomandibular disorders. In: Sessle BJ, Bryant PS, Dionne RA, eds. *Temporomandibular Disorders and Related Pain Conditions, Progress in Pain Research and Management*. Seattle, WA: IASP Press; 1995:211–226.

12. Dimitroulis G. Temporomandibular disorders: a clinical update. *Br Med J*. 1998;317:190–194.

13. McNeill C. *Temporomandibular Disorders—Guidelines for Classification, Assessment and Management*. 2nd ed. Chicago, IL: Quintessence Books; 1993.

14. Kaplan AS. Examination and diagnosis. In: Kaplan AS, Assael LA, eds. *Temporomandibular Disorders Diagnosis and Treatment*. Philadelphia, PA: WB Saunders, 1991:284–311.

15. Orsini MG, Kuboki T, Terada S, et al. Clinical predictability of temporomandibular joint disc displacement. *J Dent Res*. 1999;78:650–660.

16. Barclay P, Hollender LG, Maravilla KR, et al. Comparison of clinical and magnetic resonance imaging diagnosis in patients with disk displacement in the temporomandibular joint. *Oral Surg Oral Med Oral Pathol Oral Radiol Endod*. 1999;88:37–43.

17. Green CS, Laskin DM. Long term status of TMJ clicking in patients with myofascial pain dysfunction. *J Am Dent Assoc*. 1988;117:461–465.

18. Dolwick MF. Clinical diagnosis of temporomandibular joint internal derangement and myofascial pain and dysfunction. *Oral Maxillofac Surg Clin North Am.* 1989;1:1–6.
19. Marbach JJ, Lipton JA. Treatment of patients with temporomandibular joint and other facial pain by otolaryngologists. *Arch Otolaryngol.* 1982;108: 102–107.
20. Brazeau GA, Gremillion HA, Widmer CG, et al. The role of pharmacy in the management of patients with temporomandibular disorders and orofacial pain. *J Am Pharm Assoc (Wash).* 1998;38:354–361; quiz 362–363.
21. Cholitgul W, Nishiyama H, Sasai T, et al. Clinical and magnetic resonance imaging findings in temporomandibular joint disc displacement. *Dentomaxillofac Radiol.* 1997;26:183–188.
22. Cholitgul W, Petersson A, Rohlin M, et al. Clinical and radiological findings in temporomandibular joints with disc perforation. *Int J Oral Maxillofac Surg.* 1990;19:220–225.
23. Cholitgul W, Petersson A, Rohlin M, et al. Diagnostic outcome and observer performance in sagittal tomography of the temporomandibular joint. *Dentomaxillofac Radiol.* 1990;19:1–6.
24. Magnusson T, List T, Helkimo M. Self-assessment of pain and discomfort in patients with temporomandibular disorders: a comparison of five different scales with respect to their precision and sensitivity as well as their capacity to register memory of pain and discomfort. *J Oral Rehabil.* 1995;22: 549–556.
25. Clark GT, Seligman DA, Solberg WK, et al. Guidelines for the examination and diagnosis of temporomandibular disorders. *J Craniomandibular Disord Facial Oral Pain.* 1989;3:7–14.
26. Duinkerke AS, Luteijn F, Bouman TK, et al. Relations between TMJ pain dysfunction syndrome (PDS) and some psychological and biographical variables. *Community Dent Oral Epidemiol.* 1985;13:185–189.
27. Keith DA. Differential diagnosis of facial pain and headache. *Oral Maxillofac Surg Clin North Am.* 1989;1:7–12.
28. Dvorak J. Epidemiology, physical examination, and neurodiagnostics. *Spine.* 1998;23:2663–2673.
29. Bush K, Hillier S. Outcome of cervical radiculopathy treated with periradicular/epidural corticosteroid injections: a prospective study with independent clinical review. *Eur Spine J.* 1996;5:319–325.
30. Maigne J-Y, Maigne R, Guerin-Surville H. Upper thoracic dorsal rami: anatomic study of their medial cutaneous branches. *Surg Radiol Anat.* 1991;13: 109–112.
31. Bogduk N, Valencia F. Innervation and pain patterns of the thoracic spine. In: Grant R, ed. *Physical Therapy of the Cervical and Thoracic Spine.* 2nd ed. Melbourne: Churchill Livingstone; 1994:77–88.
32. Hardin J Jr. Pain and the cervical spine. *Bull Rheum Dis.* 2001;50:1–4.
33. Jull G, Bogduk N, Marsland A. The accuracy of manual diagnosis for cervical zygapophyseal joint pain syndromes. *Med J Aust.* 1988;148:233–236.
34. Mohn A, di Ricco L, Magnelli A, et al. Celiac disease--associated vertigo and nystagmus. *J Pediatr Gastroenterol Nutr.* 2002;34:317–318.

35. Dvorak J, Dvorak V. Differential diagnosis of vertigo. In: Gilliar WG, Greenman PE, eds. *Manual Medicine: Diagnostics*. 2nd ed. New York, NY: Thieme Medical Publishers; 1990:67–70.
36. Hohl M. Soft-tissue injuries of the neck in automobile accidents. *J Bone Joint Surg*. 1974;56A:1675–1682.
37. Jamieson DRS, Ballantyne JP. Unique presentation of a prolapsed thoracic disk: Lhermitte's symptom in a golf player. *Neurology*. 1995;45:1219–1221.
38. Kanchandani R, Howe JG. Lhermitte's sign in multiple sclerosis: a clinical survey and review of the literature. *J Neurol Neurosurg Psychiatry*. 1982;45:308–312.
39. Ventafridda V, Caraceni A, Martini C, et al. On the significance of Lhermitte's sign in oncology. *J Neurooncol*. 1991;10:133–137.
40. Youdas JW, Carey JR, Garrett TR. Reliability of measurements of cervical spine range of motion: comparison of three methods. *Phys Ther*. 1991;71:98–104.
41. Cyriax J. *Textbook of Orthopaedic Medicine, Diagnosis of Soft Tissue Lesions*. 8th ed. London: Bailliere Tindall; 1982.
42. Travell JG, Simons DG. *Myofascial Pain and Dysfunction—The Trigger Point Manual*. Baltimore, MD: Williams & Wilkins; 1983.
43. Viikara-Juntura E. *Examination of the Neck. Validity of Some Clinical, Radiological and Epidemiologic Methods*. Helsinki: University of Helsinki, Institute of Occupational Health; 1988.
44. Cheshire WP Jr. Trigeminal neuralgia. *Curr Pain Headache Rep*. 2007;11:69–74.
45. Cheshire WP. Trigeminal neuralgia: diagnosis and treatment. *Curr Neurol Neurosci Rep*. 2005;5:79–85.
46. Bennetto L, Patel NK, Fuller G. Trigeminal neuralgia and its management. *Br Med J*. 2007;334:201–205.
47. Magarey ME. Examination of the cervical and thoracic spine. In: Grant R, ed. *Physical Therapy of the Cervical and Thoracic Spine*. 2nd ed. New York, NY: Churchill Livingstone; 1994:109–144.
48. Meadows J. *Orthopedic Differential Diagnosis in Physical Therapy*. New York, NY: McGraw-Hill; 1999.
49. Jull GA, Treleaven J, Versace G. Manual examination: is pain a major cue to spinal dysfunction. *Aust J Physiother*. 1994;40:159–165.
50. Foreman SM, Croft AC. *Whiplash Injuries: The Cervical Acceleration/Deceleration Syndrome*. Baltimore, MD: Williams & Wilkins; 1988.
51. Feinstein B, Lanton NJK, Jameson RM, et al. Experiments on pain referred from deep somatic tissues. *J Bone Joint Surg*. 1954;36A:981–997.
52. Cyriax J. Rheumatic headache. *Br Med J*. 1982;2:1367–1368.
53. Friedman MH, Weisberg J. *Temporomandibular Joint Disorders*. Chicago, IL: Quintessence Publishing Company, Inc.; 1985.
54. Bogduk N. Cervical causes of headache and dizziness. In: Grieve GP, ed. *Modern Manual Therapy of the Vertebral Column*. New York, NY: Churchill Livingstone; 1986:289–302.
55. Radanov B, Sturzenegger M, Di Stefano G, et al. Factors influencing recovery from headache after common whiplash. *Br Med J*. 1993;307:652–655.
56. Dimitroulis G, Dolwick MF, Gremillion HA. Temporomandibular disorders. 1. Clinical evaluation. *Aust Dent J*. 1995;40:301–305.

57. Bradley JP, Tibone JE, Watkins RG. History, physical examination, and diagnostic tests for neck and upper extremity problems. In: Watkins RG, ed. *The Spine in Sports*. St. Louis, MO: Mosby-Year-Book Inc.; 1996.

58. Herkowitz HN. Syndromes related to spinal stenosis. In: Weinstein JN, Rydevik B, Sonntag VKH, eds. *Essentials of the Spine*. New York, NY: Raven Press; 1995:179–193.

59. Laskin DM. Etiology of the pain-dysfunction syndrome. *J Am Dent Assoc*. 1969;79:147–153.

60. Jull GA, Janda V. Muscle and motor control in low back pain. In: Twomey LT, Taylor JR, eds. *Physical Therapy of the Low Back: Clinics in Physical Therapy*. New York, NY: Churchill Livingstone; 1987:258.

61. Richardson CA, Jull GA, Hodges P, et al. *Therapeutic Exercise for Spinal Segmental Stabilization in Low Back Pain*. London, UK: Churchill Livingstone; 1999.

62. Janda V. Muscle strength in relation to muscle length, pain and muscle imbalance. In: Harms-Ringdahl K, ed. *Muscle Strength*. New York, NY: Churchill Livingstone; 1993:83.

63. Janda V. Muscles, motor regulation and back problems. In: Korr IM, ed. *The Neurological Mechanisms in Manipulative Therapy*. New York, NY: Plenum; 1978:27.

64. Sahrmann SA. *Diagnosis and Treatment of Movement Impairment Syndromes*. St Louis, MO: Mosby; 2001.

65. White AA, Sahrmann SA. A movement system balance approach to management of musculoskeletal pain. In: Grant R, ed. *Physical Therapy for the Cervical and Thoracic Spine*. Edinburgh, Churchill Livingstone; 1994:347.

66. Gossman MR, Sahrmann SA, Rose SJ. Review of length-associated changes in muscle. *Phys Ther*. 1982;62:1799–1808.

67. Greenman PE. *Principles of Manual Medicine*. 2nd ed. Baltimore, MD: Williams & Wilkins; 1996.

68. Bowen JE, Malanga GA, Pappoe T, et al. Physical examination of the shoulder. In: Malanga GA, Nadler SF, eds. *Musculoskeletal Physical Examination—An Evidence-based Approach*. Philadelphia, PA: Elsevier-Mosby; 2006:59–118.

69. Okeson JP. *Orofacial Pain: Guidelines for Assessment, Diagnosis, and Management*. Chicago, IL: Quintessence Publishing Co; 1996.

70. Okeson JP. Current terminology and diagnostic classification schemes. *Oral Surg Oral Med Oral Pathol Oral Radiol Endod*. 1997;83:61–66.

71. Friedman MH, Weisberg J. Screening procedures for temporomandibular joint dysfunction. *Am Fam Physician*. 1982;25:157–160.

72. Hedenberg-Magnusson B, Ernberg M, Kopp S. Symptoms and signs of temporomandibular disorders in patients with fibromyalgia and local myalgia of the temporomandibular system: a comparative study. *Acta Odontol Scand*. 1997;55:344–349.

73. Isacsson G, Linde C, Isberg A. Subjective symptoms in patients with temporomandibular disk displacement versus patients with myogenic craniomandibular disorders. *J Prosthet Dent*. 1989;61:70–77.

74. Kirk WS Jr, Calabrese DK. Clinical evaluation of physical therapy in the management of internal derangement of the temporomandibular joint. *J Oral Maxillofac Surg*. 1989;47:113–119.

75. Walsh R, Nitz AJ. Cervical spine. In: Wadsworth C, ed. *Current Concepts of Orthopedic Physical Therapy—Home Study Course*. La Crosse, WI: Orthopaedic Section, APTA; 2001.
76. Dvorak J, Antinnes JA, Panjabi M, et al. Age and gender related normal motion of the cervical spine. *Spine*. 1992;17:S393–S398.
77. Toole J, Tucker S. Influence of head position upon cerebral circulation. *Arch Neurol*. 1960;2:616–623.
78. Jacob G, McKenzie R. Spinal therapeutics based on responses to loading. In: Liebenson C, ed. *Rehabilitation of the Spine: A Practitioner's Manual*. Baltimore, MD: Lippincott Williams & Wilkins; 1996:225–252.
79. Ehrhardt R, Bowling RW. *Treatment of the Cervical Spine*. APTA Orthopedic Section, Physical Therapy Home Study Course; 1996.
80. Mitchell FL, Moran PS, Pruzzo NA. *An Evaluation and Treatment Manual of Osteopathic Muscle Energy Procedures*. Manchester, MO: Mitchell, Moran and Pruzzo Associates; 1979.
81. Lee DG. *A Workbook of Manual Therapy Techniques for the Upper Extremity*. Delta, BC, Canada: Delta Orthopaedic Physiotherapy Clinics; 1989.
82. Pettman E. Stress tests of the craniovertebral joints. In: Boyling JD, Palastanga N, eds. *Grieve's Modern Manual Therapy: The Vertebral Column*. 2nd ed. Edinburgh: Churchill Livingstone; 1994:529–538.
83. Uitvlugt G, Indenbaum S. Clinical assessment of atlantoaxial instability using the Sharp-Purser test. *Arthritis Rheum*. 1988;31:918–922.
84. Bouchaud-Chabot A, Liote F. Cervical spine involvement in rheumatoid arthritis. A review. *Joint Bone Spine*. 2002;69:141–154.
85. Viikari-Juntura E. Interexaminer reliability of observations in physical examinations of the neck. *Phys Ther*. 1987;67:1526–1532.
86. Viikari-Juntura E, Takala EP, Alaranta H. Neck and shoulder pain and disability. Evaluation by repetitive gripping test. *Scand J Rehabil Med*. 1988;20:167–173.
87. Vernon H, Mior S. The neck disability index: a study of reliability and validity. *J Manipulative Physiol Ther*. 1991;14:409–415.
88. Evans RC. *Illustrated Essentials in Orthopedic Physical Assessment*. St. Louis, MO: Mosby–Year book Inc; 1994.
89. Maitland G. *Vertebral Manipulation*. Sydney: Butterworth; 1986.
90. Ombregt L, Bisschop P, ter Veer HJ, et al. *A System of Orthopaedic Medicine*. London: WB Saunders; 1995.
91. Fast A, Parikh S, Marin EL. The shoulder abduction relief sign in cervical radiculopathy. *Arch Phys Med Rehabil*. 1989;70:402–403.
92. Uchihara T, Furukawa T, Tsukagoshi H. Compression of brachial plexus as a diagnostic test of a cervical cord lesion. *Spine*. 1994;19:2170–2173.
93. Landi A, Copeland S. Value of the Tinel sign in brachial plexus lesions. *Ann R Coll Surg Engl*. 1979;61:470–471.
94. Selke FW, Kelly TR. Thoracic outlet syndrome. *Am J Surg*. 1988;156:54–57.
95. Nichols AW. The thoracic outlet syndrome in athletes. *J Am Board Fam Pract*. 1996;9:346–355.
96. Marx RG, Bombardier C, Wright JG. What we know about the reliability and validity of physical examination tests used to examine the upper extremity. *J Hand Surg*. 1999;24A:185–193.

97. Roos DB. Congenital anomalies associated with thoracic outlet syndrome. *J Surg.* 1976;132:771–778.
98. Wright IS. The neurovascular syndrome produced by hyperabduction of the arms. *Am Heart J.* 1945;29:1–19.
99. Guide to physical therapist practice. *Phys Ther.* 2001;81:S13–S95.
100. Clair DA, Edmondston SJ, Allison GT. Physical therapy treatment dose for non-traumatic neck pain: a comparison between 2 patient groups. *J Orthop Sports Phys Ther.* 2006;36:867–875.
101. Bronfort G, Evans R, Nelson B, et al. A randomized clinical trial of exercise and spinal manipulation for patients with chronic neck pain. *Spine (Phila Pa 1976).* 2001;26:788–797; discussion 798–799; 2001
102. Chiu TT, Lam TH, Hedley AJ. A randomized controlled trial on the efficacy of exercise for patients with chronic neck pain. *Spine (Phila Pa 1976).* 2005;30: E1–E7.
103. Chiu TT, Hui-Chan CW, Chein G. A randomized clinical trial of TENS and exercise for patients with chronic neck pain. *Clin Rehabil.* 2005;19:850–860.
104. Feine JS, Lund JP. An assessment of the efficacy of physical therapy and physical modalities for the control of chronic musculoskeletal pain. *Pain.* 1997;71:5–23.
105. Medlicott MS, Harris SR. A systematic review of the effectiveness of exercise, manual therapy, electrotherapy, relaxation training, and biofeedback in the management of temporomandibular disorder. *Phys Ther.* 2006;86:955–973.
106. Kulekcioglu S, Sivrioglu K, Ozcan O, et al. Effectiveness of low-level laser therapy in temporomandibular disorder. *Scand J Rheumatol.* 2003;32:114–118.
107. Maigne R. La céphalée sus-orbitaire. Sa fréquente origine cervicale. Son traitement. *Ann Med Phys.* 1968;39:241–246.
108. Nicholson GG, Gaston J. Cervical headache. *J Orthop Sports Phys Ther.* 2001;31:184–193.
109. Sizer PS Jr, Phelps V, Brismee J-M. Diagnosis and management of cervicogenic headache and local cervical syndrome with multiple pain generators. *J Man Manip Ther.* 2002;10:136–152.
110. Lu J, Ebraheim NA. Anatomical consideration of C2 nerve root ganglion. *Spine.* 1998;23:649–652.
111. Bogduk N. An anatomical basis for the neck-tongue syndrome. *J Neurol Neurosurg Psychiatry.* 1981;44:202–208.
112. Polletti CE, Sweet WH. Entrapment of the C2 root and ganglion by the atlanto-epitrophic ligament: Clinical syndrome and surgical anatomy. *Neurosurgery.* 1990;27:288–290.
113. Welch KM. A 47-year-old woman with tension-type headaches. *JAMA.* 2001;286:960–966.
114. McDonnell MK, Sahrmann SA, Van Dillen L. A specific exercise program and modification of postural alignment for treatment of cervicogenic headache: a case report. *J Orthop Sports Phys Ther.* 2005;35:3–15.
115. Hurwitz EL, Aker PD, Adams AH, et al. Manipulation and mobilization of the cervical spine. A systematic review of the literature. *Spine.* 1996;21:1746–1759; discussion 1759–1760.
116. Schoensee SK, Jensen G, Nicholson G, et al. The effect of mobilization on cervical headaches. *J Orthop Sports Phys Ther.* 1995;21:184–196.

117. Hanten WP, Olson SL, Weston AL, et al. The effect of manual therapy and a
     home exercise program on cervicogenic headaches: a case report. *J Man Manip
     Ther*. 2005;13:35–43.
118. Cloward RB. Cervical diskography. A contribution to the etiology and mecha-
     nism of neck pain. *Ann Surg*. 1959;150:1052.
119. Dwyer A, Aprill C, Bogduk N. Cervical zygapophyseal joint pain patterns: a
     study from normal volunteers. *Spine*. 1990;15:453.
120. Stiell IG, Wells GA, Vandemheen KL, et al. The Canadian C-spine rule for radi-
     ography in alert and stable trauma patients. *JAMA*. 2001;286:1841–1848.

QUESTIONS

1. What is of the function of the uncinate process?
2. Which of the cervical levels has the most prominent cervical spinous process?
3. At what levels does cervical spondylosis most typically occur?
4. Which of the following is not a suboccipital muscle: rectus capitis lateralis, rectus capitis posterior major, rectus capitis posterior minor, obliquus
   capitis inferior, obliquus capitis superior?
5. What are the spinal cord root valves for the phrenic nerve?
6. T__ F__ The nerve supply for the platysma is the accessory nerve.
7. Which muscle has its origin from the zygomatic arch?
8. T__ F__ The trapezius rotates the glenoid cavity of the scapula downward.
9. What is the action of the SCM?
10. Which muscle inserts into the scalene tubercle of rib #1?
11. What is the extension of the posterior longitudinal ligament called?
12. Where does it attach?
13. What is the action of the rectus capitis posterior major?
14. How about the rectus capitis posterior minor?
15. Which muscle produces SB of the O-A to the same side as well as exten-
    sion and contralateral rotation?
16. A decreased anterior glide of the R occiput condyle would produce which
    movement deficits at the O-A joint?
17. How many degrees of SB occur (approx) at the O-A joint?
18. How about rotation?
19. Which of the above two motions is the primary motion?
20. Which AROM test(s) can you use for the A-A joint?
21. How about with the O-A joint?

22. Side bending of the O-A joint is limited by which ligaments?
23. R side bending at the O-A joint involves an anterior glide of the occiput condyle on which side?
24. With the O-A in EXT, a decreased L side glide would indicate a lesion on which side?
25. With flexion of the O-A in relation to the glide restriction, which side is the condyle restricted?
26. Which motions occur at the A-A joint?
27. With flexion, the inferior surface of C1 rolls and glides in which direction(s)?
28. How much flexion and extension is normal at the A-A joint?
29. How about the rotation?
30. In the mid-lower cervical spine, an ERS L would produce which motion restrictions?
31. Which process is thought to help prevent cervical disc protrusions?
33. A tight rectus capitis anterior would produce a decreased translation to which direction while in C-V extension?
34. T__ F__ At the O-A joint, side bending and rotation occur to the same side.
35. What is the function of the transverse ligament?
36. In which way could you test the integrity of the tectorial membrane?

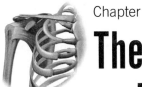

Chapter **12**

The Thoracic Spine and Ribs

OVERVIEW

In the thoracic spine, protection and function of the thoracic viscera take precedence over segmental spinal mobility. Although a significant source of local and referred symptoms, differential diagnosis of the thoracic region can be difficult. This is due to the complicated biomechanics and function of the region, the proximity to vital organs, and the many articulations.

Anatomy

The thoracic spine forms a kyphotic curve between the lordotic curves of the cervical and lumbar spines. The curve begins at T1–2 and extends down to T12, with the T6–7 disk space as the apex.[1]

 Clinical Pearl

The thoracic kyphosis is a structural curve that is present from birth.[2] Unlike the lumbar and cervical regions, which derive their curves from the corresponding differences in intervertebral disk heights, the thoracic curve is maintained by the wedge-shaped vertebral bodies, which are about 2 mm higher posteriorly than anteriorly.

At the thoracolumbar junction, typically located between T11 and L1, the changes in curvature from one of kyphosis to one of lordosis vary quite widely according to posture, age, and previous compression fractures and resulting deformity.[3,4]

The cervicothoracic junction anatomically comprises the C7–T1 segment and functionally includes the seventh cervical vertebra, the first two thoracic vertebrae, the first and second ribs, and the manubrium.

Examination

Pain arising from the thoracic spinal joints has considerable overlap and can refer symptoms to distal regions (groin, pubis, and lower abdominal wall).

 Clinical Pearl

Apart from musculoskeletal lesions, the thoracic spine is also a common source of systemic pain, and the phenomenon of referred pain poses more diagnostic difficulties in the thoracic spine than in any other region of the vertebral column (Figure 12-1).[5]

The algorithm outlined in Figure 12-2 can serve as a guide to the examination of the thoracic spine and ribs (Figure 12-2).

History

The history should include the chief complaints and a pain drawing. Determining the location of the pain can provide some clues as to the cause, as many of the thoracic structures are superficial. It is common for a patient with thoracic symptoms to have stiffness in the morning. However, sharp pain and stiffness that persist for greater than 30 minutes may indicate inflammation.

 Clinical Pearl

Morning stiffness is a moderately sensitive and specific finding (0.64 and 0.59, respectively) for ankylosing spondylitis.[6]

 Clinical Pearl

The clinician must determine whether the symptoms are provoked or alleviated with movement or posture (musculoskeletal pain), respiration (rib dysfunction or pleuritic pain), eating or drinking (gastric pain), or exertion (rib dysfunction or cardiac pain).

Visceral pain tends to be vague and dull, and may be accompanied by nausea and sweating. To help differentiate between visceral pain and musculoskeletal pain, the clinician should focus on the relationship of specific movements or activities.

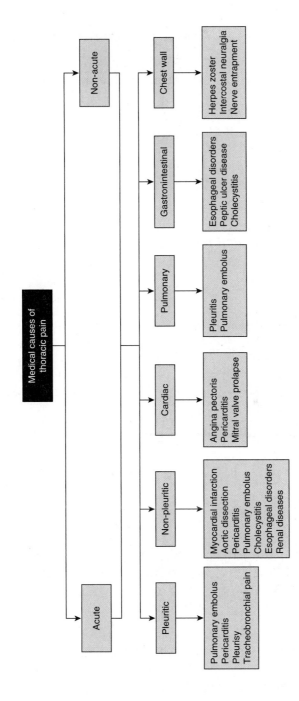

Figure 12-1 Medical causes of thoracic pain.

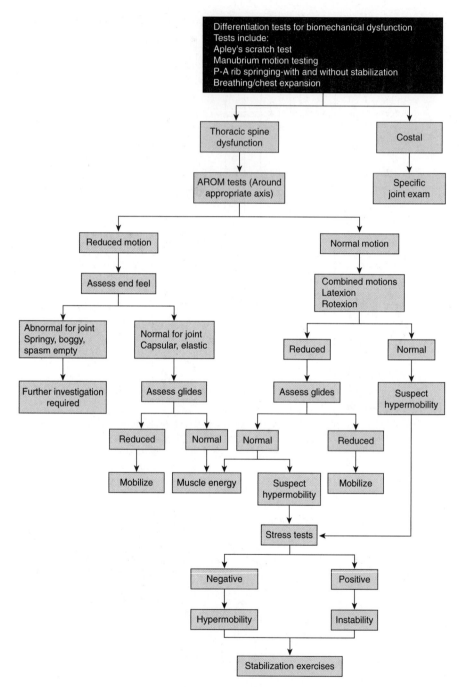

Figure 12-2 Algorithm for examination of thoracic spine and ribs.

Clinical Pearl

Scheuermann disease, which is found in approximately 10% of the population and in males and females equally, typically is seen in pubescent athletes. Although typically asymptomatic, clinical findings may include evidence of a thoracic kyphosis and pain with thoracic extension and rotation during sporting activities.

Any information regarding the onset, as well as aggravating factors, is important, especially if the pain only appears during certain positions or movements, which would suggest a musculoskeletal lesion.

 Clinical Pearl

Pulling and pushing activities typically worsen thoracic symptoms.
Deep breathing or arm elevation tends to aggravate a rib dysfunction.
Aggravation of pain by coughing, sneezing, or deep inspiration tends to implicate the costovertebral joint.
Osteoarthritic pain is typically less intense in the morning than in the afternoon or evening

Chronic problems in this area tend to result from postural dysfunctions. The patient is asked to describe the quality of the pain. Thoracic nerve root pain is often sharp, stabbing, and severe, although it can also have a burning quality. Nerve pain is usually referred in a sloping band along an intercostal space.[7] Vascular pain and visceral pain are often described as being poorly localized and achy. A sudden onset of pain related to trauma could indicate a fracture, muscle strain, or ligament sprain.

 Clinical Pearl

Although ribs are relatively flexible structures, fractures can occur anywhere blunt trauma occurs. Depending on the level, rib fractures can produce a myriad of symptoms:

- Ribs 1–4: These ribs function to protect the arteries, veins, nerves of the upper extremity. Associated problems with fractures of these ribs can include neurovascular compromise of the brachial plexus or subclavian artery and vein.

- Ribs 5–9: These ribs function to protect the lungs and heart.
- Ribs 10–12: These ribs function to protect the kidneys, diaphragm, and spleen.

The patient should be asked to point to the area of pain. If the patient has difficulty localizing the pain, the clinician should suspect referred pain as the source.

 Clinical Pearl

Symptoms that are aggravated by flexion-based activities include disk pathology, muscle strain, and ligament strain.

Symptoms that are aggravated by extension-based and side bending-based activities include facet pathology and muscle strains.

Systems Review

Thoracic pain may originate from just about all of the viscera. Both visceral and somatic afferent nerves transmit pain messages from a peripheral stimulus and converge on the same projection neurons in the dorsal horn.

Systemic illnesses such as rheumatoid arthritis and malignancy, and those conditions causing referred pain must be included in the differential diagnosis (Table 12-1). Non-musculoskeletal causes of thoracic symptoms can include, but are not limited to[8]:

- A dissecting aortic aneurysm.
- A myocardial infarction.
- Intercostal neuralgia.
- Pleural irritation. When the tissues of irritated pleura are stretched, chest pain can result. This pain can be increased both by breathing, as well as by trunk movements, a situation that could lead the clinician to believe that the problem is musculoskeletal.
- Tumor (unexplained weight loss, fever, chills, and night pain). The night pain must be differentiated from mechanical pain, which may just be

Table 12-1 Symptoms and Possible Causes

Indication	Possible Condition
Severe bilateral root pain in elderly	Neoplasm (most common areas for metastasis are the lung, breast, prostate, and kidney)
Wedging/compression fracture	Osteoporotic (estrogen deficiency) or neoplastic fracture
Onset–offset of pain unrelated to trunk movements	Ankylosing spondylitis, visceral
Decreased active motion contralateral side flexion painful with both rotations full	Neoplasm
Severe chest wall pain without articular pain	Visceral
Spinal cord signs and symptoms	Spinal cord pressure or ischemia
Pain onset related to eating or diet	Visceral

because the patient has an increased, and fixed, kyphosis, and needs a softer bed to accommodate the deformity.[9]

- An acute thoracic disk herniation. In the thoracic spine, the segmental nerve roots are situated mainly behind the inferior–posterior aspect of the upper vertebral body rather than behind the disk, which reduces the possibility of root compression in impairments of the thoracic disk.[7] Because the intervertebral foramina are quite large at these levels, osseous contact with the nerve roots is seldom encountered in the thoracic spine,[7] and, as the dermatomes in this region have a fair amount of overlap, they cannot be relied upon to determine the specific nerve root involved.

- T4 syndrome.[10–12] The T4 syndrome has an unknown etiology, although it is believed to result from a sympathetic reaction to a hypermobile segment, because the symptoms appear to resolve in response to manual therapy techniques to the thoracic segments. In the thorax, the sympathetic trunks lie on or just lateral to the costovertebral joints. These trunks may undergo mechanical deformation with abnormal posture (forward head, accentuated thoracic kyphosis, and protracted shoulder girdle), trauma, or pulling and reaching activities, producing pain, and sympathetic epiphenomena.[13] Clinical findings include local tenderness of bony points, positive slump test, positive upper limb tension tests, depression or prominence of one or more spinous processes, and local thickening and stiffness of one segment,[14] although gross cervical and thoracic motions are usually normal. Nocturnal symptoms are common, usually occurring in side lying or the supine position. More women are affected by this condition than men, in a ratio of more than 3:1.[14]

- Osteoporosis. The most common sites of osteoporosis are the hip, lumbar spine, and forearm, but vertebral compression fractures can occur in the thoracic spine resulting in increased spinal deformities (kyphosis, Dowager hump, and scoliosis).

 Clinical Pearl

Questions should be asked with regard to bowel and bladder function, upper and lower extremity numbness, tingling, or weakness, and visual or balance disorders. These symptoms may indicate compromise to the spinal cord, cauda equina, or central nervous system.

Tests and Measures

Observation

The patient should be suitably disrobed to expose as much of this region as is necessary. As a quick orientation to the relationship of the bony structures, the clinician should confirm the following:

- The spine of the scapula is level with the spinous process of T 3.
- The inferior angle of the scapula is in line with the T 7–9 spinous processes.
- The medial border of the scapula is parallel with the spinal column and about 5 cm lateral to the spinous processes.
- The iliac crests are level and symmetrical. One crest higher than the other could suggest a leg length discrepancy, an iliac rotation, or both. A significant leg length discrepancy (greater than ½ an inch) can alter the lateral curvature of the spine, and result in compensation.
- The shoulder heights are level. A normal variant is that individuals carry their dominant shoulder slightly lower than the nondominant side.
- The motion of the ribs during quiet breathing.
- Asymmetry in muscle bulk, prominence, or length.
- Any lesions, swellings, or scars on the back and chest. This is a common area for the characteristic lesion pattern of herpes zoster (shingles), which follows the course of the affected nerve.

- The degree of thoracic kyphosis. As elsewhere in the spine, posture has an important influence on the available range of motion of the neighboring joints. Conversely, changes in the lumbar posture, such as an excessive lordosis, and changes in the cervical spine such as those rendered by a forward-head position, can affect the thoracic spine.

 Clinical Pearl

Two terms, *scoliosis* and *rotoscoliosis*, are used to describe the lateral curvature of the spine. Scoliosis is the older term and refers to an abnormal side bending of the spine, but gives no reference to the coupled rotation that also occurs. Rotoscoliosis is a more detailed definition, used to describe the curve of the spine by detailing how each vertebra is rotated and side-flexed in relation to the vertebra below.

- The amount of lateral curvature of the thoracic spine. Scoliosis can be classified as functional, neuromuscular, or degenerative. Scoliosis is never normal, although most cases are idiopathic, manifesting in the preadolescent years.[1,15] An abnormal lateral thoracic curve is described as being structural or functional, and can produce a fixed deformity or a changeable adaptation, respectively, with the rib hump occurring on the convex side of the curve. Persistent scoliosis during forward bending (Adam sign) is indicative of a structural curve.

On the anterior aspect of the thoracic region, the clinician should look for evidence of deformity.

- Barrel chest. A forward and upward projecting sternum increases the anterior–posterior diameter. The barrel chest results in respiratory difficulty, stretching of the intercostal and anterior chest muscles, and adaptive shortening of the scapular adductor muscles.

- Pigeon chest. A forward and downward projecting sternum, which increases the anterior–posterior diameter. The pigeon chest results in a lengthening of the upper abdominal muscles and an adaptive shortening of the upper intercostal muscles.

- Funnel chest. A posterior projecting sternum secondary to an outgrowth of the ribs.[16] The funnel chest results in adaptive shortening of the upper abdominals, shoulder adductors, pectoralis minor, and intercostal muscles, and lengthening of the thoracic extensors, middle and upper trapezius.

Gait

The analysis of the patient's gait pattern can provide valuable information as to whether their condition originates in the spine or lower extremities, and discloses gross weakness of the muscles that affect gait.[17] For example, a decreased arm swing during gait can indicate stiffness of the thoracic segments.

Palpation of the Thoracic Spine

The spinous processes of the thoracic vertebrae are readily palpated (Figure 12-3), as they are not covered by muscle or thick connective tissue.[17]

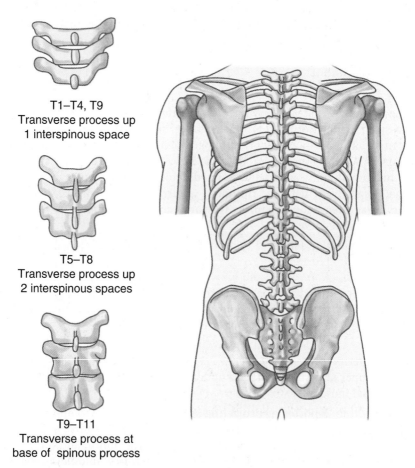

T1–T4, T9
Transverse process up
1 interspinous space

T5–T8
Transverse process up
2 interspinous spaces

T9–T11
Transverse process at
base of spinous process

Figure 12-3 Spinous process locations and the rule of 3.

Table 12-2 Anterior and Posterior Palpation Points

Anterior Aspect	Posterior Aspect
Suprasternal notch	Spinous and their associated transverse processes
Sternomanubrial angle	T 2—level with base of spine of scapula
Xiphoid process	Spinal gutter (rotatores)
Infrasternal angle	Erector spinae
Sternochondral junctions	Rib angles
Costal cartilage	Rib shafts
	Rib shafts and rib joint line of costotransverse joint
	C6—locate the largest spinous process at the base of the neck, have patient extend their neck. The first spinous process to move anteriorly under your finger is C6

The landmarks outlined in Table 12-2 may be helpful to determine the segmental level involved.

The spinous processes have varying degrees of obliquity and if they are used as landmarks, this obliquity must be understood and exploited. The areas of spinous process obliquity may be divided into four regions by the so-called "rule of threes" (Figure 12-3).[18]

- 1st group of three spinous processes (T 1–T4) and T 9. These spinous processes are level with vertebral body of the same level, and their respective transverse processes are one interspinous space above
- 2nd group of three spinous processes (T 5–T8). These spinous processes are level with the disk of the inferior level, and their respective transverse processes are two interspinous spaces above
- 3rd group of three spinous processes (T 9–11). These spinous processes are level with the vertebral body of the level below, and their respective transverse processes are level with the base of the spinous process
- The 4th group of three spinous processes reverse the obliquity.

Palpation of the soft tissues of the region is important. The clinician should note the presence of any tenderness, temperature changes, and muscle spasm. A comparison should be made between the firmness and tenderness of the paravertebral muscles, and their relationship from side to side.

Screening Tests

A few simple screening tests can help differentiate between a rib dysfunction, and a thoracic joint dysfunction.

Rib Spring Test

The patient is positioned in prone and the clinician stands on one side of the patient. Reaching over the patient, the clinician spreads the length of the thumb over the right rib in question and applies a posterior–anterior force. This is the equivalent of a left rotation of the thoracic spine. The clinician then repeats the posterior–anterior force on the rib, except this time, he blocks the rotation of the thoracic spine by placing the ulnar border of his other hand over a group of left transverse processes. Pain produced with this maneuver implicates the rib as the thoracic spine is stabilized.

Thoracic Spring Test

The patient is positioned as above. Spring testing in a posterior–anterior direction is applied with the palm of the hand with the elbows locked over the spinous processes of the thoracic spine. These spring tests are provocative for pain, but may also be used for a gross assessment of mobility.

Cervical Rotation–Side Bending Test[19–22]

This test, also known as the cervical rotation lateral flexion test, may be used to test the presence of first rib hypomobility. The patient is seated and the clinician stands behind the patient. The test is in two parts. In the first part, the patient's head is rotated to one side. From this position the patient's head is flexed forward, and an end-feel assessment is made. The test is then repeated by first rotating the patient's head to the other side and then flexing the head forward. A hard end-feel at the position of forward flexion indicates an elevated hypomobile first rib on the side opposite to the rotation. This can be confirmed by performing a spring test of the first rib.

 Clinical Pearl

> Egan and Flynn found the diagnostic accuracy (reliability) of the cervical rotation lateral flexion test as kappa = 1.0.[23]

Reflex Hammer Test

The patient is prone and the clinician uses a reflex hammer to tap over each spinous process. If tenderness is encountered, especially with a history of trauma to the area, a fracture must be ruled out.

Neck Flexion

The patient is seated and is asked to fully flex the neck. Neck flexion in this position stretches the dura of the cervical and thoracic regions. Pain with neck flexion may suggest such diagnoses as dural irritation, or meningitis.

Chest Expansion Measurement

A decreased expansion can highlight the presence of ankylosing spondylitis. It can also be the result of diaphragm palsy (C 4), intercostal weakness, pulmonary (pleura) problems, old age, a rib fracture, or a chronic lung condition. Respiratory excursion is measured at three levels using a tape measure placed circumferentially around the chest: at the level of the axilla, the xiphoid level, and at 10th rib level. Comparisons are made between the measurements taken at the position of maximum expiration and the measurement taken at full inspiration.

 Clinical Pearl

The normal circumferential difference between inspiration and expiration is 3 to 7.5 cm (1 to 3 inches).[24]

T1–2 Dural Stretch

The patient is seated and is asked to protract and retract the shoulders. Scapular approximation pulls on the thoracic extent of the dura mater via the first and second thoracic nerves.[17] A positive response of symptom reproduction should lead the clinician to suspect an upper thoracic disk protrusion, or a space-occupying lesion, such as a tumor.[25]

Deep Breathing and Flexion

This test can be used for patients who complain of pain with thoracic flexion. The patient is seated with the thoracic spine positioned in neutral. The patient is asked to inhale fully and then to flex the thoracic spine until the pain is felt. At this point, the patient maintains the position of flexion and slowly exhales. If further flexion can be achieved after exhalation, the source of the pain is likely to be the ribs rather than the thoracic spine.[26]

Active Motion Testing

Active range of motion tests are used to determine the osteokinematic function of two adjacent thoracic vertebrae during active motions, to determine which joints are dysfunctional, and the specific direction of motion loss.[27] Active range of motion is initially performed globally, looking for abnormalities, such as asymmetrical limitations of motion. A specific examination is then performed on any region that appeared to have either excessive or reduced motion. Various techniques are used to correctly assess each area of the thoracic spine.

Movement restriction of the upper thoracic spine may be secondary to pain or due to adaptive shortening of connective tissue or muscle.[28]

> ### ⚪ Clinical Pearl
>
> Physiological movement in the thoracic spine decreases with age. Midthoracic hypomobilities are the most common thoracic presentation,[29] with the movement restrictions being more common in the sagittal and frontal planes, particularly extension and side bending.[28] Most of the trunk rotation below the level of C 2 occurs in the thoracic spine.

The clinician should look for capsular or noncapsular patterns of restriction, pain, and/or painful weakness (possible fracture or neoplasm) (Figure 12-4). The capsular pattern of the thoracic spine appears to be symmetrical limitation of rotation and side bending, extension loss, and least loss of flexion.

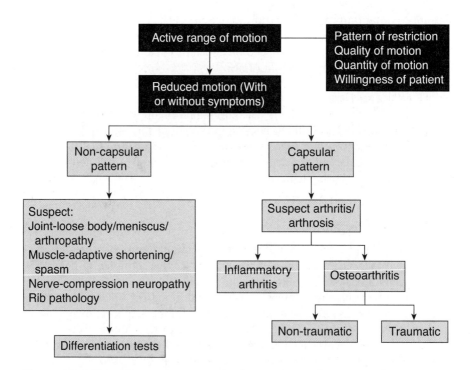

Figure 12-4 Examination sequence in the presence of symptom-free or incomplete active range of motion for the thoracic spine.

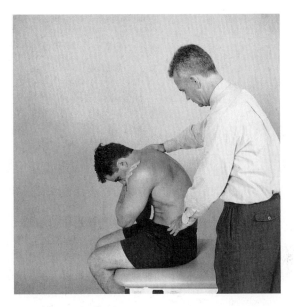

Figure 12-5 Active thoracic flexion.

☻ Clinical Pearl

Joint capsular lesions demonstrate a capsular pattern as equal and grossly severe limitation of movement in every direction.[17] With an asymmetrical impairment, such as trauma, the capsular pattern appears to be an asymmetrical limitation of rotation and side bending, extension loss, and a lesser loss of flexion.

The motions of flexion (Figure 12-5), extension (Figure 12-6), rotation (Figure 12-7), and side bending (Figure 12-8) are assessed. Overpressure applied at the end of the available range of motion is used to take the joint from its physiological barrier to its anatomical barrier. During overpressure, an increase in resistance to motion should be felt. The end feels should be noted.

Because of the length of the spine in this region, it is important to ensure that all parts of the thoracic spine are involved in the range of movement testing. Motion in the thoracic spine requires a synchronous movement between the intervertebral and zygapophyseal joints, and the rib articulations. Thus, the presence of joint dysfunction or degeneration, or structural

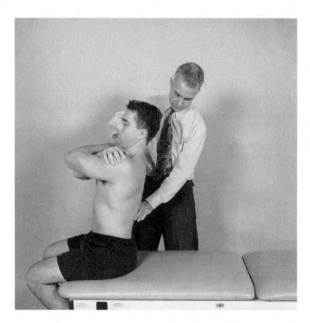

Figure 12-6 Active thoracic extension.

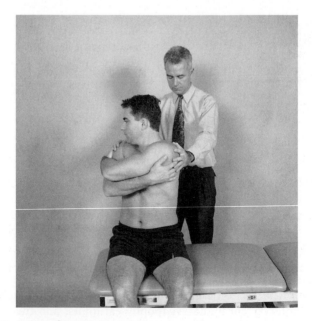

Figure 12-7 Active thoracic rotation.

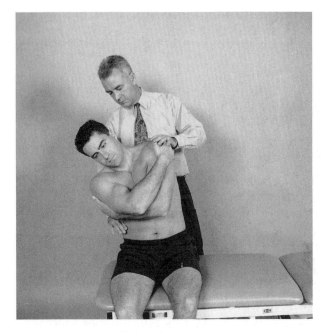

Figure 12-8 Active thoracic side bending.

changes in the spinal curvature, will influence the amount of available range of motion, and the pattern of these coupled motions.[30]

Inspiration/Expiration
The motions of the ribs are palpated during breathing.

 Clinical Pearl

If a rib stops moving in relation to the other ribs during inspiration, it is classified as a *depressed rib*.[18,31] If a rib stops moving in relation to the other ribs during expiration, it is classified as an *elevated rib*.[18,31] Due to the interrelationship of all of the ribs, if a depressed rib is implicated, it is usually the most superior depressed rib that causes the most significant dysfunction. In contrast, if an elevated rib is implicated, it is usually the most inferior restricted rib that causes the most significant dysfunction.[18,31]

Resisted Testing

Resistance applied at the point of overpressure can give the clinician an indication as to the integrity of the musculotendinous units of this area. Resistance is applied at the end range of flexion, extension, rotation, and side bending, while the clinician looks for pain, weakness, and/or painful weakness. Pain that is exacerbated with motion, but not with resisted isometric contraction suggests a ligamentous lesion.[27]

Static Postural Testing

Thoracic pain of a postural origin is difficult to provoke with active motion and resistive testing. McKenzie[32] recommends placing the patient in a position for approximately 3 minutes to load the structures sufficiently to provoke postural pain.

Differing Philosophies

The next stage in the examination process depends on the clinician's background. For those clinicians heavily influenced by the muscle energy techniques of the osteopaths, position testing is used to determine which segment to focus on. Other clinicians omit the position tests and proceed to the combined motion and passive physiological tests.

Position Testing—Spinal

The vertebrae may be tested for positional symmetry. If an ERS (extended, rotated, side-bent) or FRS (flexed, rotated, side-bent) is present, passive mobility testing will definitively diagnose the movement impairment. The upper thoracic joints (C 7–T 4) can be assessed using cervical techniques. The following techniques can be used for the T 4–T 12 levels.

Example T 7–8. The patient is positioned in sitting with the clinician standing behind the patient. Using the thumbs, the clinician palpates the transverse processes of the T 7 vertebra. The joint is tested in the following manner:

• The joint complex is flexed and an evaluation is made as to the position of the T 7 vertebra relative to T 8 by noting which transverse process is the most posterior. A posterior left transverse process of T 7 relative to T 8 is indicative of a left rotated position of the T 7–8 complex in flexion

• The joint complex is extended and an evaluation is made as to the position of the T 7 vertebra in relation to T 8 by noting which transverse process is the most posterior. A posterior left transverse process of T 7 relative to T 8 is indicative of a left rotated position of the T 7–8 joint complex in extension.

Once a segment has been localized by one of the above techniques, the arthrokinematics of the segment can be tested using the following passive mobility tests, which incorporate specific symmetrical or asymmetrical motions.

 Clinical Pearl

Care in the interpretation of the passive mobility tests is important, as local tenderness in the thoracic region is common, especially over the spinous processes due to the proximity of the dorsal rami over the apex of these bony prominences.[30,33]

Passive Mobility Testing
The upper thoracic joints (C 7–T 4) can be assessed using cervical techniques. The following techniques can be used for the T 4–T 12 levels.

Flexion of the Zygapophyseal Joints
The patient is seated at the end of the table with their arms folded and hands resting on their shoulders (Figure 12-9). The clinician stands by the side of the patient, and reaches around the front of the patient with one arm and hand. The clinician then applies a slight pressure with the sternum against the patient's shoulder so that the patient is gently squeezed. Using the other hand to monitor intersegmental motion between the spinous processes, the clinician flexes the thoracic spine (Figure 12-9). The quantity and quality of motion is noted and is compared with the levels above and below.

Extension of the Zygapophyseal Joints
The patient sits against the raised end of the treatment table, with their arms folded, and with the superior segment of the joint to be treated over the edge of the table (Figure 12-10). The clinician stands to the side of the patient. With one arm, the clinician supports the patient's head, neck, and upper thoracic spine, with the tip of the monitoring finger in contact with the spinous process of the superior segment of the joint being treated. With the other hand, the clinician grasps the points of the patient's elbows and exerts a slight pressure through the patient's arms in a superior–posterior direction, which produces a distraction at the joint being treated. While maintaining the distraction, the thoracic spine is extended by pushing gently with the hand that is behind the patient's back and applying the extension force through the clinician's sternum on the lateral aspect of the patient's shoulder (Figure 12-10).

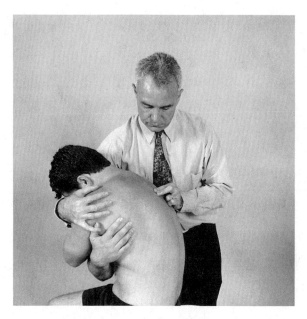

Figure 12-9 Passive mobility testing—flexion.

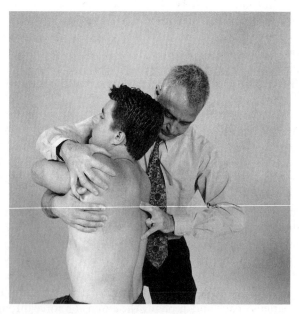

Figure 12-10 Passive mobility testing—extension.

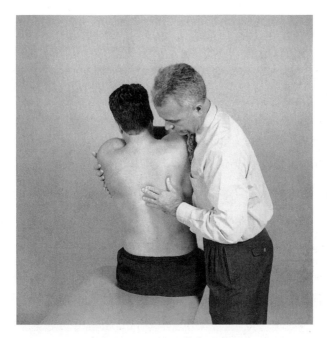

Figure 12-11 Passive mobility testing—side bending/rotation.

The quantity and quality of motion is noted and is compared with the levels above and below.

Combined Motions of the Zygapophyseal Joints
The patient is seated with one hand on top of one of their shoulders and their other hand under the opposite axilla. The clinician stands to the side of the patient. While palpating the interspinous spaces or the transverse processes of each level with one hand, the clinician wraps the other arm around the front of the patient, under their crossed arms, resting their hand on the patient's contralateral shoulder. Crouching slightly, the clinician then places their anterior shoulder region against the lateral aspect of the patient's shoulder. Side bending and rotation of the patient's thoracic spine is then performed away from the clinician (Figure 12-11) as the clinician lifts with their body. The palpating hand palpates the concave side of the curve.

Costal Examination

As mentioned, it is well worth postponing the costal (rib) examination until after the thoracic spinal joints have been examined and treated, or the testing of which proved negative.

All of the ribs move with complex combinations of what is often described as 'pump handle', 'bucket handle', and/or caliper motion.

 Clinical Pearl

Pump handle (anterior) motion is analogous to flexion/extension.

Bucket handle (lateral rib) motion is analogous to adduction/abduction, and caliper motion is analogous to internal and external rotation.

The first rib has an equal proportion of pump and bucket handle motion, whereas the sternal ribs have a greater proportion of pump handle motion. Ribs 8 through 10 have a greater proportion of bucket handle motion.

 Clinical Pearl

Although rarely seen in the outpatient physical therapy clinic, first rib fractures or subluxations can result in neurological or vascular symptoms in the upper quarter region that are exacerbated with breathing. A common subject of report with such an injury is avoidance of activities that involve arm abduction.

Palpation of the Ribs

The first rib is located 45° medially to the junction of the posterior scalene and trapezius. Palpation of the first rib during respiration can detect the presence of asymmetry. Palpation of the first rib can also be performed during the active motions of cervical rotation and side bending test in patients with suspected brachialgia. The clinician passively rotates the patient's cervical spine away from the involved side. From this position, the neck is side-bent as far as is comfortable, moving the ear to the chest. A restriction occurring in the second part of the test indicates a positive test for brachialgia. The transverse processes are roughly level with their own body. The costal cartilages of the second rib articulate with the junction between the sternum and manubrium. The remainder of the ribs should be palpated (Table 12-2). Surface landmarks can be used to locate the other ribs. For example, the fifth rib passes directly under, or slightly inferior to, the male mammary nipples. To palpate the rib angles of the interscapular ribs, the shoulders are positioned in horizontal adduction. The rib angles of 3 through 10 can then be felt about 1 to 2 inches lateral to the spinous processes.

When palpating anteriorly, on the sternum, a rib dysfunction will be highlighted by the presence of asymmetry, and should be compared with the posterior findings.

 Clinical Pearl

A prominent rib angle on the back and a depression of that rib at the sternum would indicate a posterior subluxation, the reverse occurring in an anterior subluxation, whereas a rib that is prominent both anteriorly and posteriorly indicates a single rib torsion.

Passive Mobility Examination of Ribs 2–10

Bucket and Pump Handle Motion

For rib elevation, the overpressure is applied by grasping the patient's arm above the elbow and rocking the arm into hyper-abduction for the lower ribs (bucket), and flexion for the upper seven ribs (pump).

Neurological Tests

Sensation should be tested over the abdomen; the area just below the xiphoid process is innervated by T 8, the umbilicus area is innervated by T 10, and the lower abdominal region, level with the anterior superior iliac spines, is innervated by T 12.[9] Too much overlap exists above T 8 to make sensation testing reliable.

 Clinical Pearl

A neurological deficit is very difficult to detect in the thoracic spine. In this region, one dermatome may be absent with no loss of sensation.[34]

Because of the proximity and vulnerability of the spinal cord in this region, long tract signs (Babinski, Oppenheim, clonus, DTR) should be routinely assessed. A number of tests have been devised to help assess the integrity of the neurological system in this area, and they include:

Beevor sign (T 7–12)

The patient is positioned in supine, with the knees flexed, and both feet flat on the bed. The patient is asked to raise the head against resistance, to cough or to attempt to sit up with the hands resting behind their head.[35] The clinician observes the umbilicus for motion, which should remain in a straight line. If it deviates diagonally, this suggests a weakness in the diagonally opposite abdominal muscles. If it moves distally, weak upper abdominal muscles are suggested, whereas its moving proximally suggests weak lower abdominal muscles. For example, if the umbilicus moves upwards and to the right, the muscles in the lower left quadrant must be weak. The weakness may be due to spinal nerve root palsy, in this case the tenth, eleventh, and twelfth thoracic nerves on the left.[36]

Slump Test

The slump test, a combination of other neuromeningeal tests; namely, the seated SLR, neck flexion, and lumbar slumping is considered to be a general test of neurodynamic mobility.

Abdominal Cutaneous Reflex

To test the abdominal cutaneous reflex, deep stroking over the abdominal muscles is performed using the handle of a reflex hammer. Etching diagonal lines around the patient's umbilicus tests each quadrant. Symmetry of skin rippling and/or umbilicus displacement is observed for.

Lhermitte Symptom

Although normally associated with a lesion to the cervical spinal cord (see Chapter 11), the Lhermitte's symptom may also be present in the thoracic spine in the presence of compression of the thoracic cord by metastatic malignant deposits,[37] impairments of the thoracic vertebrae,[38] and thoracic spinal tumor.[39]

Brown-Séquard Syndrome

This syndrome is characterized by an ipsilateral flaccid segmental palsy, an ipsilateral spastic palsy below the impairment, and an ipsilateral anesthesia and loss of proprioception, and loss of appreciation of the vibration of a tuning fork (dysesthesia). Contralateral discrimination of pain sensation and thermoanesthesia may be present and are both noted below the impairment. If a neurological impairment is suspected, the clinician must first exclude a neoplastic process, infectious process or fracture, and then consider a disk protrusion. A nondiskal disorder of the thoracic spine could include a neurofibroma. Some of the signs to help confirm its presence are:

- The patient reports preferring to sleep sitting up
- The pain, which slowly increases over a period of months, is felt mainly at night and is uninfluenced by activities.
- The patient reports a band-shaped area of numbness that is related to one dermatome
- The patient reports the presence of pins and needles in one or both feet, or reports any other sign of cord compression

Functional Outcomes

The reader is recommended to use the Neck Disability Index for those dysfunctions that originate above the level of the T 4 disk, and the Roland Morris Disability Scale[40,41] for pain originating below the T4 disk level.[42]

Imaging Studies

Thoracic spine injuries are difficult to detect on chest radiographs but dedicated thoracic spine radiographs should be obtained if a fracture is suspected. Lateral radiographs show details of the vertebral bodies in profile, the intervertebral foramen, and the spinous processes. Oblique radiographs show the zygapophyseal joints. Three types of fractures are recognized in the thoracic spine:

1. Wedge compression. This type involves the anterior two thirds of the vertebral body and is a stable fracture.
2. Sagittal slice. This type of fracture consists of an anterior fracture/dislocation with compression of the vertebral body below. This injury is unstable and is frequently associated with neurological compromise.
3. Posterior dislocation. This type usually results from a high-energy force and is an unstable injury.

Computed tomography (CT), especially multidetector CT, is currently the most effective method for examining the extent of the bony injury in the spine. In conjunction with sagittal reconstruction, CT is very useful in demonstrating retropulsed fragments and spinal canal compromise.

MRI is the imaging modality of choice in patients with a suspected neurological deficit.

Examination Conclusions—The Evaluation

Following the examination, and once the clinical findings have been recorded, the clinician must determine a specific diagnosis or a working hypothesis, based on a summary of all of the findings. This diagnosis can be structure related (medical diagnosis), or a diagnosis based on the preferred practice patterns as described in the *Guide to Physical Therapist Practice*.[43]

INTERVENTION

There is a lack of quality research studies investigating the effects of physical therapy on thoracic spine pain. The rehabilitation procedures chosen to progress the patient will depend on the type of tissue involved, the extent of the damage, and the stage of healing (see Chapter 3). The intervention must be related to the signs and symptoms present rather than the actual diagnosis. Posture plays a key role in the prognosis of thoracic spine injuries.

COMMON ORTHOPEDIC CONDITIONS

COMPRESSION FRACTURE OF THE VERTEBRAL BODY

Diagnosis

Compression fracture of the vertebral body—ICD-9: 805.2.

Description

- Often the result of hyperflexion or axial loading injuries—less commonly attributable to rotational stresses, side bending, horizontal shear, and hyperextension.
- Approximately two thirds of patients with thoracic spine fracture–dislocations have complete neurological deficits.

 Clinical Pearl

The most common fractures seen in the thoracic spine are anterior wedge compression fractures and burst fractures. Most thoracic spine fractures occur between the 9th and 11th vertebral bodies. Osteoporotic fractures are most common in the mid to low thoracic spine and result from an inability of the vertebral body to sustain the compression forces involved with everyday activities.

Subjective Findings

- Sudden, intense pain in the spine based on the location of the fracture.
- Pain is localized and activated by movement.
- History of osteoporosis/osteopenia.

 Clinical Pearl

A clinically silent form of osteoporotic vertebrae exists where the patient's vertebrae undergo a gradual series of microfractures over a protracted time period. These patients are asymptomatic or at most complain of chronic back pain.

Objective Findings

- Lateral view of the torso may suggest hyperlordosis of the cervical and lumbar spine.
- Point tenderness over the area of pain with possible muscle guarding.
- Both passive and active range of motion of the torso is painful beyond midrange of motion.

Confirmatory/Special Tests

The diagnosis is typically confirmed using radiographs.

Imaging Studies

Radiographs reveal a definite pattern of bone atrophy characterized by a striking deficiency of horizontal trabeculae and preservation of vertically oriented trabeculae. Radiographs may also indicate anterior thoracic wedging and ballooning of the lumbar vertebral interspaces.

Differential Diagnosis

- Rib fracture.
- Stress fracture.
- Intercostal neuritis.
- Costochondritis.
- Ankylosing spondylitis.

- Osteoarthritis.
- Pleuropulmonary conditions.

Intervention

Medical intervention involves the use of hormone replacement therapy, smoking cessation, and encouraging the patient to eat a diet with adequate protein, calcium, and vitamin D. Conservative intervention includes the following:

- Occupation modification as appropriate.
- Introduction of walking and gentle weight-bearing activities (e.g. tai chi).
- Proprioception and balance training.
- Core strengthening.
- Back-muscle strengthening exercises, which have been shown to slow the rate of bone loss associated with osteoporosis.

Prognosis

The long-term prognosis for patients with osteoporosis depends on the severity, comorbidity, and the age of the patient.

COSTOCHONDRITIS

Diagnosis

Costochondritis—ICD-9: 733.6.

Description

Costochondritis (Tietze disease) is a local inflammation of the costal cartilage, specifically at the junction of the rib and costal cartilage. It most commonly affects the second and third costochondral junctions. Sternochondritis is the term applied to the inflammation that occurs at the junction of the sternum and the costal cartilage.

 Clinical Pearl

Tietze syndrome is often used synonymously with costochondritis, although it is a distinct form of it. This condition most commonly affects the second and third costochondral junctions, but also may affect any of the cartilaginous articulations of the chest wall, including the sternoclavicular joints. The clinical findings include a localized swelling of the costosternal cartilage.

Subjective Findings

Typical complaints include a gradual or sudden onset of pain in the anterior chest region, which is increased with deep inspiration, coughing, and/or sneezing, and eased with decreased movement, quiet breathing and position changes.

Objective Findings

Many patients remain undiagnosed and present with symptoms such as back pain and increased kyphosis. Typical findings include:

- Localized swelling of the costosternal cartilage. The intercostal spaces should be nontender.
- Chest wall/costochondral joint tenderness that is aggravated by chest wall compression.

Confirmatory/Special Tests

Diagnosis is based on a history of chest pain with associated anterior chest wall tenderness that is localized to the costochondral junction of one or more ribs. The physician may confirm using local anesthetic block.

Imaging Studies

Routine radiographs of the ribs are often normal.

Differential Diagnosis

- Hiatus hernia (associated with eating, lying supine)
- Myocardial infarction (Pallor, sweating, dyspnea, nausea, or palpitations, associated risk factors)
- Angina (Chest pain or pressure that occurs with predictable levels of exertion)
- Pleurisy (Severe, sharp knife-like pain with inspiration)
- Pulmonary embolus (Chest, shoulder, or upper abdominal pain; dyspnea; history of a recent or coexisting respiratory disorder [e.g., infection, pneumonia, tumor, or tuberculosis])
- Aortic aneurysm (pulsing sensation in abdomen)

- Pneumonia (Fever, chills, headache, malaise, or nausea)
- Rib fracture (pain with chest compression, positive chest x-ray)
- Cholecystitis (Colicky pain in the right upper abdominal quadrant with accompanying right scapula pain; symptoms may worsen with ingestion of fatty foods)

Intervention

The intervention involves rest for a few days while avoiding lying on the sides, heavy lifting, and strenuous activities. Local injections of corticosteroid may be combined with a rib binder. Electrotherapeutic modalities and thermal agents should be considered with a focus on cryotherapy. The patient should be instructed on the use of ice (15 minutes every 1 to 2 hours). Specific joint mobilizations to the costovertebral articulations are recommended, as are gentle breathing exercises.

Prognosis

This is a benign, self-limiting condition, which can last from several days to several weeks.

SCOLIOSIS

Diagnosis

Scoliosis—ICD-9: 737.30 (idiopathic). Includes three categories: infantile, juvenile, and adolescent; all of which can present in adulthood.

Description

Scoliosis is defined as a lateral deviation (>10 degrees) and rotation deformity of the spine.

 Clinical Pearl

Right thoracic curves are more common, followed by double major (right thoracic and left lumbar) curves.

In adults, the condition is classified as either a deformity that developed during childhood or a deformity that developed after skeletal maturity, usually secondary to degenerative spondylosis and/or degenerative spondylolisthesis.

Subjective Findings

An accurate history includes the description of the onset of symptoms, duration and progression of pain, history of a traumatic event, activities that worsen the pain, and previous treatments and outcomes.

- Pain localized to the region of the deformity.
- Complaints of feeling shorter or noticing the appearance of a rib hump.

Objective Findings

The entire spine should be inspected and palpated with the patient standing. The relative height of the shoulders and iliac crests should be noted, as should any asymmetry at the waist. The neurological examination should include evaluation of reflexes as well as motor and sensory function of the lumbosacral nerve roots.

 Clinical Pearl

Forward bending exaggerates the asymmetry of the posterior rib cage and thoracolumbar junction.

Positive findings typically include:

- shoulder elevation
- waistline asymmetry
- rib rotational deformity (rib hump)
- trunk shift
- leg length inequality
- Neurological changes are infrequent but most commonly involve the extensor hallucis longus muscle.

 Clinical Pearl

Symptoms related to pulmonary compromise are associated with more severe thoracic curves, including both idiopathic and neuromuscular curves.

Confirmatory/Special Tests

Leg length discrepancy and forward-bending tests, otherwise the diagnosis is based on the results of radiographic studies.

Medical Studies

The diagnosis is made by standing AP and lateral radiographs of the entire spine. Electromyography is rarely indicated but occasionally may be helpful to distinguish radiculopathy from neuropathy.

Differential Diagnosis

- Hormonal disorder.
- Congenital scoliosis—vertebral body abnormalities, childhood or adolescent presentation.
- Degenerative disk disease with asymmetrical disk collapse.
- Severe disk herniation with sciatic scoliosis and radiculopathy.
- Brainstem dysfunction.
- Proprioception disorder.
- Neuromuscular scoliosis—neurological abnormalities and weakness.
- Marfan syndrome.
- Osteogenesis imperfecta.
- Neurofibromatosis.

Intervention

The most important factor in effective management remains an accurate early detection. Appropriate exercises include chest retraction, asymmetrical exercises, push-ups, knee bends, deep breathing (emphasizing diaphragmatic breathing during abdominal strengthening exercises and during bilateral stretch of the pectoralis muscles), segmental breathing (to expand the lungs on the concave side of the curve during unilateral trunk stretching), and encouragement to participate in noncontact athletic activities.

 Clinical Pearl

Several muscle groups become adaptively shortened in scoliotic patients and include sternocleidomastoids, scalenes, pectorals, erector spinae, as well as the hip flexors and hamstring muscles.

Clinical Pearl

Surgical intervention is considered in adults with curves greater than 40 degrees to 50 degrees, as these patients are at risk for progression, as well as in those with documented progression of greater than 5 degrees.

 Clinical Pearl

Bracing will not reduce the magnitude of the deformity. However, bracing serves to stabilize the curve and may prevent worsening of the curve.

Prognosis

Increased pain and deformity with diminished functional activity if left untreated.

 Clinical Pearl

Progressive neurological deterioration requires emergency management.

REHABILITATION LADDER

THORACIC SPINE

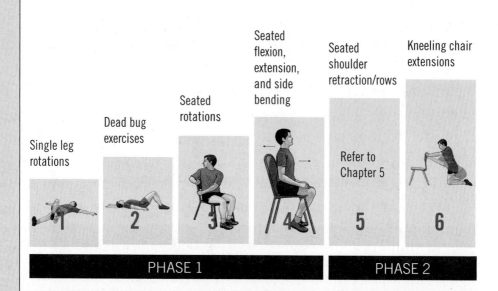

The purpose of these training ladders is to provide the clinician with a safe and progressive framework of exercises that are designed to allow the patient to improve in an efficient manner. The patient begins at the appropriate step, which is based on the stage of healing and the goal of intervention.

- Phase 1: Acute—pain management, restoration of full passive range of motion, and restoration of normal accessory motion.

- Phase 2: Subacute—active range of motion exercises and early strengthening.

- Phase 3: Chronic—specific strengthening with a strong emphasis on enhancing dynamic stability.

The degree of movement and the speed of progression are both guided by the signs and symptoms. Once the patient is able to perform an exercise for

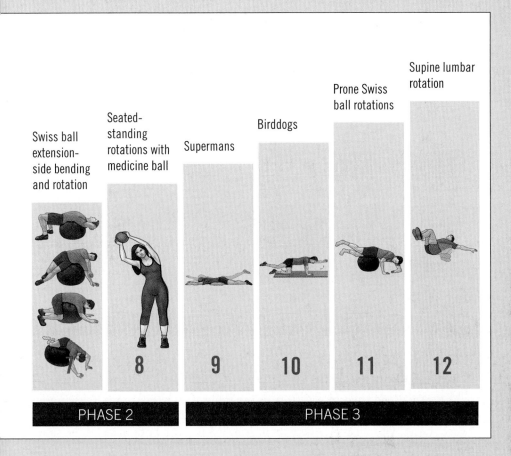

Swiss ball extension-side bending and rotation

Seated-standing rotations with medicine ball

Supermans

Birddogs

Prone Swiss ball rotations

Supine lumbar rotation

8

9

10

11

12

PHASE 2

PHASE 3

8–12 reps without pain, he or she progresses up to the next exercise step. This continues until the patient attempts an exercise that reproduces the pain. At this point, the patient returns to the last exercise that he or she was able to perform without pain and performs that exercise five times per day for 1 to 2 days before attempting to progress again. The patient is advanced through the training ladders to the appropriate point, with particular attention paid to patient response to treatment in terms of changes in symptoms, swelling, degree of irritability, or motion. In addition, muscle imbalances are addressed with appropriate flexibility exercises.

Once the patient is able to perform the last exercise of Phase 3 (Step 12 of the ladder), he or she can move on to functional and sport-specific training (Phase 4) as appropriate, which focus on power and higher-speed exercises similar to sport-specific demands.

1. Single leg rotations

The patient is positioned in supine with one hip and knee flexed so that the foot is flat on the table, and the other leg is lying flat against the table. The patient is asked to place the foot of the flexed leg on the lateral aspect of the straight leg and then to rotate toward the bed (1). The exercise is repeated to the other side by crossing the other leg.

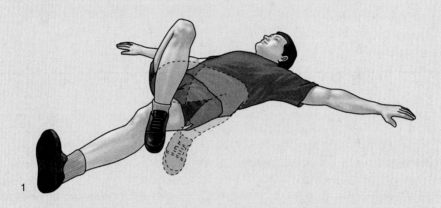

2. Dead bug exercises

The patient is positioned in supine with the hips and knees flexed and the feet flat on the table. The patient is asked to raise one arm as high above the head as possible and then to return it to the table. The patient repeats the same movement with the other arm. Once the patient is able to perform unilateral arm raises without pain, the patient is asked to raise both arms at the same time (2).

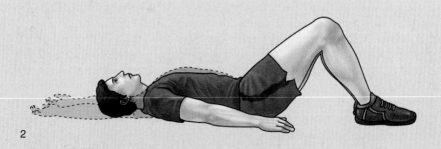

3. Seated rotations

The patient is positioned in sitting on a hardback chair. The patient is asked to reach around to one side by turning at the waist. When able to, the patient grasps the back of the chair and pulls with the arms into further rotation (3).

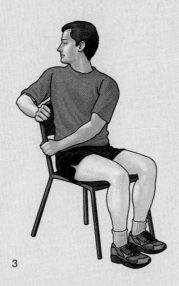

3

4. Seated active range of motion (AROM)
The patient is positioned in sitting. Ensuring that all motion occurs from above the waist, the patient is asked to perform thoracic flexion and extension (4a), and side bending (4b).

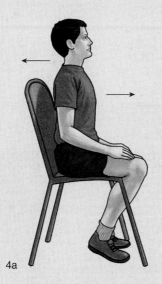

4a

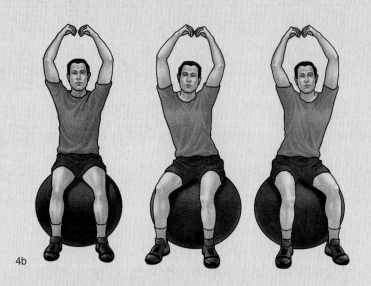

4b

5. Resistive exercises with combined shoulder motions
Refer to chapter 5 for full description.

6. Kneeling chair extension
The patient is positioned in kneeling, facing a hardback chair. The patient is asked to grasp the top of the chair and to slowly lean into the chair to create thoracic extension (6).

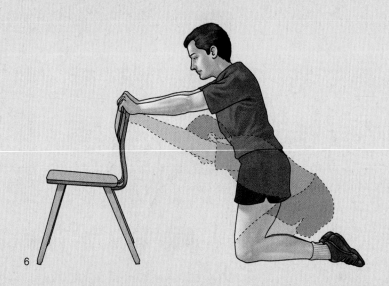

6

7. Swiss Ball exercises
The patient is instructed on how to use a Swiss Ball to increase thoracic extension (7a), side bending (7b), flexion (7c), and rotation (7d).

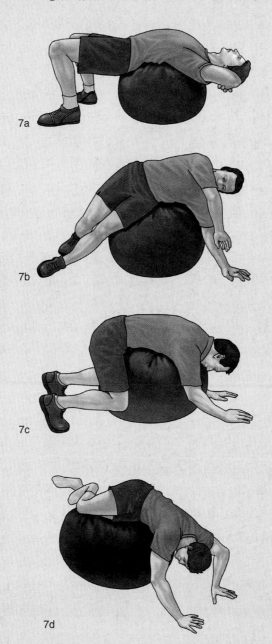

7a

7b

7c

7d

8. Seated-standing rotations with medicine ball
The patient is positioned in sitting while holding a medicine ball. The patient is asked to raise a medicine ball above the head and then to make circular motions with the arms. The patient is then progressed to performing the exercise in standing (8) so that wider arcs of motion can be acquired.

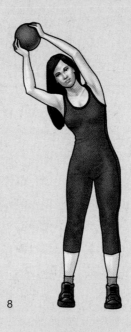

8

9. Superman
The patient is positioned in prone with the arms above the head. The patient is asked to raise one arm and the contralateral leg up toward the ceiling (e.g., right arm and left leg). The exercise is then repeated using the other arm and leg. The exercise can be made more difficult by asking the patient to raise both arms and both legs simultaneously.

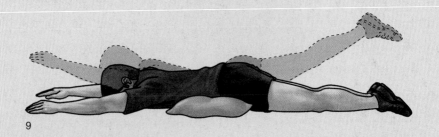

9

10. Bird dogs

The patient is positioned in the quadruped position. The patient is asked to raise one leg and the opposite arm up toward the ceiling (10). The exercise is then repeated using the other arm and leg.

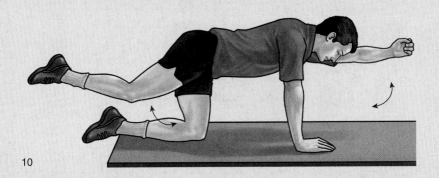

10

11. Prone Swiss Ball

The patient is positioned in prone over a Swiss Ball so that both hands and both feet are on the floor. The patient is asked to raise one arm and the opposite leg off the ground toward the ceiling. The exercise is then repeated using the other arm and leg. The exercise could be made more difficult by asking the patient to raise both legs off the ground and to induce trunk rotations (11).

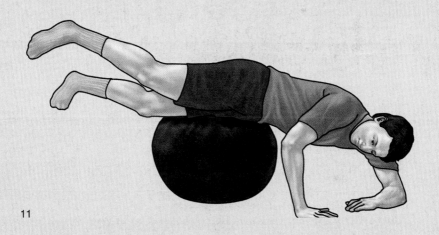

11

12. Supine lumbar rotations

The patient is positioned in supine. The patient is asked to raise both legs off the bed and to flex the hips and knees to 90 degrees (12). The patient is then asked to rotate the hips and knees down toward the bed in one direction and then the other.

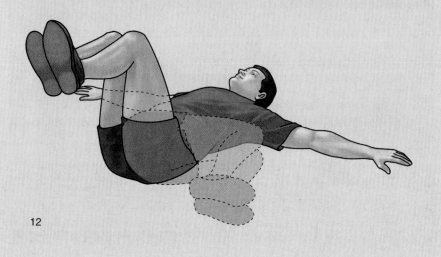

12

REFERENCES

1. Bradford S. Juvenile kyphosis. In: Bradford DS, Lonstein JE, Moe JH, et al. eds. *Moe's Textbook of Scoliosis and Other Spinal Deformities*. Philadelphia, PA: W.B. Saunders; 1987:347.
2. Frazer JE. *Frazer's Anatomy of the Human Skeleton*. London, UK: Churchill Livingstone; 1965.
3. Singer KP, Jones T, Breidahl PD. A comparison of radiographic and computer-assisted measurements of thoracic and and thoracolumbar sagittal curvature. *Skel Radiol*. 1990;19:21–26.
4. Willen J, Anderson J, Tomooka K, et al. The natural history of burst fractures in the thoracolumbar spine T12 and L1. *J Spinal Disord*. 1990;3:39–46.
5. Bogduk N, Valencia F. Innervation and pain patterns of the thoracic spine. In: Grant R, ed. *Physical Therapy of the Cervical and Thoracic Spine*. 2nd ed. Melbourne: Churchill Livingstone; 1994:77–88.
6. Bauer RL, Deyo RA. Low risk of vertebral fracture in Mexican American women. *Arch Intern Med*. 1987;147:1437–1439.
7. Lyu RK, Chang HS, Tang LM, et al. Thoracic disc herniation mimicking acute lumbar disc disease. *Spine*. 1999;24:416–418.
8. Grieve GP. *Common Vertebral Joint Problems*. New York, NY: Churchill Livingstone Inc; 1981.
9. Meadows J. *Orthopedic Differential Diagnosis in Physical Therapy*. New York, NY: McGraw-Hill; 1999.
10. DeFranca GG, Levine LJ. The T4 syndrome. *J Manipulative Physiol Ther*. 1995;18:34–37.

11. McGuckin N. The T 4 syndrome. In: Grieve GP, ed. *Modern Manual Therapy of the Vertebral Column*. New York, NY: Churchill Livingstone; 1986:370–376.

12. Maitland G. *Vertebral Manipulation*. Sydney: Butterworth; 1986.

13. Butler DL, Slater H. Neural injury in the thoracic spine: a conceptual basis for manual therapy. In: Grant R, ed. *Physical Therapy of the Cervical and Thoracic Spine*. New York, NY: Churchill Livingstone; 1994:313–338.

14. Grieve GP. Thoracic musculoskeletal problems. In: Boyling JD, Palastanga N, eds. *Grieve's Modern Manual Therapy of the Vertebral Column*. 2nd ed. Edinburgh, UK: Churchill Livingstone; 1994:401–428.

15. McKenzie RA. Manual correction of sciatic scoliosis. *N Z Med J*. 1972;76: 194–199.

16. Sutherland ID. Funnel chest. *J Bone Joint Surg*. 1958;40B:244–251.

17. Bland JH. Diagnosis of thoracic pain syndromes. In: Giles LGF, Singer KP, eds. *Clinical Anatomy and Management of the Thoracic Spine*. Oxford, UK: Butterworth-Heinemann; 2000:145–156.

18. Mitchell FL, Moran PS, Pruzzo NA. *An Evaluation and Treatment Manual of Osteopathic Muscle Energy Procedures*. Manchester, MO: Mitchell, Moran and Pruzzo Associates; 1979.

19. Lindgren KA. Thoracic outlet syndrome with special reference to the first rib. *Ann Chir Gynaecol*. 1993;82:218–230.

20. Lindgren KA, Leino E. Subluxation of the first rib: a possible thoracic outlet syndrome mechanism. *Arch Phys Med Rehabil*. 1988;69:692–695.

21. Lindgren KA, Leino E, Manninen H. Cervical rotation lateral flexion test in brachialgia. *Arch Phys Med Rehabil*. 1992;73:735–737.

22. Lindgren KA, Manninen H, Rytkonen H. Thoracic outlet syndrome—a functional disturbance of the thoracic upper aperture? *Muscle Nerve*. 1995;18: 526–530.

23. Egan WJ, Flynn TW. Thoracic spine—Physical therapy patient management using current evidence. LaCrosse, WI: APTA - Orthopedic sections home study course; 2006.

24. Moll JMH, Wright V. Measurement of spinal movement. In: Jayson MIV, ed. *The Lumbar Spine and Back Pain*. New York, NY: Grune and Stratton; 1981: 93–112.

25. Winkel D, Matthijs O, Phelps V. Thoracic Spine. In: Winkel D, Matthijs O, Phelps V, eds. *Diagnosis and Treatment of the Spine*. Maryland, MD: Aspen; 1997:389–541.

26. Evjenth O, Gloeck C. *Symptom Localization in the Spine and Extremity Joints*. Minneapolis, MN: OPTP; 2000.

27. Lawrence DJ, Bakkum B. Chiropractic management of thoracic spine pain of mechanical origin. In: Giles LGF, Singer KP, eds. *Clinical Anatomy and Management of Thoracic Pain*. Oxford, UK: Butterworth-Heinemann; 2000:244–256.

28. Singer KP, Edmondston SJ. Introduction: the enigma of the thoracic spine. In: Giles LGF, Singer KP, eds. *Clinical Anatomy and Management of Thoracic Spine Pain. The Clinical Anatomy and Management of Back Pain Series*. Oxford, UK: Butterworth-Heinemann; 2000.

29. Maigne R. *Diagnosis and Treatment of Pain of Vertebral Origin*. Baltimore, MD: Williams & Wilkins; 1996.

30. Edmondston SJ, Singer KP. Thoracic spine: anatomical and biomechanical considerations for manual therapy. *Man Ther.* 1997;2:132–143.
31. Stoddard A. *Manual of Osteopathic Practice.* New York, NY: Harper & Row; 1969.
32. McKenzie RA. *The Cervical and Thoracic Spine: Mechanical Diagnosis and Therapy.* Waikanae, NZ: Spinal Publications; 1990.
33. Maigne J-Y, Maigne R, Guerin-Surville H. Upper thoracic dorsal rami: anatomic study of their medial cutaneous branches. *Surg Radiol Anat.* 1991;13: 109–112.
34. Magee DJ. Cervical Spine. In: Magee DJ, ed. *Orthopedic Physical Assessment.* 2nd ed. Philadelphia, PA: Saunders; 1992:34–70.
35. Post M. *Physical Examination of the Musculoskeletal System.* Chicago, IL: Year Book Medical Publishers; 1987.
36. Hoppenfeld S. *Orthopedic Neurology—A Diagnostic Guide to Neurological Levels.* Philadelphia, JB Lippincott; 1977.
37. Ventafridda V, Caraceni A, Martini C, et al. On the significance of Lhermitte's sign in oncology. *J Neurooncol.* 1991;10:133–137.
38. Ongerboer de Visser BW. Het teken van Lhermitte bij thoracale wervelaandoeningen. *Ned Tijdschr Geneeskd.* 1980;124:390–392.
39. Broager B. Lhermitte's sign in thoracic spinal tumour. Personal observation. *Acta Neurochir (Wien).* 1978;106:127–135.
40. Hudson-Cook N, Tomes-Nicholson K, Breen A. A revised Oswestry disability questionnaire. In: Roland M, Jenner J, eds. *Back Pain: New Approaches to Rehabilitation and Education.* New York, NY: Manchester University Press; 1989:187–204.
41. Roland M, Morris R. A study of the natural history of back pain, part I: the development of a reliable and sensitive measure of disability of low back pain. *Spine.* 1986;8:141–144.
42. Flynn TW. Thoracic spine and chest wall. In: Wadsworth C, ed. *Current Concepts of Orthopedic Physical Therapy—Home Study Course.* La Crosse, WI: Orthopaedic Section, APTA; 2001.
43. Guide to physical therapist practice. *Phys Ther.* 2001;81:S13–S95.

QUESTIONS

1. How many articulations are present on the typical thoracic vertebra?
2. T__ F__ The external intercostal muscles run downward and posteriorly.
3. T__ F__ The external intercostals are muscles of exhalation.
4. What are the three major types of scoliosis?
5. What would be a working hypothesis with a 40-year-old patient who presents with pain and stiffness in the thoracic region, which is worse in the morning, and who demonstrates limited chest expansion?
6. What is Scheuermann disease?
7. In the thoracic region, how are the facet joints oriented?
8. Which are the atypical ribs and why?

9. At a typical thoracic segment, what does the rib articulate with?
10. What is this joint called?
11. Which levels contain the typical thoracic vertebra?
12. At the costovertebral joint, where are the demi facets located?
13. Which structures modify and restrict rotation in the thoracic region?
14. Which of the thoracic vertebrae is the smallest?
15. The typical vertebra articulates with which two vertebrae?
16. Which ribs demonstrate bucket handle movement and which display pump handle?
17. Which ribs articulate with the sternum directly?
18. How do the ribs 8–10 articulate with the sternum?
19. Describe the sternomanubrial joint.
20. In the rule of 3s, the 2nd set of spinous processes (T4–6) are level with what?
21. How about levels T7–9?
22. What about T11?
23. Which levels are known as the vertebrosternal region?
24. How about the vertebromanubrial region?
25. How about the vertebrochondral?
26. What are the coupling motions for latexion at the T3–T10 levels?
27. How about with rotexion?
28. What is the lowest thoracic level that can be treated as a cervical lesion?
29. Which thoracic levels are treated as in the lumbar spine?
30. What are the four areas for concern with patient history in the thoracic spine?
31. With thoracic forward flexion, which motions occur at the head of the rib in the vertebrosternal region?
32. How does the tubercle of the rib move?
33. In the vertebrochondral region (T8–10), which way does the rib tubercle glide in flexion?
34. In a stiff thorax, what motions occur at the head and tubercle of the rib from T1-T10?
35. How many concave facets does the sternum have to articulate with the costocartilage of ribs 3–6?
36. In which directions do the facets of the superior vertebrae move with FWB?
37. During inspiration, in which direction do the rib tubercles glide?
38. With unilateral elevation of the arm, which motions occur in the vertebromanubrial region with a mobile thorax?

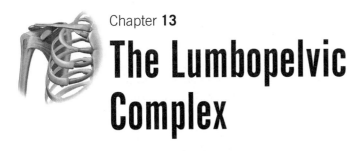

Chapter **13**

The Lumbopelvic Complex

OVERVIEW

The lumbopelvic complex consists of the lumbar spine and sacroiliac joint (SIJ). This complex can be the source of many symptoms, both serious and benign. Any clinician examining and treating this region must have a sound understanding and knowledge of the anatomy and biomechanics as abnormalities of the lumbar spine and SIJ may lead to compensatory or secondary abnormalities in other portions of the spine, pelvis, or hip.

 Clinical Pearl

Because there is no gold standard for diagnosis of SIJ dysfunction by physical exam, the diagnosis often becomes one of exclusion.

ANATOMY

The lumbar spine consists of five lumbar vertebrae, which, in general, increase in size from L1 to L5 in order to accommodate progressively increasing loads. Between each of the lumbar vertebrae is the intervertebral disc (IVD). Anatomically, the SIJ is a large diarthrodial joint that connects the spine with the pelvis. Three bones comprise the SIJ: two innominates and the sacrum. The motions at the lumbar spine predominantly occur around the sagittal plane and comprise flexion and extension, whereas the motions occurring at the hip occur in three planes and include the one motion that the lumbar spine does not tolerate well, i.e., rotation. Thus, the pelvic area must function to absorb the majority of the lower extremity rotation. In addition, when the body is in an upright position, the SIJ is subjected to considerable shear force as the mass of the upper body must be transferred to the lower limbs via the ilia.[1-3]

EXAMINATION

Low back and leg pain can arise from both local and distal structures. The Agency for Health Care Policy and Research (AHCPR) has grouped back pain into three categories: nonspecific back symptoms, sciatica, and potentially serious spinal conditions (Table 13-1).[4,5]

Clinical Pearl

Most investigators agree that no single test can be used confirm the diagnosis of SIJ dysfunction.

Table 13-1 The Agency for Health Care Policy and Research (AHCPR) Three Categories of Back Pain

Nonspecific Back Symptoms	Examples	Clinical Findings
Nonspecific low back pain (strains, sprains facet joint dysfunction, osteoarthritis)	Ligamentous strain Muscle strain or spasm Facet joint disruption or degeneration Intervertebral disc degeneration or herniation Vertebral compression fracture Vertebral end-plate microfractures Spondylolysis/spondylolisthesis spinal stenosis Diffuse idiopathic skeletal hyperostosis Scheuermann's disease (vertebral epiphyseal aseptic necrosis)	Typically no nerve root compromise, localized pain over lumbosacral area
Sciatica	Herniated disc Lateral recess spinal stenosis	Back-related lower extremity symptoms and spasm in radicular pattern, positive straight leg raising test
Potentially serious spinal conditions	Connective tissue disease	Fever, increased erythrocyte sedimentation rate, positive for antinuclear antibodies, scleroderma, rheumatoid arthritis

(continued on following page)

Nonspecific Back Symptoms	Examples	Clinical Findings
	Vertebral compression fracture	History of trauma (can be nontraumatic), osteoporosis, localized pain over spine
	Malignant/metastatic disease	Unexplained weight loss, fever, abnormal serum protein electrophoresis pattern, history of malignant disease
	Infection (disc space, spinal tuberculosis)	Fever, parenteral drug abuse, history of tuberculosis or positive tuberculin test
	Abdominal aortic aneurysm	Pulsatile mass in abdomen. Inability to find position of comfort, back pain not relieved by rest
	Cauda equina syndrome	Saddle anesthesia, urinary retention, bladder or bowel incontinence, severe and progressive weakness of lower extremities
	Hyperparathyroidism	Insidious onset, associated with hypercalcemia, renal stones, constipation
	Ankylosing spondylitis (morning stiffness)	Mostly men in their 20–40s, positive for HLA-B27 antigen, positive family history, increased erythrocyte sedimentation rate

The physical examination of this region must include a thorough assessment of the neuromuscular, vascular, and orthopedic systems of the hip, lower extremities, thoracic, low back, and pelvic regions.[6] Figure 13-1 depicts a simple algorithm for decision-making during the examination of the lumbar spine. A similar one for the SIJ is depicted in Figure 13-2.

 Clinical Pearl

In general, the SIJ can be the origin for unilateral pain with no referral below the knee, whereas irritation of a spinal nerve may cause radicular symptoms below the knee.[7]

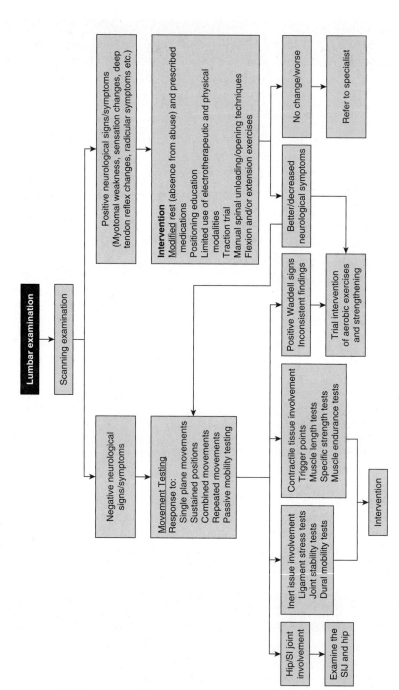

Figure 13-1 Algorithm for examination of the lumbar spine.

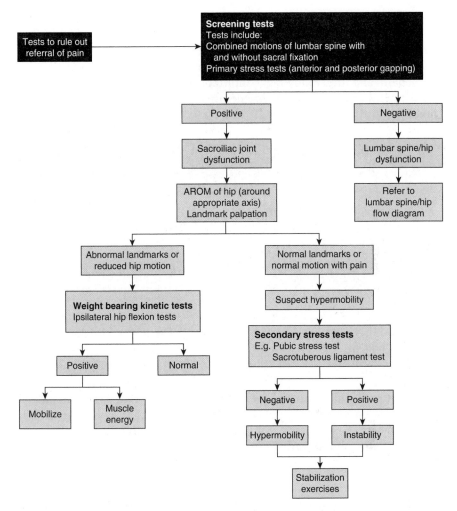

Figure 13-2 Algorithm for examination of the SIJ.

History

Correct diagnosis of low back and SIJ dysfunction requires a careful history to determine whether the causes are mechanical, or secondary and more threatening. Although dysfunctions of this region can be very difficult to diagnose, the history can provide some very important clues. To aid in the provisional diagnosis, the clinician should determine the following:

- The patient's age: Below 20 years old, low back pain is fairly rare. Possible causes include spondylolisthesis, ankylosing spondylitis, and disc pathology. Between 20 and 50 years old, pathologies to consider include disc pathology (see Common Conditions section), capsular impingement, instability, muscle strains, and capsular entrapment. About 50 years old, degenerative changes to bodily tissue are the primary source of lumbar pain and the following conditions should be considered: central and lateral recess stenosis, degenerative disc disease, and degenerative spondylolisthesis.

 Clinical Pearl

Degenerative changes to the lumbar spine typically result from daily wear and tear in combination with various injuries sustained throughout life. These changes lead to a thickening and sclerosis of the subchondral bone and development of osteophytes.

Lumbar spinal stenosis is a leading cause of impaired mobility and spinal surgery in the geriatric population.

- The patient's occupation: Occupations that involve heavy lifting, vibration, and prolonged bending are associated with low back injuries. Factors such as job satisfaction and job stress are not predictive of return to work potential.
- The patient's chief complaint: Pain and stiffness that lasts for only a short time on awakening indicates a dysfunction that is more mechanical in nature (degenerative joint disease, disc pathology, spondylolisthesis, instability, and stenosis). Pain and stiffness that persists for a longer period of time occurs when inflammation is the primary source of the symptoms.

Clinical Pearl

Lumbar segmental instability can be caused by several factors including degenerative changes, spondylolisthesis, fracture, trauma, or a previous surgical procedure. The symptoms of instability are typically aggravated with end range positions, sustained postures, and rapid movements.

- The mechanism of injury: The forces applied to the lumbar spine vary according to the task or position of the body. The mechanism of injury plays a large role in the differential diagnosis of patients with acute low back pain and a lesser role for chronic low back pain. A traumatic onset could implicate fractures, muscle strains, ligament strains, disc pathology, and facet pathology. An insidious onset could indicate degenerative disc disease and visceral pain.

- The onset of the symptoms, how long the patient has had the problem, and whether they have had similar episodes in the past.
- The location of the pain at present: Back pain may be localized centrally, unilaterally or bilaterally. Determining the location of the pain can provide some clues as to the cause (Figure 13-3).
- The type and behavior of symptoms. Questions related to the type and behavior of symptoms can help determine the structure involved and the stage of healing. It is important to determine whether the condition is improving or worsening.
  - Constant pain indicates an inflammatory process.
  - Steadily increasing pain, especially in elderly patients may indicate malignancy.[8]
  - Pain that is gradually expanding and increasing is associated with a lesion that is increasing in size such as a neuroma or neoplasm.[8]

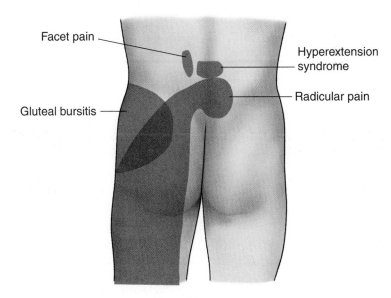

Figure 13-3 Pain location and possible causes.

- Pain with movement suggests a mechanical cause of pain.[9]
- Whether there is a diurnal or nocturnal variation in the symptoms. Complaints of morning stiffness may indicate an IVD lesion, osteoarthritis, ankylosing spondylitis, or Scheuermann's disease (see Chapter 12).
- Positions or activities that have been found to aggravate or relieve the symptoms (Table 13-2). Classically, the symptoms of lumbar canal stenosis begin or worsen with the onset of ambulation or by standing, and are promptly relieved by sitting or sidelying.[10] The symptoms of vascular and neurogenic claudication are also provoked with activity.

 Clinical Pearl

The presence of the following findings likely suggests SIJ dysfunction: [11–14]

- A history of sharp pain awakening the patient from sleep upon turning in bed.
- Pain with walking, ascending, or descending stairs, standing from a sitting position, or with hopping or standing on the involved leg.
- Sometimes limitation, on extension and ipsilateral side bending of the trunk.

Table 13-2 Relieving Positions or Movements

Relieving Position or Movement of the Lumbar Spine	Probable Cause
Flexion	Facet joint involvement
	Low back strain
	Lateral stenosis
Extension	Disc involvement
	Nerve root irritation (disc herniation)
Rest	Neurogenic claudication

Table 13-3 Preferred Sleeping Positions and Potential Diagnosis

Preferred Sleeping Position	Potential Diagnosis
Sidelying with hips and knees flexed	Lumbar canal stenosis
	Lumbar hyperextension syndrome
	Spondylolisthesis
Prone or supine with legs straight	Intervertebral disc pathology

- The patient's sleeping position (Table 13-3).
- The patient's general health and past medical history: This includes checking for a family propensity for rheumatoid arthritis, IVD lesions,[15] diabetes, osteoporosis, and vascular disease.
- The affect the symptoms have on the patient's work, daily activities, and recreational pursuits.
- Whether the patient is taking any medications. Pain medications can mask symptoms. If the patient reports taking pain medication prior to the examination, the clinician may not get a true response to pain from the patient.

Systems Review

It must always be remembered that pain can be referred to the lumbar spine and pelvis from pathologies in other regions. For example, reports of pain in the upper lumbar region could suggest the possibility of aortic thrombosis, neoplasm, dental caries, chronic appendicitis,[16] ankylosing spondylitis, or visceral disease (Table 13-1). The clinician should determine whether there has been any recent and unexplained weight loss, night pain that is unrelated to movement, and any changes in bowel and bladder dysfunction.

 Clinical Pearl

High forces and repetitive loads can lead to ligamentous, muscle, and bone injuries within the pelvis especially if those forces are asymmetrical.

Tests and Measures

Observation

Observation involves an analysis of the entire patient as to how they sit, stand, move, and respond in addition to the positions of comfort they adopt. The patient's posture and gait should be examined.

 Clinical Pearl

> Although spinal alignment provides some valuable information, a positive correlation has not been made between abnormal alignment and pain.[17,18]

A number of important bone landmarks can be used to help guide the clinician with palpation (Table 13-4). Observing the patient from the front, the clinician should confirm that

- The head sits straight on the shoulders.
- The shoulder heights are equal (the dominant side may be slightly lower in an athletic individual).
- The iliac crest heights are equal.
- The patellas are both pointing anteriorly.

Table 13-4 Important Bone Landmarks of the Lumbosacral Spine

Bone Landmark	Description
Anterior superior iliac spine (ASIS)	At the level of the sacral promontory
Posterior superior iliac spine (PSIS)	At the level of the spinous process of the second sacral vertebra
The spinous process of the fourth lumbar vertebra	In line with the highest points of the iliac crests
The body of the fifth lumbar vertebra	In line with a transtubercular plane through the tubercles on the iliac crests
The spinous process of the third sacral vertebra	Opposite the upper margin of the greater sciatic notch
Posterior inferior iliac spine	5 cm below the PSIS
Ischial spine	10 cm below the PSIS

Observing the patient from behind, the clinician should note any:

- Shifting of the pelvis or shoulders—may indicate nerve root injury (with a disc herniation lateral to the nerve roots, the patient will list away from the side of the irritated nerve root, whereas when the herniation is medial to the nerve root, the patient may list toward the side of the lesion[19]) or gluteus medius weakness.

- Underlying scoliotic curves—compare the relative heights of the shoulders, scapulae, and iliac crests.

- Differences in the angles between the spines of the scapula on each side— the spine of the scapula begins at the level of the thoracic vertebrae, while the inferior angle is in line with T7-8. The inferior angles should be equidistant from the spine.

- Scapular winging—indicates a serratus anterior weakness, or the presence of a rib hump deformity (will become more prominent with forward flexion of the trunk).

- Differences in iliac crest height—may indicate a functional leg length discrepancy.

- Differences in height of the gluteal folds and popliteal creases.

Observing the patient from the side, the clinician should note the following:

- The earlobe should be in line with the tip of the shoulder, and the peak of the iliac crest.

- The extent of the lumbar lordosis—an exaggerated lordosis may indicate a hip flexor contracture, weak hip extensors, or spondylolisthesis.[19]

The skin should be inspected for the presence of any ecchymosis, erythema, rashes, or cutaneous signs of occult spinal dysraphisms.

 Clinical Pearl

Occult spinal dysraphisms, or occult spina bifida, are failures in the complete closure of the neural (vertebral) arches, which often have external signs indicating their presence. These signs may include patches of hair, nevi, hemangiomas, or dimples on the lower back in the midline.

Palpation

Palpation of the lumbar spine area should be performed in a systematic manner, and should be performed in conjunction with palpation of the pelvic area. The clinician should move superiorly from the L5 spinous process, carefully palpating each segmental level. Evidence of tenderness, altered temperature, muscle spasm, or abnormal alignment during palpation can highlight an underlying impairment.

 Clinical Pearl

It is important to note that while palpation of soft tissue and bony tenderness has been found to have poor reproducibility ($k = 0.40$) and specificity, bony tenderness may be suggestive of spinal infection.[20]

Palpation usually begins with the patient in the standing position with an assessment of iliac crest height and palpation of the spinous processes to evaluate a possible step off from one level to the next (may be an indication of spondylolisthesis).

 Clinical Pearl

If a pelvic obliquity is found, it may be the result of a deformity within the spine, such as scoliosis or an anomalous vertebra, or it may be secondary to a leg length discrepancy.

Posterior Aspect

Palpation of the posterior aspect of the lumbar spine is best achieved by asking the patient to bend over the treatment table or lie prone.

- The clinician moves the index and middle finger quickly down the spine feeling for any abnormal projections or asymmetries of the spinous processes. Any alterations in the alignment of the spinous processes in a posterior–anterior direction, particularly at the L4–5 or L5–S1 segmental level may indicate the presence of a spondylolisthesis.[21] Specific pain elicited with posterior–anterior pressure over the segment serves as further confirmation. Asymmetry of the spinous processes in a posterior–anterior direction may also indicate wedging of a vertebral body or a complete loss of two adjacent IVD spaces.[22] Absence of a spinous process may be associated with spina bifida. Side to side alterations in the spinous process may indicate the presence of a rotational asymmetry of the vertebra.[23]

  - The supraspinous and interspinous ligaments should be palpated. The ligament is usually supple, springy, and nontender. Because this ligament is the most superficial of the spinal ligaments and farthest from the axis of flexion, it has a greater potential for sprains.[24]

- Palpation of the transverse processes (TP) of T12 and L5 present difficulties. That of L3 is easy to feel, being usually the longest of all TPs; it is usually possible to feel those of L1, L2, and L4. That of L5 is covered by the posterior ilium.[25]

- The lumbar zygapophyseal joints of each motion segment are located approximately 2 to 3 cm (0.8–1.2 inches) lateral from the spinous processes. Patients with localized tenderness over the zygapophyseal joints without other root tension signs or neurologic signs may have zygapophyseal joint pain.[26]

- A well-localized and tender point at the gluteal level of the iliac crest, 8 to 10 cm from the midline, may indicate the presence of Maigne's syndrome.[27] Maigne's syndrome is characterized by SIJ, low lumbar, and gluteal pain, with occasional referral to the thigh, laterally or posteriorly.

- Palpation of the paraspinal musculature is essential to determine whether any tender or trigger points can be appreciated or whether muscle spasm is present.[19]

- Normally the skin can be rolled over the spine and gluteal region with ease. Tightness or pain produced with the skin rolling may indicate some underlying pathology.[28] The source of the signs and symptoms is an irritation of the medial cutaneous branch of the dorsal rami of the T12 or L1 spinal nerves as it passes through a fibro-osseous tunnel at the iliac crest.[27]

Anterior Aspect

- The inguinal area, located between the anterior superior iliac spine and the symphysis pubis should be carefully palpated for evidence of tenderness, which may be indicative of a hernia, abscess, sprain of the ligament, or an infection if the lymph nodes are swollen and tender.

- In some patients, the anterior aspect of the vertebral bodies may be palpable with the patient positioned in supine with their hips flexed and feet flat on the bed. Tenderness of the anterior aspect of the vertebral bodies over the anterior longitudinal ligament may indicate the presence of an anterior instability.[29]

Lateral Aspect

Observing the patient from the side, the clinician should observe the degree of tilt at the pelvis. The question of cause and effect should be raised.

- An anterior pelvic tilt causes an increase in the lumbar lordosis and thoracic kyphosis. The anterior pelvic tilt results in a stretching of the abdominals, sacrotuberous, sacroiliac, and sacrospinous ligaments, and an adaptive shortening of the hip flexors.

- A posterior pelvic tilt results in a stretching of the hip flexors and lower abdominals, and adaptive shortening of the hamstrings.

Active Movement Testing

Normal active motion (Table 13-5) involves fully functional contractile and inert tissues, and optimal neurological function.[30–34] When examining range of motion, it is important to document any side to side differences as asymmetric movement may be one of the first findings in those with underlying disease entities.[19]

 Clinical Pearl

Because active range of motion of the lumbar spine demonstrates considerable variability and may be affected by age and sex, the evaluation of the quantity of spinal range of motion has limited diagnostic use. Instead more emphasis should be placed on the quality of motion and the symptoms provoked. However, the direction of the available pain-free range of motion may be helpful in planning the intervention.

A good view of the spine is essential during motion testing and the patient should be disrobed appropriately.

Table 13-5 Normal Active Range of Motion of the Lumbar Spine*

Direction of Motion	Mean Degrees
Flexion	59 ± 9
Extension	19 ± 9
Side bending	Right: 31 ± 6; Left: 30 ± 6
Axial rotation	Right: 32 ± 9; Left: 33 ± 9

*Data from Ng JK, Kippers V, Richardson CA, Parnianpour M. Range of motion and lordosis of the lumbar spine: reliability of measurement and normative values. *Spine.* 2001;26:53–60.

Clinical Pearl

The capsular pattern for the lumbar spine is normal trunk flexion, a decrease in lumbar extension with rotation and side bending equally limited bilaterally.[35]

From the standing position, the patient performs flexion (Figure 13-4A), extension (Figure 13-4B), and side bending to both sides (Figure 13-4C and D).

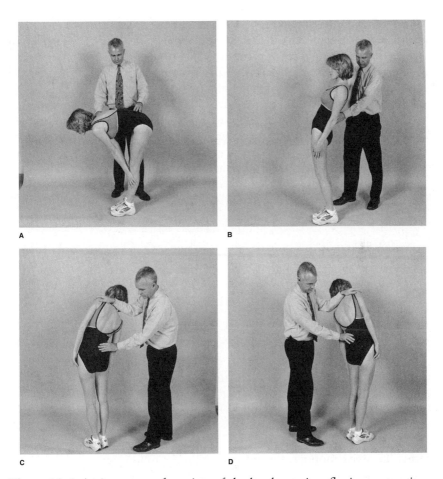

A   B

C   D

Figure 13-4 Active range of motion of the lumbar spine: flexion, extension, right sidebending, and left side bending.

Clinical Pearl

Although it is commonly taught that the first 60 degrees of forward flexion takes place in the lumbar spine, and that any further motion takes place at the hips, there have been no studies to validate this issue. Indeed, the initial 45 degrees of trunk flexion is largely due to the reversal of the lumbar lordosis.

If these motions fail to reproduce the symptoms, combined motions are introduced (see next section). At the end of each of the active motions, passive over pressure is applied to assess the end-feel, and resistance tests are performed with the muscles in the lengthened positions. The clinician should consider having the patient remain at the end range of each of the motion tests for 10 to 20 seconds, if sustained positions were reported to increase the symptoms. If repetitive or combined motions were reported in the history to increase the symptoms, McKenzie[36] advocates the use of sustained or repeated movements of the spine in an attempt to affect nuclear position. These movements are performed to either peripheralize the symptoms, lateral from the midline, or distally down the extremity, or to ideally centralize the symptoms to a point more central or near mid-line.

 Clinical Pearl

Motion at the SIJ s can occur around three axes[37]:

- X-axis: corresponds with sacral rotation in the sagittal plane. Rotation around this axis ranges from −1.1 degrees to 2.2 degrees with translation in this plane from −0.3 to 8 mm.

- Y-axis: corresponds with sacral rotation in the horizontal plane. Rotation around this axis ranges from −0.8 degrees to 4 degrees with translation in this plane from −0.2 to 7 mm.

- Z-axis: corresponds with sacral rotation in the coronal plane. Rotation around this axis ranges from −0.5 degrees to 8 degrees with translation in this plane from −0.3 to 6 mm.

During the active motions, the clinician notes the following:
- The affect the movement has on the natural curves of the spine.
- The presence of any deviations during or at the end of range.

- The provocation and distribution of symptoms.
- Any gross limitations of motion.
- Any compensatory motions.

 Clinical Pearl

The majority of published data concerning normal ranges of motion exists without concomitant data on the subjects' demographic background, specifically with respect to age, gender, and occupation.

Combined Motion Testing. The combined motion tests of the lumbar spine are used to detect biomechanical impairments. Although combined motion tests do not provide information as to which segment is at fault, they may provide information as to which motion or position reproduces the pain.[38] Combined motion tests can reproduce the pain in a structure that is either being compressed or stretched[39]:

- A reproduction or increase in symptoms with flexion and side bending away from the side of the symptoms may implicate pain in a structure that is being stretched.
- A reproduction or increase in symptoms with extension and side bending toward the side of the symptoms may implicate pain in a structure that is being compressed.

Combined motions can be performed as repetitive motions or as sustained positioning. For example, the patient can be asked to repetitively perform the combined motion of flexion and right side bending to assess for what McKenzie describes as a derangement syndrome, or the clinician can position the patient in flexion and right side bending (Figure 13-5) to assess for what McKenzie describes as a dysfunction syndrome. Alternatively, the clinician can ask the patient to maintain the position of flexion and right side bending to assess for a postural dysfunction.[36]

 Clinical Pearl

The lunge, active straight leg raise, and thigh thrust (see Special Tests for the Sacroiliac Joint) are all motions that can reproduce pain from a SIJ dysfunction.[37,40]

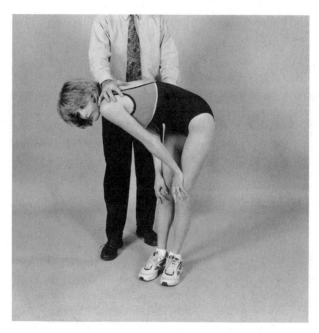

Figure 13-5 Combined motion—lumbar flexion and right sidebending.

The 6-position Test

The 6-position test is a screening tool that the author has found to be particularly useful with the acute patient in helping to determine the position of comfort for the patient, and for focusing the examination and intervention. The patient is positioned in the following positions:

1. Supine with the hips and knees extended (Figure 13-6). In individuals with adaptive shortening of the rectus femoris and the iliopsoas (a common finding), this position is manifested by an inability of the posterior thighs to rest on the table. Pain in this position may indicate a lumbar extension or lumbar rotation syndrome, especially if the next position relieves the symptoms.[41]

2. Supine in the hook lying position, with the hips and knees flexed and the feet flat on the bed (Figure 13-7). This is typically the most comfortable position for the patient with acute LBP, except in cases of severe stenosis or spondylolisthesis.

3. Supine with both knees held against the chest (Figure 13-8). This position rotates the pelvis posteriorly and widens the intervertebral foramina of the lumbar segments.[42] This is normally a comfortable position for

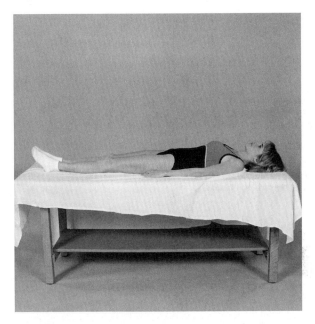

Figure 13-6 6-position test—Position 1.

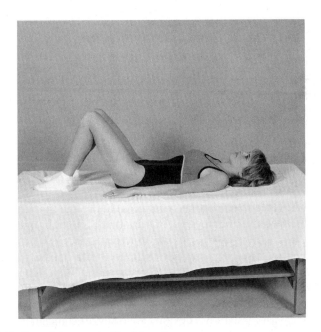

Figure 13-7 6-position test—Position 2.

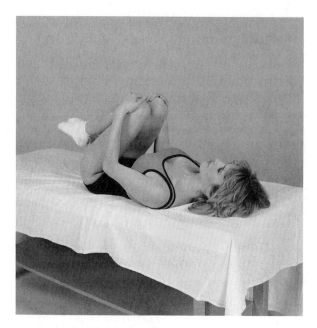

Figure 13-8 6-position test—Position 3.

patients who have spinal stenosis, lateral recess stenosis, or a lumbar extension syndrome.

4. Supine with one knee held against the chest and the other leg lying on the bed, with the hip and knee extended (Figure 13-9). Holding the left knee against the chest invokes a position of lumbar flexion and left side bending, which widens the intervertebral foramen on the right and narrows the intervertebral foramen on the left. Holding the right knee against the chest invokes a position of lumbar flexion and right side bending, which widens the intervertebral foramen on the left and narrows intervertebral foramen on the right.[42] Given the amount of rotation induced with this maneuver, this test is often positive even when the position of both knees to the chest does not provoke symptoms due to the amount of rotation it introduces to the lumbar spine. Occasionally though, one side may be pain free and can be used as an introductory exercise.

5. Prone lying with the legs straight (Figure 13-10). This is typically comfortable for patients with an IVD protrusion, but uncomfortable for patients with spinal stenosis, spondylolisthesis, and an extension or a rotation syndrome.[41]

6. Prone lying with passive knee flexion applied by the clinician (Figure 13-11). This is a confirmatory test for the previous position, if it increases the

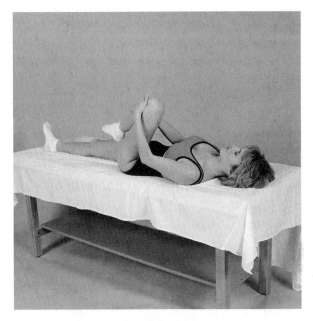

Figure 13-9 6-position test—Position 4.

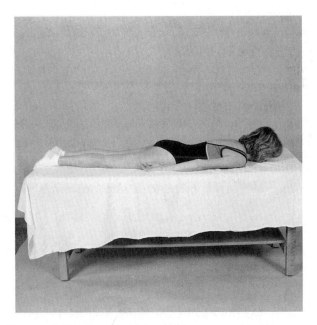

Figure 13-10 6-position test—Position 5.

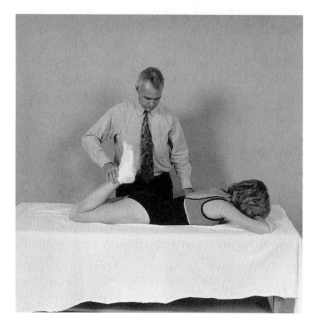

Figure 13-11 6-position test—Position 6.

symptoms in patients with spinal stenosis, spondylolisthesis, and an extension or a rotation syndrome.[41]

The results from these tests should provide the clinician with information on the affect of pelvic tilting in a nonweight bearing position has on the symptoms.

- If anterior pelvic tilting appears to aggravate the patient's symptoms, initial positions, then exercises that promote posterior pelvic tilting are advocated.

- If posterior pelvic tilting appears to aggravate the patient's symptoms, initial positions, then exercises that promote an anterior pelvic tilt are advocated.

Muscle Strength

Key Muscle Testing

The key muscle tests are used as part of the lower quarter scanning examination as they examine the integrity of the neuromuscular junction and the contractile and inert components of the various muscles (Table 13-6).[35] With the isometric tests, the contraction should be held for at least 5 seconds to demonstrate any weakness.

Table 13-6 Key Muscles of the Lumbar Quarter Scanning Examination

Myotome	Key Muscle Tested
L1–2	Hip flexion
L3–4	Knee extension
L4	Ankle dorsiflexion
L5	Great toe extension
L5–S1	Hip extension Great toe extension
S1–2	Plantar flexion Knee flexion
S3	Intrinsic muscles of the foot (except abductor hallucis)

 Clinical Pearl

The sensitivity, specificity, positive predictive value, or negative predictive value of manual muscle testing varies considerably in the peer-reviewed literature.

If the clinician suspects weakness, the test is repeated 2 to 3 times to assess for muscle fatigability, which could indicate spinal nerve root compromise.

 Clinical Pearl

The larger muscle groups, such as the quadriceps, hip extensors, and calf muscles must be tested by repetitive resistance against a sufficient load to sufficiently stress the muscle-nerve components, usually through full weight bearing.

Standing up on the toes (S1-2)
The patient raises both heels off the ground. The key muscles tested during this maneuver are the plantar flexors. These are difficult muscles to fatigue, so

the patient should perform 10 heel raises unilaterally with their arms resting on the clinician's shoulders (Figure 13-12).

Unilateral squat while supported (L3-4)
The patient performs unilateral squats while supported. The key muscles being tested during this maneuver are the quadriceps and hip extensors. Neurological weakness of the quadriceps (L3–L4) is relatively rare and often suggests a nondiscogenic lesion such as a neoplasm, especially if the weakness is bilateral.[43]

Heel walking (L4)
The patient walks toward, or away from, the clinician while weight bearing through their heels (Figure 13-13). The key muscles being tested during this maneuver are the dorsiflexors (L4).

⬤ Clinical Pearl

About 40% of IVD lesions affect the L4 level, about an equal amount as those that affect the L5 root.[44]

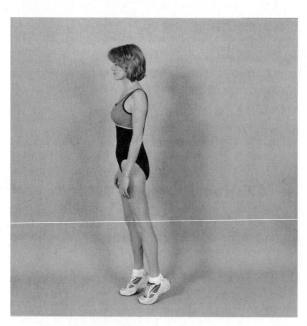

Figure 13-12 Standing up on toes.

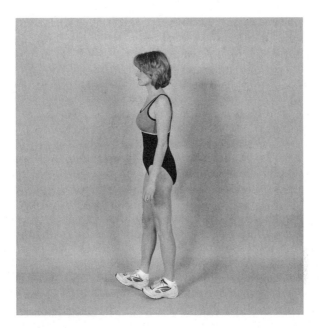

Figure 13-13 Heel walking.

Hip flexion (L1–2)
The patient is seated on the edge of a table. The patient's hip is actively raised off the treatment table to about 30 degrees to 40 degrees of flexion. The clinician then applies a resisted force proximal to the knee, into hip extension (Figure 13-14) while ensuring that the heel of the patient's foot is not contacting the examining table. Both sides are tested for comparison. An inability to raise the thigh off the table indicates palsy.

🔵 Clinical Pearl

Palsy at the L2 level should always serve as a red flag, as IVD protrusions at this level are rare, but this is a common site for metastasis.[45] Painful weakness of hip flexion may indicate the presence of a fractured transverse process, metastatic invasion, acute spondylolisthesis, acute segmental articular dysfunction, a major contractile lesion of the hip flexors (rare), or hip joint pathology.

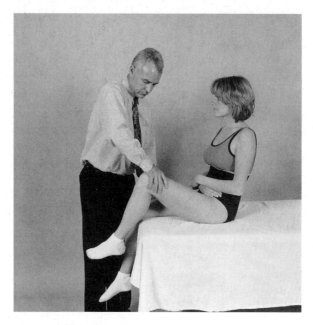

Figure 13-14 Resisted hip flexion.

Knee extension (L3–4)

The patient is seated. The clinician positions the patient's knee in 25 degrees to 35 degrees of flexion and then applies a resisted flexion force at the mid-distal shaft of the tibia (Figure 13-15). Both sides are tested for comparison. An alternate position for testing knee extension can be performed in prone. The patient's leg is positioned in about 120 degrees of knee flexion taking care to do this passively. The clinician rests the superior aspect of their shoulder against the dorsum of the patient's ankle and a superior force is applied while the clinician grips the edges of the examining table. Both sides are tested for comparison.

Hip extension (L5–S1)

The patient is prone. The patient's knee is flexed to 90 degrees and their thigh is lifted slightly off the examining table by the clinician, while the other leg is stabilized. A downward force is applied to the patient's posterior thigh while the clinician ensures that the patient's thigh is not in contact with the table. Both sides are tested for comparison.

Knee flexion (S1-2)

The patient is prone. The patient's knee is flexed to 90 degrees and an extension isometric force is applied just above the ankle (Figure 13-16). Both sides are tested for comparison.

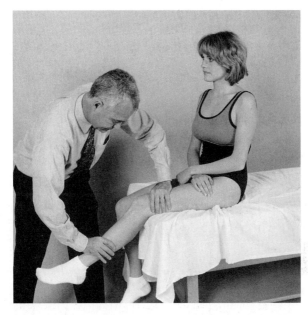

Figure 13-15 Resisted knee extension.

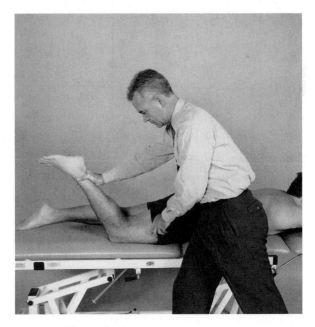

Figure 13-16 Resisted knee flexion.

Great toe extension (L5)
The patient is supine. The patient is asked to hold both big toes in a neutral position and the clinician applies resistance to the nails of both toes (Figure 13-17) and compares the two sides.

Ankle eversion (L5–S1)
The patient is supine. The patient is asked to place the feet at 0 degrees of plantar and dorsiflexion relative to the leg. A resisted force is applied to move each foot into inversion by the clinician (Figure 13-18) and a comparison is made.

 Clinical Pearl

In those patients complaining of symptoms near the adductor origin on the pubic bone, pain in the ipsilateral anteroposterior iliac spine, and symptom provocation during exercise, the clinician should consider and abductor strain or an obturator neuropathy. Although far less common than an adductor strain, a lesion to the obturator nerve can result in the following findings:

- Impaired sensation along the areas innervated by the obturator nerve.

- Weakness with manual muscle testing of hip adduction, especially following exercise.

- Pain with a resisted external rotation of the hip.

- Pain with passive stretching of the pectineus muscle.

- A positive Howship–Romberg sign (see Special tests of the lumbar spine).

Core Stability
The term *core* when used with reference to the lumbar spine, describes a point from where the center of gravity for all movement is initiated.[46-50] The static and dynamic structures of the "core" serve to maintain postural alignment and dynamic equilibrium during functional activities.[51] Thus, it is important to examine the core musculature for weakness and adaptive shortening. Of the core muscles, the rectus abdominis has a tendency to become weak, and the quadratus lumborum has a tendency to become adaptively shortened and overactive.[52]

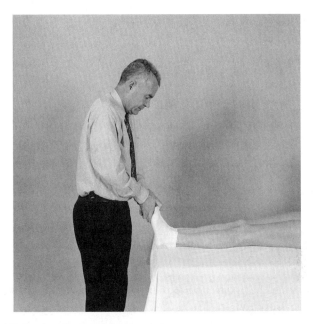

Figure 13-17 Resisted great toe extension.

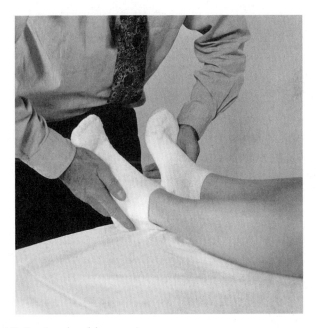

Figure 13-18 Resisted ankle eversion.

Deep Tendon Reflexes

The reflexes should be assessed and graded accordingly, with any differences between the two sides noted. The tendon should be struck directly once the patient's muscles and tendons are relaxed.

Patellar Reflex (L3)

The patient is positioned in sitting with their legs hanging freely. Alternatively, both knees can be supported in flexion with the patient positioned in supine (Figure 13-19).

Hamstring Reflex (Semimembranosus: L5, S1, and Biceps Femoris: S1–2)

The patient is positioned in prone with the knee flexed and the foot resting on a pillow. The clinician places a thumb over the appropriate tendon and taps the thumbnail with the reflex hammer to elicit the reflex.

Achilles Reflex (S1-2)

The patient should be positioned so that the ankle is slightly dorsiflexed with passive overpressure (Figure 13-20).

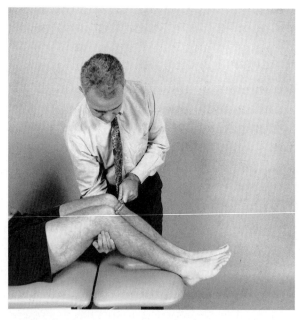

Figure 13-19 Patellar reflex.

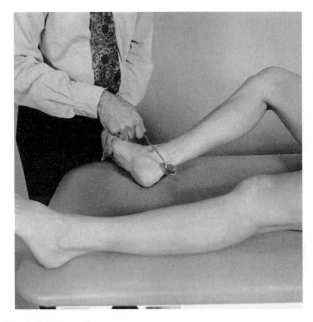

Figure 13-20 Achilles reflex.

Pathological Reflexes

- Babinski
- Clonus
- Oppenheim

Sensory Testing

The clinician checks the dermatome patterns of the nerve roots, as well as the peripheral sensory distribution of the peripheral nerves. Dermatomes vary considerably between individuals.

Differing Philosophies

The next stage in the examination process depends on the clinician's background. For those clinicians heavily influenced by the muscle energy techniques of the osteopaths, position testing is used to determine which segment to focus on. Other clinicians omit the position tests and proceed to the combined motion and passive physiological tests.

> ### ● Clinical Pearl
>
> Given the questionable reliability and validity of the tests for the SIJ, a diagnosis of SIJ dysfunction needs to be based on the results from a thorough history and a physical examination that includes both pain provocative tests and a biomechanical examination. The algorithm depicted in Figure 13-12 should serve as a guide.

Position Testing

Position testing is performed with the patient positioned in three positions: neutral (Figure 13-21), flexion (Figure 13-22), and extension (Figure 13-23). The transverse processes are then layer palpated. The findings and possible causes for the position testing are outlined in Table 13-7 and Table 13-8.

Passive Physiological Intervertebral Mobility Testing (PPIVM)[53,54]

These tests are most effectively carried out if the combined motion tests locate a hypomobility, or if the position tests are negative, rather than as the

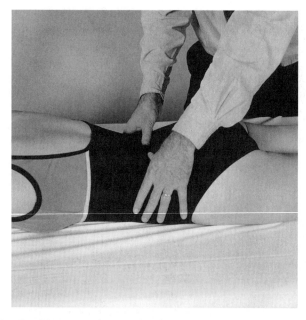

Figure 13-21 Position testing in neutral.

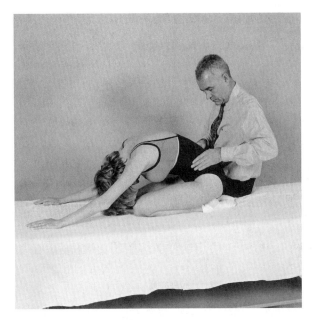

Figure 13-22 Position testing in flexion.

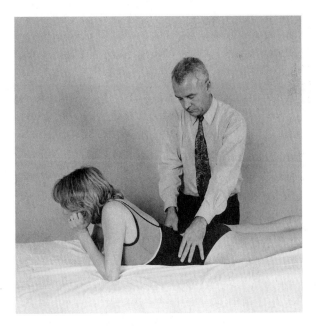

Figure 13-23 Position testing in extension.

Table 13-7 Causes and Findings of an ERSL

Causes of an ERSL	Associated Findings
Isolated left joint flexion hypomobility	PPIVM and PPAIVM tests in the right flexion quadrant are reduced
Tight left extensor muscles	PPIVM test in the right flexion quadrant is decreased, while the PPAIVM is normal
Arthrosis/itis left joint/Capsular pattern	PPIVM and PPAIVM tests are equally reduced in the right flexion and left flexion quadrants
Fibrosis left joint	PPIVM and PPAIVM tests equally reduced in the right and left flexion quadrants
Right posterior–lateral disc protrusion	PPIVM tests in the right extension quadrant reduced with a springy end-feel. Both flexion quadrants appear normal

PPIVM = passive physiological intervertebral motion; PPAIVM = passive physiological accessory intervertebral motion.

entry tests for the lumbar spine. Judgments of stiffness made by experienced physical therapists examining patients in their own clinics have been found to have poor reliability.[55]

Table 13-8 Causes and Findings for an FRSR

Causes of an FRSR	Associated Findings
Isolated left joint extension hypomobility	PPIVM and PPAIVM tests in the left extension quadrant are reduced
Tight left flexor muscles	PPIVM test in the left extension quadrant is decreased PPAIVM test is normal
Arthrosis/itis left joint/capsular pattern	PPIVM and PPAIVM tests in the right flexion quadrant are more reduced than in the left extension quadrant
Fibrosis left joint	PPIVM and PPAIVM tests equally reduced in the right flexion and left extension quadrants
Left posterior–lateral disc protrusion	PPIVM tests in the left extension quadrant are reduced with a springy end-feel. Both flexion quadrants are normal

PPIVM = passive physiological intervertebral motion; PPAIVM = passive physiological accessory intervertebral motion.

The passive physiological movement tests are performed into

- Flexion
- Extension
- Rotation
- Side bending

The adjacent spinous processes of the segment are palpated simultaneously, and movement between them is assessed as the segment is passively taken through its physiological range.

Unfortunately, the passive physiological intervertebral mobility tests do not completely exclude such intersegmental impairments as minor end range asymmetrical hypomobilities, or hypermobilities, because the application of side bending or rotation in neutral does not fully flex or extend the zygapophyseal joints, nor is it possible to fully flex or extend both zygapophyseal joints simultaneously. The findings and possible causes for the PPIVM are outlined in Table 13-7 and Table 13-8.

Passive Physiological Accessory Intervertebral Movement Test (PPAIVM)

Passive physiological accessory intervertebral movement tests investigate the degree of linear or accessory glide that a joint possesses, and are used on segmental levels where there is a possible hypomobility, to help determine if the motion restriction is articular, periarticular or myofascial in origin. In other words, they assess the amount of joint motion, as well as the quality of the end-feel. The motion is assessed, in relation to the patient's body type and age and the normal range for that segment, and the end-feel is assessed for

- Pain
- Spasm/hypertonicity
- Resistance

Spinal locking techniques may be used to help localize these techniques to the specific level, or to a specific side of the segment. The findings and possible causes for the PPAIVM are outlined in Table 13-7 and Table 13-8.

Special Tests for the Lumbar Spine

Neurodynamic Mobility Testing

These include the straight leg raise (SLR) test, slump test, the Bowstring tests, the double straight leg raise, and the femoral nerve stretch (prone knee flexion) test. The SLR test should be a routine test during the examination of the lumbar spine among patients with sciatica or pseudoclaudication.

Clinical Pearl

Ipsilateral straight-leg raising has sensitivity (72%–97%) but not specificity (11%–66%) for a herniated IVD, whereas crossed straight-leg raising is insensitive but highly specific.[56]

The femoral nerve stretch test is not pathognomonic for upper lumbar disc herniation as it is likely to be positive in several conditions including all forms of femoral neuropathy, adaptive shortening of the ilopsoas and rectus femoris muscles, or pathology in or about the hip joint.[57]

A leg elevation of less than 60 degrees is abnormal, suggesting compression or irritation of the nerve roots. A positive test reproduces the symptoms of sciatica, with pain that radiates below the knee, not merely back or hamstring pain.[56]

H and I Tests

These are biomechanical tests for the spine, testing both the range and the function of the joint complex using combined motions.[43,53,58] The tests get their name from the pattern produced by the motions that make up each test, and are used to detect biomechanical impairments in the chronic or subacute stages of healing.

The *H* test involves the patient initiating with side-flexion of the lumbar spine, followed by extreme forward flexion of the lumbar spine. From this position, the patient maintains the side-flexion, and moves into extreme extension of the lumbar spine. The test is then repeated using side-flexion to the other side, and repeating the flexion and extension motions while maintaining the side-flexion.

The *I* test involves the patient initiating with extreme forward flexion of the lumbar spine, before moving into side-flexion of the lumbar spine. From this position the patient side-flexes the trunk to the other side. The test is then repeated using extreme extension and side-flexion to both sides, and the range of motion and end-feels are compared.

Posterior–anterior Pressures

Posterior–anterior pressures, advocated by Maitland,[59] are applied over the spinous, mammillary and transverse processes of this region. The clinician should apply the posterior–anterior force in a slow and gentle fashion using the index and middle finger of one hand, while monitoring the paravertebrals with the other hand.

Hoover

The Hoover test may be performed to assess the patient's voluntary effort. The patient's heels are cupped by the clinician, and the patient is instructed to individually raise his or her legs. Increased pressure should be felt on the untested cupped heel if true volitional effort is provided. There are no studies in the literature that discuss the sensitivity, specificity, positive predictive value, or negative predictive value of this maneuver.

The Bicycle Test of van Gelderen[60]

This test is designed to stress the lower extremity vascular system without causing any central canal or foraminal stenosis that could be misinterpreted as intermittent neurogenic claudication. The patient is instructed to cycle at a moderate pace (90 rpm) for 5 minutes or until symptoms are felt. A position of lumbar flexion (high seat height with low handle bars) is used to help minimize any effect from a neurogenic claudication, which would be exacerbated in lumbar extension and relieved by lumbar flexion.

- A patient with lateral spinal stenosis tolerates this position well.

- A patient with intermittent claudication of the lower extremities typically experiences an increase in symptoms with continued exercise, regardless of the position of the spine.

- A patient with intermittent cauda equina compression typically has an increase of symptoms with an increase in lumbar lordosis.

- A patient with a disc herniation usually fairs well if the lumbar spine remains extended.

- A positive test is indicated by a reproduction of some or all of the patient's symptoms in the same extremity that demonstrates a decrease in the pulse amplitude of a particular arterial branch.

Howship–Romberg Sign[61,62]

Compression of the obturator nerve by an obturator hernia produces the pathognomonic Howship–Romberg sign—pain along the medial aspect of the thigh to the knee and, less often, the hip that is relieved by flexion of the thigh and exacerbated by abduction, extension, and medial rotation. Confirmation is made using ultrasonography and CT.

 Clinical Pearl

The loss of the adductor reflex due to compression of the obturator nerve has been termed the Hannington-Kiff sign.[63]

Special Tests for the Sacroiliac Joint

It is estimated that the incidence rate for SIJ pathology is 15%. While these maneuvers are capable of eliciting pain, restricted movement and/or muscle spasm, they are fairly nonspecific in determining the exact level involved, or the exact cause of the symptoms, and have been found to have poor inter-rater reliability in the absence of corroborating clinical data.[64]

 Clinical Pearl

It is important to remember when examining the SIJs that altered motion is not always synonymous with pain.

The Standing Flexion Test

This test is performed with the patient standing, facing away from the clinician, with his/her feet approximately 12 inches apart so that the patient's feet are parallel and approximately acetabular distance apart. The examiner then places his/her thumbs on the inferior aspect of each PSIS. The patient is asked to bend forward keeping both knees extended. The extent of the superior movement of each PSIS is monitored by the clinician. Normally, the PSIS should move equally. If one PSIS moves more superiorly and anteriorly than the other, this is the side of restriction and hypomobility. Despite the fact that this test is still widely used, studies have shown that the test has a high false positive rate and poor reliability.[65,66]

Ipsilateral Hip Flexion Test in Standing

This test assesses the ability of the sacrum to nutate (tilt anteriorly) relative to the innominate on both the weight-bearing and nonweight-bearing side. With the patient standing, the clinician palpates the pelvis and asks the patient to transfer load to one lower extremity, retain balance, and flex the contralateral hip (Figure 13-24). The load transfer should occur smoothly with minimal adjustments of the lower extremity, and the pelvis should remain in its original coronal and transverse plane.

The Seated Flexion Test (Piedallu's Sign)

The patient is sitting with their legs over the end of the table and feet supported.[67] In this position, the innominate motion is severely abbreviated as the sitting position places the innominates near the end of their extension range. The test is performed as follows. Each posterior superior iliac spine (PSIS) is palpated with the thumb placed under it caudally. The patient then bends forward at the waist. Providing there is no impairment in the SIJ or the lower lumbar spine, as the patient bends forwards, both thumbs should move

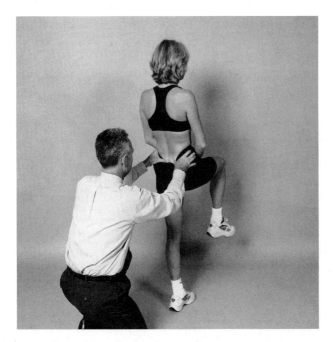

Figure 13-24 Ipsilateral hip flexion in standing.

cranially. If the joint is "blocked," it moves upward further in relation to the other side.[66] The test is purported to help distinguish between a sacroiliac lesion and an iliosacral lesion.[68–70] However, as with the standing flexion test, studies have questioned the usefulness of this test, reporting great disparity in terms of reliability, specificity, and sensitivity.[66,71]

The Long Sit Test

The long sit test is used to indicate the direction of the rotation that the innominate has adopted, and is used in conjunction with the standing flexion test. The patient is asked to raise themselves off the bed from a supine position into a long sit position (Figure 13-25) without any twisting or use of the arms, while the clinician monitors the medial malleoli. After noting the side of the impairment obtained from the standing flexion test, the clinician observes whether the medial malleolus on that side moves distally or proximally during the long sit test. Rotation about a coronal axis, whose resultant movement leads to an increase in the length of a limb, is defined as extension. If it shortens the length of the limb, it is defined as flexion. Thus, if the apparent shorter leg becomes longer during the test, the innominate on that side is purportedly held in a posteriorly rotated malposition, while if the apparent longer leg becomes shorter

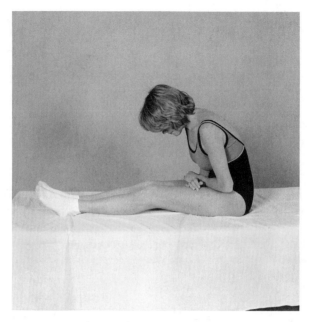

Figure 13-25 Long sit end position.

during the test, the innominate on that side is allegedly held in an anteriorly rotated malposition.

The problems with this test involve the maneuver itself. To ask a patient who is some degree of discomfort to rise off the bed from a supine position into a long-sit position without any twisting, or use of the arms is unnecessarily painful. In addition, for the successful completion of the maneuver, the patient needs 90 degrees of hip flexion/hamstring length.

Sign of the Buttock Test

The patient lies supine and the clinician performs a passive unilateral straight leg raise. If there is a unilateral restriction, the clinician flexes the knee and notes whether the hip flexion increases. If the restriction was due to the lumbar spine or hamstrings, hip flexion increases. If the hip flexion does not increase when the knee is flexed, it is a positive sign of the buttock test. The sign of the buttock is not a single sign as the name would suggest, but is a collection of signs indicating a serious pathology present posterior to the axis of flexion and extension in the hip. Among the causes of the syndrome are osteomyelitis, infectious sacroiliitis, and fracture of the sacrum/pelvis, septic bursitis, ischiorectal abscess, gluteal hematoma, gluteal tumor, and rheumatic bursitis. If the sign of the buttock is encountered, the patient must be immediately returned to the physician for further investigation.

Gaenslen's Test

The patient is positioned in supine at the edge of the bed. The leg furthest from the edge of the bed (nontested leg) is flexed at the hip and knee and held by the patient with both arms. The clinician stabilizes the pelvis and passively positions the upper leg (test leg) into hyperextension at the hip, so that it hangs over the edge of the table.[72] The clinician applies a further stretch to the test leg into hip extension and adduction. Pain with this maneuver is considered a positive test for a SIJ lesion, hip pathology, or an L4 nerve root lesion. The test also stresses the femoral nerve.

Yeoman's Test

This test[73] is performed with the patient positioned in prone. The clinician stabilizes the sacrum with the palm of one hand. With the other hand, the clinician grasps the patient's distal thigh and extends the patient's hip. At the end of the available motion, the hip is hyperextended so that the innominate is forced into anterior rotation. A positive test produces pain over the SIJ. Other structures that are stressed with this maneuver include the lumbar spine, the hip joint, and the psoas muscle.

Gillet Test

The patient is positioned in standing, facing away from the clinician, with his/her feet approximately 12 inches apart. Once each PSIS is localized by the clinician's thumbs, the patient is asked to stand on one leg while flexing the contralateral hip and flexing his/her knee to his/her chest. A positive finding, which indicates a so-called partial iliosacral dysfunction, occurs when the thumb on the side of the hip being flexed does not move at all or moves cranially (toward the head) in relation to the other thumb.

Fortin Finger Test

The patient is asked to point to the region of pain with one finger. Considered a positive sign if the patient can localize the pain with one finger, the area pointed to is immediately inferomedial to the PSIS within 1 cm, and the patient consistently points to the same area over at least two trials.

Patrick's (Faber or Figure-four) Test

The patient is positioned in supine. The test leg is positioned so that the sole of the foot rests against the medial side of the other knee (or on top of the knee of the opposite leg). This position flexes, abducts, and externally rotates the femur at the hip joint. The clinician slowly lowers the knee of the test leg toward the bed. At the end of available motion, the pelvis is stabilized, and overpressure is applied. Pain with this maneuver indicates hip joint pathology, SIJ dysfunction, or an iliopsoas muscle spasm.[74]

Active Straight Leg Raise (ASLR) Test

When performed passively, the straight leg raise test is usually associated as a test of neurodynamic mobility, or hamstring length. When performed actively, the straight leg raise test has been recommended as a disease severity scale for patients with posterior pelvic pain after pregnancy.[75-77] The patient is positioned in supine with the straight legs 20 cm apart, relaxed and externally rotated. The patient is asked to raise one leg at a time about 5 cm above the bed without bending the knee. If pain is reproduced with this maneuver, the patient is fitted with a pelvic belt and the test is repeated. If the addition of the belt removes the pain, the test is positive. It seems that the integrity of the function to transfer loads between the lumbosacral spine and legs is tested by the ASLR test.

Anterior Gapping (Distraction) Test

The anterior gapping stress test is performed with the patient supine with their legs extended. The clinician stands to one side of the patient and, crossing their arms, places the palm of their hands on the patient's anterior superior iliac spines. The clinician then applies a laterally directed force with both hands, thereby gapping the anterior aspect of the SIJ. The stress is maintained for 7 to 10 seconds, or until an end-feel is felt.

In addition to being sensitive for severe arthritis, this test and its posterior counterpart (see below) are also believed to be sensitive to ligament tears,[35] although they have been shown to be poorly reproducible.[66]

 Clinical Pearl

> Provocation testing of this joint has better reliability than other measures and is most indicative of SIJ diagnosis. Active movement tests lack reliability as do positional palpation tests.

Posterior Compression Test

The patient is positioned in side lying and the clinician applies pressure to the lateral side of the ilium, thereby compressing the anterior aspect of the joint, and gapping its posterior aspect. The posterior and interosseus ligaments are among the strongest in the body and are not usually torn by trauma, but may be attenuated by prolonged, or repeated, stress. This test is less sensitive for arthritis due to the reduced leverage available to the clinician. Thus, if it is positive, it indicates severe arthritis. This test also indirectly tests the ability of the sacrum to counternutate.

Thigh Thrust

The patient lies supine with the hip and knee flexed where the thigh is at right angles to the table and slightly adducted. One of the examiner's hands cups the sacrum and the other arm and hand wraps around the flexed knee. The pressure applied is directed posteriorly along the line of the vertically oriented femur. The procedure is carried out on both sides. The presumed action is a posterior shearing force to the SIJ of that side.

Shear Test

The patient is positioned in prone and the clinician stands near the patient's feet. While stabilizing the patient's ilium through the hip joint by applying traction through the leg, the clinician applies a pressure to the sacrum near the coccygeal end, directed cranially. The test is considered positive if the maneuver aggravates the patient's typical pain.

Imaging Studies

Plain radiographs are not recommended for the routine evaluation of acute low back pain within the first month unless a finding from the history and clinical examination raises concern. A major diagnostic problem with LBP is that many anatomic abnormalities seen on imaging tests including myelography, computed tomography (CT), and magnetic resonance imaging (MRI) are common in healthy individuals.[78,79] However, if red flags suggest cauda equina syndrome or progressive major motor weakness, the prompt use of CT, MRI, myelography or combined CT, and myelography is recommended.[5] In the absence of red flags after one month of symptoms, it is reasonable to obtain an imaging study if surgery is being considered.

Laboratory Studies

Laboratory tests generally are not necessary in the initial evaluation of low back pain. However, if tumor or infection is suspected, the physician may order a complete blood cell count and erythrocyte sedimentation rate. Other blood studies, such as testing for HLA-B27 antigen (present in ankylosing spondylitis) and serum protein electrophoresis (results abnormal in multiple myeloma), are performed as warranted.[10]

Examination Conclusions—The Evaluation

Following the examination, and once the clinical findings have been recorded, the clinician must determine a specific diagnosis or a working hypothesis, based on a summary of all of the findings. This diagnosis can be structure related (medical diagnosis), or a diagnosis based on the preferred practice patterns as described in the Guide to Physical Therapist Practice.[80] Tables 13-9 and 13-10 summarize the typical findings in a patient with a

Table 13-9 Reduced Movement

Reduced Movement	
Myofascial	**Joint/Pericapsular**

Cause:
• Muscle shortening (scars, contracture, adaptive)
	Cause:
	• Capsular or ligamentous shortening due to
	   • Scars
	   • Adaptation to a chronically shortened position
	• Joint surface adhesions

Findings: Reduced movement or hypomobility may have an insidious or sudden onset. The presence or absence of pain depends on the level of chemical and/or mechanical irritation of the local nociceptors, which in turn is a function of the stage of healing. Pain is usually aggravated with movement and alleviated with rest Negative scan	Findings: Reduced movement or hypomobility may have an insidious or sudden onset. The presence or absence of pain depends on the level of chemical and/or mechanical irritation of the local nociceptors which in turn is a function of the stage of healing. Pain is usually aggravated with movement and alleviated with rest Negative scan
PPIVM and PAIVM Findings: Reduced gross PPIVM but PPAIVM normal	PPIVM and PAIVM Findings: Reduced gross PPIVM and PPAIVM
Intervention: Muscle relaxation techniques Transverse frictions Stretches	Intervention: a. Joint mobilizations at specific level
Pericapsular/Arthritis	**Disc Protrusion**
Cause: Degenerative or degradative changes	Cause: Cumulative stress Low level but prolonged over-use Sudden macro-trauma
Findings: Negative scan Reduces gross PPIVM in all directions except flexion Active motion restricted in a capsular pattern (decreased extension and equal limitation of rotation and side-flexion)	Findings: Positive scan Key muscle fatigable weakness Hyporeflexive DTRs Sensory changes in dermatomal distribution Subjective complaints of radicular pain
PPIVM and PAIVM Findings: Reduced gross PPIVM but PPAIVM normal	PPIVM and PAIVM Findings: Reduced gross PPIVM and PPAIVM
Intervention: Capsular/muscle stretching Active exercises/PREs Anti-inflammatory modalities if necessary Joint protection techniques	Intervention: 1. Traction 2. Active exercises in to spinal extension Positioning

Table 13-10 Excessive Movement

Excessive Movement	
Hypermobility	Instability
Causes:	Causes:
Cumulative stress due to neighboring hypomobility	Sudden macrotrauma (ligamentous)
Low level but prolonged over-use	Hypermobility allowed to progress (ligamentous)
Sudden macro-trauma that is not enough to produce instability	Degeneration of interposing hyaline or fibrocartilage (articular)
Findings:	Findings:
Subjective complaints of "catching". Good days and bad days. Symptoms aggravated with sustained positions	Subjective complaints of "catching". Good days and bad days. Symptoms aggravated with sustained positions
Negative scan	Negative scan
PPIVM Findings:	PPIVM Findings:
Increase in gross PPIVM with pain at end range	Increase in gross PPIVM with pain at end range
	Presence of nonphysiological movement (positive stress test)
	Recurrent subluxations
Intervention:	Intervention: falls into three areas:
1. Educate the patient to avoid excessive range	• Global stabilization
2. Take stress off joint (mobilize hypomobility)	• Educate patient to stay out of activities likely to take him/her into the instability
3. Anti-inflammatory modalities if necessary	• Total body neuromuscular movement pattern re-education
4. Stabilize if absolutely necessary	• Work or sports conditioning and rehabilitation
	• Local stabilization
	• Muscular splinting of the region (lifting techniques, twisting on feet, chin tucking when lifting)
	• Bracing with supports (collars, corsets, splints, and braces)
	• Regional neuromuscular movement pattern re-education
	• Segmental stabilization
	• PNF and active exercises to the segment

biomechanical diagnosis, highlighting both the similarities and the differences between each.

INTERVENTION

At present, there is no evidence that physical therapy treatment for chronic low back pain is more effective than placebo treatment.[81] The rehabilitation procedures chosen to progress the patient will depend on the type of tissue involved, the extent of the damage, and the stage of healing (See Chapter 3). The intervention must be related to the signs and symptoms present rather than the actual diagnosis.

COMMON ORTHOPEDIC CONDITIONS

ACQUIRED SPONDYLOLISTHESIS

Diagnosis

Acquired (degenerative) spondylolisthesis—ICD-9: 738.4. Other types of spondylolisthesis include congenital spondylolisthesis (ICD-9: 756.12).

Description

Spondylolysis is a fracture of the region of the pars interarticularis. Spondylolisthesis is a diagnostic term that identifies anterior slippage and inability to resist shear forces of a vertebral segment in relation to the vertebral segment immediately below it. Frequently, spondylolisthesis leads to spinal instability—the inability of the spine to maintain its normal pattern of displacement when placed under physiological load.

 Clinical Pearl

The most common site for spondylolysis (a defect of the pars interarticularis of the spine) and spondylolisthesis is L5 to S1.

Subjective Findings

The symptoms, if they do occur, usually begin in the second decade. The subjective findings typically include the following:

- Complaints of pain with activities involving lumbar extension and twisting.
- Symptoms are typically eased with flexion postures (reduction of the lumbar lordosis).
- Depending on the extent and severity, neurologic symptoms (radiculopathy, neurogenic claudication) may be present.

 Clinical Pearl

The four grades of spondylolisthesis are as follows:

Grade 1—0% to 25% slippage.

Grade 2—25% to 50% slippage.

Grade 3—50% to 75% slippage.

Grade 4 -- greater than 75% slippage.

It is important to remember that there is often no correlation with the degree of slip and the severity of symptoms.

 Clinical Pearl

If neurogenic claudication is present, the patient may complain of bilateral thigh and leg tiredness, aches, and fatigue.

Clinical Pearl

Questions regarding bicycle use versus walking (see Confirmatory/ Special tests) can help the clinician to differentiate neurogenic from vascular claudication. Both cycling and walking increase symptoms in vascular claudication due to the increased demand for blood supply. However, patients with neurogenic claudication worsen with walking but are unaffected by cycling due to the differing positions of the lumbar spine adopted in each of these activities.

Objective Findings

The physical examination typically reveals little in the way of findings unless the patient has reported symptoms of a neurologic nature. However, the following findings may be present:

• Pain with posterior anterior pressure on the vertebral body of the involved level.

• Painful and limited trunk extension.

• Adaptively shortened hamstrings.

• Weakness in one or both lower extremities.

• Palpable "step-off" deformity of spinous process if significant spondylolisthesis is present.

Confirmatory/Special Tests

The van Gelderen bicycle test (see chapter text).

Medical Studies

AP and lateral radiographs are important.

• The oblique plane will show a fracture in the region of the pars interarticularis (Scottie dog collar fracture).

• The lateral view will show slippage of the superior vertebra on the inferior vertebra. However, in a lateral view, taken while the patient is supine, the forward displacement often appears trivial, because it is only when the patient is standing that the true degree of slip is appreciated. Consequently, if spondylolisthesis is suspected, a lateral spot view of the lumbosacral junction must be taken while the patient stands upright, and during flexion and extension of the trunk.

Clinical Pearl

Spondylolisthesis is graded according to the percentage of slip. Slip percentage is the distance from a line extended along the posterior cortex of the S1 body to the posteroinferior corner of the

L5 vertebra, divided by the anteroposterior diameter of the sacrum. Grading is then performed using the Meyerding classification, as follows: grade I, 1% to 25%; grade II, 26% to 50%; grade III, 51% to 75%; grade IV, 76% to 100%; and grade V (spondyloptosis) more than 100%.

Differential Diagnosis

- Coexisting osteoarthritis of the hip
- Spinal stenosis
- Degenerative joint disease
- Myelopathy
- Spinal tumors
- Infections

Intervention

The intervention for spondylolisthesis depends on the severity of the slip and the symptoms, and ranges from conservative to surgical. Conservative intervention is more likely to be successful in the case of a limited slip and sparse clinical findings. Such an approach includes pelvic positioning initially to provide symptomatic relief, followed by an active lumbar stabilization program, and stretching of the rectus femoris and iliopsoas muscles to decrease the degree of anterior pelvic tilting.

Prognosis

Most patients benefit from a conservative intervention. In those cases where conservative measures do not provide adequate relief, surgery in the form of decompression and fusion with or without instrumentation, may be required.

ANKYLOSING SPONDYLITIS

Diagnosis

Ankylosing spondylitis—ICD-9: 720.0. Also referred to as also known as spondyloarthropathy, Bekhterev's disease, or Marie-Strümpell disease.

Description

Ankylosing spondylitis (AS), a member of the seronegative spondyloar-thropathies group of arthritides, is a chronic rheumatoid disorder that affects males and females equally, although females tend to get the milder form of the disease. Those who have the HLA-B27 antigen are more likely to be diagnosed than those without. A familial history is a strong risk factor.

 Clinical Pearl

The disease includes involvement of the anterior longitudinal liga-ment and ossification of the disc, thoracic zygapophysial joint joints, costovertebral joints, and manubrio sternal joint.

Subjective Findings

Back pain, particularly at night, may be the presenting complaint. Patients often awaken in the early morning (between 2 and 5 AM) with back pain and stiffness, and usually either take a shower or exercise before returning to sleep. Patients also reported difficulties with spinal rotation movements, and coughing or sneezing. Calin and colleagues describe five screening questions for AS:

1. Is there morning stiffness?
2. Is there improvement in discomfort with exercise?
3. Was the onset of back pain before age 40 years?
4. Did the problem begin slowly?
5. Has the pain persisted for at least 3 months?

Using at least four positive answers to define a "positive" result, the sensitivity of these questions was 0.95 and specificity, 0.85.[76]

Objective Findings

The physical examination can often reveal following positive findings:

- A flattening of the normal lumbar lordosis.
- An increase in the thoracic kyphosis in advanced cases.
- Limited lumbar flexion range of motion initially progressing to limited lumbar and thoracic flexion.
- Decreased chest expansion.

- Positive sacroiliac stress tests (anterior and posterior compression, Gaenslen's test, Fabere).

 Clinical Pearl

Extra skeletal manifestations such as iritis, conjunctivitis, and urethritis may occur.

Confirmatory/Special Tests

The multijoint involvement of the thoracic joints makes the checking of chest expansion measurements a required test in this region.

Rib springing may give a hard end-feel.

Medical Studies

The HLA-B27 antigen remains one of the strongest known associations of the disease, but other diseases are also associated with the antigen.

Early radiographic findings in the spine include squaring of the superior and anterior margins of the vertebral bodies. Later findings include ossification of the anterior longitudinal ligament and autofusion of the facet joints (bamboo spine).

Differential Diagnosis

- Degenerative disc disease/lumbar disc pathology
- Gluteal strain
- Ligament sprain
- Tendonitis/synovitis
- Rheumatoid arthritis
- Lumbopelvic instability

Intervention

An exercise program is particularly important for these patients to maintain functional spinal outcomes. The goal of exercise therapy is to maintain the mobility of the spine and involved joints for as long as possible, and to prevent the spine from stiffening in an unacceptable kyphotic position. A strict regimen of daily exercises, which include positioning and spinal extension/postural exercises, breathing exercises, and exercises for the peripheral joints, must be followed. Several times a day, patients should lie prone for 5 minutes, and they should be encouraged to sleep on a hard mattress and avoid the side lying position. Swimming is the best routine sport.

Prognosis

In time, AS may progress to involve the whole spine and results in spinal deformities, including flattening of the lumbar lordosis, kyphosis of the thoracic spine, and hyperextension of the cervical spine. These changes, in turn, result in flexion contractures of the hips and knees, with significant morbidity and disability.

LOW BACK STRAIN-SPRAIN

Diagnosis

Low back strain/sprain—ICD-9: 846.0 (lumbosacral (joint/ligament) sprain), 847.2 (lumbar sprain), and 724.2 (lumbago). The term *lumbago* is used to describe local back pain of a discogenic origin but also can be used to describe a sudden onset of persistent LBP, marked by a restriction of lumbar movements and reports of "locking."

Description

The terms lumbar sprain (injury to a ligamentous structure) and lumbar strain (injury to a musculotendinous structure) are often used interchangeably, although they are separate entities. Muscle injuries are associated with a history of trauma and are capable of producing a significant degree of discomfort. As with elsewhere in the body, ligament tears of the lumbar spine are normally traumatically induced—when forces exceed the tissues' physiological capacities, rather than the result of overuse. Knowledge of the various restraints to the various motions of the lumbar spine can aid in determining which ligament has the potential to be sprained with a given mechanism

Subjective Findings

- Pain, which varies in severity, is based on the location and extent of the injury.
- Usually a history of traumatic episode (lifting, twisting, etc.).
- Difficulty in finding a comfortable position. The pain is increased with stretching of the involved structure and with sustained positions.
- The symptoms are typically eased with the rest and neutral postures.

Clinical Pearl

Red flags indicating high risk include unexplained weight loss, pain > 1 month, failure to improve with conservative therapy, pain unrelieved by bed rest, or previous history of cancer.

Objective Findings

The goal is often to rule out systemic causes of pain or neurologic compromise requiring surgical intervention.

- Active range of motion of the lumbar spine, particularly flexion, is typically reduced and painful. The other motions may be full and pain-free.
- Resisted hip motions may elicit the pain.
- Selective tissue tension testing of the specific structure elicits pain.
- Neurologic exam is negative.
- If the ligament is involved, stability tests will be positive.

Confirmatory/Special Tests

No examine maneuver is unique or specific to low back pain. Confirmation is made through an in-depth evaluation of neurologic and musculoskeletal systems and, if necessary, imaging studies.

Medical Studies

Plain radiographs are generally not recommended in the first month of symptoms in the absence of significant injury.

Differential Diagnosis

- Musculoskeletal injuries to the lumbar pelvic and hip musculature
- Degenerative changes in intervertebral discs and facet joints
- Herniation of nucleus pulposus of intervertebral disc with irritation of adjacent nerve roots
- Spinal stenosis
- Anatomic abnormalities (e.g., scoliosis)
- Underlying systemic diseases (primary or metastatic cancer, infection, ankylosing spondylitis)
- Visceral diseases unrelated to spine (e.g., diseases of aorta, kidneys)

Intervention

The optimal intervention for patients with acute back pain remains largely enigmatic, and a number of clinical studies have failed to find consistent evidence for improved intervention outcomes with many intervention approaches. However, it is generally agreed that in the acute phase of rehabilitation for the lumbar spine, the intervention goals are to

- Decrease pain, inflammation, and muscle spasm. Pain relief may be accomplished initially by the use of modalities such as cryotherapy, and electrical stimulation, gentle exercises, and occasionally the temporary use of a spinal brace. Thermal modalities, especially ultrasound, with its ability to penetrate deeply, may be used after 48 to 72 hours.

- Promote healing of tissues.

- Increase pain-free range of segmental motion. Range of motion for the lumbar spine is regained initially in the unloaded position of the spine, depending on patient response, in prone lying, the quadruped position, or supine lying. Initially, the exercises prescribed are those that were found to provide relief during the examination.

- Regain soft tissue extensibility. Manual techniques during this phase may include myofascial release, grades I and II joint mobilizations, massage, gentle stretching, and muscle energy techniques.

- Regain neuromuscular control.

- Allow progression to the functional phase. The exercises must challenge muscle and enhance performance but be performed in such a way as to minimize loading of the spine to reduce the risk of injury exacerbation.

- Patient education. Information about activities to avoid should be given, in addition to advice about positions of comfort.

Prognosis

The prognosis for this diagnosis is typically excellent but the number of physical therapy sessions required to provide relief for nonspecific low back pain varies widely. The factors provided to explain this variance include the medical diagnosis, duration of the complaint, prior therapy, and the patient's age and gender.

LUMBAR DISC HERNIATION

Diagnosis

Lumbar disc herniation—ICD-9: 722.1.0; (without myelopathy), 722.73 (with myelopathy), 724.3 (sciatica).

Description

A lumbar disc herniation usually develops over time as the weaker postero-lateral portion of the annulus fibrosis develops fissures that permit contents of the disc to herniate into the lumbar canal adjacent to the existing lumbar nerve root.

 Clinical Pearl

- Peak incidence at ages 30 to 55 years.
- Lumbar much more common than thoracic disc herniation.
- Lower lumbar much more common than upper lumbar.
- 98% of clinically important lumbar disc herniations occur at L4–L5 or L5–S1.
- Radiculopathy is such a sensitive finding (95%) that its absence almost rules out a clinically important disc herniation, although it is only 88% specific for herniation.

Subjective Findings

- Back pain and/or leg pain.
- Paresthesia: Paresthesia, a symptom of direct involvement of the nerve root, can be defined as an abnormal sensation of pins and needles, numbness, or prickling.
- Coughing, sneezing, or a Valsalva maneuver typically exacerbates the symptoms.

 Clinical Pearl

Cauda equina: signs and symptoms include urinary retention, unilateral or bilateral sciatica, sensory and motor deficits, saddle anesthesia, anal sphincter tone decreased and sensory deficit over buttocks, posterior–superior thighs, and perineal regions.

Objective Findings

- Patients with disc-related low back pain commonly present with a pelvic shift or list when acute sciatica is present.

- Muscle weakness and reduced walking capacity are among several functional deficits associated with a lumbar herniated nucleus pulposus.
- Neurologic examination (motor, reflex, sensation) positive for lower motor neuron lesion.

 Clinical Pearl

The characteristics of an LMN include muscle atrophy and hypotonus, diminished or absent deep tendon reflex (DTR) of the areas served by a spinal nerve root or a peripheral nerve, and absence of pathologic signs or reflexes. Hyporeflexia, if not generalized to the whole body, indicates a lower motor neuron or sensory paresis, which may be segmental (root), multisegmental (cauda equina), or nonsegmental (peripheral nerve).

 Clinical Pearl

Weakness of the gastrocnemius is a clinical sign associated with involvement of the L5–S1 disc (neurologic level S1), whereas weakness of the extensor hallucis longus is a positive sign for involvement of the L4–5 disc (neurologic L5).

Confirmatory/Special Tests

- Straight leg raise: Positive test reproduces symptoms in the leg between 30° and 60° elevation.
- Crossed straight leg raise.
  - Patient raises the uninvolved leg between 30° and 60° elevation.
  - Pain occurs in the symptomatic (other) leg.
- Sit-to-stand test (upper vs. lower lumbar involvement): Patient attempts to rise from chair using only one leg—detects quadriceps weakness (L3-L4).

Medical Studies

Radiographs are mandatory, but MRI is exam of choice for diagnosis. In addition, other tests including nerve conduction velocity (NCV), electromyographic (EMG) studies, discogram, myelogram, and CT scan may be ordered.

Differential Diagnosis

The differential diagnosis can be aided by a description of the distribution of the patient's symptoms and the results of the physical examination. These include:

- Hip joint pathology (degenerative joint disease, bursitis, avascular necrosis, synovitis, etc.).
- Meralgia paresthetica (entrapment of the lateral cutaneous nerve of the thigh).
- Irritation of the spinal nerve root by osteophytic spurs.
- Sacroiliac or pelvic dysfunction.
- Intermittent claudication of the iliac or iliofemoral arteries.
- Spondylolisthesis.
- Lateral recess stenosis.
- Muscle strain.
- Stress fracture of the lumbar/thoracic vertebra (burst and compression).
- Neoplasm.
- Isolated peripheral nerve injury or neuritis.
- Diabetic neuropathy/amyotrophy, the latter of which is relatively uncommon but can occasionally be the presenting symptom of uncontrolled diabetes mellitus.

Intervention

Intervention focuses on a return to normal activities as soon as possible by decreasing inflammation, patient education and involvement, a trial of mechanical traction, and therapeutic exercises with an emphasis on core strengthening. The McKenzie program can be valuable to the overall intervention strategy and, if centralization of pain occurs, a good response to physical therapy can be anticipated.

Prognosis

The natural history of radiculopathy and disc herniation is not quite as favorable as for simple low back pain, but it is still excellent, with approximately 50% of patients recovering in the first 2 weeks, and 70% recovering in 6 weeks.

SACROILIAC JOINT DYSFUNCTION

Diagnosis

Sacroiliac joint dysfunction—ICD-9: 724.6 (disorders of the sacrum), 846.9 (unspecified site of sacroiliac region sprain).

Description

Although still somewhat controversial, the sacroiliac joint (SIJ) is generally accepted as an anatomic structure within the lumbar complex that if injured can be a cause of lower back pain. Mechanical dysfunction, pregnancy, inflammation, infection, trauma, and degeneration all have been attributed to the cause of SIJ pain and dysfunction.

 Clinical Pearl

The iliac joint surfaces are formed from fibrocartilage, and the sacral surfaces are formed from hyaline cartilage.

Subjective Findings

Patients often relate that pain especially worsens when they have been sitting for long periods or when they perform twisting or rotary motions. The symptoms do not typically travel distally to or beyond the knee. Specific activities that seem to aggravate SIJ pathology include:

- Heavy lifting
- Cycling
- Sit to stand transfers

Objective Findings

- Inspection often reveals a pelvis with asymmetric height. This finding can be an indication of unilateral restriction in motion of one or both SIJs.
- The patient usually places a thumb directly over the dimple of the PSIS (sacral sulcus) (Fortin finger sign).
- Motor strength tests, the sensory examination, and reflexes in the lower extremities are typically normal.

- One or more of the pain provocation tests for the SIJ (see chapter text) are positive. Unfortunately, although systematic, these tests have not proven reliable in controlled studies.

 Clinical Pearl

The configuration of the SIJs is extremely variable from person to person, and between genders in terms of morphology and mobility. However, it has been determined that these differences are not pathological, but are normal adaptations.

Confirmatory/Special Tests

- Sacral Compression Test
- Anterior Gapping Test
- Posterior Distraction Test
- Pubic Stress Tests
- Patrick's (FABER or Figure-Four) Test: Pain with this maneuver indicates hip joint pathology, pubic symphysis instability, SIJ dysfunction, or an iliopsoas muscle spasm.

 Clinical Pearl

Unfortunately, to date, no manual diagnostic tests have shown reliability for determining how much an individual's SIJ is moving in either symptomatic or asymptomatic subjects. Thus, rather than relying on manual motion testing to determine SIJ dysfunction, the clinician should focus more on the symmetry, or asymmetry, of the motions palpated or observed, and combine these results with all of the findings from the examination.

Medical Studies

Use of imaging studies when evaluating sacroiliac pathology is a source of controversy among clinicians because whether normal and abnormal radiographic studies can help differentiate symptomatic versus nonsymptomatic patients is unclear. The usual SIJ examination is performed using anteroposterior pelvis/lumbar spine radiography.

 Clinical Pearl

Specific sacroiliac views (taken at a 25° to 30° angle to the antero-posterior plane) superimpose the anterior and posterior joint margins, which may increase the sensitivity for detecting abnormalities.

Differential Diagnosis

The SIJ can be the site of manifestation for several disease processes, and referred symptoms. Conditions to consider include:

* Sacroiliac tuberculosis
* Spondyloarthropathy (ankylosing spondylitis)
* Crystal arthropathies
* Pyogenic arthropathies
* Lumbosacral radiculopathy
* Piriformis syndrome.
* Gluteal strain

 Clinical Pearl

In a patient with sacroiliitis, inflammatory origins (e.g., ankylosing spondylitis (AS), psoriatic arthritis) must be considered.

Intervention

The exercises prescribed must challenge and enhance muscle performance while minimizing loading of the SIJ to reduce the risk of injury exacerbation. The exercise program should include normalization of hip range of motion, core strengthening, and pelvic floor strengthening.

 Clinical Pearl

The body has two mechanisms to overcome this shear force; one dependent on the shape and structure of the joint surfaces of the

SIJ s (form closure) which is wedge shaped with a high coefficient of friction, and the other mechanism involving generation of compressive forces across the SIJ via muscle contraction (force closure).

 Clinical Pearl

In addition to the exercise program, the patient should be educated on the trunk and lower extremity positions to avoid (those that produce an excessive or sustained sacral counternutation) and those to adopt (the positions that enhance sacral nutation).

Prognosis

SIJ dysfunction usually improves significantly, relatively quickly. Surgical intervention is rarely used for nontraumatic SIJ pain and is only considered in patients with chronic pain that has lasted for years, has not been effectively treated by other means, and has led to an extremely poor quality of life.

 Clinical Pearl

Radiofrequency denervation has shown some promise for the treatment of especially recalcitrant sacroiliac dysfunction although further study is needed.

SPINAL STENOSIS

Diagnosis

Spinal stenosis—ICD-9: 724.02 (spinal stenosis of lumbar region). Synonyms include neurogenic claudication and myelopathy.

Description

Degenerative spinal stenosis (DSS) is defined as narrowing of the spinal canal (central stenosis), or intervertebral foramina (lateral recess) of the lumbar spine.

It is predominantly a disorder of the elderly and is the most common diagnosis associated with lumbar spine surgery in patients older than 65 years.

 Clinical Pearl

The causes for DSS include facet joint hypertrophy, loss of IVD height, IVD bulging, and spondylolisthesis.

Subjective Findings

- Pain in legs, when walking (+/– neurologic defects) with/without gait abnormalities
- Symptoms relieved by rest ("pseudo-claudication")
- Symptoms can occur anytime the spine is extended (such as standing or lying)
- +/– Worse with coughing/sneezing
- Symptoms relieved by flexing the spine

Objective Findings

- Normal arterial pulses
- +/– Motor, sensory, reflex changes

Confirmatory/Special Tests

In addition to a thorough neurologic and vascular examination, the following special tests may be of help:
- The bicycle test of van Gelderen (see chapter text)
- Straight leg raise test

Medical Studies

AP and lateral radiographs.

Differential Diagnosis

- Abdominal aortic aneurysm—palpable pulsatile mass
- Arterial insufficiency—distance walked to claudication remains constant
- Diabetes mellitus

- Infection
- Tumor
- Multiple sclerosis (MS)

Intervention

Therapeutic exercise is one of numerous interventions that have been proposed for the conservative management of patients with lumbar spinal stenosis. Several authors advocate only the use of Williams flexion exercises because of the neuroforaminal narrowing that occurs with lumbar extension. However, the prescribed program may need to be modified so that it does not exacerbate any coexisting orthopedic conditions, such as osteoarthritis of the hips or knees, while still being effective. The therapeutic exercise progression is based on the underlying impairments and should include postural education; hip flexor, rectus femoris, and lumbar paraspinal stretching; lumbar (core) stabilization exercises targeting the abdominals and gluteals; aerobic conditioning; and positioning through a posterior pelvic tilt.

Prognosis

The rate of progression varies widely depending on the stage and severity of the condition.

ZYGAPOPHYSIAL JOINT DYSFUNCTION

Diagnosis

Zygapophysial joint dysfunction—ICD-9: 721.3.

Description

In the intact lumbar vertebral column, the primary function of the zygapophysial joint is to protect the motion segment from anterior shear forces, excessive rotation, and flexion. The intra-articular meniscoids of the zygapophysial joints have been inculpated in the cause of some types of LBP, when they fail to return to their original position on recovery from a flexion or extension movement and block the joint toward the neutral position.

Clinical Pearl

Facet joint syndrome is a term used to describe a pain-provoking dysfunction of the zygapophysial joint. This pain is the result of a lesion to the joint and its pain-sensitive structures. Zygapophysial movement dysfunctions can result from a hypomobility, or a hypermobility-instability.

Subjective Findings

The subjective examination typically reveals the following findings:
- History of bending, reaching
- Complaints of pain with lumbar extension. Side bending toward or away from the side of the symptoms may provoke pain.

Objective Findings

An in-depth evaluation of neurologic and musculoskeletal system helps exclude other diagnoses and identify facet joint pathology.

Confirmatory/Special Tests

No exam maneuver is unique or specific to facet-mediated low back pain.

Medical Studies

Plain radiographs are generally not recommended in the first month of symptoms in the absence of significant injury.

Differential Diagnosis

- Lumbosacral disc injuries
- Discogenic pain syndrome
- Acute bony injuries of the lumbosacral spine
- Lumbosacral sprain or strain
- Lumbosacral spondylolysis or spondylolisthesis
- Piriformis syndrome
- Sacroiliac joint injury

Intervention

- Soft tissue techniques applied to the area
- Specific mobilization of the involved segment
- Exercises to strengthen the abdominals, gluteals, multifidus, and erector spinae (lumbar stabilization progression)
- Aerobic exercises using a stationary bike and an upper body ergonometer

Prognosis

The prognosis for this condition is typically very good with conservative management.

REHABILITATION LADDER

LUMBAR SPINE AND SIJ

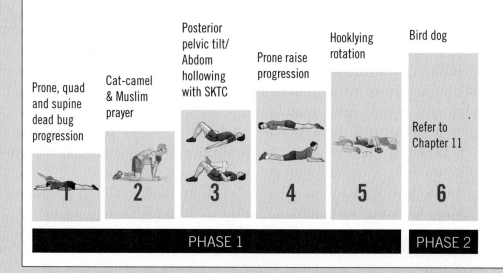

The purpose of these training ladders is to provide the clinician with a safe and progressive framework of exercises that are designed to allow the patient to improve in an efficient manner. The patient begins at the appropriate step, which is based on the stage of healing and the goal of the intervention.

- Phase 1: Acute—pain management, restoration of full passive range of motion, and restoration of normal accessory motion.
- Phase 2: Subacute—active range of motion exercises and early strengthening.
- Phase 3: Chronic—specific strengthening with a strong emphasis on enhancing dynamic stability.

The degree of movement and the speed of progression are both guided by the signs and symptoms. Once the patient is able to perform an exercise

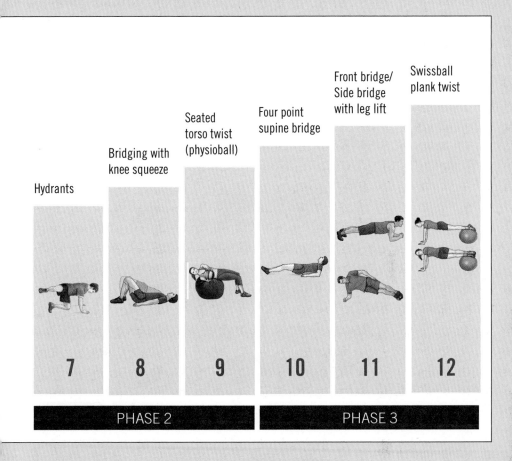

Hydrants

Bridging with
knee squeeze

Seated
torso twist
(physioball)

Four point
supine bridge

Front bridge/
Side bridge
with leg lift

Swissball
plank twist

7   8   9   10   11   12

PHASE 2   PHASE 3

for 8–12 reps without pain, he/she progresses up to the next exercise step. This continues until the patient attempts an exercise that reproduces the pain. At this point, the patient returns to the last exercise that he/she was able to perform without pain and performs that exercise 5 times/day for 1 to 2 days before attempting to progress again. The patient is advanced through the training ladders to the appropriate point, with particular attention paid to patient response to treatment in terms of changes in symptoms, swelling, degree of irritability, or motion. In addition, muscle imbalances are addressed with appropriate flexibility exercises.

Once the patient is able to perform the last exercise of Phase 3 (Step 12 of the ladder), he or she can move on to functional and sport-specific training (Phase 4) as appropriate, which focus on power and higher-speed exercises similar to sport specific demands.

1. Prone, quad, and supine dead bug progression

The patient is instructed on the dead bug progression, starting in prone (1a-d), and progressing to the quadruped position (e–f).

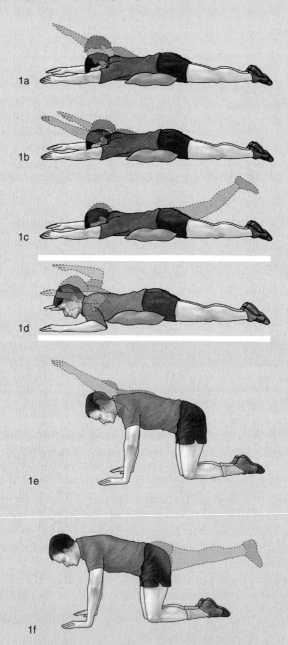

2. Cat-camel and Muslim prayer exercises

The patient is positioned in quadruped and is instructed on the cat–camel exercise (2a) and the Muslim prayer exercise (2b).

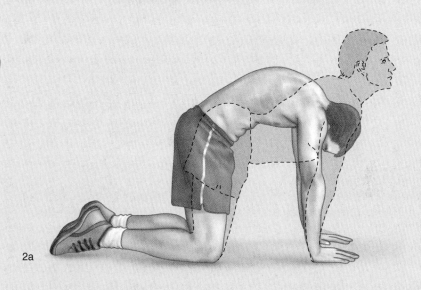

2a

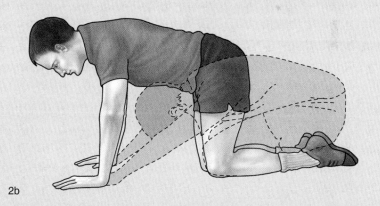

2b

3. Posterior pelvic tilt and single knee to chest

The patient is positioned in supine. Instructions are provided as to how to perform a posterior pelvic tilt by flattening the lumbar spine (3a). The patient is then asked to perform a single knee to chest one leg at a time.

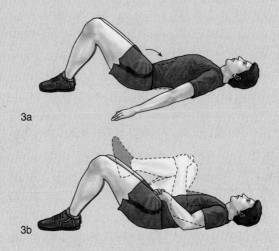

3a

3b

4. Prone raise progression

The patient is positioned in prone lying (4a). A pillow may be positioned under the abdomen if the patient is unable to tolerate prone lying. Once the patient is able to tolerate prone lying, instructions are given on how to perform prone on elbows (4b). This position is maintained for up to 30 seconds. Once the patient is able to tolerate prone elbows, the prone push-up (4c) is taught to the patient.

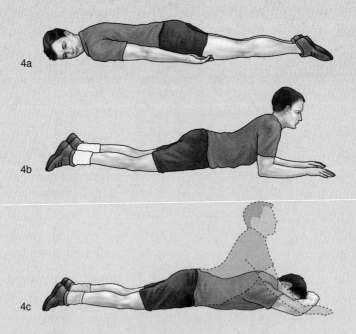

4a

4b

4c

5. Hooklying rotations
The patient is positioned in supine with the hips and knees flexed and the feet flat on the table. The patient is asked to slowly rotate the hips and knees toward the bed in one direction and then the other (5).

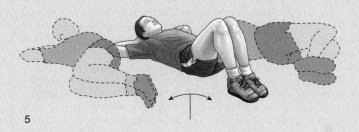

5

6. Bird-dog exercise
Refer to chapter 11 for full description.

7. Hydrant
The patient is positioned in the quadruped position. Using one leg at a time, the patient is asked to raise the bent leg out to the side (7). The exercise is then repeated on the other side. To make this exercise more difficult, the patient can be asked to raise the opposite arm and leg out to the side.

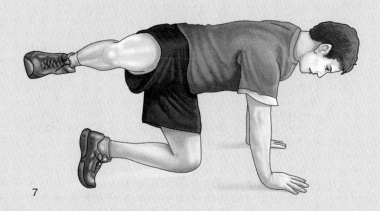

7

8. Bridging with knee squeeze

The patient is positioned in supine with the hips and knees flexed and the feet flat on the table. A pillow is placed between the knees. The patient is asked to squeeze the knees together while performing a bridge (8).

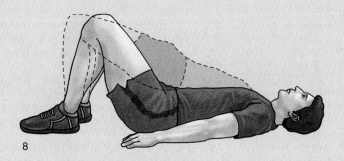

8

9. Seated torso twist (Swiss ball)

The patient is positioned sitting on a Swiss ball and holding a medicine ball. The patient is asked to lean back slightly, while engaging the abdominals and keeping the back straight and the chest lifted. Once in the correct position, the patient is asked to rotate to the right (9). The patient then returns to the start position and rotates to the left.

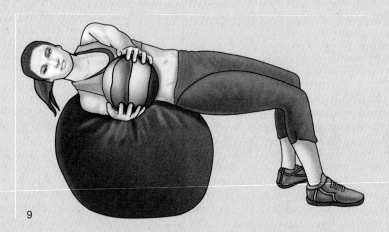

9

10. Four point supine bridge

The patient is positioned in supine propped up on the elbows and feet are about shoulder-width apart with the back of the shoes on the ground and legs almost completely extended. The patient is asked to look up to the ceiling, while lifting the hips by contracting the hamstrings, gluteal muscles, and lower back (10). The position is held for up to 30 seconds.

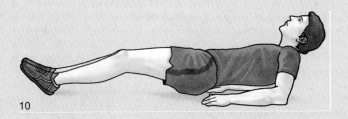

11. Front and side bridge
The patient is taught how to perform a front bridge (11a) and the side bridge (11b). Each position is held for up to 30 seconds.

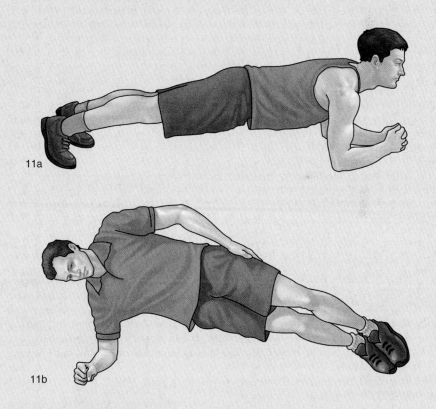

12. Swiss ball Plank twist
The patient is positioned in the push-up position with their feet and lower leg resting on a Swiss ball (12a). Once correct balance is maintained, the patient

is asked to twist the trunk in one direction and then the other while maintaining balance (12b).

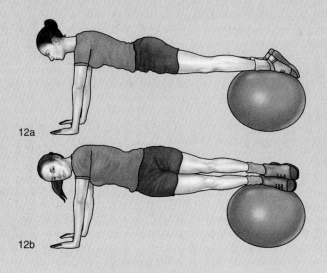

12a

12b

REFERENCES

1. Snijders CJ, Vleeming A, Stoeckart R. Transfer of lumbosacral load to iliac bones and legs. Part 1: Biomechanics of self bracing of the sacroiliac joints and its significance for treatment and exercise. *Clin Biomech.* 1993;8:285–294.
2. Snijders CJ, Vleeming A, Stoeckart R, et al. Biomechanical modelling of sacroiliac joint stability in different postures. *Spine State Art Rev.* 1995;9:419–432.
3. Basmajian JV, Deluca CJ. Muscles Alive: Their Functions Revealed by Electromyography. Baltimore: Williams & Wilkins; 1985.
4. Bigos S, Bowyer O, Braen G, et al. Acute low back problems in adults. *Clinical Practice Guideline No. 14.* Rockville, MD: Agency for Health Care Policy and Research; 1994.
5. Bigos S, Bowyer O, Braen G, et al. *Acute Low Back Problems in Adults. AHCPR Publication 95-0642.* Rockville, MD: Agency for Health Care Policy and Research, Public Health Service, U.S. Department of Health and Human Services; 1994.
6. Jermyn RT. A nonsurgical approach to low back pain. *JAOA.* 2001;101(suppl): S6–S11.
7. Hall H. A simple approach to back pain management. *Patient Care.* 1992;15: 77–91.
8. Ombregt L, Bisschop P, ter Veer HJ, et al. *A System of Orthopaedic Medicine.* London: WB Saunders; 1995.

9. Donelson R. The McKenzie approach to evaluating and treating low back pain. *Orthop Rev*. 1990;19:681–686.

10. Bratton RL. Assessment and management of acute low back pain. *Am Fam Physician*. 1999;60:2299–2308.

11. Alderink GJ. The sacroiliac joint: Review of anatomy, mechanics, and function. *J Orthop Sports Phys Ther*. 1991;13:71–84.

12. DonTigny RL. Function and pathomechanics of the sacroiliac joint: a review. *Phys Ther*. 1985;65:35–44.

13. Dreyfuss P, Michaelson M, Pauza K, et al. The value of medical history and physical examination in diagnosing sacroiliac joint pain. *Spine*. 1996;21:2594–2602.

14. Schwarzer AC, Aprill CN, Bogduk N. The sacroiliac joint in chronic low back pain. *Spine*. 1995;20:31–37.

15. Matsui H, Terahata N, Tsuji H, et al. Familial predisposition, clustering for juvenile lumbar disc herniation. *Spine*. 1992;17:1323–1328.

16. Drezner JA, Harmon KG. Chronic appendicitis presenting as low back pain in a recreational athlete. *Clin J Sport Med*. 2002;12:184–186.

17. Biering-Sorenson F. Low back trouble in a general population of 30-, 40-, 50- and 60 year old men and women: study design, representiveness and basic results. *Dan Med Bull*. 1982;29:289–299.

18. Magora A. Investigation of the relation between low back pain and occupation: 4. Physical requirements: bending, rotation, reaching and sudden maximal effort. *Scand J Rehabil Med*. 1973;5:186–190.

19. Soloman J, Nadler SF, Press J. Physical examination of the lumbar spine. In: Malanga GA, Nadler SF, eds. *Musculoskeletal Physical Examination—An Evidence-based Approach*. Philadelphia: Elsevier-Mosby; 2006:189–226.

20. Deyo RA, Rainville J, Kent DL. What can the history and physical examination tell us about low back pain? *JAMA*. 1992;268:760–765.

21. Nachemson A, Bigos SJ. The low back. In: Cruess RL, Rennie WRJ, eds. *Adult Orthopaedics*. New York: Churchill Livingstone; 1984:843–938.

22. Ombregt L, Bisschop P, ter Veer HJ, et al. Clinical examination of the lumbar spine. In: Ombregt L, Bisschop P, ter Veer HJ, et al., eds. *A System of Orthopaedic Medicine*. London: WB Saunders; 1995:577–611.

23. Sahrmann SA. *Diagnosis and Treatment of Movement Impairment Syndromes*. St Louis: Mosby; 2001.

24. Kapandji IA. *The Physiology of the Joints, The Trunk and Vertebral Column*. New York: Churchill Livingstone; 1991.

25. Bourdillon JF. *Spinal Manipulation*. 3rd ed.. London, England: Heinemann Medical Books; 1982.

26. Fukui S, Ohseto K, Shiotani M, et al. Distribution of referred pain from the lumbar zygapophyseal joints and dorsal rami. *Clin J Pain*. 1997;13:303–307.

27. Maigne R. *Diagnosis and Treatment of pain of Vertebral Origin*. Baltimore: Williams & Wilkins; 1996.

28. Greenman PE. *Principles of Manual Medicine*. 2nd ed.. Baltimore: Williams & Wilkins; 1996.

29. O'Sullivan PB. Lumbar segmental 'instability': clinical presentation and specific stabilizing exercise management. *Man Ther*. 2000;5:2–12.

30. Allbrook D: Movements of the lumbar spinal column. *J Bone Joint Surg.* 1957;39B:339–345.

31. Ng JK, Kippers V, Richardson CA, et al. Range of motion and lordosis of the lumbar spine: reliability of measurement and normative values. *Spine.* 2001;26:53–60.

32. Pearcy M, Portek I, Shepherd J. Three-dimensional analysis of normal movement in the lumbar spine. *Spine.* 1984;9:294–297.

33. Pearcy M, Tibrewal SB. Axial rotation and lateral bending in the normal lumbar spine measured by three-dimensional radiography. *Spine.* 1984;9:582.

34. Troup JDG, Hood CA, Chapman AE. Measurements of the sagittal mobility of the lumbar spine and hips. *Ann Phys Med.* 1967;9:308–321.

35. Cyriax J. *Textbook of Orthopaedic Medicine, Diagnosis of Soft Tissue Lesions.* 8th ed.. London: Bailliere Tindall; 1982.

36. McKenzie RA. *The Lumbar Spine: Mechanical Diagnosis and Therapy.* Waikanae NZ, ed. Spinal Publication; 1981.

37. Goode A, Hegedus EJ, Sizer P, et al. Three-dimensional movements of the sacroiliac joint: a systematic review of the literature and assessment of clinical utility. *J Man Manip Ther.* 2008;16:25–38.

38. Edwards BC. Combined movements of the lumbar spine: examination and clinical significance. *Aust J Physiother.* 1979;25.

39. Edwards BC. Combined movements of the lumbar spine: examination and treatment. In: Palastanga N, Boyling JD, eds. *Grieve's Modern Manual Therapy of the Vertebral Column.* Edinburgh: Churchill Livingstone; 1994: 561–566.

40. Laslett M, Young SB, Aprill CN, et al. Diagnosing painful sacroiliac joints: a validity study of a McKenzie evaluation and sacroiliac provocation tests. *Aust J Physiother.* 2003;49:89–97.

41. Sahrmann SA. Movement impairment syndromes of the lumbar spine. In: Sahrmann SA, ed. *Diagnosis and Treatment of Movement Impairment Syndromes.* St Louis: Mosby; 2001:51–119.

42. Jull GA. Examination of the lumbar spine. In: Grieve GP, ed. *Modern Manual Therapy of the Vertebral Column.* Edinburgh: Churchill Livingstone; 1986:553.

43. Meadows J. *Orthopedic Differential Diagnosis in Physical Therapy.* New York: McGraw-Hill; 1999.

44. Saal JA. Natural history and nonoperative treatment of lumbar disc herniation. *Spine.* 1996;21:2S–9S.

45. Seichi A, Kondoh T, Hozumi T, et al. Intraoperative radiation therapy for metastatic spinal tumors. *Spine.* 1999;24:470–473; discussion 474–475.

46. Gracovetsky S, Farfan HF. The optimum spine. *Spine.* 1986;11:543.

47. Gracovetsky S, Farfan HF, Helleur C. The abdominal mechanism. *Spine.* 1985;10:317–324.

48. Aaron G. The use of stabilization training in the rehabilitation of the athlete. Sports Physical Therapy Home Study Course, APTA, Sports Physical Therapy Section; 1996.

49. Panjabi M, Abumi K, Duranceau J, et al. Spinal stability and intersegmental muscle forces: a biomechanical model. *Spine.* 1989;14:194–199.

50. Panjabi MM. The stabilizing system of the spine. Part 1. Function, dysfunction adaption and enhancement. *J Spinal Disord.* 1992;5:383–389.
51. Clark MA. *Integrated Training for the New Millenium.* Thousand Oaks, CA: National Academy of Sports Medicine; 2001.
52. Vasilyeva LF, Lewit K. Diagnosis of muscular dysfunction by inspection. In: Liebenson C, ed. *Rehabilitation of the Spine: A Practitioner's Manual.* Baltimore: Lippincott Williams & Wilkins; 1996:113–142.
53. Meadows JTS. The principles of the Canadian approach to the lumbar dysfunction patient. *Management of Lumbar Spine Dysfunction—Independent Home Study Course.* La Crosse, WI: APTA, Orthopaedic Section; 1999.
54. Lee DG, Walsh MC. *A Workbook of Manual Therapy Techniques for the Vertebral Column and Pelvic Girdle.* 2nd ed.. Vancouver: Nascent; 1996.
55. Maher C, Latimer J, Adams R. An investigation of the reliability and validity of posteroanterior spinal stiffness judgments made using a reference-based protocol. *Phys Ther.* 1998;78:829–837.
56. Deyo RA, Weinstein JN. Low back pain. *N Engl J Med.* 2001;344:363–370.
57. Nadler SF, Campagnolo DI, Tomaio AC, et al. High lumbar disc: diagnostic and treatment dilemma. *Am J Phys Med Rehabil.* 1998;77:538–544.
58. Dutton M. *Manual Therapy of the Spine: An Integrated Approach.* New York: McGraw-Hill; 2002.
59. Maitland G. *Vertebral Manipulation.* Sydney: Butterworth; 1986.
60. Dyck P, Doyle JB. "Bicycle test" of van Gelderen in diagnosis of intermittent cauda equina compression syndrome. *J Neurosurg.* 1977;46:667–670.
61. Mantoo SK, Mak K, Tan TJ. Obturator hernia: diagnosis and treatment in the modern era. *Singapore Med J.* 2009;50:866–870.
62. Bjork KJ, Mucha P, Jr., Cahill DR: Obturator hernia. *Surg Gynecol Obstet.* 1988;167:217–222.
63. Hannington-Kiff JG. Absent thigh adductor reflex in obturator hernia. *Lancet.* 1980;1:180.
64. Binkley J, Stratford PW, Gill C. Interrater reliability of lumbar accessory motion mobility testing. *Phys Ther Rev.* 1995;75:786–792; discussion 793–795.
65. Dreyfuss P, Dryer S, Griffin J, et al. Positive sacroiliac screening tests in asymptomatic adults. *Spine* (Phila Pa 1976) 1994;19:1138–1143.
66. Potter NA, Rothstein JM. Intertester reliability for selected clinical tests of the sacroiliac joint. *Phys Ther.* 1985;65:1671.
67. Mitchell FL, Moran PS, Pruzzo NA. *An Evaluation and Treatment Manual of Osteopathic Muscle Energy Procedures.* Manchester, MO: Mitchell, Moran and Pruzzo Associates; 1979.
68. Fryette HH. *Principles of Osteopathic Technique.* Colorado: Academy of Osteopathy; 1980.
69. Hartman SL. *Handbook of Osteopathic Technique.* 2nd ed.. London, England: Unwin Hyman Ltd., Academic Division; 1990.
70. DiGiovanna EL, Schiowitz S. *An Osteopathic Approach to Diagnosis and Treatment.* Philadelphia: JB Lippincott; 1991.
71. Levangie PK. Four clinical tests of sacroiliac joint dysfunction: the association of test results with innominate torsion among patients with and without low back pain. *Phys Ther.* 1999;79:1043–1057.

72. Hoppenfeld S. Physical examination of the hip and pelvis. *Physical Examination of the Spine and Extremities*. East Norwalk, CT: Appleton-Century-Crofts; 1976:143.
73. Yeoman W. The relation of arthritis of the sacro-iliac joint to sciatica, with an analysis of 100 cases. *Lancet*. 1928;2:1119–1122.
74. Evans RC. *Illustrated Essentials in Orthopedic Physical Assessment*. St. Louis: Mosby-Year book Inc; 1994.
75. Mens JM, Vleeming A, Snijders CJ, et al. Validity of the active straight leg raise test for measuring disease severity in patients with posterior pelvic pain after pregnancy. *Spine*. 2002;27:196–200.
76. Mens JMA, Vleeming A, Snijders CJ, et al. Validity and reliability of the active straight leg raise test as diagnostic instrument in posterior pelvic pain since pregnancy. *Spine*. 2001;26:1167–1171.
77. Mens JMA, Vleeming A, Snijders CJ, et al. The active straight-leg-raising test and mobility of the pelvic joints. *Eur Spine J*. 1999;8:468–473.
78. Boden SD, Davis DO, Dina TS, et al. Abnormal magnetic resonance scan of the lumbar spine in asymptomatic subjects: a prospective investigation. *J Bone Joint Surg*. 1990;72A:403–408.
79. Weisel SE, Tsourmas N, Feffer H, et al. A study of computer-assisted tomography, I: the incidence of positive CAT scans in an asymptomatic group of patients. *Spine*. 1984;9:549–551.
80. Guide to physical therapist practice. *Phys Ther*. 2001;81:S13–S95.
81. Badke MB, Boissonnault WG. Changes in disability following physical therapy intervention for patients with low back pain: dependence on symptom duration. *Arch Phys Med Rehabil*. 2006;87:749–756.

QUESTIONS

1. How many degrees of freedom are available in the spine?
2. How many natural curves are contained within the spine?
3. Which of the lumbar levels has the smallest spinous process?
4. Name the bony structures of the pelvic ring.
5. What are the anatomic differences between a male and a female pelvis?
6. At what levels does lumbar disc prolapse most commonly occur?
7. Which is more serious, a disc protrusion or a disc herniation?
8. What are the two anatomic classifications of lumbar spinal stenosis?
9. What causes neurogenic claudication?
10. What type of exercise is recommended for patients with lumbar stenosis?
11. What two common medical conditions affect the sacroiliac joint?
12. What is the sign of the buttock?

Answers

CHAPTER 1

1. Smooth, striated (skeletal), and cardiac
2. A muscle that has a parallel fiber arrangement.
3. Synergist muscles are muscle groups that work together to produce a desired movement.
4. An agonist muscle contracts to produce the desired movement while synergistic muscles are groups of muscles that work together to cause the same movement.
5. Flexor pollicis longus, extensor digitorum longus
6. Rectus femoris
7. The deltoid
8. Meissner
9. Pacinian
10. Type II
11. Type IIb
12. To provide sensory information concerning changes in the length and tension of the muscle fibers.
13. Annulospiral, and flower spray
14. Nuclear bag and nuclear chain
15. To provide support, enhance leverage, protect vital structures, provide attachments for both tendons and ligaments, and store minerals.
16. Tendons that wrap around a convex surface or the apex of a concavity, those that cross two joints, those with areas of scant vascular supply, and those that are subjected to repetitive tension, are particularly vulnerable to overuse injuries.
17. The term tendinitis implies inflammation, whereas tendinosis results from a degenerative process.
18. Fascia

19. The erect standing position with the feet just slightly separated and the arms hanging by the side, the elbows straight and with the palms of the hand facing forward.
20. Sagittal
21. The sagittal axis
22. Flexion of the hip or knee
23. The glenohumeral joint
24. The hip joint
25. Full elbow extension
26. Full elbow extension, full forearm supination
27. Slide (glide), roll/rock, spin
28. False: male surface *(female, rocks)*
29. The motion of a bone in space
30. The motion of joint surfaces
31. The forces acting upon a joint
32. If the joint surface is convex relative to the other surface, the slide occurs in the opposite direction to the osteokinematic motion. If, on the other hand, the joint surface is concave, the slide occurs in the same direction as the osteokinematic motion.
33. Flexion of the shoulder/hip
34. Glenohumeral abduction/adduction
35. An unmodified sellar joint is also referred to as a saddle joint. Two examples include the trapeziometacarpal joint, and the calcaneocuboid joint
36. A modified sellar joint is a saddle-shaped joint whose surface convexity is not perpendicular to its concavities (a hinge joint). Two examples include any of the interphalangeal joints.

CHAPTER 2

1. Examples include any structure within the central nervous system, nerve roots, nerve trunks, and peripheral nerves.
2. The brain and the spinal cord
3. Cerebrospinal
4. The corticospinal tracts
5. The corticospinal tracts

6. The spinothalmic tract
7. The dorsal column lemniscal
8. Alpha and gamma
9. Innervation of muscle fibers
10. They supply the small intrafusal muscle fibers of the muscle spindle.
11. The C5 nerve root
12. T4.
13. L4 and L5
14. Gait ataxia, pathological reflexes, spasticity, hyperreflexia.
15. 8
16. L4–S2
17. Calcium, potassium, and sodium
18. CN XI
19. CN IV
20. CN IX (glossopharyngeal) and CN X (vagus)
21. Biceps, brachialis, supinator, and extensor carpi radialis
22. The phrenic nerve
23. Radial
24. Median
25. Median
26. Ulnar
27. Ulnar
28. Median
29. D
30. E
31. D
32. A
33. C
34. A
35. C
36. A
37. D
38. D
39. C

40. E

41. E

42. D

43. E

44. D

45. C

46. Lower

CHAPTER 3

1. Examination, evaluation, diagnosis, prognosis, and intervention.

2. The history, systems review, and tests and measures.

3. Any five of the following: changes in mental status, fever, changes in bowel or bladder, nausea, night sweats, dyspnea, unexplained weight loss, visual disturbances, diaphoresis, and hematuria.

4. Referred symptoms.

5. Any two of the following: joint capsule, the ligaments, the bursa, the articular surfaces of the joint, and the synovium, the dura, bone and fascia.

6. Muscle belly tendon, the tenoperiosteal junction, any sub muscular/tendinous bursa, and bone.

7. A capsular pattern of restriction is a limitation of pain and movement in a joint specific ratio, which is usually present with arthritis, or following prolonged immobilization.

8. Arthritis, osteoarthrosis, prolonged immobilization, or acute trauma

9. Internal derangement, adhesion, or muscle tightness

10. Gross limitation of flexion, abduction and internal rotation; slight limitation of extension.

11. Plantarflexion more limited than dorsiflexion

12. External rotation > abduction > internal rotation (3:2:1)

13. Flexion > extension (± 4:1)

14. Between 15 and 60 seconds

15. The physiological barrier is the point at which voluntary range of motion of a joint is limited by soft tissue tension, whereas the anatomic barrier is the point at which passive range of motion is limited by bone contour or soft tissues (ligaments), or both.

16. Slow, large amplitude movements performed to the limit of the range

17. Any three of the following: pathological end feel, fracture, infectious arthritis, acute inflammatory disorders, tumor, joint ankylosis.

18. Bone to bone: abrupt end feel felt when two hard surfaces meet; soft tissue approximation: the end feel felt when the soft tissues surrounding a joint are compressed; capsular: the end feel described as an immediate stop of movement with some give.

19. Spasm, springy, and empty.

20. A weak and painful finding could indicate any one of the following: fracture, metastases, hyperacute arthritis, and grade II tear.

21. A weak and painless finding could indicate any of the following: complete rupture of contractile tissue, nerve palsy, or weakness caused by disuse, inhibition.

22. L2–4

23. The foot evertors (fibularis muscles); or the hamstrings.

24. Stride length and cadence

25. Excessive hip and knee flexion, poor foot clearance during swing on the involved side, foot slap immediately after initial contact.

26. A contralateral pelvic drop during single limb support

27. C3–T1, L2–S3

28. Patellar

29. To reinforce a deep tendon reflex during testing.

30. The clinician applies noxious stimuli to the crest of the patient's tibia by running a fingernail along the crest. A positive test, demonstrated by the Babinski sign, is indicative of an UMN impairment.

31. The CORs and VORs work together to maintain the position and *visual fixation* of the eyes during movements of the head and neck.

32. Neurodynamic mobility tests

33. The minimum number of films needed is usually two, the AP and lateral.

34. Infection, malignancy, chronic inflammation

35. Factors associated with certain autoimmune diseases

36. ESR is the rate at which erythrocytes precipitate out of unclotted blood in one hour. Increases in ESR are related to inflammation, infections, malignancy, and various collagen vascular diseases.

37. The initial response is the inflammation phase and it is manifested by erythema, swelling, elevated tissue temperature, and pain.

38. Histamine and serotonin

39. Stress

40. The decrease in tissue temperatures produces a decrease in metabolic rate
41. 15°C to 25°C
42. For pain relief or to decrease muscle guarding or spasm
43. 41°C to 45°C
44. Cryotherapy produces a relative slowing down of nerve conduction.
45. Any five from the following: cardiac pacemaker, history of seizures, placement of electrodes over a pregnant uterus, placement of electrodes over the carotid sinus, placement of electrodes over the pharyngeal area, placement of electrodes over an area suspected of arterial or venous thrombosis.
46. Slack (stage 2)

CHAPTER 4

1. Isometric contraction
2. Eccentric
3. Eccentric
4. Extensibility, elasticity, irritability, and the ability to develop tension
5. False. More force
6. The strength gains are developed at a specific point in the range of motion and not throughout the range; not all of a muscle's fibers are activated
7. b
8. Type/mode of exercise, intensity, duration, and frequency
9. b
10. c
11. b
12. c
13. b
14. a
15. a
16. a
17. Exercise of low intensity and long duration
18. c
19. a
20. c
21. b

22. b
23. c
24. c
25. c
26. Any three of the following—incontinence, urinary tract infections, un-protected open wounds, heat intolerance, severe epilepsy, uncontrolled diabetes, unstable blood pressure or severe cardiac and/or pulmonary dysfunction
27. 92°F to 95°F
28. a
29. b
30. a

CHAPTER 5

1. It is the capsular tissue in the interval between the subscapularis and the supraspinatus tendons.
2. 2 (glenohumeral joint):1 (scapulothoracic joint)
3. The rotator cuff depresses the humeral head to counteract the superior pull of the deltoid muscle.
4. The circumflex scapular artery
5. Eight degree of retroversion
6. The glenohumeral joint, the acromioclavicular joint, the sternoclavicular joint and the scapulothoracic articulation
7. Pneumonia, cardiac ischemia, and peptic ulcer disease
8. 90 degree of glenohumeral abduction and full external rotation; or full abduction and external rotation
9. Trapezius, serratus anterior, rhomboid major and minor, and levator scapulae
10. The long thoracic nerve
11. A rupture of the supraspinatus, or deltoid
12. Abduction
13. A failure of the distal end of the acromion to ossify
14. The axillary nerve
15. A tear of the supraspinatus, or injury to the suprascapular nerve

ANSWERS

16. It occurs when the infraspinatus and supraspinatus muscles are pinched between the posterior superior aspect of the glenoid with the upper limb is in a position of elevation and external rotation, such as the cocked position of a pitcher.

17. An excision of the distal 2 cm of the clavicle, typically used to provide pain relief for patients suffering from acromioclavicular dislocation

18. Impingement of a subacromial structure

CHAPTER 6

1. The ulnohumeral and radiohumeral joints, and the proximal radioulnar joint.

2. The normal carrying angle of the elbow varies with flexion and extension, ranging from 6 degrees of varus with full flexion to 11 degrees of valgus in full extension. In men the mean value is between 11 degrees and 14 degrees (full extension), and in women it is between 13 degree and 16 degree.

3. The coracoid ligament, the lateral ulnar collateral ligament, and the anterior band of the medial collateral ligament.

4. Brachialis

5. The radial nerve

6. The musculocutaneous nerve

7. The ulnar nerve

8. The deep branch of the radial nerve

9. Olecranon impingement or an olecranon stress fracture

10. Wrist flexion and forearm pronation

11. It is a generic term referring to several overuse injuries in young throwers.

12. Lateral epicondylitis

13. Fracture of the epicondyle

14. Fracture of the trochlea

15. Posterolateral

16. The median nerve

17. The median nerve

18. Saturday night palsy

19. 80 degree to 90 degree

20. Flexion > extension (±4:1)

21. 35 degree supination, 70 degree elbow flexion.

CHAPTER 7

1. Extensor pollicis longus
2. Thumb
3. The ulnar artery and the ulnar nerve
4. Scaphoid, lunate, triquetral, and pisiform
5. The tip of the little finger is innervated by the ulnar nerve, the dorsal thumb-index web space is innervated by the radial nerve, and the palmar tip of the index finger is innervated by the median nerve.
6. 10 degree of supination
7. Bunnell–Littler
8. Mallet finger
9. Full wrist extension
10. De Quervain disease
11. Greater loss of flexion than extension
12. An avulsion fracture of the flexor digitorum profundus tendon from the distal phalanx.
13. Gamekeeper thumb
14. A Colles fracture is extra-articular with dorsal angulation, and displacement, whereas a Barton fracture is an intra-articular shear fracture that may be dorsal or volar.
15. The superficial radial nerve
16. The ulnar nerve
17. Undisplaced (require immobilization in a below-elbow cast for four weeks), displaced (one main transverse fracture with little cortical comminution), and unstable (having gross comminution of cortical bone and pronounced crushing of cancellous bone).
18. A radial fracture with disturbance of the distal radioulnar joint
19. Primary pulmonary hypertension, thoracic outlet syndrome, atherosclerosis, and drug ingestion or exposure.
20. Scaphoid fracture, radial nerve neuritis, and basal joint arthritis of the thumb CMC joint.
21. C6 radiculopathy, pronator syndrome, Raynaud phenomenon, complex regional pain syndrome (CRPS), and diabetic neuropathy.
22. Phalen and Tinel
23. *Fall On an Out Stretched Hand*
24. A benign, slowly progressive fibroproliferative disease of the palmar fascia.
25. PIP joint hyperextension with concurrent DIP joint flexion

26. Transverse furrows that begin at the lunula (the crescent-shaped whitish area of the bed of the fingernail) and progress distally as the nail grows. They result from a temporary arrest of growth of the nail matrix occasioned by trauma or systemic stress.

27. Median nerve

CHAPTER 8

1. Ilium, ischium, and pubis.

2. It is the angle between the axis of the femoral head and neck and the axis of the femoral shaft in the frontal plane.

3. Ober's test is used to determine the length of the iliotibial band/tensor fascia lata.

4. A cane can decrease force loads by 40%.

5. The lateral cutaneous nerve of the thigh.

6. A hip pointer is a contusion of the lateral hip.

7. Myositis ossificans.

8. Piriformis syndrome is caused by inflammation or spasm of the piriformis muscle resulting in irritation of the sciatic nerve.

9. A double vertical fracture of the pelvis.

10. Osteonecrosis, sciatic nerve injury, and femoral head fracture.

11. Trochanteric.

12. Legg–Calve–Perthes disease.

13. Psoas bursitis.

14. Superior gluteal nerve palsy, osteoarthritis of the hip, or an L5 disk protrusion.

15. Piriformis, superior gamellus, obturator internus, inferior gamellus, obturator externus, quadratus femoris, adductor magnus, and iliopsoas.

16. External rotation.

17. The hip flexors.

CHAPTER 9

1. The medial meniscus.

2. Superior tibiofibular—modified ovoid; inferior tibiofibular—neither *(syndesmosis)*; tibiofemoral—bicondylar; and patellofemoral—pseudo-joint (sesamoid).

3. Anterior cruciate ligament, posterior cruciate ligament, and the coronary ligament.

4. The outer third.

5. The POL, the predominant ligament structure on the posterior medial corner of the knee joint, functions to control anterior medial rotatory instability and to provide static resistance to valgus loads when the knee moves into full extension.

6. To prevent posterior translation of the tibia on the femur during open kinetic chain activities, and to prevent anterior translation of the femur on the fixed tibia during closed kinetic chain activities.

7. The most common symptom is pain along the medial side of the knee that is exacerbated with prolonged sitting.

8. 12 degrees to 18 degrees.

9. The medial meniscus.

10. The Q-angle is formed by the intersection of two lines: a line through the center of the patella to the anterior superior iliac spine and another line from the tibial tubercle to the center of the patella

11. A bipartite patella still has an intact ossification center.

12. Inflammation of the infrapatellar fat pad.

13. Weight-bearing as tolerated—most total knee arthroplasty uses cement fixation.

14. Deep vein thrombosis.

15. In the popliteal space behind the knee, at the fibular head, in the anterior compartment of the leg (deep fibular nerve), and in the lateral compartment of the leg (superficial fibular nerve).

16. A decrease in flexion greater than that of extension.

17. The posterior horn.

18. The medial meniscus is oval, whereas the lateral meniscus is round

19. Full extension and external rotation of the tibia.

20. Weight bearing.

21. The collaterals.

22. The anterior fibers.

23. Genu recurvatum.

24. Approximately 90 degrees.

25. The common fibular (peroneal) nerve.

26. The semimembranosus muscle.

CHAPTER 10

1. The rear foot (talus and calcaneus), the midfoot (navicular, cuboid, and cuneiform), and the metatarsals and phalanges
2. Abductor hallucis, flexor digitorum brevis, and abductor digit minimi
3. The calcaneonavicular ligament
4. Between the talus and calcaneus
5. The navicular, cuboid, and the three cuneiforms
6. The medial, intermediate, and lateral cuneiforms, and the cuboid
7. Posterior tibialis
8. Calcaneus
9. Talus
10. The ligaments of the calcaneocuboid joint include the long plantar ligament and a portion of the bifurcate ligament dorsally.
11. The cuneiforms, together with articulations with the metatarsal bones, form Lisfranc joint.
12. The primary function of the tibialis posterior muscle is to invert and plantar flex the foot.
13. The fibular (peroneal) muscles serve as both plantar flexors and evertors of the foot.
14. The saphenous nerve
15. Abduction in the transverse plane, dorsiflexion in the sagittal plane, and eversion in the frontal plane
16. The close-packed position is weight-bearing dorsiflexion
17. Full inversion
18. Entrapment of the neurovascular bundle comprised of the posterior tibial nerve and tibial artery at the medial ankle
19. In the third web space between the third and fourth metatarsals.
20. An intra-articular fracture of the distal tibia
21. A fracture of the fifth metatarsal base at the metaphyseal–diaphyseal junction
22. By changing the position of the knee and then dorsiflexing the ankle, the clinician can differentiate between the lengths of the gastrocnemius and the soleus muscle—flexing the knee and passively dorsiflexing the ankle joint tests the gastrocnemius length, whereas the soleus is tested by dorsiflexing the ankle joint with the knee extended.
23. Thomson test—squeezing the gastrocnemius in a nonweight-bearing position should produce.

CHAPTER 11

1. The uncinate processes are considered to be a guiding mechanism for flexion and extension in the cervical spine and to resist posterior translation as well as some degree of the side bending.
2. C7
3. C5–6
4. Rectus capitis lateralis
5. C3–5
6. false
7. masseter
8. false
9. ipsi SB, contra rot
10. scalenus anterior
11. tectorial membrane
12. body of C2
13. ipsilateral side bending and contralateral rotation and extension of the OA joint
14. as above
15. obliquus capitis superior
16. decreased extension, **right** side bending and **left** rotation
17. 5 degrees
18. 8 degrees
19. Side bending *(rotation is conjunct)*
20. Max flexion of lower cervical spine followed by rotation of the head
    Max SB of lower cervical spine followed by rotation of the head
21. Max rotation of lower cervical spine then nodding of the head
22. Alar
23. **R**
24. Right (↓d **L** glide = ↓d **R** SB = ↓d ability of **R** condyle to extend *(move anteriorly)*
25. same side
26. flexion/extension; rotation
27. rolls anteriorly and glides posteriorly
28. 10 degree
29. 40 degree

30. flexion, rotation **right** and SB **right**

31. uncinate

33. Left translation

34. false *(opp. sides)*

35. prevents anterior translation of C1 on C2

36. A combination of traction and neck flexion

CHAPTER 12

1. A typical thoracic vertebra has 12 separate articulations

2. False, downward and laterally

3. False

4. Functional, structural, and congenital

5. Ankylosing spondylitis.

6. Anterior wedging and vertebral endplate irregularity in the thoracic spine associated with kyphosis

7. coronally *(facilitate rotation)*

8. 1, 10, 11, 12 *(only articulate with their own vertebra and do not possess inferior demi facets)*

9. two adjacent vertebra and the intervening disk

10. Costovertebral

11. T2–9

12. On the centrum

13. Ribs

14. T3

15. Own level and one above

16. T1–6 = pump handle
T7–12 = bucket handle

17. T1–7

18. Via the one above them *(11th & 12th are free at their lateral ends)*

19. Symphysis with fibrocartilaginous disk

20. Disk below

21. Level with vertebral body below

22. disk below

23. T3–7

24. T1–2

25. T8–10

26. SB and rotation occur to opposite sides

27. Rotation and SB occur to same side

28. T3

29. T10 and below

30. elderly patient with no causal factor *(tumor)*
gallbladder disease
cardiac disease
osteoporosis

31. Anterior rotation *(conjunct)*

32. Superior glide *(tubercle is at proximal or medial end of rib)*

33. PMS *(posteromediosuperiorly)*

34. Inferior glide of tubercle (T1–7)
ALI of tubercle (T8–10)

35. 8

36. Superolaterally

37. T1–7 glide inferiorly
T8–10 glide ALI
T11–T12 remain stationary

38. Posterior rotation, SB and slight extension to side of elevated arm

CHAPTER 13

1. 6 (flexion/extension, right and left rotation, right and left side bending, superior and inferior translation, anterior and posterior translation, and right and left lateral translation).

2. 4 (two lordotic curves and two kyphotic curves).

3. L5.

4. The ilia, sacrum, coccyx, femora, and pubis.

5. The male pelvis is heavy and thick with large joint surfaces, whereas the female pelvis is light and thin with small joint surfaces. In addition the male sacrum is long and narrow, whereas the female sacrum is short and wide.

6. L4–5.

7. A disk herniation in which the annular fibers are disrupted, whereas in a disk protrusion the annular fibers remain intact.

8. Lateral stenosis (occurs within the lumbar intervertebral foramina and/or nerve root canal), and central stenosis (occurs within the spinal canal).

9. Mechanical irritation of the cauda equina.

10. Flexion oriented exercises and deweighted treadmill ambulation.

11. Ankylosing spondylitis and Reiter syndrome.

12. The sign of the buttock is not a single sign, as the name would suggest, but rather a collection of signs indicating that a serious pathology is present posterior to the axis of flexion and extension in the hip. The sign of the buttock test is positive if the hip flexion does not increase when the knee is flexed during a straight leg raise. Among the causes of the syndrome are osteomyelitis, infectious sacroiliitis, fracture of the sacrum or pelvis, septic bursitis, ischiorectal abscess, gluteal hematoma, gluteal tumor, and rheumatic bursitis.

Index

Page numbers followed by italic *f* or *t* denote figures or tables, respectively.